OXFORD MEDICAL PUBLICATIONS

Textbook of community psychiatry

Textbook of
Community Psychiatry

GRAHAM THORNICROFT AND GEORGE SZMUKLER

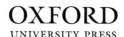

OXFORD

UNIVERSITY PRESS

OXFORD

UNIVERSITY PRESS

Great Clarendon Street, Oxford OX2 6DP

Oxford University Press is a department of the University of Oxford.
It furthers the University's objective of excellence in research, scholarship,
and education by publishing worldwide in

Oxford   New York

Athens   Auckland   Bangkok   Bogotá   Buenos Aires   Calcutta
Cape Town   Chennai   Dar es Salaam   Delhi   Florence   Hong Kong   Istanbul
Karachi   Kuala Lumpur   Madrid   Melbourne   Mexico City   Mumbai
Nairobi   Paris   São Paulo   Singapore   Taipei   Tokyo   Toronto   Warsaw
with associated companies in
Berlin   Ibadan

Oxford is a registered trade mark of Oxford University Press
in the UK and in certain other countries

Published in the United States
by Oxford University Press, Inc., New York

© Thornicroft & Szmukler, 2001

A catalogue record for this title is available from the British Library

Library of Congress Cataloging in Publication Data
(Data available)
1   3   5   7   9   10   8   6   4   2

ISBN 0 19 262997 2

Typeset by
Florence Production Ltd, Stoodleigh, Devon
Printed in Great Britain on acid free paper by
The Bath Press, Avon

We wish to dedicate this book to
Judel Szmukler, Linnet Szmukler, Rachel Szmukler,
Heidi Lempp, Amalia Thornicroft, Calum Thornicroft and Eric Byers

Contents

II   Psychiatry *in* the community: the service system

Values into practice

Integration of components into a system of care

Service components

List of contributors

Wolfram an der Heiden
Department of Psychiatry, Zentralinstitut für Seelische Gesundheit, J5 68159 Mannheim, Germany

Paul Appelbaum
University of Massachusetts Medical School, Worcester, MA 01655, USA

Patricia Backlar
Department of Philosophy, Portland State University, P.O.B. 751, Portland, OR 97207, USA

Sube Banerjee
Health Sciences Research Department Institute of Psychiatry, Kings College London, De Crespigny Park, Denmark Hill, London SE5 8AF, UK

Karen Barfoot
Royal North Shore Hospital and Community Mental Health Services, 55 Hercules Street, Chatswood, NSW 2067, Australia

Diana Barnes
Centre for Applied Social Studies, University of Durham, 15 Old Elvet, Durham DH1 3HL, UK

Thomas Becker
Department of Psychiatry, University of Leipzig, Liebigstrasse 22b, D-04103 Leibzig, Germany

Nick Bouras
York Clinic, Guy's Hospital, 47 Weston Street, London SE1 3RR, UK

Paul Bowden
South London and Maudsley NHS Trust, Denmark Hill, London SE5 8AZ, UK

Richard E. Breslow
Capital District Psychiatric Center, 75 New Scotland Avenue, Albany, NY 12208, USA

Tom Burns
St. George's Hospital Medical School, Jenner Wing, Cranmer Terrace, London SW7 0RE, UK

Mary Cannon
Institute of Psychiatry, King's College, De Crespigny Park, Denmark Hill, London SE5 8AF, UK

John Carpenter
Centre for Applied Social Studies, University of Durham, 15 Old Elvet, Durham DH1 3HL, UK

Martin Gittelman
New York Medical College-Lincoln Medical and Mental Health Center, 100 West 94th St., New York, NY 10025, USA

Gyles Glover
Centre for Applied Social Studies, University of Durham, 15 Old Elvet, Durham DH1 3HL

David Goldberg
Health Services Research Department Institute of Psychiatry, King's College, De Crespigny Park, London SE5 8AF, UK

Kevin Gournay
Health Services Research Department, Institute of Psychiatry, King's College, De Crespigny Park, Denmark Hill, London SE5 8AF, UK

Susan Grey
South London and Maudsley NHS Trust, Denmark Hill, London SE5 8AZ, UK

Lars Hansson
Department of Clinical Neuroscience, Division of Psychiatry, Lund University, University Hospital, SE-221 85 Lund, Sweden

Frank Holloway
Croydon Mental Health Services, South London & Maudsley NHS Trust, Bethlem Royal Hospital, Monks Orchard Road, Beckenham, Kent BR3 3BX, UK

Jeremy Holmes
Department of Psychotherapy, North Devon District Hospital, Barnstaple, Devon EX 31 4JB, UK

Geraldine Holt
York Clinic, Guy's Hospital, 47 Weston Street, London SE1 3RR, UK

David Hunter
University of Durham, Durham, UK

Rachel Jenkins
Health Services Research Department, Institute of Psychiatry, King's College, De Crespigny Park, Denmark Hill, London SE5 8AF, UK

Sonia Johnson
Department of Psychiatry and Behavioural Sciences, University College London, Gower Street, London WC1E 6BT, UK

Peter Jones
Department of Psychiatry, University of Cambridge, Addenbrooks Hospital, Cambridge

Martin Knapp
Centre for the Economics of Mental Health, Institute of Psychiatry, King's College, De Crespigny Park, Denmark Hill, London SE5 8AF, UK

Harriet Lefley
Department of Psychiatry and Behavioral Sciences, University of Miami School of Medicine, Mental Health Building, Jackson Memorial Hospital, Miami, FL 33101, USA

Margaret Leggatt
World Fellowship for Schizophrenia and Allied Disorders, 29 Mary Street, North Carlton, Victoria 3054, Australia

Anthony Lehman
Department of Psychiatry, Centre for Mental Health Services Research, University of Maryland, 645 West Redwood Street, Baltimore, MD 21201, USA

Glynn Lewis
Department of Psychological Medicine, University of Wales College of Medicine, Heath Park, Cardiff, UK

Anthony Mann
Institute of Psychiatry, King's College, De Crespigny Park, Denmark Hill, London SE5 8AF, UK

Patrick McGorry
Centre for Young People's Mental Health, University of Melbourne, Department of Psychiatry, Royal Melbourne Hospital, Grattan Street, Parkville, Victoria 3050, Australia

David Mechanic
Institute for Health, Health Care Policy and Aging Research, Rutgers University, 30 College Avenue, New Brunswick, NJ 08903 USA

I. Harry Minas
Centre for International Mental Health, University of Melbourne, Level 2, Bolte Wing, St. Vincent's Hospital, Nicholson Street, Fitzroy, Victoria 3065, Australia

Richard Mollica
Harvard Program in Refugee Trauma, 8 Story St, Third Floor, Cambridge, MA 02138, USA

Alison Murray
Unit for Social and Community Psychiatry, Department of Psychiatry, St Bartholomew's and the Royal London Hospital Medical School, London, UK

Richard Øvretveit
Bergen University School of Medicine, The
Nordic School of Public Health, Box 12133,
Goteborg, Sweden

David Pilgrim
National Primary Care Research and
Development Centre, University of Manchester,
5th Floor Williamson Building, Oxford Road,
Manchester M13 9PL, UK

Shulamit Ramon
School of Community Health and Social Studies,
Anglia Polytechnic University, East Road,
Cambridge CB1 1PT, UK

M. Susan Ridgely
RAND Health, 1700 Main Street, PO Box 2138,
Santa Monica, CA 90407–2138, UK

Ann Rogers
National Primary Care Research and
Development Centre, University of Manchester,
5th Floor Williamson Building, Oxford Road,
Manchester M13 9PL, UK

Nikolas Rose
Department of Sociology, Goldsmiths College,
University of London, New Cross, London
SE14 6NW, UK

Alan Rosen
Royal North Shore Hospital, 55 Hercules Street,
Chatswood, NSW 2067, Australia

Norman Sartorius
Departement Psychiatric, Hopitaux Universitaires
de Geneve, 6–18 Bd. De St. Georges, 1205
Geneva, Switzerland

Aart Schene
Department of Psychiatry, Academic Medical
Centre, University of Amsterdam, Meibergdreef
9, 1105 AZ Amsterdam, The Netherlands

Jack Scott
Centre for Mental Health Services Research,
University of Maryland, 645 West Redwood
Street, Baltimore, MD 21201, USA

Geoff Shepherd
The Health Advisory Service (HAS), 46–48
Grosvenor Gardens, London SW1W 0EB, UK

Bruce Singh
University of Melbourne, Department of
Psychiatry, Royal Melbourne Hospital, Grattan
Street, Parkville, Victoria 3050, Australia

Mike Slade
Section of Community Psychiatry (PRiSM),
Health Services Research Department, Institute
of Psychiatry, King's College, De Crespigny Park,
Denmark Hill, London SE5 8AF, UK

George Szmukler
South London & Maudsley NHS Trust,
Maudsley Hospital, Denmark Hill, London
SE5 8AZ, UK

Michele Tansella
Department of Medicine and Public Health,
Section of Psychiatry, University of Verona,
Ospedale Policlinico, 37134 Verona, Italy

Hollie Thomas
Department of Psychological Medicine,
University of Wales College of Medicine, Heath
Park, Cardiff, UK

Graham Thornicroft
Section of Community Psychiatry (PRiSM),
Health Service Research Department, Institute of
Psychiatry, King's College, De Crespigny Park,
Denmark Hill, London SE5 8AF, UK

Andre Tylee
Health Services Research Department, Institute
of Psychiatry, King's College, De Crespigny Park,
Denmark Hill, London SE5 8AF, UK

Peter Tyrer
Imperial College School of Medicine, St Mary's
Campus, Paterson Centre, London W12 1PD,
UK

Richard Warner
University of Colorado and Medical Health
Centre of Boulder County, 1333 Iris Avenue,
Boulder, CO 80304-2296, UK

1 | What is 'community psychiatry'?

George Szmukler and Graham Thornicroft

Introduction

"Science is built up of facts, as a house is built of stones; but an accumulation of facts is no more a science than a heap of stones is a house"

Henri Poincaré (1905) *Science and Hypothesis*

"It could be said of me that in this book I have only made up a bunch of other men's flowers, providing of my own only the string that ties them together"

Montaigne (1580) *Essais* bk. 3, ch. 12

When does a subject reach sufficient maturity for its principles to be presented systematically as one expects in a traditional textbook, as opposed to a loose collection of observations, essays or opinions? We asked ourselves this question in relation to the subject of 'community psychiatry' when approached by our publisher to consider preparing a textbook. After some delay, we felt that the time had arrived for an initial foray.

The practice of psychiatry in the second half of the 20th century, and especially in its last decade, has changed fundamentally. Mentally ill people have been moved out of the relative 'simplicity' of the large institution, with its clear structures and hierarchies, and into the community. This necessitated new types of relationships between 'health' and 'social' care. A range of new facilities has been required for the treatment, care and support for people with mental health problems in the community, replacing many of the functions previously provided in hospitals. More agencies and staff (professional and non-professional) have declared an interest and entered the scene, often bringing new and quite different perspectives on the needs of those with mental disorders. Among these new voices in the community have been those of service users themselves. Increasing cultural diversity and respect for social difference have added to the range of value systems to be taken into account. At the same time, governments have taken increasing direct interest in mental health issues, formulating ever more specific strategies, guidance, directives and legislation.

These changing relationships between health and other forms of care in the community are reflected in the evolving definitions of community psychiatry over the past 40 years or so, as illustrated in Table 1.1.

These definitions show a progression to ever more complex ideas about the nature of community psychiatry, starting from a simple relocation of old structures and hierarchies outside hospital, to professionally defined and controlled treatment arrangements in the community, to concepts of treatment provided within systems involving many agencies and people. These trends are portrayed in finer grain detail by a series of texts which have charted this evolving field (see Levine, 1981; Henderson, 1988; Mosher and Burti, 1989; Bennett and Freeman, 1991; Bhugra and Leff, 1993; Breakey, 1996; Levin and Petrila, 1996).

As doctors, we have edited this textbook within the discipline of psychiatry. Psychiatry refers to the application of knowledge from the biological and social sciences to the care and treatment of patients suffering from disorders of mental activity and behaviour [its etymological roots stem from *psyche* (breath, life, soul) and *iatreia* (healing)]. The term is sometimes taken to refer only to the work of medically qualified practitioners, but we use it in its wider sense to cover the other mental health professions, including, amongst others, nurses, psychologists, social workers and

Table 1.1 *Evolving definitions of community psychiatry*

Rehin and Martin (1963)

"any scheme directed to providing extra-mural care and treatment to facilitate the early detection of mental illness or relapse and its treatment on an informal basis, and to provide some social work service in the community for support or follow-up." (quoted in Bennett and Freeman, 1991).

Sabshin (1966)

"the utilisation of the techniques, methods, and theories of social psychiatry, as well as those of the other behavioural sciences, to investigate and meet the mental health needs of a functionally or geographically defined population over a significant period of time, and the feeding back of information to modify the central body of social mental health and other behavioural science and knowledge."

Freudenberg (1967)

"community psychiatry assumes that people with mental health disorders can be most effectively helped when links with family, friends, workmates and society generally are maintained, and aims to provide preventive, treatment, and rehabilitative services for a district which means that therapeutic measures go beyond the individual patient."

Serban (1977)

"community psychiatry has three aspects: first, a social movement; second a service delivery strategy, emphasising the accessibility of services and acceptance of responsibility for mental health needs of a total population; and third, provision of best possible clinical care, with emphasis on the major mental health disorders and on treatment outside total institutions."

Bennett (1978)

"community psychiatry is concerned with the mental health needs not only of the individual patient but of the district population, not only of those who are defined as sick, but those who may be contributing to that sickness and whose health or well-being may, in turn, be put at risk."

Tansella (1986)

"a system of care devoted to a defined population and based on a comprehensive and integrated mental health service, which includes outpatient facilities, day and residential training centres, residential accommodation in hostels, sheltered workshops and in-patient units in general hospitals, and which ensures, with multi-disciplinary team-work, early diagnosis, prompt treatment, continuity of care, social support and a close liaison with other medical and social community services and, in particular, with general practitioners."

Strathdee and Thornicroft (1997)

"the network of services which offer continuing treatment, accommodation, occupation and social support and which together help people with mental health problems to regain their normal social roles."

Thornicroft and Tansella (1999)

"A community-based mental health service is one which provides a full range of effective mental health care to a defined population, and which is dedicated to treating and helping people with mental disorders, in proportion to their suffering or distress, in collaboration with other local agencies."

Adapted from Thornicroft and Tansella (1999).

occupational therapists. As we shall see, the practice of psychiatry in the community requires an understanding which goes far beyond that offered by the traditional medical and behavioural sciences.

Community psychiatry and social psychiatry

How does community psychiatry differ from 'social psychiatry'? The latter has rarely been defined formally and the term seems to be used less commonly. Leff (1993) defined it as follows: "social psychiatry is concerned with the effects of the social environment on the mental health of the individual, and with the effects of the mentally ill person on his/her environment". Most texts on 'social psychiatry' and the work of 'social psychiatry' units have focused on identifying and elucidating the operation of social influences on mental disorder (Bebbington, 1990; Bhugra and Leff, 1993). Most research has been directed at establishing causal mechanisms relating to the onset or course of mental illness. While drawing implications for treatment has been important, evaluation of complex interventions has received little attention. Community psychiatry, in contrast, focuses on service delivery. Common to both is a dependency on epidemiological methods. Findings from studies within the domain of social psychiatry inform our thinking about needs for care of populations, about environmental influences that may affect these and about treatments which services should offer.

Definition of 'community psychiatry'

Our definition of community psychiatry is shown in Table 1.2. In this definition, we choose to highlight several fundamental issues. First, we wish to emphasize that community psychiatry needs to be concerned with the provision of treatment and care to all segments of the population

Table 1.2 *Definition of community psychiatry*

'Community psychiatry comprises the principles and practices needed to provide mental health services for a *local population* by:

(i) establishing *population-based needs* for treatment and care

(ii) providing a service system linking a wide *range of resources* of adequate capacity, operating in *accessible locations* and

(iii) delivering evidence-based treatments to people with mental disorders.'

in proportion to need. Secondly, we envisage services as a type of wide area network, whose adequacy reflects the strength of the component parts (including health as well as social care, state as well as voluntary, formal as well as informal provision) and the degree of inter-connectedness between these elements. Thirdly, we consider that community psychiatry is an approach that accords priority to the delivery of effective treatments wherever they are needed; thus it is not confined to any particular location or site. Treatment aims to take place in locations accessible and acceptable to patients.

Essential to an understanding of community psychiatry is a recognition that it is shaped by a variety of often conflicting *values*. Some values derive from the *larger community*—especially those expressed through a state's *social policy* on the one hand, and through *science* on the other; while others derive from the *smaller groups* of participants directly engaged in mental health issues—those of service users, carers—informal and formal, and health professionals (Banton, 1985; Dear and Wolch, 1987; Furedi, 1997; Perkins and Repper, 1998). This means that an analysis of community psychiatry requires an examination of health care simultaneously from multiple perspectives. It also requires the application of the methods of a variety of academic disciplines, including the behavioural and social sciences, history, politics and, since questions of value are so central, moral philosophy and ethics.

At the core of this book is our view that the treatments and services which constitute community psychiatry need to be understood as the surface manifestations of undercurrents of underlying beliefs and values. Figure 1.1 presents what we term an 'ensemble–schism' model emphasizing these two major levels. The underlying values held by the various parties to mental health services often pull in different or even opposing directions. Their influence on the role and shape of mental health services can be schismatic, leading to disharmony, disunion or division. At the same time, effective services have the qualities of an 'ensemble'—individuals, teams and service components, like the building blocks of an orchestra, together creating a totality greater than the sum of their parts.

Viewed, as it were from above, the service system and its interfaces are shown more clearly in Figure 1.2.

Figure 1.1 shows the major value bases introduced above. There are others, and, within each group, there may be striking differences (e.g. between psychiatrists, psychologists and social workers among the professionals alone), but these are generally the most significant.

By *social policy*, we refer to central and local government policies and legislation which affect the lives of individuals and communities. Such policies are usually implemented to solve social problems. In the introduction to a text on social policy, the editors state that "in the past few years social policy has risen to the top of the political agenda ... The nature of the welfare state, having once seemed uncontroversial and even dull, is now deeply contested and its institutions subject to a seemingly permanent revolution" (Ellison and Pierson, 1998). Deinstitutionalization has resulted in a vastly more complex set of interfaces between health services (and within health, between mental health services and the others), social services, housing, employer organizations and the criminal justice system. Changes in each may have a serious impact on the care of the mentally ill. The details of social policy in any place are shaped by history, politics, economics and a wide range of other social forces. Social change results in changing problems, for example those associated with drug abuse, an ageing population, new patterns of

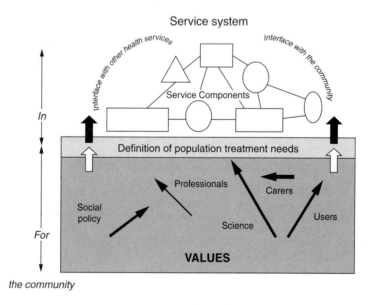

Figure 1.1 *'Ensemble—schism' model of community psychiatry.*

family configuration and changing attitudes and expectations to matters such as 'need', social welfare or civil liberties. Furthermore, today's solutions may become tomorrow's problems (e.g. how housing estates are planned, or how benefits are redistributed). Multi-culturalism adds an extra dimension.

Science should provide a more stable values base. Its fundamental principles, for example objectivity and the rigorous testing of hypotheses, win widespread respect. However, when applied to complex health care interventions, there are many uncertainties about the right methods—the randomized controlled trial may not always be

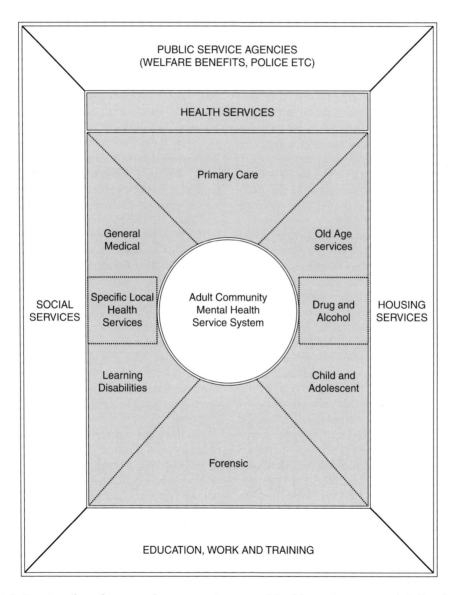

Figure 1.2 *Key interfaces between the community mental health service system and (i) other health services and (ii) other public service agencies.*

the most appropriate method for assessing effectiveness (Black, 1996; Taylor and Thornicroft, 1996); there is little consensus on the status of 'qualitative' methods (Mays and Pope, 2000); and methods for evaluation of 'systems' are in their infancy. Because societies change quite rapidly in relation to the pace of scientific inquiry, findings may be quickly out of date. The salience today of substance abuse co-occurring with psychotic disorders and the consequent need to rethink treatment strategies is a good example. Science is also subject increasingly to government regulation. The research agenda is being taken out of the hands of scientists, who are now required to be more accountable for the way in which they use research monies. Users and other parties with an interest in mental health issues, for example the criminal justice system, increasingly influence what should be researched. Models of the fundamental nature of 'mental health problems' and their implications may vary dramatically.

Professionals offer a range of treatments which may be evidence based and congruent with their models of mental illness, but *users* and *carers* may see these as not relevant to their needs, or even as unhelpful. Users wish to determine the shape of services that, after all, are intended primarily to serve them, and they wish to achieve outcomes which are of their choosing. So too do carers. The voices of both are now being heard to an unprecedented extent. Several examples of common conflicts between values espoused by the participants in mental health care are shown in Table 1.3.

The schema in Figure 1.1 can be used in relation to two other related schemata—pathways individuals take into and through care developed by Goldberg and Huxley (1980, 1992) (see also Chapter 34) and the matrix identified by Thornicroft and Tansella (1999) which locates elements in the mental health services system at three distinct levels: national, local and patient, and at three time phases: inputs, processes and outcomes (see also Chapter 13 and glossary).

The core of the *'ensemble–schism' model* can be expressed in a metaphor which the reader may find not too fanciful, that of a 'life-raft'.

The raft may be made of parts, of wood or other materials, according to what is made available, and which represent the separate service components. These component parts are of varying quality and fitness for purpose, according to whether the craft is intended to sail the high seas or calmer coastal waters, about which there may be dispute among the owners, builders and designers of the vessel. The buoyancy of the components changes over time with wear and tear. Separately, they are insufficient for the whole enterprise to float, but jointly they may succeed.

The strength of the whole depends as much upon the linkages between the components as upon the quality of the components themselves. If a linkage is weak, it may place an unbearable strain on the rest of the structure. Long-term viability depends on the quality of original materials used, the skill of construction and the care expended in ongoing maintenance. This metaphor also emphasizes that, on occasions, the treatment and care offered by mental health services may have life or death consequences.

In terms of those aboard the raft, we can distinguish, among others, between the crew (staff) and passengers (service users). The former needs to be well trained and competent to deal with routine and emergency tasks, and to effect leadership. There is a degree of mutual interdependence between these two groups, and all may need to contribute to decisions on the direction of the vessel for rowing to be co-ordinated to make headway. Similarly, the leadership will need to pay careful attention to the morale of both passengers and crew.

The direction and speed of travel will be influenced by several factors: the purposive propulsion of those on board, continuing sea changes (in popular opinion about mental illness), the tides (of political priorities), occasional storms (of outcry over scandals or violent incidents) and underwater currents (of values held by key stakeholders). There is always the possibility of drift (from a lack of movement in an agreed direction) or even regression (where counter-vailing forces overpower forward movement). Over time, those aboard may well develop increasingly sophisticated positioning and navigation systems, to

Table 1.3 *Examples of competing values in community psychiatry*

Value domains		Examples of common conflicts
Social policy versus	Science	Direction of research determined by government policy (e.g. of value to NHS; particularly problematical patient groups) versus scientific curiosity of researchers
		Evidence-based treatments versus state priorities for funding, limited resources
	Professionals	'Unacceptable' variations in clinical care versus clinical autonomy, judgement, innovation
		Demand by state for control or containment of disturbing persons versus professional desire to provide treatment and care
	Users	Users' demand for services of their choice versus services which are affordable and regulated
		Users' demand for less 'coercion' versus state's need to exercise control over risky persons
	Carers	Carers unacknowledged providers of care previously provided by state
		Services provided for users versus rights to services for carers
Science versus	Professionals	Evidence-based treatments versus professional judgement (especially where evidence base is inadequate or controversial)
		Treatments efficacious under controlled experimental conditions versus effectiveness in the 'real world'
	Users	Disagreement over fundamental nature of 'mental disorder'
		Disagreement over what 'outcomes' should be assessed in evaluation of treatment interventions, and their relative importance (e.g. user satisfaction versus effects on symptoms)
	Carers	Research focuses on outcomes for users, not on implications for carers
Professionals versus	Users	Professionals' views of goals of treatment (e.g. symptom reduction, reduction of 'disability', 'compliance' with medication) versus users' views (e.g. decent accommodation, meaningful daytime activities)
		Where the balance should be struck between professional 'paternalism' versus patient 'autonomy'; or between 'coercion' versus care
	Carers	Duty of care to patient versus addressing the needs of carers (especially if patient objects)
		Professionals' perspective on nature of patient's problem versus carers', and whose should be accepted
Users versus	Carers	User's right to confidentiality versus carer's need to know so proper care can be provided, or for carer's own well-being
		If patient and family are seen by treatment team, whose interests are primary, and when might this change

know both where they are and where they intend to go.

The size of the life-raft is important because it indicates the ability of the whole enterprise to offer support or even survival to the requisite number of people (the capacity of the system), quite separate from the question of whether the raft is well built and durable. Finally, it is important to distribute the load over the entire structure, to avoid unbalancing the system with dire consequences for all.

Values constantly change, especially those expressed in social policy. While such value shifts often follow predictable paths, the consequent temporality of community psychiatry can be both frustrating and fascinating. Thus, this textbook, while attempting to define *principles* underlying the provision of psychiatric care for a local population, for the most part gives *examples of solutions* to problems of service delivery, and their evaluation.

The structure of this book

As a consequence of another conceptual basis for this book, namely the distinction between defining community psychiatry *for* the community, and its *operational* delivery *in* the community (see Fig 1.1), we have organized the content of this book into the same two overall components:

(i) Psychiatry *for* the community, in which population needs for psychiatric care are considered; and

(ii) Psychiatry *in* the community, in which we examine service systems designed to meet those needs.

Our primary focus has not been on the effectiveness of treatment interventions at the individual patient level, for example drug treatments or cognitive behaviour therapy (for which many outstanding texts already exist), but rather on how they can best be delivered to those who may gain benefit. In short, we are concerned essentially with the service system which delivers treatment and care.

Section I. Psychiatry for the community

The *value base* of community psychiatry as expressed in **social policy** is examined in this first section of the book. Social policy is examined from a historical point of view (Chapter 2) and in relationship to notions of 'community' (Chapter 3), a central idea both politically and sociologically. Multiple meanings can be discerned which have implications for the organization of community psychiatric services. Ideologies may dictate, among other matters, what is considered to be a mental disorder, what types of causes should be given salience, who should be treated, by whom, where, using what kinds of treatments, what counts as evidence of usefulness and what are the desired outcomes.

The **scientific background** is discussed in terms of the scope of its overall contribution in community psychiatry (Chapter 4), epidemiological methods as applied to mental disorder (Chapter 5) and methods for evaluation of treatments in the community (Chapter 6), as well as evaluation strategies for more complex services (Chapter 7). These approaches provide the 'evidence base' underlying the treatment and care provided by mental health services. We have seen, however, that what comprises 'evidence' may be contested by different participants engaged in defining what should be provided by mental health services.

The **extent and impact of mental disorders** define the problems that are the business of mental health services. These can be conceptualized at a number of levels. Firstly, we can determine the incidence, prevalence and distribution of mental disorders in the population. Epidemiological methods also lead to the identification and estimation of the effect size of risk factors for these disorders and to causal hypotheses (Chapter 8). The next level considers these disorders in relation to the social environment, leading to notions of disability and handicap, as well as quality of life (Chapter 9). Next is a level of conceptualization of more recent origin, that of 'needs'. Here mental disorders are viewed in relation not only to the social environment, but also to care and treatment which is available, appropriate or necessary (Chapter 10). The economic costs to the community of mental disorder are then examined (Chapter 11), as well as the psychological and social impact on those closest to sufferers (Chapter 12).

Section II. Psychiatry in the community

We move on to a consideration of the translation of **values into practice** at the planning stage—how the values expressed through the scientific approach, social policy and the perspectives of those engaged locally in mental health services are translated into principles defining what a service should provide (Chapter 13); how values are balanced against finite resources which almost invariably are insufficient for the practical attainment of the endorsed principles (Chapter 14); and how accepted principles are translated into service planning (Chapter 15). Most of the larger communities in the industrially developed world today are multi-cultural. A key question is how mental health services, imbued as they are with values, should respond to ethnic diversity. What are the key principles and how can they be translated into services that ensure that care and treatment are delivered fairly to minority groups? (Chapter 16).

Next we consider methods for **integrating service components into a system of care**. Fundamental to community care is the multi-disciplinary team (Chapter 17). Sectorization is a device employed in a number of regions to provide a framework for integrating the components of a service within the service, as well as with other community agencies (Chapter 18). Next we examine how service elements might be balanced within the service system (Chapter 19), and the related question of striking an appropriate balance between 'generic' and 'specialist' teams or services (Chapter 20). Finally, we recognize that training occupies a central role in enabling a service system to function effectively (Chapter 21).

The main **service components** are then described together with estimations of their place within community mental health services and their effectiveness. These are case management and assertive community treatment (Chapter 22), emergency services (Chapter 23), out-patient services (Chapter 24), partial hospitalization (Chapter 25), day care and occupation (Chapter 26), residential care (Chapter 27) and in-patient services (Chapter 28).

If local community mental health services are to function effectively, they need to establish effective links and means to negotiate **the boundaries with specialist services**. The latter provide treatments across larger geographical areas requiring skills infrequently exercised at a local level (e.g. forensic), or which deal with groups of patients or clients whose care requires a very different orientation (e.g. learning disabilities or mental handicap). We consider, in turn, forensic services (Chapter 29), drug and alcohol services, particularly with respect of co-occurring substance abuse with mental disorders (Chapter 30), specialist psychotherapies (Chapter 31), older adult services (Chapter 32) and learning disability services (Chapter 33). Children's services have been omitted because they involve very different approaches; they are essentially 'local' as well as 'specialist', and they entail interfaces in the community, for example with education and social services, which are very different from adult services. They require a separate text.

The **interfaces between mental health services and the wider community** are then examined. The vast majority of persons with mental disorders, especially the so-called 'minor mental disorders', are in fact treated in primary care. The balance of care between primary and secondary services for these patients as well as shared care for those with 'serious mental illness' is considered in Chapter 34. The crucial interface with social welfare services is examined in Chapter 35. Alliances with other agencies and bodies in the wider community are discussed in Chapter 36.

Next we consider a growing population for whom the surrounding community itself is unfamiliar and constitutes a major challenge—immigrants, including refugees (Chapter 37). Finally we consider a pervasive element which often regulates relationships between the mentally ill and the community and, by a form of association, between mental health services and the community—stigma (Chapter 38).

The next section examines **service users and carers**. Service users play an increasingly powerful role in determining how they should be treated, but their role within (or perhaps without) mental health services can be conceptualized in a variety of ways (Chapter 39). At the same time, carers, mainly through self-help organizations, have also insisted on having their contributions acknowledged and can prove valuable partners in developing better services (Chapter 40).

The next section deals with **prevention of mental disorder**. Most of this subject, especially primary and secondary prevention, should properly be treated within the sections on principles and the integration of components of care into a system. However, we believe that the development of ideas and services related to prevention remains rudimentary, and that at this stage it is more helpful to consider the subject separately. Although new thinking challenges the traditional division into primary (Chapter 41), secondary (Chapter 42) and tertiary (Chapter 43) prevention, they still have widespread usage so we have persevered with them.

The final section of the book discusses **ethical issues and dilemmas** of special relevance to community psychiatry. We are well and truly in the realm of values again and this discussion should of course have been located in Section I. However, we have placed it at the end for two reasons. First, although the dilemmas we present are not new, the advent of community psychiatry has added new layers of complexity requiring us to see them in a new light. We believe that these chapters are appreciated better following a presentation of the details of the practice of community psychiatry. Secondly, we exemplify an important circular process, the constant moving back and forth between the domains of values and practice. Three key issues are presented: rationing, priorities and targeting (Chapter 44); treatment pressures, coercion and compulsion (Chapter 45); and privacy and confidentiality (Chapter 46).

The contributions to this book have been written by an international group of authorities for an international audience. Recognizing that each country has its own particular health care context, institutions, policies and practices, we decided to help readers by including a **glossary** of terms that generally are limited to use in one country.

Pragmatism to theory

From this discussion, it will be clear that we *do* consider that the field of community psychiatry has reached a sufficient level of maturity for its principles and practices to be presented systematically in a traditional textbook format. Nevertheless, as a set of scientific paradigms relevant to the domain of psychosocial phenomena (Lief, 1948; Kuhn, 1962), it is still far from fully elaborated. While some key themes have a rapidly developing scientific base, for example the tools of evidence-based medicine as applied to treatments for individual patients (Cochrane, 1971; Geddes and Harrison, 1997), at the same time methods for the evaluation of whole service systems are largely absent (Lawrence and Lorsch, 1986; Wing, 1989; Knudsen and Thornicroft, 1996). However, perhaps the greatest deficit in this field of enquiry is that knowledge is largely atheoretical. We offer two illustrations. 'Quality of life' is a humanistic concept which attempts to examine the effect of illness from the patient's point of view—"on what they have, how they are doing, and how they feel about their life circumstances" (Lehman, 1996). All are agreed that there is something very important in the notion. However, a number of measures have been developed, each examining something different. A clear conceptual framework is lacking, for example, to help us understand how 'quality of life' is related to 'subjective well-being' or how it fits into an integrated model of mental health outcome evaluation. Another example is 'family burden', referring to the impact of mental disorders on carers. Rarely is the concept located within a theoretical framework (such as the 'stress–appraisal–coping' paradigm) which opens the door to generating hypotheses and systematically studying relationships to other key variables (Szmukler *et al.*, 1996). 'Burden' is also an example where terminology itself may limit conceptual development. It implies that care-giving is restricted to negative aspects only, and that the patient's illness is like a passive load to be borne by others. This one-sided conception leads to a neglect of broader aspects of interactions and relationships between carer and patient, amenable to study, for example within a family systems framework (Stern *et al.*, 1999).

An increasing appreciation of the 'burden' of mental disorders on all countries of the world is evident (Robins and Regier, 1991; Desjarlais *et al.*, 1995; Meltzer *et al.*, 1995; Murray and Lopez, 1996). At the same time, the contributors to this volume show that significant ground has been gained in tackling the problem. Advances include a strengthening of the evidence base, a growth of theory across a broad range of areas, improving links between policy and evidence, better models for collaboration within and between services and other agencies, and a focus on the role of values and ethics in a community context. Despite the complexity of community psychiatry, there is every reason to feel confident that its principles and practice will continue to develop apace.

References

Banton, R., Clifford, P., Frosch, S., Lousada, J. and Rosenthall, J. (1985) *The Politics of Mental Health*. London: Macmillan

Bebbington, P.E. (ed.) (1990) *Social Psychiatry: Theory, Methodology and Practice*. New Brunswick, NJ: Transaction Publishers.

BeBennett, D. and Freeman, H (1991) *Community Psychiatry. The Principles*. Edinburgh: Churchill Livingstone.

Black, N. (1996) Why we need observational studies to evaluate the effectiveness of health care. *British Medical Journal*, 312, 1215–1218.

Bhugra, D. and Leff, J. (1993) *Principles of Social Psychiatry*. Oxford: Blackwell Scientific Publications.

Breakey, W. (1996) *Integrated Mental Health Services*. Oxford: Oxford University Press.

Cochrane, A. (1971) *Effectiveness and Efficiency: Random Reflections on Health Services*. Leeds: The Nuffield Provincial Hospitals Trust.

Dear, M. and Wolch, L. (1987) *Landscapes of Despair*. Polity: Cambridge.

Desjarlais, R., Eisenberg, L., Good, B. and Kleinman, A. (1995) *World Mental Health. Problems and Priorities in Low-income Countries*. Oxford: Oxford University Press

Ellison, N. and Pierson, C. (1998) *Developments in British Social Policy*. Basingstoke: Macmillan Press.

Freudenberg, R. (1976) Psychiatric care. *British Journal of Hospital Medicine*, 19, 585–592.

Furedi, F. (1997) *Culture of Fear: Risk-Taking and the Morality of Low Expectation*. London: Cassell Academic.

Geddes L. and Harrison, P. (1997) Closing the gap between research and practice. *British Journal of Psychiatry*, 171, 220–225.

Goldberg, D. and Huxley, P. (1992) *Common Mental Disorders. A Bio-social Model*. London: Routledge.

Goldberg, D. and Huxley, P. (1980) *Mental Illness in the Community*. Tavistock: London.

Henderson, A.S. (1988) *An Introduction to Social Psychiatry*. Oxford: Oxford University Press.

Knudsen, H.C. and Thornicroft, G. (1996) *Mental Health Service Evaluation*. Cambridge: Cambridge University Press.

Kuhn, T. (1962) *The Structure of Scientific Revolutions*. Chicago: University of Chicago Press.

Lawrence, P. and Lorsch, J. (1986) *Organisation and Environment*. Boston: Harvard Business School Press.

Leff, J. (1993) Principles of social psychiatry. In: Bhugra, D. and Leff, J. (eds), *Principles of Social Psychiatry*. Oxford: Blackwell Scientific Publications.

Lehman, A.F. (2000) Measures of quality of life among persons with severe and persistent mental disorders. In: Thornicroft, G. and Tansella, M. (eds), *Mental Health Outcome Measures*. Berlin: Springer.

Levin, B. and Petrila, J. (1996) *Mental Health Services. A Public Health Perspective*. Oxford: Oxford University Press.

Lief, A. (1948) *The Commonsense Psychiatry of Dr. Alfred Meyer*. New York: McGraw-Hill.

Mays, N. and Pope, C. (2000) Qualitative research in health care: assessing quality in qualitative research. *British Medical Journal*, 320, 50–52.

Meltzer, H. *et al.* (1995) *The Prevalence of Psychiatric Morbidity Among Adults Living in Private Households*. London: HMSO.

Mosher, L. and Burti, L. (1989) *Community Mental Health. Principles and Practice*. New York: Norton.

Murray, C.J.L. and Lopez, A.D. (eds) (1996) *The Global Burden of Disease, Volume 1. A Comprehensive Assessment of Mortality and Disability from Diseases, Injuries and Risk Factors in 1990, and Projected to 2020*. Cambridge, MA: Harvard University Press.

Perkins, R. and Repper, J. (1998) *Dilemmas in Community Mental Health Practice*. London: Radcliffe Medical Press.

Rehin, G. and Martin, F. (1963) Some problems for research in community care. In: Freeman, H.L. and Farndale, J. (eds), *Trends in the Mental Health Service*. Oxford: Pergamon Press, pp. 34–43.

Robins, L.N. and Regier, D.A. (1991) *Psychiatric Disorders in America*. New York: The Free Press.

Sabshin, M. (1966) Theoretical models in community and social psychiatry. In: Roberts, L.M., Halleck, S.L. and Loeb, M.B. (eds), *Community Psychiatry*. Madison, WI: University of Wisconsin Press, pp. 78–92.

Serban, G. (1977) *New Trends of Psychiatry in the Community*. Cambridge, MA: Ballinger.

Stern, S., Doolan, M., Staples, E., Szmukler, G. and Eisler, I. (1999) Disruption and reconstruction: narrative insights into the experience of family members caring for a relative diagnosed with serious mental illness. *Family Process*, 38, 353–369.

Strathdee, G. and Thornicroft, G. (1997) Community psychiatry and service evaluation. In: Murray, R., Hill, P. and McGuffin, P. (eds), *The Essentials of Psychiatry*. Cambridge: Cambridge University Press, pp. 234–257.

Szmukler, G.I., Burgess, P., Herrman, H., Benson, A., Colusa, S. and Bloch, S. (1996) Caring for relatives with serious mental illness: the development of the 'Experience of Caregiving Inventory'. *Social Psychiatry and Psychiatric Epidemiology*, 31, 137–148.

Tansella, M. (1986) Community psychiatry without mental hospitals—the Italian experience: a review. *Journal of Royal Society of Medicine*, 79, 664–669.

Taylor, R.. and Thornicroft, G. (2000) Uses and limits of randomised controlled trials in mental health services research. In: Tansella, M. and Thornicroft, G. (2000) *Mental Health Outcome Measures*, 2nd edn. London: Royal College of Psychiatrists (Gaskell). (In press).

Thornicroft, G. and Tansella, M. (1999) *The Mental Health Matrix. A Manual to Improve Services*. Cambridge: Cambridge University Press.

Wing, J. (ed.) (1989) *Health Services Planning and Research. Contributions from Psychiatric Case Registers*. London: Gaskell.

2 | Historical changes in mental health practice

Nikolas Rose

Introduction

However we define 'community psychiatry', it is clear that, in contemporary societies, practices addressed to the mental troubles of individuals have proliferated across everyday life. Psychiatric medicine is practised in mental hospitals, psychiatric wards in general hospitals, special hospitals, medium secure units, day hospitals, out-patient clinics, child guidance clinics, prisons, children's homes, sheltered housing, drop-in centres, community mental health centres, domiciliary care by community psychiatric nurses and, of course, in the GP's surgery. Connected up to these sites of psychiatry are a whole variety of social workers and care workers and a plethora of psychotherapies practised in consulting rooms. No phase of life is unknown to these practices: infertility, pregnancy, birth and the post-partum period; infancy; childhood at home and at school; sexual normality, perversion, impotence and pleasure; family life, marriage and divorce, employment and unemployment, mid-life crises and failures to achieve; old age, terminal illness and bereavement.

Wherever problems arise—in our homes, on the streets, in factories, schools, hospitals, the army, courtroom or prison—experts with specialist knowledge of the nature, causes and remedies of mental distress are on hand to provide its diagnoses and propose remedial action. In addition, of course, there is a wider penetration of psychiatry, broadly defined, into popular culture, as psychiatrists, mental hospitals, the mentally ill and the problems of mental health feature daily in political and social debates, in our newspapers, in television documentaries, exposés, talk shows and soap operas. The languages that have been disseminated have given us new vocabularies in which to think and talk about our problems—stress, trauma, depression, neuroses, compulsions, phobias. They have also provided us with new ways of explaining, judging and accounting for our personal miseries, of distinguishing the normal and the abnormal, identifying what is illness, when to seek assistance and from whom. It would not, therefore, be too much of an exaggeration to say that we live in a 'psychiatric society'.

'Community psychiatry', then, is one dimension of the 'psychiatric societies' that have taken shape over the course of the 20th century. There have been many international variations in the historical paths followed in different national contexts, but the rationalities and practices that have taken shape are remarkably similar across the western world. In this chapter, focusing upon the UK, I want to sketch out some of the key moments in this history (except where stated specifically, reference is to developments in England and Wales).

The territory of psychiatry

The early decades of the 20th century are usually understood as a period when 'organicism' in psychiatry was in its heyday, when therapeutic pessimism dominated and when psychiatry and its practitioners, like their patients, were entrapped in the enclosed institutional spaces that were the legacy of the asylum movement of the previous 100 years; asylums that had now become little more than vast warehouses for containment of those thought to be of unsound mind. At the outbreak of the First World War, there were nearly 140 000 patients in mental hospitals and other institutions in England and Wales, and the average county asylum housed over 1000 inmates. These figures were to increase over the subsequent four decades, reaching a peak of more than 150 000 inmates by 1954 (Jones, 1972, Appendix 1). Conventional psychopathology by and large saw mental pathology in terms of a relationship between an inherited constitution and the life stresses to which it was subject. The inherited nervous system might be insufficiently equipped with nerve cells, association fibres or be otherwise organically flawed. After conception, including during the *in utero* period, the nervous system might be damaged by stress. The brain might be injured, or harmed by toxins such as alcohol or by lack of nutrition or defects in the blood supply. In addition to such direct stress, the nervous system was also subject to the effects of indirect stress. Anxiety, inappropriate or overdemanding education, worries about employment or finance, intemperance or sexual excess, even religious fanaticism could adversely affect the nervous system (Rosen, 1959; Rose, 1985, pp. 177–179).

However, this organicism still allowed psychiatry a role outside the asylum. Epilepsy, alcoholism, mental defect, mania, melancholia and other personal and social ills were regarded as expressions of an inherited neuropathic constitution which might lead to antisocial and immoral conduct. Such undesirable behaviour might also provoke the onset of explicit pathology in those with such a predisposition, and thus could be criticized on medical as well as moral grounds. Careful management of infants was essential. For those children whose families had shown pathology, this would strengthen the constitution and build up habits which would minimize the risk of onset. It was also vital in other families, for not even the strongest constitution was immune to damage. In addition, of course, the profligate breeding of those with severely tainted constitutions could lead to a swamping of the nation with neuropaths and a decline in national efficiency and the quality of the race. Hence the involvement of many key figures from the field of mental medicine in eugenic campaigns for the medical inspection, sterilization or permanent segregation of mental defectives and others of the social problem group (Rose, 1985).

The wider socio-political role for psychiatry here was largely reactive and defensive: to help minimize and control the threat posed by insanity. However, in the period following the First World War, a number of psychiatrists developed a more positive strategy. This modelled itself on the arguments of the new public health that claimed to be able to address large-scale problems concerning the size and quality of the population and its consequences (Armstrong, 1983). In this preventive medicine, the political fortunes of the nation came to be seen as dependent upon the physical health of each individual; simultaneously, individuals were thought to play an active part in the spread of ill health through their personal conduct. Hence reform of this conduct could actively promote social well-being. A complex apparatus of medical inspection, education in domestic hygiene, registration of births, infant welfare clinics, health visitors, school milk and meals, health clinics and so forth was established to investigate these habits and to educate citizens to conduct their personal lives in a hygienic manner and, indeed, to encourage them to want to be healthy. The new social psychiatry adopted many of these principles, and tried actively to promote mental welfare and mental hygiene. The first focus of this strategy was 'the neuroses'. This term was applied to conditions that were considered to be mild mental disturbances: they did not disable the individual completely, but were sufficient to cause social inefficiency and personal unhappiness. If left untreated, these minor troubles were thought likely to develop into more serious mental problems. It was also argued that many of those in workhouses and prisons—vagrants, criminals, delinquents and others who were socially or industrially inefficient—suffered from mental pathology which had probably begun in a small way in treatable neurosis. Hence the neuroses of childhood were of particular concern. They provided a fortunate early warning of troubles to come and, given the malleability of the child, it was thought that, in the majority of cases, they could be treated successfully.

The neuroses came to light in all those sites where individuals could now be seen to fail in relation to institutional norms and expectations—

in the production line routines of factory labour, in the expectations of universal schooling, in the newly established juvenile courts and, especially, in the unprecedented demands upon the military in the First World War. Shell shock accounted for 10% of officer casualties in the 1914–1918 war, and for 4% of casualties from other ranks. More than 80 000 such cases were estimated to have occurred over the course of the war, and some 65 000 ex-servicemen were still receiving disability pensions in 1921 because of shell shock. While senior military officers frequently regarded shell shock as merely a disguise for cowardice, organicist physicians considered the condition to be a genuine one resulting from minute cerebral haemorrhages caused by the blast (Hearnshaw, 1964, pp. 245–246; Rose, 1985, pp. 182–183). However, doctors working in the shell shock clinics and specialized hospitals that were set up to deal with these cases were unconvinced by such organic explanations, especially given the lack of independent evidence of the postulated lesions. Versions of the therapeutic methods invented by Janet in Paris and Freud in Vienna were tried out on the shell-shocked with some success. Shell shock appeared to respond to a variety of approaches ranging from occupational training, through persuasion and a form of rational re-education, the use of suggestion, to a type of psychotherapy using hypnosis or free association. Experience with this treatment converted many to a kind of dynamic theory of the will, using concepts such as instinct and repression, and attentive to the intermixing of physical and mental symptoms. These beliefs played a key role in the mental hygiene movement: for the first time, psychiatrists would collaborate with other professionals in a strategy for the prevention, early detection and voluntary treatment of mental ill-health

The rationale of mental hygiene, with its belief in a continuity between minor and major mental disorders and in the importance of early intervention for individual adjustment and social efficiency, underpinned the argument made in a series of official reports from the 1920s to the outbreak of the Second World War (discussed in detail in Rose, 1985, pp. 197–209). Poor mental

hygiene was thought to be the cause of all sorts of social ills, preventable by education in proper techniques for mental welfare and mental hygiene, and by early detection of the signs of trouble followed by prompt and efficient treatment. It was believed that this was hampered by the stigma which surrounded lunacy, by the isolation of the asylum from other medical facilities and by the legal procedures of 1890 which allowed asylums only to take patients certified through a cumbersome legal process. This discouraged individuals with mild problems from seeking help, and discouraged doctors from utilizing asylums, turning them into institutions for the incarceration of those considered beyond hope. Not only was this a counter-productive method of organizing services, it was also conceptually unwarranted. As the Royal Commission on Lunacy and Mental Disorder put it in 1926 "insanity is, after all, only a disease like other diseases . . . a mind deranged can be ministered to no less effectively than a body deranged . . . The problem of insanity is essentially a public health problem to be dealt with on modern public health lines" (1926, pp. 16–22).

Treatment should not require certification, compulsion or incarceration. Facilities should be available in hospitals for out-patient and voluntary treatment to encourage easy access to help at an early stage of the disease (Rees, 1945, p. 29). This was the rationale that led to the establishment of the Maudsley Hospital, which was completed in 1915 and the Cassel Hospital, which opened in 1919 (Barnes, 1968, pp. 10–15; Jones, 1972, pp. 235–236). It was for similar reasons that the Mental Treatment Act 1930 renamed asylums 'mental hospitals' and stipulated that, in the majority of cases, lunatics should be termed simply 'persons of unsound mind'. Patients could now be received for in-patient treatment on voluntary application, and local authorities were to make provision for the establishment of psychiatric out-patient clinics at general and mental hospitals. (The responsibilities of local authorities for lunacy and mental deficiency services and aftercare had already been widened by provisions of the Local Government Act of 1929 which followed the recommendations of the Royal Commission on

Lunacy and Mental Disorder; cf. Rose, 1985, pp. 158–163.)

Disturbed individuals could come to the clinics themselves, once they or others were educated in the signs of mental disturbance, and now free of the fears of stigma or incurability. Others were to be referred to them from school, court and elsewhere by statutory and voluntary agencies. In the clinics, assessment and treatment would be carried out, reports would be supplied to courts or schools, individuals would be referred to other institutions. However, the clinics would also provide the base for a system of mental hygiene which could act more widely on the lives of patients, ex-patients and potential patients. Social workers, psychiatric social workers, probation officers, school attendance officers and others would operate between the clinic and home, school or courtroom, conveying information, advice and education. The new mental hygiene was to provide the basis of a project of general public education as to the habits likely to promote mental welfare. Mental health was to be a personal responsibility and a national objective.

Community as therapy

Despite these developments, in practice the pre-Second World War psychiatric population was split between the 'neurotics', i.e. maladjusted and delinquent children, inefficient workers, shell-shocked soldiers and the like, and the 'psychotics'. These latter were those certified under mental health legislation, segregated from the sufferers of physical illness and confined in the large, isolated, custodial mental hospitals. The provision of out-patient clinics was confined to a few geographical areas; only a small number of the more recently built asylums had established separate facilities for new acute patients; very few beds for in-patient treatment were provided in wards of general hospitals; some, but not all, municipal hospitals had set up 'observation wards' where mental patients could be confined under short sections for limited periods for assessment and diagnosis before being discharged or committed to a mental hospital.

In the 1930s, mental hospitals in England and Wales had an average population of around 1200, but some contained up to 3000 patients. The majority were there for long periods, if not permanently, and active therapeutic intervention was spasmodic. It was accepted that the majority of patients were suffering from psychoses which were often hereditary in origin and mostly incurable. The old ideals of moral treatment had largely been discarded; however, for the most fortunate patients, asylums did operate as communities where they "lived a life of contented servitude, working as orderlies, storemen, or domestic servants in a cosier world than that outside" (Clark, 1964). With the melancholic, paraphrenic or deluded, certain attachments formed between staff and patients; for others, the regime varied from neglect, through surveillance and containment, to degradation and brutality.

However questionable their claims to efficacy, the new physical treatments developed in the 1930s did disrupt this stasis. They offered asylum doctors an image of themselves as healers of the sick and not merely superintendents of the institution. Waves of enthusiasm for these treatments swept through the hospitals. Physical treatments—from removal of tonsils to varieties of convulsion therapy—were selected according to the latest reports in the medical literature or the predilections of the medics. As with the claims for bleedings and purgings of the 18th century and for the use of sedatives such as chloral hydrate and bromides in the 19th century, such hopes were usually short lived. However, despite limited experimentation in asylums, or in units attached to them, the principal task of asylum doctors remained the containment of chronic patients; it often required the use of coercion and offered few prospects for innovation other than more efficient administration.

Within mental medicine, hostility was growing between the long established sector of asylum superintendents who dominated the Board of Control, defenders of the need for separate and distinct institutions for the treatment of the mentally ill, and physicians who sought the integration of the practice, training and facilities of psychiatry with those of the general hospital. The future of psychiatry was being shaped outside the asylum mainstream, in specialist units in general hospitals, in out-patient clinics, in private practice, in psychotherapy and psychoanalysis. The Second World War was to shift the balance decisively between these two wings of psychiatry (cf. Baruch and Treacher, 1978).

John Rawlings Rees, Director of the Tavistock Clinic, was appointed consulting psychiatrist to the Army, perhaps because the problems at issue in wartime were precisely those of functional nerve disorder over which the Tavistock had established its jurisdiction. In any event, the consequence was that the new tasks of psychiatry were to be thought from within the rationale of mental hygiene. Psychiatrists tried to develop methods of selection, both for the weeding out of potential problem cases and in the selection of those suitable for promotion. They tried to adjust military training techniques in order to enhance the fit between the mental and the organizational, and sought to maximize morale by methods of man-management which would promote solidarity through acting on the psychiatrically important aspects of group life. Whilst each of these developments would have significance for the expanded role of the 'psy' professions in the postwar period, most important for psychiatry itself was the issue of treatment. [On the concept of the psy professions (psychiatrists, psychologists, psychiatric social workers and many more), see Rose (1996).]. Psychiatrists were involved in the treatment of casualties: in the army alone, they saw almost a quarter of a million cases during the Second World War, even discounting those referred from army intakes, those seen in selection testing and patients seen in psychiatric hospitals (Rees, 1945, p. 46). Whilst only about 8000 of these were diagnosed as psychotics, about 130 000 were considered to be neurotics. The invaliding rate for psychiatric disabilities was more than 30% of all discharges for medical causes. Whilst military neurosis centres did manage to return about 80% of their cases to duty, the results of treatment overall were poor. This emphasized the need for new treatment techniques. More fundamentally, it confirmed that psychiatry should not focus upon the confinement of the small number

of psychotically deranged persons. To fulfil the task that society required, it needed to shift its attention to the detection and treatment of those large numbers of the population who were now known to be liable to neurotic breakdown, maladjustment, inefficiency and unemployability on the grounds of poor mental health (cf. Jones, 1972, pp. 262–282).

Perhaps the most significant invention in treatment concerned the institution itself. At the start of the Second World War, whilst confinement might have been a condition for certain types of treatment, it was not in itself considered to be therapeutic. However, in the course of the war, for the first time since the heyday of moral treatment, some at least began to argue that the institution itself could be a therapeutic technology. Maxwell Jones credits Wilfred Bion with the first recognition of the principle underlying the social therapies that "social environmental influences are themselves capable of effectively changing individual and group patterns of behaviour" (Jones, 1952, p. 519; cf. Kraüpl Taylor, 1958; Manning, 1976). In 1943, Bion tried an experiment in which he treated the unruly conduct of the inmates of the Training Wing of Northfield Military Hospital through manipulating authority relationships, believing that if the men themselves had to take responsibility for organizing tasks, and for defining and disciplining miscreants, they would learn that the disruption was not grounded *in* authority but in their psychological relationships *to* authority.

Although the authorities terminated this experiment after 6 weeks, it was followed by a second 'Northfield experiment' in which Thomas Main sought to produce what he referred to as a 'therapeutic community' in which the hospital was to be used "not as an organisation run by doctors in the interests of their own greater technical efficiency, but as a community with the immediate aim of full participation of all its members in its daily life and the eventual aim of the resocialisation of the neurotic individual for life in ordinary society . . . a spontaneous and emotionally structured (rather than medically dictated) organisation in which all staff and patients engage" (Main, 1946, p. 67). At the same time, Maxwell Jones became joint director of the Mill Hill Neurosis Unit, set up by the Ministry of Health for the treatment of 'effort syndrome', and concluded that the patient's reactions to the hospital community mirrored his reactions to the community outside, and hence that the hospital itself might be an instrument to be used to explore and improve the patients condition.

At the end of the war, Jones was put in charge of one of the units for labour resettlement set up by the Ministry of Labour with the aim of rehabilitating ex-prisoners of war for civilian life. The techniques deployed in these 'transitional communities' for 'social reconnection' were those which had been developed in the community treatment of neurotic soldiers, with the addition of attempts to connect up the 'transitional community' with the local community which surrounded it (Curle, 1947; Wilson *et al.*, 1947; cf. Kraüpl Taylor, 1958). Where rehabilitation previously had been a mere adjunct to therapy conducted by other means—mediating between life under the dominance of medicine and life as a private matter—it was now seen as the essence of the therapeutic intervention itself. The patient was one who had lost his or her capacity to function as an adjusted social individual; treatment was to reinvest them with the rights, privileges, capacities, moralities and responsibilities of personhood. This way of thinking, in which mental ill-health is identified in terms of a failure to cope, and treatment becomes a matter of the restoration of coping capacities, would spread widely through psychiatric practice in the post-war period, and indeed would become the practical rationale of much of community psychiatry in the 1970s and beyond.

In the immediate post-war period, Jones argued that the techniques he had developed could be applied to any other socially maladjusted individuals—in particular to 'psychopaths' (Jones, 1952). In 1947, he moved to the Industrial Neurosis Unit at Belmont Hospital and applied these methods to the 'chronic unemployed neurotics' it received from all over England including inadequate and aggressive psychopaths, schizoid personalities, early schizophrenics, various drug addicts, sexual perverts and chronic psychoneurotics. Through a

variety of discussion groups, intense small groups and psychodrama, sexual, criminal, industrial or social deviants, whose behaviour was now construed as a manifestation of an underlying personality disorder, were to be managed back to a state of adjustment in which they could function smoothly within the institutional regimes which they previously had disrupted.

It required only a simple shift of perspective to see that the traditional mental hospital violated all these therapeutic maxims. Hence, in the 1950s, a two-pronged attack on such institutions was mounted under the banner of the 'therapeutic community'. On the one hand, a series of research studies of psychiatric institutions confirmed the pathogenic features of their organization and management (e.g. Stanton and Schwartz, 1954; Caudill, 1958). On the other, a series of 'adventures in psychiatry' were undertaken, notably at the Cassel, Claybury and Fulbourn, which sought to reorganize the mental hospital more or less according to the new rationale and to incorporate some or all of the new techniques of administrative therapy into their institutions, sometimes in combination with chemotherapy or psychoanalytically inspired individual therapy (Clark, 1960; Martin, 1962; Barnes, 1968, pp. 4–15). These developments were isolated and short lived. Many psychiatrists were scandalized by the reported 'goings on' in such hospitals. They criticized the therapeutic efficacy of these attempts to use the institution as a positive element in the production of the cure, and they used arguments about the negative effects of mental hospital life in order to support their case. However, in fact, this new 'social' vision of the psychiatric institution reverberated through the system, leading to the widespread unlocking of wards throughout the 1950s, coupled with reductions in the regimentation of the lives of confined patients, and a policy of accelerated discharge. T.P. Rees at Warlingham Park Hospital opened the doors of 21 out of his 23 wards in the early 1950s; by 1956, 22 out of 37 wards at Netherne Hospital were opened and 60% of patients were allowed out on parole within the boundaries of the estate; MacMillan opened the doors at Mapperly Hospital Nottingham in 1954, Stern did likewise at the

Central Hospital Warwick in 1957, as did Mandelbrote at Coney Hill, Gloucester (for details see Kräupl Taylor, 1958, pp. 155–156).

This attention to the organizational and interpersonal features of the psychiatric setting offered new opportunities for psychiatric nurses. The new therapeutic vision of the interpersonal relationships of the hospital enabled them to stake a claim for a more autonomous type of expertise. Doctors could not claim special skills in the manipulation of the dynamic relationships between members of the institutional community; yet these were now to be utilized systematically in the construction of a normal identity for the patient. At its high point, which was probably in the 1970s, this underpinned a new 'psychotherapeutic' vision of psychiatric nursing as an activity which could itself be curative through working upon the patient's relationships with situations in the everyday life of the ward.

In the psychiatric wards of old mental hospitals and new psychiatric units, and in the day hospitals and halfway houses that began to proliferate, new techniques of nursing were developed and deployed. Nurses, in psychiatric and in general nursing, gradually altered their view of the patient: no longer merely a series of tasks, the patient was a sick person who needed to be engaged actively in the process of getting better. [Developments in nursing can be traced through the articles and letters in *Nursing Mirror* and *Nursing Times* over this period. See also Meacher (1979) and Barnes (1968). These developments in nursing are consonant with the shift in medical perception noted in Armstrong (1984).] These developments in nursing were accompanied by the growth of other forms of institutional therapy that owed something to the therapeutic community idea. Occupational and industrial therapies sought not only to increase muscular co-ordination and, hence, self-confidence, but also to encourage the habits of labour. As mental disorder began to be seen, at least in part, as an inability to cope with the demands of employment, work itself began to be seen as a vital element in the treatment of mental disorder (Miller, 1986). The developing programme of hospital closure allowed these practices to develop in new psychiatric spaces—in day

hospitals run by the hospital service, day centres run by local authorities, halfway houses, hostels, group homes and a variety of other residential and non-residential institutions. In the 1970s and 1980s, these professionals and their techniques would find their homes in the new institutions of the psychiatric community.

A place would also be found for the authentic therapeutic communities. There was not only Belmont, now known as Henderson Hospital, and the Cassel, but also 'mini'-therapeutic communities (Clark, 1970; Manning and Hinshelwood, 1979). These were characterized by such techniques as large and small group meetings, projective and expressive therapies involving art and drama, occupational therapies and individual therapies—developed in psychiatric units in general hospitals, in rehabilitative institutions in the prison system, in institutions for maladjusted, delinquent and criminal youths, in houses for drug users and alcoholics often run by ex-patients, in the work of Richmond Fellowship and in many other residential establishments in the public, grant-aided, charitable and private sectors. These institutions provide a therapeutic rationale for the confinement of young neurotics and the personality disordered, the persistently self-damaging, the repetitively suicidal, the ostentatiously antisocial, those who continually act out and those who are continually manipulated by others: those whose illness appears to consists only of a disruptive failure of social adjustment and whose treatment can thus be seen as co-extensive with, and exhausted by, a systematic programme of resocialization.

Accounting for community psychiatry

Conventional accounts of the move of psychiatry 'into the community' in the second half of the 20th century in the UK, the USA and much of Europe stress two factors: the discovery of genuinely effective psychotropic drugs and the recognition that confinement could be damaging. On the one hand, drugs offered the possibility of amelioration of symptoms if not cure, and did away with the necessity for long periods of institutional confinement, whilst also validating the medical mandate over problems of mental health. On the other hand, the discovery of the poor conditions within mental institutions and the pathogenic effects of confinement itself led to a view that long periods of confinement were damaging and antitherapeutic. In the USA, Albert Deutsch documented conditions in the asylums that were reminiscent of those in the concentration caps, and Erving Goffman published his sociological account of the effects of the 'total institution' in stripping away the personality and identity of the inmate (Deutsch, 1948; Goffman, 1962). In Britain, Russell Barton diagnosed a condition he christened 'institutional neurosis', i.e. a form of illness produced by the institution itself, and John Wing demonstrated that institutionalism—apathy, resignation, dependence, depersonalization and reliance on fantasy—was common to long-stay inmates of even well-run mental hospitals, and that reforms centring upon enriching the institutional environment were difficult to maintain in the face of institutional exigencies (Barton, 1959; Wing, 1962; see also Lomax, 1921). It appeared that the pathogenic effects of the mental hospital were, themselves, intractable; the solution was not to reform the institution but to do away with it. Such accounts suggest that these developments led to changes in policy, based on the view that mental hospitals did little good but much harm, and consumed scarce resources which were better directed to more effective forms of provision. Wherever possible, hospitalization should be avoided, where necessary it should be in the ordinary medical system, the length of stay should be minimized, and individuals should be maintained 'in their communities' where, rather than suffering the pathogenic consequences of institutionalization, they would be subject to the benign influences of normality.

Critics of this account of psychiatric progress point out that critiques of 'museums of madness' were nothing new, and so other factors must account for their effects at this particular moment in psychiatric history (e.g. Baruch and Treacher, 1978; Treacher and Baruch, 1981; Scull, 1985). They also dispute the significance accorded to the new discoveries in psychopharmacology, pointing to the repetitious history of enthusiastic claims for the efficacy of physical treatments of mental disorder followed by disillusionment occasioned by relapse, side effects or other disappointments. Further, there is little correlation between patterns of hospital bed use and discharge rates and the use of such drugs in different areas and countries; for example, the early use of phenothiazine drugs in the 1950s was as much for control within the hospital as to facilitate discharge. Thus sociologists and historians have suggested that the determinants of the move away from custodial responses to mental disorder must be found elsewhere. They have suggested that what was at stake was not a desegregation of the mentally ill, but a desegregation of psychiatry—a desire of psychiatrists to end their isolation and gain access to the power, careers and status of other medical specialties.

From this perspective, the 'drug revolution' is regarded not as the origin of the move away from the mental hospital but as a pseudoscientific legitimation for it (Treacher and Baruch, 1981). Critics also suggest that the political rationale for a shift away from the custodial institution lay in a 'fiscal crisis of the state': the costs of incarceration, of maintaining the buildings and paying the increased wages won by the unions were harder and harder to justify, in a situation where the state was finding it increasingly difficult to fund its welfare activities through the taxation system without unacceptable demands upon private profit (Scull, 1985).

The truth probably lies somewhere between these two narratives. Whilst the cost of maintaining mental hospitals, which were built largely in the 19th century, was a significant factor, as we have seen, the events that led to unlocking the wards and the run-down of the mental hospital system began much earlier, certainly before any 'fiscal crisis'. Indeed, cross-national comparisons show no correlation between moves away from incarceration and economic prosperity or crisis. Of course, the development of post-war welfare states provided crucial conditions for this shift in policy. Whilst in the 19th century, institutional confinement was seen as the condition for social support, in the era of the welfare state and social insurance this was no longer the case. Social insurance made it possible for individuals without wage labour to be maintained without incarceration. Public housing facilities provided the conditions for such persons to be physically sheltered outside institutions, as did the development of private and charitable housing schemes. The foundation of a comprehensive system of primary medical care enabled GPs to play a key role in the dispensing of the pharmaceutical treatments which would enable treatment to be maintained without custodial institutions. The consolidation of medical and psychiatric social work within the local authorities and the hospitals enabled supervision of the patients outside hospitals. However, the changes in psychiatry have been an intrinsic element in the new rationale of welfare, not a fortunate beneficiary. The post-war modernization of psychiatry was neither a mere rationalization for financial savings nor a consequence of psychopharmacology: it was the generalization of a socio-political strategy whose rudiments had been put in place over a 50-year period.

Blurring the boundaries of the institution

Official discussions of psychiatry in the post-Second World War period appear merely to reiterate and extend the themes concerning the need for early and voluntary treatment and the organizational and clinical similarities and interdependencies between mental and physical ills. The Royal Commission on Mental Illness and Mental Deficiency, which was set up in 1954 and reported in 1957, posed the issues in a similar way, as did the Mental Health Act 1959 which followed on from its recommendations. As the Minister put it, what was involved was a "re-orientation of mental health services away from institutional care towards care in the community". Hence the Act extended the open-door policy, established informal admissions as the norm, extended local authority powers, encouraged liaison between health and social services, and so forth (see, for the above, Jones, 1972, p. 307). This strategy

linked up with developments in the post-war apparatus of the welfare state. Psychiatric social work had extended from the child guidance clinics and mental hospitals into the heart of social casework (Younghusband, 1978). Psychiatric social workers were employed not only in the prison and Borstal services, in care committees and so forth, but also in the extensive work of rehabilitation of ex-service men and women, working in the mental health advisory services set up for this purpose under the National Health Service Act of 1946. Furthermore, psychiatrically trained social workers were now operating as Children's Officers under the Children Act of 1948: all social work now attended, to a greater or lesser extent, to the psychological investments and conflicts which underpinned even those presenting problems which were apparently entirely practical.

While the Mental Health Act of 1959 allocated considerable discretionary powers to doctors with respect to involuntary admission to mental hospital and the administration of treatment without the patient's consent, this was neither an extension of the coercive powers of the authorities nor a triumph of organicist medicine over other theories of the origin of mental disorder or other professional claims for a role in a mental health system. On the contrary, the strategy sought to minimize the role of incarceration in the social responses to mental distress, to establish links, relays and alliances between medicine and other social agencies, to facilitate the movement of individuals amongst and between the different branches of the mental health system, and to encourage each of us to take responsibility for the preservation and promotion of mental health.

However, despite these conceptual continuities, the transformations of the psychiatric system in the 1950s and 1960s do mark a significant shift in the spatial dispensation of psychiatry. Whilst neither criticisms of the asylum nor claims for the efficacy of physical treatments were new, in the context of the new rationale for psychiatry as a part of public health, they enabled an extension of psychiatric modernization to those sectors of the psychiatric system which previously had been most difficult to access. On the one hand, it was now argued that the closed asylums with their populations of chronic and psychotic patients were not only sucking in social resources which were more usefully deployed in the other sectors of the system, but were also actively damaging in their effects. On the other hand, whatever their real efficacy, the new pharmacological technologies of treatment made it possible to imagine that people with severe psychiatric problems could nonetheless be managed outside the hospital. The medical complex of GPs, out-patients departments and ordinary general hospitals could administer the drug-based therapeutics without the segregative institution. Social insurance and social workers could service the ill person without confinement. In addition, madness—understood now merely as illness, unhappiness and inefficiency—no longer constituted a fundamental threat to reason and order which required incarceration. The asylum had become unnecessary.

The policy landmarks of the new configuration are clear enough (Jones, 1972, pp. 321–334). Enoch Powell, Minister of Health, in his 1961 speech to the National Association of Mental Health, announced the objective of halving the number of places in hospitals for mental illness over the next 15 years, and the closure of the majority of the existing mental hospitals. The Ministry circular following this speech confirmed the decline in bed spaces, urged planning for closure of "large, isolated and unsatisfactory buildings", and laid out the four kinds of accommodation to be provided in the new system: acute units for short-stay patients, usually in general hospitals; medium-stay units for medium-stay patients; units for long-stay patients, often in hostels or annexes of general hospitals; and secure units provided on a regional basis. In 1962, the Hospital Plan for the next 15 years envisaged the phasing out of all specialist hospitals, such as those for the mentally ill and the chronically sick, and their incorporation into district general hospitals. In 1963, *Health and Welfare: The Development of Community Care* urged the desirability of 'community care', but did not specify what this entailed. By 1971, *Hospital Services for the Mentally Ill* proposed the complete abolition of the mental hospital system, with all in-patient,

day-patient and out-patient services provided by departments of district general hospitals, linked in to services provided by the local authority social services, GPs and in consultation with the Department of Employment.

This policy was continued throughout the 1970s, irrespective of the political complexion of the government or minister of the day. The lines of argument were similar in *Better Services for the Mentally Ill*, produced by Barbara Castle's Labour ministry in 1975, and in *Care in Action* and *Care in the Community*, produced in 1981 under the aegis of the monetarist conservatism represented by Patrick Jenkin. The strategy was now more clearly developed: articulated in terms of the creation of a comprehensive psychiatric service, a continuum of care and a community psychiatric system; prevention through education and the encouragement of practices to promote mental health; early treatment entailing the removal of stigma, ease of access, minimization of legal formalism and the education of professionals so that they may pick up the early signs of mental disorder; out-patient treatment in clinics, sheltered housing, through domiciliary services and with social work support; in-patient treatment to be minimized, for as short a period as possible and within the district general hospital; and aftercare on discharge provided by the out-patient services. Despite the controversies over the passage of the 1983 Mental Health (Amendment) Act, its emphases on care in the community, on the minimization of hospitalization and compulsory detention, and so forth, were entirely consonant with the direction of psychiatric modernization.

The psychiatric system which had taken shape in England, Europe and the USA by the 1980s was not primarily an apparatus of coercion and segregation, delineated by the mental hospital and monopolized by the medical profession. At the programmatic level, it aspired towards a 'continuum of care' which would run from custodial measures for those with major mental derangements, through voluntary treatment for minor mental troubles, to prophylactic work by propaganda, advice and the reform of personal life in the interests of mental health. The psychiatric population was highly differentiated and distributed across a range of specialized sites: secure units, local authority group homes, specialized units for children, alcoholics, anorexics, drug users, and so forth. Relationships had also been established between such institutions and other sites where psychiatric expertise was deployed: the child guidance clinic, the courtroom, the counselling centre, the prison and the classroom. In this 'advanced' psychiatric system, key roles were played by non-medical professions—nursing, social work, probation, psychology, education, occupational therapy—and increasingly by quasi-professional 'voluntary' or self-help organizations.

Nor was this psychiatric complex dominated by a socially blind organicism at the level of theory or treatment. Most psychiatric professionals allowed a key role for 'social factors' in the precipitation and prevention of mental distress, sought to inject psychiatric considerations into debates over social policies, and established collaborative relationships between medical treatment in hospital and the aid of other social agencies. A practical eclecticism enabled the co-existence of therapeutic ideologies and techniques which appear fundamentally opposed: from individual psychotherapy to co-counselling, from dynamic group therapy to behaviour modification, from drug treatment to family therapy. Hospitals using psychotropic medications, therapeutic communities, feminist self-help groups, social work group homes, community nurses and many other strange bedfellows combined to chart the domain of mental health and develop technologies for its management. The move away from the asylum extended the range of social ills seen to be flowing from psychiatric disturbance and simultaneously psychiatrized new populations. Children, delinquents, criminals, vagrants and the work shy, the aged, unhappy marital and sexual partners all became possible objects for explanation and treatment in terms of mental disturbance. In the majority of cases, such treatment was not imposed coercively upon unwilling subjects but sought out by those who had come to identify their own distress in psychiatric terms, believed that psychiatric expertise would help them and were thankful for the attention they received.

Community and control

The shifts in psychiatric policy over the closing two decades of the 20th century entailed a critique of many of these assumptions, and a reshaping of the practices to which they were linked. Many of the treatments that had been developed over the previous 50 years fell into disrepute, as expensive, lengthy and unproven: the demand for 'evidence-based treatments' was a key factor in displacing psychodynamically inspired therapies with interventions that sought rapid and measurable transformations in specific pathologies of thought or conduct. In this and other ways, the conceptual and practical boundaries between minor and severe mental illness were reconfigured. Many psychiatrists questioned the conception of a continuum of mental distress and argued for the need to concentrate on the severe conditions—which were increasingly thought to have an organic basis—which should be the principal target of treatment and the principal concern of publicly funded psychiatric services. 'Care in the community' was criticized from all sides (see N. Rose, 1998). Critics drew attention to the neglect, homelessness and degradation that had been produced in the name of an unrealistic policy of reduction of hospitalization, which was, in any event, hampered by inadequate funding, incompetent management and service rivalry. Newspaper headlines focused on the despairing plight of former mental patients isolated in bedsitters, vagrancy, homelessness, despair and suicide, and claimed that this was a policy which, under the guise of reform, amounted to abandonment. Many psychiatrists began to argue that the key factor for a successful life in the community for those with mental health problems was the maintenance of psychotropic medication: community psychiatry required not so much 'a continuum of care' but effective measures to ensure drug compliance outside the hospital.

By the close of the 20th century, assertions that care in the community had 'failed' no longer focused on the neglect of the vulnerable in the community but on the supposed threat to 'the community' by the mentally ill in their midst. A concerted campaign of 'scare in the community' had generated a new popular conception of 'mental illness' in terms of the propensity to violence (Philo, 1996; D. Rose, 1998). Hence a new socio-political demand is placed on psychiatry: it should take as its principal objective the surveillance and control of the mentally ill in the name of the protection and security of 'the community' (cf. Crichton, 1995). The little phrase 'care in the community patient' came to identify certain persons who, because illness had stripped them of their normal moral safeguards, posed a threat to the tranquillity, order and safety of 'the public'. The issue of homicides by those suffering from mental illness, previously a matter for a small number of forensic psychiatrists concerned with a small minority of 'dangerous individuals' who were 'mentally abnormal offenders', has come to shape arguments about the socio-political obligations of psychiatrists and other mental health professions to secure the security of 'the public'. One word characterizes the new demands placed on psychiatry and the new strategies for its spatial reconfiguration: risk (N. Rose, 1998; cf. Castel, 1991; Steadman *et al.*, 1993; Duggan, 1997). Mechanisms for the control of risk are now seen as central to the operation of all psychiatry—identification of risk factors, risk assessment, risk schedules, risk registers and risk management (Royal College of Psychiatrists, 1996).

The role of mental health professionals is now less that of cure or care than of the administration of dangerous, damaged or desperate individuals across a complex institutional field comprising institutions of various levels of security, halfway houses of various types, day centres, drop-in centres, hospital hostels, clinics, sheltered housing, assertive outreach teams and much more. The failures of psychiatry are now posed in terms of the failure of prediction and control of risky individuals, and hence the placing of 'the community' at risk. The demand is growing for the extension of coercive powers of mental health law—measures to secure drug compliance, provisions for preventive detention, etc.—in the belief that this is the only way to mitigate the dangers posed by the severely mentally ill to themselves, their families, psychiatric professionals and 'the public' (cf. Pratt, 1995; Simon, 1998).

As concerns about security come to the fore, a new spatialization of psychiatry is taking shape. We can describe this roughly in terms of the tripartite division that is becoming standard within British psychiatric policy and legislation: low risk, medium risk and high risk. In the zone of low risk, quasi-therapeutic techniques of control have proliferated across everyday life, regulating and reshaping individual conduct according to norms of autonomy, responsibility, competence and self-fulfilment. Here one finds counselling, mediation, conciliation, cognitive therapies, behavioural techniques and the like within the school, the factory, the training programme for the unemployed, and in hospital clinics, tutors' studies, the work of health visitors and social workers, and in GPs' surgeries. These practices of control operate in a much broader therapeutic habitat: a culture in which radio, television and cinema offer us psychologized images of ourselves, and a whole range of practices of life are shaped and organized in therapeutic terms (on control, see Rose, 1999).

In the zone of medium risk, state-funded and provided facilities have been drastically reduced. There are public psychiatric wards, social workers, quasi-public provision from 'voluntary agencies' and the like. Alongside this public provision, a private market has opened up for the management of acute mental health problems which do not appear immediately linked to danger to others. The new private arrangements are supported by the growth of private health insurance and by the emergence of market style arrangements for the purchase of care by publicly funded health services. In this zone of medium risk, mental health is increasingly governed through the family. That is to say, through strategies that seek to enhance, intensify and instrumentalize the apparently 'natural' bonds of obligation between members of domestic units: the self-governing family is urged, educated and obliged to take on itself the socio-political responsibility of managing its own mental health problems and its own problematic members.

However, in line with more general trends to the residualization of state welfare, the work of public agencies and state institutions has come to focus on the issue of 'high risk'. Mental health professionals have been given a key role within an extending apparatus charged with the obligation (which it inevitably fails to live up to) of the continuous and unending management of permanently problematic persons in the name of community safety. Different tactics are involved: 24 h nursed care, community treatment orders, assertive outreach, crisis intervention and the like. Spaces of psychiatric confinement are reassessed. On the territory of 'the community at risk', the different types of psychiatric institutions are virtually defined in terms of the need for security rather than those of therapy or care (Grounds, 1995). We are beginning to see the construction of a new archipelago of islands of confinement: special hospitals, medium secure units, re-locked wards in psychiatric hospitals. At the same time, new proposals are formulated for the confinement of certain 'monstrous individuals: those who, although they may have served a sentence for their crimes, and have not been diagnosed with a treatable mental illness, are considered too risky to the general public to be allowed to go free. Across the English-speaking world, strategies are debated for the preventive detention of sexual predators, paedophiles, the incorrigibly antisocial—of those thought to pose a risk to the community on the basis not so much of what they have done, but of what they are and what they might do (e.g. for Australia, Greig, 1997; for New Zealand, Pratt, 2000; for the USA, Scheingold *et al.*, 1994).

The assessment and management of risk has become part of the political obligation of psychiatry and the professional obligation of all those working with issues of mental health (Alberg *et al.*, 1996; Snowden, 1997). Psychiatry and law are intrinsically bound together within these new strategies of regulation, and the mechanisms of law play a key role in shaping the conduct of psychiatric professionals. The shadow of the law—the real or imagined fear of prosecution or of censure by quasi-judicial public inquiries—shapes professional conduct, and provides the legitimization for the relentless task of documentation intrinsic to these new risk-based psychiatric technologies. Psychiatric judgement has become enwrapped in a grid of legal and quasi-legal obligations (such as codes of practice, notes of guidance, and so forth) within a new regime of blame,

in which mental health professionals operate under the threat of being held accountable for any harm to 'the community' which might result from the actions of those with whom they have been involved.

'Madness' has come to be emblematic of all the threats that are ascribed by those who think of themselves as 'normal' to those who they marginalize or exclude. Within this perception, difference is recoded as danger, and a constant labour is required to mark out and police those differences that are no longer demarcated by the walls of an asylum or the closed doors of the hospital ward. In this new problems space, not merely those with mental health problems, not only psychiatric professionals, but everyday life itself is 'governed through madness', i.e. regulated and shaped in terms of the fear of those with mental health problems and the need to reduce risks (on governing, see Rose, 1999; cf. Simon, 1997 on 'governing through crime'). At a time when the 'users', 'consumers' and 'survivors' of psychiatry are, at last, demanding their own say in the practices of mental health, the challenge for psychiatrists 'in the community' over the next decades lies in their capacity to manage these new tensions between their obligations to their patients and these sociopolitical demand for control.

Acknowledgements

This is a revision and update of a chapter entitled 'Psychiatry: the discipline of mental health, which appeared in *The Power of Psychiatry* edited by Peter Miller and Nikolas Rose, Cambridge, Polity Press, 1986. More detailed references to original texts can be found there, and in Rose (1985). Thanks to Diana Rose for her advice in preparing this version.

References

Alberg, C., Hatfied, B. and Huxley, P. (1996) *Learning Materials on Mental Health: Risk Assessment*. Manchester: University of Manchester.

Armstrong, D. (1983) *Political Anatomy of the Body: Medical Knowledge in Britain in the Twentieth Century.* Cambridge: Cambridge University Press.

Armstrong, D. (1984) The patient's view. *Social Science and Medicine*, 18, 737–744.

Barnes, E. (ed.) (1968) *Psychosocial Nursing: Studies from the Cassel Hospital.* London: Tavistock.

Barton, R. (1959) *Institutional Neurosis.* Bristol, UK: Wright.

Baruch, G. and Treacher, A. (1978) *Psychiatry Observed.* London: Routledge and Kegan Paul.

Castel, R. (1991) From dangerousness to risk. In: Burchell, G., Gordon, C. and Miller, P. (eds), *The Foucault Effect: Studies in Governmentality.* Hemel Hempstead, UK: Harvester Wheatsheaf, pp. 281–298.

Caudill, W. (1958) *The Psychiatric Hospital as a Small Society.* Cambridge, MA: Harvard University Press.

Clark, D.H. (1964) *Administrative Psychiatry.* London: Tavistock.

Clark, D.H. (1970) The therapeutic community: concept, practice, future. *British Journal of Psychiatry*, 117, 375–388.

Crichton, J. (ed.) (1995) *Psychiatric Patient Violence: Risk and Response.* London: Duckworth.

Curle, A. (1947) Transitional communities and social reconnection. A follow-up study of the civil resettlement of British prisoners of war. *Human Relations*, 1, 42–68.

Deutsch, A. (1948) *The Shame of the States.* Reprinted New York: Arno, 1973.

Duggan, C. (ed.) (1997) *Assessing Risk in the Mentally Disordered. British Journal of Psychiatry Supplement 32.* London: Royal College of Psychiatrists.

Goffman, E. (1962) *Asylums.* New York: Doubleday.

Greig, D. (1997) Shifting the boundary between psychiatry and law. *Liberty: Journal of the Victorian Council of Civil Liberties.* February 1997.

Grounds, A. (1995) Risk assessment and management in a clinical context. In: Crichton, J. (ed.), *Psychiatric Patient Violence: Risk and Response.* London: Duckworth, pp. 43–59.

Hearnshaw, L.S. (1964) *A Short History of British Psychology, 1840–1940.* London: Methuen.

Jones, K. (1972) *A History of the Mental Health Services.* London: Routledge and Kegan Paul.

Jones, M. (1952) *Social Psychiatry.* London: Tavistock.

Jones, M. (1972) Therapeutic communities past, present and future. In: Pines, M. and Rafelson, L. (eds), *The Individual and the Group, Vol. 1.* London: Plenum.

Kräupl Taylor, F. (1958) A history of group and administrative therapy in Great Britain. *British Journal of Medical Psychology*, 31, 153–173.

Lomax, M. (1921) *Experiences of an Asylum Doctor.* London: Allen and Unwin.

Main, T. (1946) The hospital as a therapeutic institution. *Bulletin of the Menninger Clinic*, 10, 66–70.

Manning, N.P. (1976) Innovation in social policy—the case of the therapeutic community. *Journal of Social Policy*, 5, 265–279.

Manning, N, and Hinshelwood, R. (eds) (1979) *The Therapeutic Community: Reflections and Progress.* London: Routledge and Kegan Paul.

Martin, D. (1962) *Adventure in Psychiatry.* Oxford: Cassirer.

Meacher, M. (ed.) (1979) *New Methods of Mental Health Care.* Oxford: Pergamon.

Miller, P. (1986) The psychotherapy of employment and unemployment. In: Miller, P. and Rose, N. (eds), *The Power of Psychiatry*, Cambridge: Polity, pp. 143–176.

Philo, G. (1996) *Media and Mental Distress.* London: Longmans.

Pratt, J. (1995) Dangerousness, risk and technologies of power. *Australia and New Zealand Journal of Criminology*, 28, 3–31.

Pratt, J. (2000) Sex crime and the new punitiveness. *Behavioral Sciences and the Law*, 18(2–3): 135–151.

Rees, J.R. (1945) *The Shaping of Psychiatry by War.* London: Chapman and Hall.

Rose, D. (1998) Television, madness and community care. *Journal of Community and Applied Social Psychology*, 8, 213–228.

Rose, N. (1985) *The Psychological Complex: Psychology, Politics and Society in England, 1869–1939.* London: Routledge and Kegan Paul.

Rose, N. (1989) *Governing the Soul: The Shaping of the Private Self.* London: Routledge (2nd edn. London: Free Associations, 1999).

Rose, N. (1996) *Inventing Ourselves: Psychology, Power and Personhood.* Cambridge: Cambridge University Press.

Rose, N. (1998) Governing risky individuals: the role of psychiatry in new regimes of control. *Psychiatry, Psychology and Law*, 5, 177–195.

Rose, N. (1999) *Powers of Freedom: Reframing Political Thought.* Cambridge: Cambridge University Press.

Rosen, G. (1959) Social stress and mental disease from the 18th century to the present: some origins of social psychiatry. *Millbank Memorial Fund Quarterly*, 37, 5.

Royal College of Psychiatrists (1996) *Assessment and Clinical Management of Risk of Harm to Other People.* London: Royal College of Psychiatrists.

Royal Commission on Lunacy and Mental Disorder (1926) *Report.* Cmd. 2700 London: HMSO.

Scheingold, S., Pershing, J. and Olson, T. (1994) Sexual violence, victim advocacy and Republican criminology. *Law and Society Review*, 28, 729–763.

Scull, A. (1985) *Decarceration*, 2nd edn. Cambridge: Polity.

Simon, J. (1997) Governing through crime. In: Friedman, L. and Friedman, G. (eds), *The Crime Conundrum: Essays on Criminal Justice.* Boulder, CO: Westview Press.

Simon, J. (1998) Managing the monstrous: sex offenders and the new penology. *Psychology, Public Policy and Law*, 4, 1–16.

Snowden, P. (1997) Practical aspects of clinical risk assessment and management. In: Duggan, C. (ed.), *Assessing Risk in the Mentally Disordered. British Journal of Psychiatry Supplement 32.* London: Royal College of Psychiatrists, pp. 32–34.

Stanton, A.H. and Schwartz, M.S. (1954) *The Mental Hospital.* London: Tavistock.

Steadman, H.J., Monahan, J., Clark Robbins, P., Appelbaum, P. Grisso, T. Klassen, D., Mulvey, E.P. and Roth, L. (1993) From dangerousness to risk assessment: implications for appropriate research strategies. In: Hodgins, S. (ed.), *Mental Disorder and Crime.* Newbury Park, CA: Sage, pp. 39–62.

Treacher, A. and Baruch, G. (1981) Towards a critical history of the psychiatric profession. In: Ingleby, D. (ed.), *Critical Psychiatry.* Harmondsworth: Penguin, pp. 120–159.

Wilson, A.T.M., Doyle, M. and Kelnar, J. (1947) Group techniques in a transitional community. *Lancet*, 1, 735–738.

Wing, J. (1962) Institutionalism in mental hospitals. *British Journal of Social and Clinical Psychology*, 1, 38.

Younghusband, E. (1978) *Social Work in Britain: 1950–1975.* London: George Allen and Unwin.

3 | Defining 'community': meanings and ideologies

Shulamit Ramon

Introduction

The concept of 'community' is at the core of social and personal identity, policy and action (Payne, 1998). This chapter will examine, especially within a British and West European context: the definitions and meanings attached to 'community' and related concepts; issues of belonging and solidarity (social inclusion and exclusion, tolerance and stigma); issues which relate to the links between the community, the family and individual citizens; and the significance of these interlinked issues for all stakeholders in mental health services (e.g. empowerment, self-help, therapeutic communities, ghettoization and media approaches).

Multiple meanings of 'community'

Although in use since the 14th century, the concept of community was first used for analytical purposes by Toennies (1887/1963) the German sociologist. He distinguished between community of *shared meaning* ('*gemeineschaft*'— rural or traditional relationships characterized by intimacy and durability, and made meaningful by a shared culture) and that of *shared interest* ('*geselleschaft*'—urban or modern relationships characterized by impersonality, temporariness, competition and a contractual quality). In both cases, the community was perceived as a large group of people located near each other physically. Toennies assumed that rural communities valued an emotional, particularizing kind of human will, whereas urban communities reflected

a preference for the reduction of everything to abstract calculations. This historical development, representing a breakdown of traditional society, authority and sense of 'community', was viewed by him as a loss.

Indeed, the community provides a convenient level at which to look at the greater differentiation which has taken place with the industrial revolution. It is smaller than a whole society, yet larger than the primary unit of the family, while concrete enough to provide an image of the combined *sense of belonging, shared frame of reference and solidarity within a lived social framework.*

Durkheim, the French social psychologist and sociologist and contemporary of Toennies, focused on *social solidarity* in his attempt to understand what makes societies work and explained the different social patterns we see around us (Durkheim, 1889/1978). He argued that we once operated on the basis of *mechanical* solidarity focused on an intense morality generated by a small, homogeneous group of people in a simply organized society. We are now on our way towards *organic* solidarity, which is more abstract, universalistic, based on a division of labour and the organization of complementary differences. Durkheim's analysis of suicide as the ultimate rejection of social membership indicated to him the existence of anomie in the modern world (Durkheim, 1888/1952). Interestingly, the ideal type of 'solidarity' to which he hoped we would move in the future would be to go back to the past model of *guild-based* groups. Guilds are groups joined according to shared interest and expertise, where relative equality of power reigns by preventing 'unsuitable' people from entering.

'Solidarity' in its current sense is polarized: one end of the range is focused on defending the rights of those less able than oneself to do so, and on creating larger alliances based on shared interests of people unequal in power (e.g. the new social movements, the disability alliance). The other end of the range is represented by the re-emergence of nationalism, ethnocentricity and religious fundamentalism.

There are other conceptualizations of community which are noteworthy at this point. Community could denote belonging to a *status group*, 'a group of people who have a common lifestyle and share a sense of group identity' (Collins, 1988, p. 152); or a *consciousness community*, a group of people who happen to share the same economic interest, without necessarily sharing a common lifestyle or identity. This led Anderson (1983) to propose that we live with *imagined* communities, a suggestion which becomes almost concrete with the introduction of virtual realities—and communities—on the Internet. Willmott (1986) proposed that we consider place communities (shared location), communities of interest (without a geographical base) and communities of attachment (where people identify with particular social preferences).

An astonishing feature of both the sociological debate about communities and the related empirical research has been the tendency to describe such entities in a positive light, even when the evidence itself is mixed. Usually communities are portrayed as high on solidarity, with poor, worthy individuals, surviving against the odds and demonstrating instances of community spirit. While these qualities doubtless exist, the subtext of this description of working class communities–often referred to as *the* prototype of all urban communities—is littered with conflicts between children and their mothers, men and women, young and old, families and sub-neighbourhoods, apart from the conflict between classes. Yet with few exceptions (notably Samuel and Thompson, 1990), these issues are left unexamined. In part, this is likely to be an outcome of absorption in major class struggles, or awe at those so engaged. The timing of interest in the 'community'—at the end of the 19th century and after each of the world wars—reflects the longing for a more trustworthy and welcoming world, where uncertainty is not a key concern and consequently everyone knows their place (Jodelet, 1991).

'Neighbourhood' and 'network'

These two terms have been proposed as either replacements or additions to the concept of community since the 1970s.

Neighbourhood

Neighbourhoods are entities well known to most of us, with specific boundaries, a few specific features and a number of 'made-up' features, conjured to create distinctions in the description of one neighbourhood versus another. Neighbourhoods, i.e. the geographical proximity of people who have not chosen to live next to each other, and who are (at least in the beginning) strangers, are less embedded with mythical qualities than communities. Often people are there accidentally, with very few expectations of the neighbourhood *per se*, apart from those built up gradually on the basis of their relationships with the few people with whom they have developed a closer tie. Closer relationships develop out of shared interests (e.g. having school-aged children, or local religious congregations).

While these are interests which may change with time, a number of writings on 'neighbourhood' take for granted the existence of a shared wish among those who live nearby for a reasonable standard of living in communal areas—in terms of safety, cleanliness and comfort. This assumption is based on the history of some communities, where during a crisis neighbours did help each other (e.g. mining communities). It is argued convincingly that in urban neighbourhoods the degree of anonymity is greater, the quest for privacy stronger (Bulmer, 1987) and the readiness to provide voluntary help less than in a rural community. Nevertheless, it is assumed that given support and leadership, most neighbourhoods will turn into informal support networks. However, projecting from the informal care which existed/exists in communities with a considerable shared interest and attachment, as well as a shared location, to other types of communities may be unwarranted.

The debate in the literature on neighbourhood care tends to range from issues such as the optimal size of a neighbourhood (from 2000 to 10 000; Barefoot, 1990); through the usefulness of top-down attempts to create local leadership and support networks (Abrams, 1989); to redefining community as a set of neighbourhoods and proposing the relocation of community care in the latter (Baldwin, 1993).

Networks

Bulmer (1987, p. 108) has proposed that the term 'social network' is better suited than 'community' to convey the sense of relationships between concepts such as 'institution' or 'groups' to the activities and relationships of actual people. For him, this term enables a better description and understanding of a wider set of informal relationships which most of us have in different spheres of our lives.

Networks have been defined as a specific set of linkages (Mitchell, 1969) in which groups and individuals develop closer relationships around specific shared interests. Membership in one does not stand in opposition to membership in another, nor does membership in one exclude membership in another. Networks are less constrained by geographical boundaries than either communities or neighbourhoods, and their elasticity, in principle, allows for greater inclusion than exclusion. They provide an intermediary level between the state and its citizens, or society and its members.

Froland (1981) further argues that the concept of network has the advantage of putting together *the structure* of relationships among a set of actors "... the specific *exchanges* which take place among them and the *roles* they play with each other" (pp. 19–20). He and colleagues in Portland, Oregon, proposed types of networks and strategies needed to build up the helping network:

- a personal network strategy;
- a voluntary linking strategy;
- mutual aid networks;
- neighbourhood helping networks;
- community empowerment networks.

These may help us to focus on creating helping networks by professionals. The parallel British attempt to follow a neighbourhood-based ('patch') network approach in social work also took place in the early 1980s. The Barclay Committee on the roles and tasks of social workers defined 'community' as 'local networks of formal and informal relationships, together with their capacity to mobilise individual and collective responses to adversity' (Barclay, 1982, p. xiii). A decade later, Trevillion (1992) applied the concept specifically to the practice of community care, focusing on building up and connecting networks in the community as the key to the successful implementation of this policy.

Both the Barclay Report and Trevillion ignored the non-technical obstacles which have militated against the application of the network concept in social work and community care practice. These include:

- a prevailing, politically motivated ideology based on individualization and the denial of the need to invest in building community networks and collectives;
- fear of creating collectives, seen as synonymous with 'socialism' or 'communism', leading to anarchy and riots;
- blaming individuals for being poor rather than attributing some of the reasons for becoming poor to social structural factors;
- the sense of defeat and despair pervasive in poor estates;
- dismantling existing community work teams and settings in the late 1970s and early 1980s; and
- losing the expertise which the workers in these settings had. These may lie at the root of the failure to offer seamless and valued services in mental health too, a finding of many inquiry

committees and governmental reports (e.g. *Building Bridges*, 1995).

In summary, the 'neighbourhood' and 'network' concepts are easier to understand and work with, they pay due attention to issues of scale, and they are less pretentious than the concept of 'community'. However, both terms lack the emotional and moral appeal of the concept of community, and the sense of *lived* social space.

Definitions of community and modern ideologies of family values/communitarianism

The emergence of large urban areas and the debate on the nature of communities is closely related to the decrease in some key functions carried out previously by families, namely economic production and education, and informal socialization (Morgan, 1985). However, families are expected to rely mainly on their own emotional, financial and physical support. Until the 1980s, this support tended to be given mainly by parents to their children and to each other. Increasingly, middle-aged adult children care for their elderly parents and elderly adults care for their sick and long-term disabled partners.

Since the 1970s, there has been a greater proportion of single parent families, mostly headed by women. The majority are poorer than the average, and live on state benefits. There is an open social debate as to whether such a family provides sufficient support for its children. No similar debate is taking place as to the level of support a single parent receives in her/his own right. Regardless of the large proportion of single parent families, and the considerable increase in non-married partnerships, the dominant ideology remains one of a married, two-parent family. A social polarization in Britain is suggested by the increase in the average age of having a first child, while simultaneously the country heads the European league in the numbers of teenage pregnancies.

In Britain, the increase in support to elderly parents and partners, and the burden linked to it on middle-aged and elderly adults are perceived as the outcome of both the increase in longevity and health of elderly people, and the decrease in state welfare provisions taking place in the 1980s and 1990s. The majority of carers are women (Ungerson, 1995), but an increasing number of elderly carers are men. Research evidence (Ungerson, 1995; Shephered; 1996; Hill *et al.*, 1998) indicates that:

- Care by relatives saves the public/the state considerable sums of money.
- The burden of caring is reflected in a lower level of income than for comparable families, and a higher rate of physical and psychological symptoms of ill-health among carers.
- Carers do not receive either the quantity or the quality of attention and support they need from professional service providers. This is particularly the case in the field of mental health.
- Carers offer care from a variety of motives, such as love, duty, conviction; formal services (either within the state or the private sector) provide inferior and impersonal care; however, carers would like to be supported, and for their efforts to be valued positively by others, including their community.
- Male carers receive more support from formal care providers than women carers, perhaps in response to the relative novelty of having men in the caring role, as well as following stereotypes of women's domestic abilities.

The Carers Recognition Act, 1996, in the UK gives relatives the right to assessment. It falls short of meeting the issues just outlined, although offering a symbolic recognition of carers' needs.

One of the unwritten norms of western societies today is that families, and their individual members, should not be only passive recipients of rights but also should actively take responsibility for social action in the community where they live. Fulfilling this norm does not carry with it any specific sanctions. The latter point has been emphasized particularly by the *communitarian movement*. This movement originated in the USA at the beginning of the 1990s. Its prime spokesperson is Etzioni, who has researched professionalism and social change (Etzioni, 1995). The movement sees itself responding to the sense of crisis in American communities, urban and rural. Indicators of the crisis include the very low level of participation in national elections and in local civic activities, the high rate of killings of teenagers by other teenagers in schools and outside them, and the high rate of single parent families, crime and substance misuse.

In his analysis, Etzioni argues that the core issues are neither structural nor economic, nor are they about power differentials between powerful (e.g. the gun owners lobby) and powerless social groups (e.g. the victims of a shooting in a school). Instead, responsibility rests with the prevailing ideological preference for a right to receive from others (especially those anonymous others, such as the state) and the relative absence of any commitment to give to others. The movement proposes a reversal of these preferences, demonstrating the value of taking responsibility not only for oneself and one's family, but also for other people in the community. Aware of the risk of being branded as 'majoritarian' in a society in which individualism and the safeguarding of formal citizen's rights are the ruling ideologies, communitarians state they are not against minorities, but against 'selfish' people and groups. 'Neighbourhood watch' schemes, parent-established play groups and mothers against guns/drugs are good examples of communitarian activities. None of the examples cited relates to people who are disadvantaged, or who are both disadvantaged and stigmatized by the majority (such as those suffering from mental illness). Tellingly, self-help groups are not cited as examples of communitarianism, as *social inclusion* is not part of the communitarian agenda.

Etzioni's analysis has been welcomed by British governments as relevant to the felt crisis of its communities. The wish that citizens should take individual and collective social responsibilities is reflected in a large number of government policies, such as the 'Back to Work' policy. However, communitarianism does not provide adequate solutions to some central communal difficulties such as social exclusion and discrimination against ethnic minorities and the disabled.

Community integration versus fragmentation and atomization of modern society

It is taken for granted in lay perception today that modern urban life is typified by greater fragmentation than in the past, due to: the greater spatial separation of different life spheres (e.g. work, family, education, leisure); the very different roles and tasks we perform and undertake in these spheres; the increased focus on individuality and the parallel decrease in the focus on collective activities; and the more hectic pace of life. Increasingly it is argued that this state of affairs also applies to rural living, formerly portrayed idyllically. Wellman (1982) suggests that the degree of isolation is greater today in rural than in urban settings, due to the lack of variety of groups and activities available in towns (but not in villages). Furthermore, it is suggested that this fragmentation increases emotional and physical stress, and that those more isolated are more likely to suffer from mental distress, which may—or may not—develop into full-blown mental illness. Combined with being perceived as socially deviant or different, social isolation may be an additional risk factor, signifying that the person is both unwanted and devalued. It is proposed that discrimination against members of black ethnic minorities, which often leads to higher levels of unemployment and poverty, is the main reason for higher rates of identified severe mental illness in this group in comparison with the white majority (Fernando, 1991; Bhui and Olajide, 1999).

American researchers in the period from the 1930 to 1960s focused on the hypothesis that poor people, living in run-down areas, were more likely to become mentally ill, due to the accumulation of such stresses and the development of 'anomie'. Alternatively, it has been proposed that people already suffering from mental illness drift into poorer urban areas and become part of the population of such an area (Dunham and Faris, 1939; Hollingshead and Redlich, 1958). The two mechanisms may interact.

Universally, the prevalence of people in poor areas suffering from mental illness significantly exceeds that of people in less poor areas. This suggests that poverty is a risk factor (Thornicroft, 1991). Townsend's analysis of poverty highlights that its effect is not limited to poor health and insufficient income, but that it acts as an effective barrier to *participation in civic activities*, thus increasing isolation and exclusion, as well as social and personal devaluation (Townsend, 1996). Interestingly, proponents of psychiatric hospitals argued consistently that hospitals were *the community* and home for the in-patients (Carrier and Tomlinson, 1996). That this is an unsustainable argument is demonstrated by the high degree of lack of choice in such hospitals and the limitations on developing close relationships. The common observation that most in-patients did not know the first names of other patients on the same ward, let alone of workers, and that they hardly used verbal language to communicate with others (although quite able to talk), highlights that far from being a community, the mental hospital as a social institution represents an impoverished form of communal life (Copperman and McNamara, 1999; Williams and Keating, 1999). Mental hospitals have been severely criticized as total institutions in which both segregation from participation in ordinary community activities and a unidimensional identity of patienthood is fostered (Goffman, 1961).

Such thinking has motivated professionals and politicians to close these institutions. It is now accepted that an active stance to overcome the isolation of service users is necessary. The range of the attempts to overcome isolation, enable people to lead a valued life in the community, and to empower them, has included:

- Self-care and social skills training (Trower, 1978).
- Vocational training and employment initiatives (Beard *et al.*, 1982; Nehring, 1993).

- Therapeutic communities (Jones, 1952; Baruch and Treacher, 1978).
- Self-help groups (Ernst and Goodison, 1981; Adams and Lindenfield, 1985).
- The active pursuit towards the re-acquisition of socially valued roles *in* the community and *for* the community. This has been the hallmark of the normalization/social role valorization (SRV) approach (Wolfensberger, 1983; Brown and Smith, 1991; Ramon, 1991; Brandon *et al.*, 1995).

Of these measures, therapeutic communities and self-help groups merit special attention, as they attempt to *recreate* a *mini-community*, and to better understand the core of community living in its application to people suffering from mental illness (and at times for their relatives/carers). The regime in wards designated as therapeutic communities was much more democratic than on other wards, with more openness and *interdependency*. This setting offered opportunities to share painful issues as well as enjoyable activities, together with everyday responsibilities for maintaining a pleasant environment. At best, these settings provided a supportive network, rather than a community; at worse, they became a ghettoized environment. The discussion of the benefits of therapeutic communities continues. The Henderson hospital in Surrey, England (which works in this way with people labelled as having 'personality disorder') has been given a large grant by the Department of Health to enable it to develop two similar facilities elsewhere following research evidence concerning the efficacy of this type of intervention (Dolan *et al.*, 1997). Therapeutic communities have also been established outside hospitals by organizations such as the Richmond Fellowship and the Arbours Association, as a major tool for rehabilitation and resettlement in the community of young people with mental illness. Petch (1993) compared three group homes, including one based on therapeutic community principles in Scotland. Her study illustrated a higher degree of satisfaction and ambition to move out of a protected environment by the residents in the therapeutic community in comparison with the others.

Self-help groups have always existed in some form, but came to special prominence as part of the *new social movements* of the 1960s and 1970s as a reaction by people, active about causes they care about, to the fragmentation of social life (Melluci, 1995). Typically, a new social movement focuses on one issue, works collectively using small groups dynamics, has a flattened hierarchy, is more democratic than the old social movements and values emotional expression as much as intellectual expression. (e.g. feminist groups, the Greens). Self-help groups share many of these characteristics, but additionally members share a similar major problem, as well as associated stigmatization and isolation (Ernst and Goodison, 1981; Adams, 1990). Such groups, probably better defined as *mutual support* networks, offer:

- relief through sharing;
- reduction of isolation;
- re-valuation of members by themselves as people with positive qualities;
- sharing information;
- sharing action (as a pressure group, as providers of specific types of support, by consciousness raising).

Self-help groups therefore, do not attempt to be a community, but rather to offer a haven within an existing community that is perceived as unhelpful and ostracizing.

Community regeneration

Communitarianism is one attempt at community regeneration. Other approaches include working with residents of poor housing estates to activate them as well as on improving their physical infrastructure; regeneration of areas which have become derelict due to massive unemployment (e.g. the Docklands in East London and Consett in Durham) by bringing new enterprises and housing; creating opportunities for dialogue among groups which have become suspicious of each other (e.g. the police and the black community, professionals and service users in mental health); and creating frameworks for closer collaboration. An example of the last are Health Action Zones in the UK, a special attempt to bring multiple agencies together to work to improve the health of a local population (Hoggett *et al.*, 1999). Most existing urban regeneration projects are not focused specifically on mental illness, but are likely nevertheless to impact on people with mental health problems.

The question as to whether the state (through either central or local government) can lead community regeneration remains open. Research shows that communities need their own informal leadership to ensure the success of regeneration schemes, and that state workers may stifle such leadership (Saunders, 1993). Unless the involvement of weaker groups is fostered, leaders will emerge from among the stronger groups within the community, while the former will continue to be socially excluded (Lees and Smith, 1975). Nevertheless, little has happened since the 1970s in terms of involving weaker groups (Hoggett *et al.*, 1999). The reasons are the same as the reasons for the failure of the implementation of the networks approach to social work and community care, namely the denial of issues of power and the systematic avoidance of tackling them by those in power (e.g. politicians, professionals).

Self-directed group work (Mullender and Ward, 1991) is a more updated version of professional work with deprived groups in which power issues are not denied. This focuses on empowering groups to become active in mutual support and problem solving, and has been applied to mental health service users too.

Changing meaning of social exclusion and inclusion

The issue of social inclusion and exclusion has been a theme in most writings on the community, beginning with Durkheim's concepts of solidarity and anomie outlined earlier. Comments made above about the impact of poverty on civic participation and of discrimination against black ethnic minorities are also relevant.

From 1979 to May 1997, the use of the terms social inclusion and exclusion were 'politically incorrect' in Britain. The terms have been part of the European Union language since the early 1980s, used in different antipoverty programmes, in which the then British government participated only grudgingly. The terms were shunned in Britain as they had little place within an ideology of full-blown individualism and capitalism, in which the very existence of society—as distinct from individuals and families—was doubted by a 'Thatcherite' world-view. Elsewhere in western Europe, it was acknowledged that the welfare state was in crisis, but some (always partial) solutions to the crisis required urban regeneration and the *active involvement* of welfare recipients, perceived primarily as victims of structural factors and not as 'scroungers', and likely to rebuild their lives if treated with dignity and given suitable opportunities. For the success of individual rebuilding, there is a need for rebuilding the collective of those who have been disenfranchised in many informal ways and socially excluded, as well as the need for links to those who were included.

The focus on regions recognized as economically and socially deprived, coupled with shared European partnerships across public and not-for-profit sectors, highlighted the application of these principles. Most antipoverty programmes concentrated on unemployed people without a disability (Chanan, 1992). However, a number included vocational training and employment initiatives for subgroups of people with long-term disabilities.

The underlying principle of supporting the social inclusion of those hitherto excluded was to help them to help themselves. This is the meaning of inclusion used by the current British government, as expressed in different versions of 'back to work' schemes. While disability groups, including mental health service users, are ready, in principle, to endorse this utilitarian approach to social inclusion, serious differences exist between the government's approach and those of disability groups concerning the types and scope of opportunities and support measures required for this massive 'self-help' exercise to succeed. A related

issue is whether top-down governmental initiatives, such as legislation (e.g. the Disability Discrimination Act), and the Social Exclusion Unit in the UK can lead to reduction in exclusion and stigmatization.

The 'social role valorization' (SRV) approach is wider in its connotations than social inclusion, but incorporates social inclusion and fighting exclusion as core components. SRV focuses on the need to create a multi-layered framework which includes:

- changing our everyday disability language;
- services with attractive physical appearance;
- socially positively valued opportunities for visibility and joining activities in the community; and
- ending the segregation and separate congregation of disabled people.

All of this pre-dates the current British interest in social exclusion and inclusion. The empowerment of users and of carers in a variety of ways (e.g. through self-help groups, peer and self-advocacy) is another logical outcome of this approach which so far is absent from official notions of inclusion. While SRV is not specific to users of mental health services, it has been applied to them with success when major effort has been exerted in creating this framework, including a genuine transfer of power from professionals to users and carers (Hennelly, 1990)

Ghettoization, tolerance and stigmatization of the mentally ill

'Ghettoization' occurs when a minority group wishes to live somewhat apart to defend its lifestyle and/or to defend itself physically, or when a minority group is forced to do so. Due to urban decay, some areas are more run down than others and attract people who can only afford cheap rent. The area gets the reputation of being a ghetto, and this repels some people while attracting others. There are no ghettos solely for people with mental illness but, due to poverty, they often congregate in the poorer areas of town. Drug misuse, crime, poor housing, the concentration of poorer ethnic minority groups, social exclusion and at times experimentation with alternative lifestyles, including communal living, are likely to be prominent. It is difficult to assess the level of tolerance towards people suffering from mental illness in any particular society or community, given the wide range of such categories, the heterogeneity of people thus labelled and the changeability of their state of well-being.

The follow-up of the Defeat Depression Campaign by the Royal College of Psychiatrists (Paykel *et al.*, 1998) provides us with the findings of a twice repeated measurement for a large sample of 2000 people in contemporary Britain. The findings illustrate that depression is perceived to be an illness likely to happen to most respondents, for which they believe there are useful interventions leading to likely positive outcomes. They sharply disagree that medication offers the most useful intervention. Instead, they think that counselling should be the preferred mode of intervention. These views hardly changed between 1990, 1995 and 1997, namely before and after the campaign. The substantiated and repeated lack of stigmatization towards people with depression at different points in time cannot be attributed to the campaign.

The Mind Respect Campaign (Repper *et al.*, 1997) and other studies (e.g. Rogers and Pilgrim, 1997) paint a very different picture, one of isolation and at times intimidation of people who suffer from severe mental illness. These findings are reinforced by research on media coverage of mental illness and people thus labelled (Philo, 1996). However, a much more stereotyped perspective emerges in the media research, in which people suffering from severe mental illness are often portrayed as violent (Ramon, 1996). Furthermore, this portrayal is common in Britain but not replicated in other countries in which massive hospital closure has taken place, such as Italy (Ramon and Savio, 2000). It is likely that the media and the public have people with schizophrenia and personality disorder in mind rather than those suffering from depression. Furthermore, media views, which disregard and distort factual evidence about schizophrenia and personality disorder sufferers, will influence public attitudes and behaviours towards other subgroups within the range of mental distress and illness. For example, Taylor and Gunn (1999) have demonstrated that homicides by mentally ill people have not increased in numbers as psychiatric hospital closures have proceeded. Yet the public and politicians continue to believe that hospital closure and care in the community have led to an increase. The manipulation by journalists of fears expressed by lay people, and the effect this has had on politicians, is another important issue highlighted by these studies.

A different methodological approach has been employed in community studies by anthropologists (Roosens, 1979) and social psychologists (Jodelet, 1991). They used participant observation and interviews, mostly unstructured, over long periods. Roosens looked in the 1970s at attitudes and behaviours in Gheel, a Belgian town which has housed people with mental illness and learning difficulties since the 13th century. He reported that the presence of people with mental illness living in Gheel with foster families is barely tolerated, despite the fact that they have lived with the same families for a long time and, in a number of cases, have become the main carers of their foster parents. Jodelet looked at the views, attitudes and behaviours in Dur-sur-Arun and Ainey-le Chateau, large French villages which have become small towns in which people with mental illness have lived as lodgers under psychiatric supervision since 1900. Almost 1200 lodgers lived there during the 1980s. Using the social representation approach, she showed that the lodgers were perceived as subhuman, cheap labour and a group apart not to be associated with by the majority. Ordinary villagers who transgressed these boundaries and formed close intimate relationships with a lodger usually were ostracized by the local community, and felt the need to move away with their lodger-partner.

Both studies demonstrated no attribution of violence to this group by the ordinary population. It would seem that the negative attitudes are based on fear of the unintelligible nature of mental illness and the 'strangeness' of these people. The majority of the population opted for indifference and disregard as their reaction, and not for open suspicion or hostility. It is disappointing that both studies excluded the perspective of people categorized as mentally ill.

There are very few studies, or even examples, of educational campaigns involving the general public. The Defeat Depression Campaign has already been mentioned. Cummings and Cummings' classic project in the USA (Cummings and Cummings, 1957) highlighted how difficult it was to change community attitudes through an educational project. However, Wolff *et al.*'s (1996) project in Streatham illustrates that positive results can be achieved by employing more than one method and involving people with mental illness when focusing on a neighbourhood rather than a community. The work of Psichatria Democractica, the Italian movement of professionals for the reform of the mental health system, demonstrates the positive value of mass media and neighbourhood models, in influencing local people through the joint involvement and demonstrable solidarity of professionals, users, relatives, artists, journalists, young people and politicians (Mauri, 1986; Del Guidice, 1990; Ramon, 1992).

Conclusion

The concept of 'community' has more than one definition, and many meanings and connotations. Although less clear-cut than related concepts such as 'neighbourhood' and 'network', community has a more embracing and symbolic–emotional meaning as *a lived social space* which the other concepts lack. At its core are issues of belonging, identity, solidarity and shared beliefs or interests. The concept has acquired an almost mythological, rather than an explanatory function.

This chapter has attempted to examine, especially within a British and West European context, the following:

- definitions and meanings attached to 'community' and related concepts;

- issues of belonging and solidarity (social inclusion and exclusion, tolerance, stigma);

- issues which relate to the links between the community, the family and individual citizens; and

- the significance of these interlinked issues for all stakeholders in mental health services (e.g. empowerment, self-help, therapeutic communities, ghettoization, media approaches).

The analysis has drawn a number of important implications for policy, education and training, as well as for everyday clinical practice.

References

Abrams, P., Abrams, S., Humphrey, R. and Snaith, R. (1989) *Neighbourhood Care and Social Policy.* London: HMSO.

Adams, R. (1990) *Self-help, Social Work and Empowerment.* London: Macmillan-BASW.

Adams, R. and Lindenfield, G. (1985) *Self-help and Mental Health.* Ilkley, UK: Self-Help Associates.

Anderson, B. (1983) *Imagined Communities: Reflections on the Origins and Spread of Nationalism.* London: Verso.

Baldwin, S. (1993) *The Myth of Community Care: An Alternative Neighbourhood Model of Care.* London: Chapman and Hall.

Barclay Report (1982) *Social Workers, their Role and Tasks.* London: National Institute for Social Work/ Bedford Square Press.

Barefoot, P. (1990) Community support and neighbourhood size. *Architecture and Behaviour*, 6, 225–232.

Baruch, J. and Treacher, A. (1978) *Psychiatry Observed.* London: Routledge.

Beard, J.H., Propst, R.N. and Malamud, T.J. (1982) The Fountain House model of psychiatric rehabilitation. *Psychosocial Rehabilitation Journal*, 16, 2.

Bhui, K. and Olajide, D. (eds) (1999) *Mental Health Service Provision for a Multi-cultural Society.* London: Saunders.

Brandon, D., Brandon A. and Brandon, T. (1995) *Advocacy: Power to People with Disabilities.* Birmingham: Venture Press.

Brown, H. and Smith, H. (1991) *Normalisation: A Reader for the Nineties.* London: Routledge.

Bulmer, M. (1987) *The Social Basis of Community Care.* London: Allen and Unwin.

Carrier, J. and Tomlinson, D. (1996) *Asylum in the Community.* London: Routledge.

Chanan, G. (1992) *Out of the Shadows, European Foundation for the Improvement of Living and Working Conditions*. Ireland: Shankill.

Collins, R. (1988) *Theoretical Sociology*. San Diego, CA: Harcourt.

Copperman, J. and McNamara, J. (1999) Institutional abuse in mental health settings: survivor perspectives. In: Stanley, N. Manthorpe, J. and Penhale, B. (eds), *Institutional Abuse: Perspectives Across the Life Course*. London: Routledge, pp. 152–172.

Cummings, J. and Cummings, E (1957) *Closed Ranks*. New York: Basic Books.

Del Giudice, G., Evaristo, P. and Reale, M. (1990) How can psychiatric hospitals be phased out? In: Ramon, S. (ed.), *Psychiatry in Transition: British and Italian Experiences*. London: Pluto Press, pp. 199–207.

Department of Health (1995) *Building Bridges*. London: HMSO.

Dolan, B. Warren, F. and Norton, K. (1997) Change in borderline symptoms one year after therapeutic community treatment for severe personality disorder. *British Journal of Psychiatry*, 171, 274–279.

Dunham, W. and Faris, R. (1939) *Mental Disorder in Urban Areas*. Chicago: University of Chicago Press.

Durkheim, E. (1888/1952) *Suicide: A Study in Sociology*. London: Routledge.

Durkheim, E. (1889/1978) Review of Ferdinand Toennies gemienshaft and gessleshaft. In: Traughtt, M. (ed.), *Emile Durkheim on Institutional Analysis*. Chicago: University of Chicago, pp. 115–122.

Ernst, S. and Goodison, L. (1981) *In Our Own Hands: A Book of Self-help Therapy*. London: The Women's Press.

Etzioni, A. (1995) *The Spirit of Community: Rights, Responsibilities and the Communitarian Agenda*. Glasgow: Fontana Press.

Fernando, S. (1991) *Mental Health, Race and Culture*. London: Mind Macmillan.

Froland, C., Pancoast, D.L., Chapman, N.J. and Kimboko, P.J. (1981) *Helping Networks and Human Services*. Beverly Hills: Sage.

Goffman, I. (1961) *Asylums*. Harmonsworth: Penguin.

Hennelly, R. (1990) Mental health resource centres. In: Ramon, S. (ed.), *Psychiatry in Transition: British and Italian Experiences*. London: Pluto Press, pp. 208–218.

Hill, R., Shephered, G. and Hardy, P. (1998) In sickness and in health: the experiences of friends and relatives caring for people with manic depression. *Journal of Mental Health*, 7, 6.

Hoggett, P., Stewart, M., Razzaque, K. and Barker, I. (1999) *Urban Regeneration and Mental Health in London*. London: King's Fund Publishing.

Hollingshead, H. and Redlich, F. (1958) *Social Class and Mental Illness*. New York: The Free Press.

Jodelet, D. (1991) *Social Representations of Madness*. Hemel Hempstead, UK: Wheatsheaf

Jones, M. (1952) *Social Psychiatry*. London: Tavistock.

Lees, R. and Smith, G. (1975) *Action Research in Community Development*. London: Routledge.

Mauri, D. (ed.) (1986) *La Liberta e Terapeutica?* Rome: Feltrinelli.

Melluci, A. (1995) The new social movements revisited: reflections on a sociological misunderstanding. In: Maheu, L. (ed.), *Social Movements and Social Classes*. London: Sage, pp. 107–119.

Mitchell, J.C. (1969) The concept and use of social network. In: Mitchell, J.C. (ed.), *Social Networks in Urban Situations: Analyses of Personal Relationships in Central African Towns*. Manchester: Manchester University Press.

Morgan, D. (1985) *The Family, Politics and Social Theory*. London: Routledge.

Mullender, A. and Ward, D. (1991) *Self-directed Groupwork*. London: Birch and Whiting.

Nehring, J., Hill, R. and Poole, L. (1993) *Work, Employment and Community: Opportunities for People with Long-term Mental Health Problems*. London: Research and Development in Psychiatry.

Paykel, E.S., Hart, D. and Priest, R.G. (1998) Changes in public attitudes to depression during the Defeat Depression Campaign. *British Journal of Psychiatry*, 173, 519–522.

Payne, M. (1998) 'Community' as a basis for social policy and social action. In: Ramon, S. (ed.), *The Interface between Social Work and Social Policy*. Birmingham: Venture Press, pp. 25–42.

Petch, A. (1993) *A Home in the Community: An Evaluation of Supervised Accommodation for People with Mental Health Problems*. Aldershot, UK: Avebury.

Philo, G. (ed.) (1996) *Media and Mental Distress*. London: Longman.

Ramon, S. (ed.) (1991) *Beyond Community Care: Normalisation and Integration Work*. London: Mind Macmillan.

Ramon, S. (1992) Making sense of the experience of closure: a case study of social work teams. In: Ramon, S. (ed.), *Psychiatric Hospitals Closure: Myths and Realities*. London: Chapman and Hall.

Ramon, S. (1996) A scandalous category: media representations of people suffering from mental illness. In: Ramon, S. (ed.), *Mental Health in Europe: Ends, Beginnings and Rediscoveries*. London: Mind Macmillan, pp. 186–210.

Ramon, S. and Savio, M. (2000) A scandal of the 80s and 90s. In: Ramon, S. (ed.), *A Stakeholder's Approach to Innovation in Mental Health Services: A Reader for the 21st Century*. London: Pavilion Publishing, pp. 209–227.

Repper, J., Sayce, L., Strong, S., Willmot, J. and Haines, M. (1997) *Respect: Tall Stories from the Back Yard.* London: Mind Publications.

Rogers, A. and Pilgrim, D. (1997) The contribution of lay knowledge to the understanding and promotion of mental health. *Journal of Mental Health*, 6, 1.

Roosnes, E. (1979) *The Mad in the Town Gheel and its Secular Therapy.* London: Sage.

Samuel, R. and Thompson, P. (1990) *The Myths We Live By.* London: Routledge.

Saunders, P. (1993) Citizenship in a liberal society. In: Turner, B.S. (ed.), *Citizenship and Social Theory.* London: Sage, pp. 57–90.

Shepherd, G. (1996) *Relative Values.* London: The Sainsbury Centre for Mental Health.

Taylor, P.J. and Gunn, J. (1999) Homicides by people with mental illness: myth and reality. *British Journal of Psychiatry*, 174, 9–14.

Toennies, F. (1887/1963) *Community and Sociology.* New York: Harper and Row.

Thornicroft, G. (1991) Social deprivation and rates of treated mental disorder developing statistical models to predict psychiatric service utilisation. *British Journal of Psychiatry*, 158, 475–484.

Townsend, P. (1996) *A Poor Future.* London: Lemos and Crane.

Trevillion, S. (1992) *Caring in the Community: A Networking Approach to Community Partnership.* London: Longman.

Trower, P. (1978) *Social Skills and Mental Health.* London: Methuen.

Ungerson, C. (1995) Gender, cash and informal care: European perspectives and dilemmas. *Journal of Social Policy*, 24, 31–52.

Wellman, B. (1982) Studying personal communication. In: Marsden, P.V. (ed.), *Social systems and Network Analysis.* Beverly Hills: Sage, pp. 96–117.

Williams. J. and Keating, F. (1999) The abuse of adults in mental health settings. In: Stanley, N., Manthorpe, J. and Penhale, B. (eds), *Institutional Abuse: Perspectives Across the Life Course.* London: Routledge, pp. 130–161.

Willmott, P. (1986) *Social Networks, Informal Care and Public Policy.* London, Policy Studies Institute (PSI research report 655).

Wolfensberger, W. (1983) Social role valorisation: a proposed new term for the principle of normalisation. *Mental Retardation*, 21, 235–239.

Wolff, G., Pathare, S., Craig, T. and Leff, J. (1996) Public education for community care, a new approach. *British Journal of Psychiatry*, 168, 441–447.

4 | *The scientific foundations of community psychiatry*

David Mechanic

Introduction

Community psychiatry from its inception has been as much an ideology as a scientific endeavour. Its seeds are identifiable early in the 20th century in efforts to reform the care of persons with psychiatric illnesses, prevent illness whenever possible and promote mental health. Its ideals were embodied in the USA in the founding of the Mental Health Association in 1909, the mental hygiene and child guidance movements in the 1920s and 1930s, and the creation of the National Institute of Mental Health in 1946 (Grob, 1991). However, community psychiatry as we know it today is largely a post-Second World War endeavour built around a growing appreciation of the importance of broad environmental factors and a spirit of community cohesiveness and equality associated with the battle against the Nazi threat and totalitarianism.

Experience in the war made clear how men under sustained stress could become psychiatric casualties and how prudent organizational and administrative measures could help to reduce the impact (Grob, 1991). The post-war period was also a time of great expectations that the developing social and behavioural sciences could provide the knowledge and methods to solve persistent social problems, contribute positively to personal development and help create better and healthier communities. In the UK, the development of social psychiatry and its embodiment of environmentalism was exemplified by the efforts of such persons as Aubrey Lewis, Maxwell Jones and the work of Civil Resettlement Units as transitional communities for British prisoners of war

(Wilson *et al.*, 1952; Bennett and Freeman, 1991;Grob, 1991). Social psychiatric and rehabilitative research and their practical implementation flourished in England in the 1950s and 1960s with the innovative work of T.P. Rees, Rudi Freundenberg, John Wing and his colleagues at the MRC Social Psychiatry Unit, and Douglas Bennett at the Maudsley (Watts and Bennett, 1983). Nevertheless, community psychiatry as we have come to know it has been substantially an American movement that coincided with the development of a large behavioural science research infrastructure, strong social and environmental activism, rapid and massive deinstitutionalism of the mentally ill and other institutionalized clients and the definition of mental health by its leaders as a public health problem requiring a broad population perspective.

Deinstitutionalization of public mental hospitals in the USA beginning in 1955, while largely a product of the introduction of neuroleptic drugs, changes in administrative and public attitudes, the growth of a social welfare infrastructure in the community and a strong social community ideology, was supported by a growing body of research that depicted the regimentation and dehumanization of large mental hospitals and the debilitating effects of long-term hospitalization (Mechanic, 1999). Such studies also showed the link between administrative changes and patients' behaviour.

Particularly important in helping shape public attitudes were the theoretical essays on *Asylums* by Erving Goffman based on observations made in the federal government's Saint Elizabeth's Hospital (Goffman, 1961). In presenting his conceptions of how total institutions could shape conceptions of the self and behaviour, he provided a framework for studying organizational effects that shaped the work of much sociological and social psychological work of a more quantitative and scientific character. Particularly important in England and America was the work of John Wing (1962, 1978) on 'institutionalism' and George Brown (1985) on expressed emotion, as well as joint work by Wing and Brown on other factors that affected the course of psychiatric disorder in the community (Wing and Brown, 1970). As with other advances made in the UK, these insights were adopted and implemented more quickly and widely in the USA by the mental health professions then dominated by psychodynamic and psychodevelopmental perspectives, a spirit of experimentalism, a strong community ideology and, at times, a significant measure of irresponsibility.

Many good and innovative practices were introduced, but also some that were poorly conceived, had little scientific basis and harmed patients and the community (Mechanic, 1999). Among the most ill informed view points prevalent in this period were: that mental illnesses were not real, only a response to labelling; that mental illness was simply a continuum of distress from mild to severe and did not characterize distinguishable disorders; that careful diagnosis had no value because disorders were based uniquely in personal development; that parents caused most serious mental illness in their children; that only long-term psychoanalysis brought 'real cures'; and many more (Grob, 1991; Mechanic, 1999). No doubt, many equally simplistic and invalid ideas prevail today.

An effective community psychiatry depends on identifying and implementing practices based on adequate scientific foundations. Increasingly, social psychiatric research that informs community care is subject to rigorous research evaluation, often using the methodology of randomized controlled trials.

Scientific foundations

In the past 50 years, every major discipline in the social and behavioural sciences has contributed theory and research to understanding: the occurrence of mental disorder in the community; aetiological and other factors affecting the course of disorder; processes of definition, attribution and help-seeking; and promising modes of community intervention. These areas of study range from psychiatric epidemiology to mental health services research and include such disciplines as social, clinical and professional psychology; medical sociology; medical anthropology; social work and social welfare; human ecology; medical geography; and health economics. No single chapter can cover all of the relevant areas. In the discussion that follows, this chapter focuses on 10 substantive research areas that usefully inform the practice of community psychiatry. These include: (i) the role of socio-economic differences, social inequalities and social cohesion; (ii) culture, ethnicity and mental illness; (iii) social selection processes; (iv) stress, coping and social support processes; (v) self-efficacy and mastery processes; (vi) illness behaviour and help-seeking processes; (vii) crisis intervention and preventive psychiatry; (viii) the social disability model; (ix) behaviour change processes; and (x) psychosocial rehabilitation.

Socio-economic differences, social inequalities and social cohesion

There is now a massive body of literature that documents that in all societies persons of lower socio-economic status (SES), lower educational attainment and lower occupational level are at higher risk of distress, dissatisfaction, morbidity, disability and early death (Mechanic, 1978; Bunker *et al.*, 1989; Amick *et al.*, 1995). These studies cover both physical and mental disorders, and every stage of the life cycle from perinatality to old age. Patterns may vary from one disorder to another, and there are some disease patterns associated with affluence, but, in general, the associations with SES are large and pervasive.

There are innumerable ways in which poverty, poor education and the character of work may predispose individuals to poor health outcomes, but many uncertainties remain about these processes. On the one hand, certain genetic and personality characteristics may result in risk of lower SES, or illnesses and disabilities lead individuals to fall in the stratification structure or prevent them from keeping pace with their peers in social advancement (Turner and Wagenfeld, 1967; Mechanic, 1978). Alternatively, most of the health risks associated with SES appear to be a result of the exposures, life situations and social processes that persons of lower social rank disproportionately experience. These include poor housing, exposure to toxins, nutritional inadequacies, adverse life events, low rates of positive events, crime and community disorganization, victimization, poor health habits, abuse of substances and less access to quality medical care.

The role of SES is widely recognized, but suggestions are also mounting that inequalities themselves, independent of SES levels, contribute to higher morbidity and mortality (Wilkinson, 1996; Kawachi and Kennedy, 1997). One of the mechanisms commonly suggested is that inequalities result in breakdown of social cohesion involving residential segregation, crime and violence, loss of social integration and connectedness, and erosion of vital instrumental supports (Kawachi and Kennedy, 1997; Lynch *et al.*, 1998).

Concern with social cohesion dates back to Durkheim's classic study of suicide (Durkheim, 1951) and his theories about how different types of social connectedness either predisposed to suicide or provided protection. Since Durkheim, numerous studies have examined how social isolation, weak social supports, lack of agreement about norms and weak social controls contribute to deviance, diminished well-being and poor health status (Thoits, 1995). Fewer studies, however, have followed the tradition of Durkheim that focuses less on individual responses and more on 'collective representations' that expose individuals to risk as embodied in religious norms, social conventions or strengths of social control. Although it is reasonably clear that many of the processes of importance occur at the community level, there is much that remains unknown.

In the 1960s, some community psychiatrists in the USA presumed to know more than our knowledge allowed and did much to diminish respect for community psychiatric efforts. However, within reasonable limits, and with appropriate political support, there are community development opportunities to promote conditions that reduce risk among lower SES communities (Benzeval *et al.*, 1995; Acheson, 1998).

Culture and mental illness

The scientific process seeks universals, generalizations that apply to all people and all places whenever possible. However, good science must always be vigilant for exceptions to universal observations that note differences by time, place and circumstances (Kleinman, 1988). Psychiatry has vigorously sought to define universals and to develop diagnostic systems and procedures that apply everywhere. However, there are vast cultural and ethnic differences that lead to culturally specific diagnoses, different ways of responding, varying meanings in understanding bodily indications and feelings, diverse ways of expressing distress and seeking help, and varying cultural content in symptom formulation and expression (World Health Organization, 1973; Kleinman and Good, 1985). While clients with schizophrenia in varying cultures may all express their disorder in one way or another through delusions or hallucinations, or other core symptoms, they may express them very differently with varying societal consequences. All cultures recognize persons who are blatantly psychotic (Murphy, 1976), but how they define such behaviour and what they do about it may also have profound consequences (Eaton and Weil, 1955; Sartorius *et al.*, 1986). Increasingly we all live and work in multi-cultural and multi-ethnic societies. Some reasonable level of understanding of such cultural differences is required for competent practice.

Culture can be both an impediment and a resource for the community psychiatrist. It can be an impediment in the sense that members of varying cultural groups may: reject the psychiatrist's models and conceptualizations; refuse their preferred treatments; fail to co-operate in treatment; and influence others in ways that thwart the management of the illness process. By understanding the patient's and family's perspective, clinicians may be better able to create the conditions of co-operation necessary for good treatment outcomes. Chinese clients who deny being depressed but who see themselves as suffering from neurasthenia possibly may be treated more successfully within this definitional context (Kleinman, 1986). The findings that patients with schizophrenia have a less destructive course of illness in developing than in developed countries (Sartorius *et al.*, 1986) suggests ways in which culture can be used constructively to learn how better to sustain clients in community settings. Whether an improved course results from more community support and lower criticism, more accepting kinship groups and communities, or an ecological and economic context that can more easily absorb deviance remains unclear. It is clear, however, that culture and societal reactions help shape how illness is manifested and its negative consequences. Violent behaviour sometimes associated with schizophrenic disorders may arise from internal brain processes, but it is also shaped by cultural content and how the family and community react to the mentally ill person (Eaton and Weil, 1955).

Social selection

Individuals and groups are active agents who organize their environments, plan their efforts and selectively seek out opportunities and experiences. People and their social groups select how they will be schooled, who they associate with, who they court and marry, the amount and timing of their fertility, where they live, the types of work they choose and avoid, how they recreate, where they seek medical and other assistance and even when they die. Failure to understand such selective processes in the community can lead the community psychiatrist into costly errors.

The scientific community understands the pervasiveness of such selection and no study is deemed competent or acceptable unless such selective factors are controlled, as in randomized controlled trials or through sophisticated statistical controls if randomization is not feasible. Social selection, however, is not simply a bias to be factored out but a crucial phenomenon to be understood and utilized in intervention efforts. Selection affects exposure to stressors and other risk factors and the ability to attract social support and instrumental assistance. Increasingly, we learn that risk factors which we believed were independent of individuals or their inclinations—such as attack, rape or accidental injury—are also more likely to occur to some people than others because they select to be out at times, in places or in situations that others selectively would avoid (Dohrenwend, 1998). Fully independent events are extraordinarily difficult to identify, and many events occur in developmental sequences over the life course. As Brown has illustrated nicely, independent events such as loss of a mother may lead to a lower level of care-giving by family members, motivation to escape the family environment, association with unreliable partners and early school-leaving, premature sexual activity, pregnancy, inappropriate marriages, and depression and poor mental health outcomes (Brown, 1986). However, the cycle is not inevitable and can be interrupted by a caring and supportive partner (Quinton and Rutter, 1984a,b) or perhaps by other supportive interventions. Understanding the selective dynamics also suggests opportunities for community and individual interventions to steer individuals and support them in following less damaging trajectories.

Selection is also central to processes of seeking and receiving treatment. Typically, before receiving treatment, persons must first decide that they have a problem, make inferences about the nature of the problem, choose to seek assistance and select the type of help (Mechanic, 1999). If assistance is sought from the formal system such as the family doctor, recognition of the problem will depend on how the problem is presented, and referral to specialty mental health clinicians will in part depend on the attitudes the patient expresses. These steps, or filters as some have called them (Goldberg and Huxley, 1980), characterize the multiple pathways that clients may follow at various points along the care trajectory.

The stress, coping and social support process

The stress, coping and social support process is perhaps the most important unifying framework of community psychiatric practice. It functions both to help understand the occurrence and prevalence of mental disorders in the community and to provide guidance in efforts to influence the course of disorder so as to moderate the consequences of psychiatric disturbance. It informs and guides preventive efforts, crisis response and many aspects of the social rehabilitative process.

There is a vast research literature in this area, but the basic guiding conception is that the function of individuals and groups depends on the match between the challenges of their environments and demands made on them and their instrumental and psychosocial capacities to deal with them (counter-harm or coping resources) (Lazarus, 1966; Lazarus and Folkman, 1984). When such capacities are overwhelmed, individuals become anxious and depressed, and are more likely to abuse substances, have interpersonal conflicts and get into a variety of other difficulties. Evidence is mounting that both instrumental and emotional support can buffer the impact of 'stressors' or independently contribute to reduced adverse outcomes such as depression or anxiety (Cohen and Syme, 1985; Thoits, 1995). Such processes of social support further may affect immune processes resulting in reduced susceptibility to illness and even mortality (House *et al.*, 1988; Cohen *et al.*, 1997). While support is viewed generally as a positive feature of adaptation, many questions remain about the relative role of different types of support (emotional support, intimacy, instrumental support, community involvement and participation) and the conditions under which social networks create obligations and social controls that are themselves stressful (Thoits, 1995). Areas receiving growing attention in research in the USA involve the role of religious participation and beliefs, social support groups, self-help and consumer-run community services.

The stress–coping–social support model is a primary paradigm for training social workers, psychiatric and community nurses, and many psychologists in the USA. It informs crisis intervention services, the programmes of community mental health centres, the organization of family and patient support groups and a variety of psychoeducational approaches in which clients are taught skills of everyday living and families are taught how to manage the burden of a mentally ill family member. It also provides a useful perspective for the entire mental health team, each of whom have special competencies but who share the general model.

Self-efficacy and mastery

A newer entrant into the stress–coping–social support model is the concept of individuals' sense of control over the circumstances of their lives and the extent to which they feel powerless or helpless. Increasingly, interventions and therapeutic approaches are structured to increase individuals' feelings of control. This idea is embodied in a variety of overlapping concepts that now receive a great deal of research attention. Among these concepts are self-efficacy, locus of control, learned helplessness, sense of power, health optimism and others. However defined and measured, self-efficacy is associated consistently with lower levels of demoralization, depression, anxiety and other forms of distress (Seligman, 1975; Rodin, 1986; Peterson and Bossio, 1991). Modifying such attributions has become a central aspect of cognitive therapy and counselling (Beck, 1976).

Perhaps more persuasive is the fact that experimental interventions designed to increase sense of control have been shown to be associated with improved mental health and general health outcomes (Rodin and Langer, 1977). The notion of self-efficacy is, of course, a concept characteristic of modern individualistic cultures, and most of the research has been done in the USA. Its relevance for societies with different dominant ideologies remains unclear. Nor is it clear how self-efficacy relates to other attributional processes, or generalizes to persons of varying generational cohorts and age groups. It is apparent, however, that many persons with mental disorder feel little control over their illnesses or their lives. Teaching alternative means for exercising control and increasing confidence about mastery potential is a useful treatment modality in many instances.

Illness behaviour

It is well established that individuals perceive and define problems and symptoms differently, make varying attributions about them, use diverse vocabularies of distress and have varying propensities to seek or resist care or to co-operate in treatment. The study of illness behaviour seeks to understand how people differentially define and interpret symptoms and take action including self-medication, informal care-seeking and use of formal services (McHugh and Vallis, 1985). Illness behaviour is particularly important in mental health services because of the stigma typically associated with psychiatric illness and the use of mental health services, the phenomenology of some disorders that leads to the denial of illness and refusal of help, and anti-mental health ideologies common among some elements of the public. By understanding how individuals experience and interpret psychiatric symptoms, we improve our capacities to develop meaningful and responsive services and avoid damaging errors in how we structure community programmes or respond to various social and cultural groups in the community.

Somatization is one of the more commonly studied areas of illness behaviour with respect to mental health (Smith, 1990). Somatization should be seen as a response process and vocabulary of distress, and not simply a psychiatric disorder (Mechanic, 1995). Cultures may have highly elaborate psychological vocabularies of distress or impoverished ones. Living in a highly psychological era it is easy to forget that in most cultures, and throughout most of history, somatic expressions have been the dominant way of expressing distress, and still remains typical in much of the world and particularly among persons with lower levels of modernity and educational attainment.

Disagreement persists on whether somatization reflects the limits of a psychological vocabulary, cultural differences in acceptable contexts for discussing emotional distress and interpersonal problems, feared stigma and the perceived undesirability of psychological symptoms, or different attributional processes. These considerations are important not only in how services are structured and people treated, but they also have significant implications for psychiatric nosology and how we evaluate psychiatric epidemiology. For example, epidemiological studies in the USA consistently report that elders have a lower prevalence of depression than younger respondents (Robins and Regier, 1991), observations at variance with observations of many geriatricians, other physicians and family practitioners. The difficulty may be that typically depression in the elderly is quite different, often associated with physical co-morbidity, loss of physical function, loss of cherished social networks and a tendency toward somatization. Further investigation is needed to sort these issues out.

Illness behaviour studies teach us the importance of understanding patients' perspectives on their symptoms and illnesses and to approach them in a way compatible with their belief systems and values. There is no evidence that treating Chinese patients who characterize their illness as neurasthenia (defined as a physical condition) is any less helpful than trying to convince them that they suffer from major depression and require mental health care. The insistence that the client accept the perspectives and definitions of the mental health clinician is the source of many failures in mental health care. In many circumstances, appropriate treatment and management can be provided within a definition consistent with the patient's cultural and personal needs.

Crisis intervention and preventive psychiatry

Crisis intervention has a long history in social work as a significant approach to community work. Such approaches are now used commonly by mobile mental health teams who respond to psychiatric crises in the community, evaluate the problem, provide instruction and support, make determinations about further need for service and link clients to needed treatment resources (Primm, 1996; Katschnig and Cooper, 1991; Mechanic, 1999). This is a pragmatic and valuable approach that is now routine practice in many communities. Such teams in some localities are the gate-keepers for in-patient care for public patients and make assessments of the need for holding the client temporarily and for civil commitment.

Crisis intervention and preventive psychiatry now has a more modest role than it did in the 1960s in the USA when some community psychiatrists advocated a grandiose and naive approach that ultimately did much to discredit the valuable potential of community psychiatry. In the words of one such advocate, "The psychiatrist must truly be a political personage in the best sense of the word. He must play a role in *controlling* the environment which man has created" (Duhl, 1963, p. 73). The guru of community psychiatry of the period was Gerald Caplan who advocated that psychiatry should engage in primary prevention to limit the occurrence of mental illness (Caplan, 1964). Much of the required agenda was political action, and not scientific practice, and these activities could not be sustained as the social and political environment changed. Nor was there ever any reasonable evidence that the types of programmes advocated by community psychiatrists could prevent any of the serious mental illnesses (Mechanic, 1999).

Yet there was some reasonable theory underlying Caplan's approach. He saw the challenge as one of identifying harmful influences, encouraging environmental forces to help resist them and increasing the population's resistance to future illness. Caplan believed that various crises and transitional periods were times of particular risk such as entering school, child-bearing, having surgery, moving, etc., and advocated that community psychiatrists seek out situations of social vulnerability and provide supportive help and coping techniques. He believed that mental illness could be prevented by intervening during crises and by working through such professionals as doctors, nurses, teachers and administrators who naturally were in contact with individuals in crisis, and by interventions in such contexts as divorce courts and colleges.

The view that it is possible to give people anticipatory guidance and emotional inoculation that help them to face stressors and traumatic events is a worthy hypothesis and one that informs many of the efforts already described. There is now substantial preventive intervention research that suggests that well-formulated programmes can be helpful in reducing significant levels of depression, anxiety and other forms of distress (Mrazek and Haggerty, 1994; Smedley and Syme, 2000). There is also some promising work on interventions to prevent conduct disorder, early pre-marital pregnancy and substance use.

Unfortunately, there is no persuasive evidence that any of the interventions now available can significantly affect the occurrence of the major mental disorders; but there is substantial evidence that the course of illness can be moderated, that disability can be reduced and that persons with severe and persistent mental illness in the community can be supported so that function and life satisfaction is improved (Tatum and Goldberg, 1991; Mrazek and Haggerty, 1994). There is also increasing evidence that even persons with the most severe mental illnesses successfully can work competitively with supportive employment programmes (Bond *et al.*, 1997).

Social disability

The disability rights movement that developed early in the USA has now become active throughout the world. The movement was informed by the sociological conception that disability resulted from a lack of concordance between the individuals' capacities and the physical and social environments in which they functioned (Pope and Tarlov, 1991; Albrecht, 1992). Persons with limitations, it was argued, were disabled primarily because of environmental and physical barriers, attitudes intolerant of their limitations, stigma, and discrimination and exclusion. Through social mobilization and political advocacy, disability rights groups have achieved legislation that requires physical accessibility to public facilities and employment protection.

Mental health advocacy has followed a similar course in the USA and other countries, seeking to achieve favourable legislation, reduce stigma and change public attitudes, and provide information and assistance to clients and family members. In the USA, the National Alliance for the Mentally Ill (NAMI) representing some 170 000 family members has fought aggressively for mental health parity in health insurance and increased research expenditures in the neurosciences, psychopharmacology and mental health services. Such organizations, while family based, work closely with mental health professionals to plan their agenda and to bring the latest research and understanding to its members. For example, they have taken the lead in disseminating to their members the results of the national effort to evaluate the evidence base of treatment approaches in schizophrenia and the large gaps in application (Lehman *et al.*, 1998). By helping their members to be activated and knowledgeable consumers of mental health services, they hope to change mental health practice.

Approaches to changing behaviour

Core to many of the behavioural science disciplines are theories and research programmes on changing individual and group behaviour. These programmes have long studied such basic processes as learning, cognitive processes, interpersonal influence and group dynamics. The scientific principles derived from these studies have been important in behaviour therapy, cognitive therapy, interpersonal therapy, and family and group therapies. Most advances, however, have been at the level of individual interventions and much less so at the community level.

Some of the most successful community care approaches such as assertive community treatment and related endeavours, however, incorporate insights from behaviour change research to reinforce positive behaviour and maintain co-operation in treatment and medication compliance. Many programmes have learnt how to increase social supports by constructively involving families in the treatment plan and management processes. Psychoeducational programmes built around reducing expressed emotion and developing patient management skills have used group processes successfully to achieve better outcomes than results from individual family instruction (McFarlane, *et al.* 1995). Many medical and psychiatric programmes now sponsor a variety of support groups, family groups and survivor groups. The link between theory and research and practice still remains somewhat tenuous but, increasingly, practitioners are taking useful ideas from the scientific literature as a basis for intervention programmes.

A number of behavioural change models and related research now inform efforts to influence preventive health activities, although they have not been applied widely in mental health services (Mechanic, 1994; Glanz *et al.*, 1997). Such models, however, have important implications for substance abuse prevention, for achieving compliance with medical regimens and other aspects of the treatment process. A dominant idea is that behaviour change must address parallel processes involving both instrumental and emotional aspects of behaviour (Leventhal, 1970). On the one hand, individuals must know what to do and how to do it with minimal inconvenience and disruption in their valued activities; on the other hand, they must manage their emotions to control fear, anxiety and other adverse states. Intervention programmes must address both aspects since the failure to control adverse emotional states may result in denial and reduced coping efforts. Also important to this approach is the need for continued periodic reinforcement through social support and other means and the use of cues to trigger health concern and health actions. These cues may be programmatic or internal as when patients are taught to recognize exacerbation of symptoms and to take appropriate action. Cues may be implemented practically through various devices and communications.

Psychosocial rehabilitation

Care of persons with serious mental illness in the community is focused on managing the patient and illness, co-ordinating the varying services required from various institutional sectors including housing, social services, medical care, etc., and increasing function through structuring the client's day, providing training in needed everyday skills, providing social contacts and social support, recreational activities and supportive work rehabilitation. Such care is often informed by the behavioural knowledge and disability models already described. The Program in Assertive Community Treatment (PACT), now replicated throughout the world, either in part or wholly, represents a pragmatic approach that builds on many of the conceptions reviewed (Stein and Santos, 1998). PACT and related programmes are highly complex interventions and we know relatively little about which components are most important for achieving the outcomes observed. One set of studies suggests that a major factor affecting outcomes associated with model programmes such as PACT is client empowerment (Rosenfield, 1992).

The future scientific basis of community psychiatry

Community psychiatry has evolved from a movement driven more by ideological passion than by an evidence-based perspective. It is now informed to a much greater degree by an epidemiological approach and increasingly rigorous mental health services research (Breakey, 1996), and these directions are likely to become even more evident in the future. In the last two decades, we have learned a great deal about how to manage community mental health services and what approaches work with varying kinds of patients, and such learning is accelerating. Unfortunately, the problems continue to change as well, and problems of co-morbidity associated with serious mental illness (Kessler *et al.*, 1994), particularly substance abuse, pose difficult challenges including medication adherence in the community, homelessness and the management of violence (Steadman *et al.*, 1998; Mechanic, 1999).

Mental health workers are more thoughtful about their capabilities for prevention than they were a few decades ago (Linn *et al.*, 1988). Ideas about prevention are now being developed within a sounder methodological and experimental framework and are subjected to more rigorous scrutiny. There is little evidence that we have the capacity to reduce the occurrence of serious mental illness, but there are many promising indications that community prevention can become a viable evidence-based approach. A very thorough examination of preventive opportunities by an expert committee of the Institute of Medicine of the National Academy of Sciences of the United States concluded that "the knowledge base for some mental disorders is now advanced enough that preventive intervention research programs, targeted at risk factors for these disorders, can rest on sound conceptual and empirical foundations" (Mrazek and Haggerty, 1994, p. xv).

Mental health services systems, and community efforts related to them, go through cycles influenced by ideological movements, new scientific paradigms, and changing economic conditions and political circumstances (Rochefort, 1997). Evolving service approaches are now being influenced significantly by pharmaceutical developments and advances in the neurosciences on the one hand and by deinstitutionalization, economic constraints on health care and new ways of managing services on the other (Mechanic, 1998; Mechanic *et al.*, 1998). While some of these developments push psychiatry toward a narrow medical perspective, others call for a broader community and preventive care perspective. As we move forward, community psychiatry will have to define clearly how it fits into these sometimes competing tendencies.

References

Acheson, D. (1998) *Independent Inquiry into Inequalities in Health*. London: Stationary Office

Albrecht, G.L. (1992) *The Disability Business: Rehabilitation in America*. Newbury Park, CA: Sage.

Amick, B.C., III, Levine, S., Tarlov, A.R. and Walsh, D.C. (eds) (1995) *Society and Health*. New York; Oxford University Press.

Beck, A.T. (1976) *Cognitive Therapy and the Emotional Disorders*. New York: International Universities Press.

Bennett, D.H. and Freeman, H.L. (1991) *Community Psychiatry: The Principles*. Edinburgh: Churchill Livingstone.

Benzeval, M., Judge, K. and Whitehead, M. (1995) *Tackling Inequalities in Health: An Agenda for Action*. London: King's Fund.

Bond, G.R., Drake, R.E., Mueser, K.T. and Becker, D.R. (1997) An update on supported employment for people with severe mental illness. *Psychiatric Services*, 48, 335–346.

Breakey, W.R. (ed.) (1996) *Integrated Mental Health Services: Modern Community Psychiatry*. New York: Oxford University Press.

Brown, G.W. (1985) The discovery of expressed emotion: induction or deduction? In: Leff, J. and Vaughn, C. (eds), *Expressed Emotion in Families*. New York: Guilford Press, pp. 7–25.

Brown, G. (1986) Mental illness. In: Aiken, L.H. and Mechanic, D. (eds), *Applications of Social Science to Clinical Medicine and Health Policy*. New Brunswick, NJ: Rutgers University Press, pp. 175–203.

Bunker, J.B., Gomby, D.S. and Kehrer, B.H. (1989) *Pathways to Health: The Role of Social Factors*. Menlo Park, CA: Henry J. Kaiser Family Foundation.

Caplan, G. (1964) *Principles of Preventive Psychiatry*. New York: Basic Books.

Cohen, S. and Syme, S.L. (eds) (1985) *Social Support and Health*. Orlando, FL: Academic Press.

Cohen, S., Doyle, W.J., Skoner, D.P., Rabin, B.S. and Gwaltney, J.M., Jr (1997) Social ties and susceptibility to the common cold. *Journal of the American Medical Association*, 277, 1940–1944.

Dohrenwend, B. (ed.) (1998) *Adversity, Stress and Psychopathology*. New York: Oxford University Press.

Duhl, L.J. (ed.) (1963) *The Urban Condition: People and Policy in the Metropolis*. New York: Basic Books.

Durkheim, E. (1951) *Suicide: A Study in Sociology*. New York: The Free Press.

Eaton, J.W. and Weil, R.J. (1955) *Culture and Mental Disorders*. New York: The Free Press.

Glanz, K., Lewis, F. M. and Rimer, B.R. (eds.) (1997) *Health Behavior and Health Education*, 2nd edn. San Francisco: Jossey-Bass.

Goffman, E. (1961) *Asylums: Essays on the Social Situation of Mental Patients and Other Inmates*. Garden City, NY: Doubleday Anchor.

Goldberg, D. and Huxley, P. (1980) *Mental Illness in the Community: The Pathways of Psychiatric Care*. New York: Tavistock Publications.

Grob, G. (1991) *From Asylum to Community*. Princeton, NJ: Princeton University Press.

House, J., Landis, K.R. and Umberson, D. (1988) Social relationships and health. *Science*, 241, 540–545.

Katschnig, H. and Cooper, J. (1991) Psychiatric emergency and crisis intervention services. In: Bennett, D.H. and Freeman, H.L. (eds), *Community Psychiatry: The Principles*. Edinburgh: Churchill Livingstone, pp. 517–542.

Kawachi, I. and Kennedy, B.P. (1997) Health and social cohesion: why care about income inequality? *British Medical Journal*, 314, 1037–1040.

Kessler, R.C., McGonagle, K.A., Zhao, S., Nelson, C.B., Hughes, M., Eshleman, S. *et al.* (1994) Lifetime and 12-month prevalence of DSM-III-R psychiatric disorders in the United States: results from the national comorbidity study. *Archives of General Psychiatry*, 51, 8–19.

Kleinman, A. (1988) *Rethinking Psychiatry: From Cultural Category to Personal Experience*. New York: The Free Press.

Kleinman, A. and Good, B. (eds) (1985) *Culture and Depression: Studies in the Anthropology and Cross-cultural Psychiatry of Affect and Disorder*. Berkeley, CA: University of California Press.

Kleinman, A. (1986) *Social Origins of Distress and Disease: Depression, Neurasthenia and Pain in Modern China*. New Haven, CT: Yale University Press.

Lazarus, R.S. (1966) *Psychological Stress and the Coping Process*. New York: McGraw-Hill.

Lazarus, R.S. and Folkman, S. (1984) *Stress, Appraisal and Coping*. New York: Springer.

Lehman, A.F., Steinwachs, D.M. (1998) Translating research into practice: the schizophrenia Patient Outcomes Research Treatment (PORT) recommendations. *Schizophrenia Bulletin*, 24, 1–10.

Leventhal, H. (1970) Findings and theory in the study of fear communications. In: Berkowitz, L. (ed.), *Advances in Experimental Social Psychology*, Vol. 5. Orlando, FL: Academic Press.

Linn, L.S., Yager, J. and Leake, B. (1988) Psychiatrists' attitudes toward preventive intervention in routine clinical practice. *Hospital and Community Psychiatry*, 39, 637–642.

Lynch, J.W., Kaplan, G.A., Pamuk, E.R., Cohen, R.D., Heck, K.E., Balfour, J.L. *et al.* (1998) Income inequality and mortality in metropolitan areas of the United States. *American Journal of Public Health*, 88, 1074–1080.

McFarlane, W.R., Lukens, E., Link, B., Dushay, R., Deakins, S.A., Newmark, M. *et al.* (1995) Multiple family groups and psychoeducation in the treatment of schizophrenia. *Archives of General Psychiatry*, 52, 679–687.

McHugh, S. and Vallis, T.M. (1985) *Illness Behavior: A Multidisciplinary Model*. New York: Plenum Press.

Mechanic, D. (1978) *Medical Sociology*, 2nd edn. New York: The Free Press.

Mechanic, D. (1994) *Inescapable Decisions: The Imperative of Health Reform* (especially pp. 119–135). New Brunswick, NJ: Transaction Publishers.

Mechanic, D. (1995) Sociological dimensions of illness behavior. *Social Science and Medicine*, 41, 1207–1216.

Mechanic, D. (ed.) (1998) *Managed Behavioral Health Care: Current Realities and Future Potential, New Directions for Mental Health Services, No. 78*. San Francisco: Jossey-Bass.

Mechanic, D. (1999) *Mental Health and Social Policy: The Emergence of Managed Care* (4th edn). Boston: Allyn and Bacon.

Mechanic, D., McAlpine, D.D. and Olfson, M. (1998) Changing patterns of psychiatric inpatient care in the United States, 1988–1994. *Archives of General Psychiatry*, 55, 785–791.

Mrazek, P.J. and Haggerty, R.J. (eds) (1994) *Reducing Risks for Mental Disorders: Frontiers for Preventive Intervention Research*. Washington, DC: National Academy Press.

Murphy, J.M. (1976) Psychiatric labeling in cross-cultural perspective. *Science*, 191, 1019–1028.

Peterson, C. and Bossio, L.M. (1991) *Health and Optimism*. New York: The Free Press.

Pope, A.M. and Tarlov, A.R. (eds) (1991) *Disability in America: Toward a National Agenda for Prevention*. Washington, DC: National Academy Press.

Primm, A.B. (1996) Assertive community treatment. In: Breakey, W.R. (ed.), *Integrated Mental Health Services: Modern Community Psychiatry*. New York: Oxford University Press, pp. 222–237.

Quinton, D. and Rutter, M. (1984a) Parents with children in care, 1: current circumstances and parenting. *Journal of Child Psychology and Psychiatry*, 25, 211–229.

Quinton, D. and Rutter, M. (1984b) Parents with children in care, 2: intergenerational continuities. *Journal of Child Psychology and Psychiatry*, 25, 231–250.

Robins, L.N. and Regier, D.A. (eds) (1991) *Psychiatric Disorders in America: The Epidemiologic Catchment Area Study*. New York: The Free Press.

Rochefort, D. (1997) *From Poorhouses to Homelessness: Policy Analysis and Mental Health Care*, 2nd edn. Westport, CT: Auburn House.

Rodin, J. (1986) Aging and health: effects of the sense of control. *Science*, 233, 1271–1276.

Rodin, J. and Langer, E.J. (1977) Long-term effects of a control-relevant intervention with the institutionalized aged. *Journal of Personality and Social Psychology*, 35, 897–902.

Rosenfield, S. (1992) Factors contributing to the subjective quality of life of the chronic mentally ill. *Journal of Health and Social Behavior*, 33, 299–315.

Sartorius, N., Jablensky, A., Korten, A., Ernberg, G., Anker, M., Cooper, J.E., Day, R. (1986) Early manifestations and first-contact incidence of schizophrenia in different cultures. *Psychological Medicine*, 16, 909–928

Seligman, M.E.P. (1975) *Helplessness: On Depression, Development and Death*. San Francisco: W.H. Freeman and Co.

Smedley, B.D. and Syme, S.L. (eds.) (2000) *Promoting Health: Intervention Strategies from Social and Behavioural Research*. Washington, D.C.: National Academic Press.

Smith, G.R. (1990) *Somatization Disorder in the Medical Setting*. DHHS Publication No. (ADM) 90-1631. Washington, DC: US Government Printing Office.

Steadman, H.J., Mulvey, E.P., Monahan, J., Robbins, P.C., Appelbaum, P.S., Grisso, T. *et al.* (1998) Violence by people discharged from acute psychiatric inpatient facilities and by others in the same neighborhoods. *Archives of General Psychiatry*, 55, 393–401.

Stein, L.I. and Santos, A.B. (1998) *Assertive Community Treatment of Persons with Severe Mental Illness*. New York: W.W. Norton and Co.

Tatum, D. and Goldberg, D. (1991) Primary medical care. In: Bennett, D.H. and Freeman, H.L. (eds), *Community Psychiatry: The Principles*. Edinburgh: Churchill Livingstone, pp. 361–385.

Thoits, P.A. (1995) Stress, coping and social support processes: where are we? what next? *Journal of Health and Social Behavior*, Extra Issue, 53–79.

Turner, R.J. and Wagenfeld, M.O. (1967) Occupational mobility and schizophrenia: an assessment of the social causation and social selection hypothesis. *American Sociological Review*, 32, 104–113.

Watts, E.N. and Bennett, D.H. (1983) *Theory and Practice of Psychiatric Rehabilitation*. Chichester, UK: John Wiley.

Wilkinson, R.G. (1996) *Unhealthy Societies: The Afflictions of Inequality*. London: Routledge.

Wilson, A.T. M., Trist, E.L. and Curle, A. (1952) Transitional communities and social reconnection: a study of the civil resettlement of British prisoners of war. In: Swanson, G.E. Newcomb, T.M. and Hartley, E.L. (eds), *Readings in Social Psychology*. New York: Holt, Rinehart and Winston, pp. 561–579.

Wing, J. (1962) Institutionalism in mental hospitals. *British Journal of Social and Clinical Psychology*, 1, 38–51.

Wing, J. (1978) *Reasoning About Madness*. Oxford: Oxford University Press.

Wing, J. and Brown, G.W. (1970) *Institutionalism and Schizophrenia: A Comparative Study of Three Mental Hospitals, 1960–1968*. Cambridge: Cambridge University Press.

World Health Organization (1973) *Report of the International Pilot Study of Schizophrenia*, Vol 1. Geneva: WHO.

5 | *Epidemiological methods*

Glyn H. Lewis, Hollie V. Thomas,
Mary Cannon and Peter B. Jones

What is epidemiology?

Epidemiology is the population-based study of all aspects of disease and illness. Since John Snow removed the Broad Street pump 150 years ago, the remit of epidemiology has expanded considerably. It now embraces the whole range of studies involved in human disease. Epidemiological principles underpin much medical research particularly that concerned with the planning and evaluation of health services, including community psychiatry. This chapter briefly describes some of the principles behind epidemiological methods. Our later chapter (Chapter 8) provides more information concerning the epidemiology of psychiatric disorder.

Uses of epidemiology

Aetiology of disease

One of the uses of epidemiology that has attracted most interest is the study of the aetiology of disease. There are two main reasons why the aetiology of disease is important. First, the causes of disease should be able to inform preventive policies. Prevention is better than cure, and removing causal or risk factors should reduce the incidence of disease. The provision of sewers and clean water supplies in European cities was based upon Snow's observation that contaminated water increased the risk of cholera (Snow, 1936).

Aetiology is also important for a second reason; it helps to improve understanding about the mechanisms of disease. In the long term, this could lead to better psychopathological models and inform future treatments. Studying aetiology for these aims can also be described as basic science or 'blue skies' research and has to be carried out in tandem with laboratory-based research on psychopathology. The main way in which aetiology is studied using epidemiological methods is by studying the association between exposures and onset of disease. Trying to infer cause from association is clearly a difficult task, and this will be discussed at more length below.

Public health

Epidemiology is sometimes described as the science of public health, though epidemiology is a far broader discipline than this implies. However, epidemiology is an essential component of public health. Finding the aetiology of disease should inform preventive approaches, but epidemiological methods are also available to assess the population impact of causative factors in order to estimate the likely effects of preventive interventions. The evaluation of preventive procedures and screening also requires an epidemiological approach. New, longitudinal or life-course approaches to the epidemiology of diseases underpin this emerging application of the discipline.

Description and needs assessment

Epidemiology can be used to describe the occurrence of disease in terms of person, place and time. Incidence (new cases per person–time) and prevalence (the proportion of a population with disease over a given period) are important in describing disease for both policy and planning of services. The assessment of met and unmet needs is dependent upon such descriptive data, though it also relies upon evidence of effective treatments.

Clinical effectiveness and evidence-based medicine

There is an overlap between the methods used in health service research and those used in epidemiology. Questions concerning clinical effectiveness, whether evaluated using randomized controlled trials (RCTs) or observational studies, tend to be investigated using epidemiological methods. Evidence-based medicine (Evidence-Based Medicine Working Group, 1992) grew out of the interest of applying epidemiological and statistical approaches to everyday clinical decisions. In the early days, the term clinical epidemiology described this general approach. The use of systematic reviews of the literature to generate evidence and extrapolating these to clinical situations tends to rely upon epidemiological principles and uses some of the statistical analyses familiar to epidemiologists.

Causal inference

An association between an exposure and a disease can be explained by chance, bias, confounding, reverse causality or causation. Epidemiologists are usually interested in whether an exposure is a cause for the disease.

Chance

Significance testing and estimation of confidence limits assess the probability that chance alone can explain the findings. A type 1 error occurs when a statistically significant result occurs by chance. It is a particular problem when many statistical tests are conducted within a single study in the absence of a clearly stated prior hypothesis. A type 2 error occurs when a clinically important result is obscured by chance or random error, often made more likely by inadequate sample size.

Bias

Systematic error or *bias* can distort an association in any direction, either increasing or decreasing the association. Bias is a result of defects in the design or execution of a study, and the two main types in epidemiological studies are selection bias and information bias.

Selection bias can occur in any investigation but is a particular problem in case–control studies. It arises if the sampling method used to identify cases and controls results in a poor representation of the diseased and non-diseased individuals in the same population. An example is seen in the study of Brown and Harris (1978) who identified community cases of depression using a cross-sectional survey and patient cases of depression by contact with psychiatric services. When the community cases were compared with community controls, there was an association between depression and having a young family (odds ratio 3.77), but this association was absent when comparing the patient cases and community controls. Selection bias is acting here because, for someone who is depressed, having young children might reduce the likelihood of receiving treatment from psychiatrists. Since the majority of cases of depression never get referred to a psychiatrist, a community sample would not be an appropriate control group for cases seen in psychiatric services.

Information bias in an analytical study occurs when subjects are misclassified according to their exposure status, disease status or both. If this misclassification of disease status is dependent on exposure status or vice versa, the estimate of association will be biased. Examples of such differential misclassification include recall bias, reporting bias and observer bias. *Recall bias* occurs especially in case–control studies and cross-sectional surveys when individuals with the disease may be asked about the exposure retrospectively. In cohort studies, exposure is determined before onset of the disease and so it is less likely to be biased by the presence of disease. Case–control studies may also be able to use exposure information collected before the onset of disease. *Observer bias* occurs when the observer is aware of the hypothesis and the measurement of exposure or disease is biased. Keeping the assessments blind to disease or exposure can reduce the chance of this happening.

Confounding

Confounding occurs when an estimate of the association between an exposure and disease is mingled with the real effect of another exposure on the same disease due to the two exposures being correlated. If an association results from confounding, it does not mean that this association is wrong but that there is an alternative explanation for it. An epidemiologist should identify potential confounders at the design stage of the study and collect information on them, otherwise at the time of analysis it will be difficult to reject alternative explanations for any associations found in the data. A variable is said to be a confounder if the analysis that controls for this variable produces results that are markedly different from the crude or uncontrolled analysis.

Reverse causality

This is the possibility that the exposure is the result rather than the cause of the disease. This is more likely to occur in case–control studies and cross-sectional surveys that assess exposure after the onset of disease. Cohort studies usually eliminate this possibility by selecting people without the disease at the beginning of the study. However, it can remain a problem for some conditions, such as psychosis, where the timing of the onset of disease remains a matter of debate.

Causation

An association may indicate that the exposure causes the disease. Trying to infer causation is a difficult task. It is usually helpful to review the epidemiological literature to decide whether there is a consistent finding, irrespective of the population or study design. When there is a strong association, then the likelihood that the relationship is causal is increased. For example, for relative risks greater than 3 or 4, then confounding and bias have to be quite marked to explain the findings. However, there is generally little confidence in findings when the relative risk is 1.5 or below. A dose–response relationship can also provide additional evidence for causality, depending upon the hypothesized mechanism of action. For example, one would expect that more severe obstetric complications would lead to higher rates of schizophrenia than milder forms if that were a causal

agent. Finally, the scientific plausibility of the findings has to be considered. Epidemiology, when it is investigating cause, is interested in biological and psychological relationships.

Adjusting for confounding

Confounding can be controlled for in the design of a study, but more usually it is controlled for in the analysis, providing that sufficient information on possible confounding variables has been collected.

In the design—restriction Only those individuals who are not exposed to the confounding variable are included in the study.

In the design—matching The groups to be compared are often matched on potential confounding variables (e.g. age and sex), particularly in case–control studies. Matching on confounding variables that are difficult to measure (e.g. neighbourhood) is particularly useful since it would be difficult to adjust accurately for these variables in the statistical analysis of a study. Matching on variables that are not potentially important confounders is bad practice since the researcher cannot later investigate any association between the disease and exposure to the matching variables. The disadvantages of matching are the increase in administrative effort required and the slightly more complex analysis that is required in case–control studies to take into account the matching factors and to prevent the results from the study being biased. *Overmatching* can also occur in case–control studies when there is inadvertent matching on the exposure variable(s) and the power of the study is reduced.

In the design—randomization This is the most powerful method of controlling for confounders that can be used. Random allocation of subjects from a sufficiently large sample into groups receiving different preventive or therapeutic treatments should eradicate any other underlying differences between the groups except those arising by chance. Of course, it is usually impossible to investigate aetiological agents using randomization.

In the analysis—stratification The association between the disease and exposure of interest is analysed according to different levels or strata of the confounding variable. The true relationship between disease and exposure is revealed within each stratum of the confounding variable. A weighted average or summary estimate can then be calculated across the strata of the confounding variable. The Mantel–Haenszel odds ratio gives a weighted average of the odds ratios in the different strata, the odds ratios from larger strata being given more weight. Standardized mortality ratios are a way of adjusting for the confounding effects of age and sex using a stratified analysis.

In the design–multi-variate analysis As the number of confounders increases, stratified analyses such as the Mantel–Haenszel method become impractical. Instead, multi-variate modelling techniques are used to adjust for confounding by a large number of variables. Logistic regression analysis is used when studying binary outcomes (e.g. diseased versus well) to estimate odds ratios that are adjusted simultaneously for several confounders.

Similar modelling techniques include conditional logistic regression, which estimates adjusted odds ratios in a matched case–control study, and Poisson regression which estimates adjusted rate ratios using person–time data from cohort studies. Least squares regression is used to model continuous outcomes (e.g. scores on a depression test) and assumes that the dependent variable is normally distributed; this is often not the case with many outcomes in psychiatry.

Epidemiological study designs

The main study designs used in epidemiological research can be described as either observational (ecological, cross-sectional, case–control and cohort), experimental (randomized controlled trial) or summary in nature (systematic reviews).

Ecological or aggregate studies

Ecological studies examine the association between disease and the characteristics of an aggregation of people rather than the characteristics of individuals. The main difficulty with this design is that the association between exposure and disease at an aggregate level may be highly susceptible to confounding and may not be reflected in an association at the individual level. In this context, the confounding is often termed the *ecological fallacy*. The advantages of using aggregate data are that long-term differences in lifestyle (e.g. recreation) can be detected and some community variables can only be thought of in ecological terms. For example, Sainsbury (1955) found an association between area suicide rates and the population turnover in those areas. He explained these results by suggesting that alienation in an area might increase suicide rates.

Cross-sectional surveys

This type of descriptive study relates to a single point in time and can therefore report on prevalence of a disease, but is adversely affected by the duration of illness. A cross-sectional survey is often quick and cheap. It eliminates the problems of selection bias and has been used frequently for the study of depression and other neurotic conditions. However, any association found in a cross-sectional survey could be with either incidence or duration.

Case–control studies

In a case–control study, individuals with the disease are compared with a comparison group of controls. If the prevalence of exposure is higher in the cases than in the controls, the exposure might be a risk factor for the disease, and if lower the exposure might be protective. Case–control studies are relatively cheap and quick and can be used to study rare diseases. However, great care is needed in the design of the study in order to minimize selection bias. The validity of case–control studies does not depend upon matching but upon ensuring that the cases and controls come from the same population. A useful rule is to ensure that controls, if they developed the disease, should be included in the sampling frame for your cases.

The importance of this rule can be illustrated by the case–control study of O'Callaghan and colleagues (1992). This examined the association between abnormalities in pregnancy and childbirth and the development of schizophrenia. Obstetric notes were traced for 65 people with schizophrenia attending a psychiatric hospital in Dublin; the next birth in the Dublin obstetric hospital was used as the control. The odds ratio for schizophrenia in relation to an obstetric complication was about 2.4 (95% CI 1.1–6.0). Since the study design did not dictate that control subjects must still be resident in Dublin at the time of the study, it is likely that some controls might have moved away. Therefore, even if they had developed schizophrenia, they would not have been eligible as cases. A design in which the investigators had only included cases who still lived in Dublin would have reduced the chance of a selection bias.

For a case–control study of schizophrenia, the cases could be new presentations to a service in a defined catchment area. If we assume that all cases of schizophrenia attend psychiatric services, then the appropriate control group would be general population controls. For hospital cases of depression, general population controls would be a poor choice of controls because very few cases of depression reach specialist services so selection into treatment would be important (see example of selection bias).

A *matched case–control study* involves one or more controls being selected for each case due to their similarity for a number of characteristics that are thought to be potential important cofounders. Common matching variables are age and sex.

A *nested case–control study* is one based within a cohort study or sometimes a cross-sectional survey. The cases are those that arise as the cohort is followed prospectively and the controls are all, or a sample of the non-diseased members of the cohort.

The analysis of case–control studies results in the reporting of odds ratios; case–control studies cannot estimate disease incidence rates directly. If the study is matched, a more complex matched analysis needs to be performed (conditional logistic regression).

Cohort or longitudinal studies

A cohort (or longitudinal, or follow-up) study is an observational study in which a group of persons who are exposed to a potential cause of disease, together with a group who are unexposed, are followed-up over a period of time. The incidence of the disease of interest is compared in the two groups. Ideally, the exposed and unexposed groups should be chosen to be virtually identical, with the exception of the exposure. Often the exposure of interest is a continuous variable. Such information can be subdivided into grades of exposure, and a trend of increasing disease with increasing exposure can be examined. Such dose–response relationships are often important evidence in the search for causal associations.

The ability of a cohort study to rule out reverse causality as a reason for an observed association is of great benefit. For example, Lewis *et al.* (1992) studied a cohort of 50 000 Swedish male conscripts. The incidence of schizophrenia was 1.65 times higher in those brought up in cities compared with those brought up in country areas. These results could not have occurred because of the 'geographical drift' hypothesis. This suggests that schizophrenics tend to drift into city areas because of the presence of their illness. Since this cohort study asked about upbringing before the onset of disease, the authors concluded that environmental factors found in cities increase the risk of the disorder. Drift into cities could also occur, and a genetic contribution to the explanation whereby those at genetic risk of the disorder drift into cities and have children there cannot be excluded.

Exposure definition is linked to the timing of the study. Cohort studies always look forward from the exposure to disease development; however, they can sometimes be termed 'retrospective' when they use historical data on exposure, i.e. information already collected, often for another purpose. Historical cohort studies have the major advantage of offering a short-cut to studying diseases with a long interval between exposure and disease. The disadvantage of these studies is that exposure measurement is dependent on the historical record that is available, and exposure measurement may have been more inaccurate in the past. A particularly useful historical method is where some type of biological sample has been stored which can be measured as an index of exposure at the present time.

The completeness of follow-up is particularly important in cohort studies. It is essential that as high a proportion of people in the cohort as possible are followed-up, and those who migrate, die or leave the cohort for any reason should be recorded. These reasons for leaving the cohort may be influenced by the exposure, and incomplete follow-up can therefore introduce bias.

The analysis of cohort studies involves calculation of either the incidence rate or risk of disease in the exposed cohort compared with that in the unexposed cohort. Relative and absolute measures of effect can then be calculated.

A summary comparison of the advantages and disadvantages of case–control and cohort study designs is shown in Table 5.1.

Randomized controlled trials

RCTs are usually used (when possible) to investigate the effectiveness of medical interventions. They are the strongest design to investigate causality between an intervention and outcome because confounders are allocated randomly between the groups. The study population ideally should be representative of the population to which the results will apply. However, since trials are often comprised of volunteers, this is rarely the case. The subjects are then allocated randomly into the control group who receive the standard or placebo treatment and the intervention group who receive the new treatment. This random allocation aims to prevent any underlying differences between the two groups being responsible for any differences in outcome. Even random allocation can fail in this, especially if the number of subjects being assorted is relatively small. Therefore, it is important to collect baseline information on factors that affect outcome for all subjects and to check the similarity of the randomized groups in these baseline variables. Finally, measurement bias should be minimized in the assessment of the outcome of the study by a standardized method of assessment which should be blind to the study group to which a subject belongs.

Bias can still be introduced if subjects who are lost to follow-up are different in their outcome from those who have complete follow-up and

Table 5.1 *Advantages and disadvantages of case–control and cohort studies*

Case–control	Cohort
Strengths	
Suitable for rare diseases	Suitable for rare exposures
Better for studying causes that are in the distant past	Recall bias and reverse causality are unlikely to explain an association
Can examine many risk factors for a single disease	Can examine many outcomes for a single exposure
Relatively quick and inexpensive	Can calculate incidence rates
Weaknesses	
Susceptible to selection bias	Usually unsuitable for rare diseases
Can be susceptible to recall bias and reverse causality	Can be expensive and can lead to a long delay before the results are available
Unsuitable for rare exposures and cannot calculate incidence rates directly	Losses to follow-up can affect validity

there is differential drop-out between the randomized groups. Therefore, it is important to minimize the non-compliance rate and loss to follow-up rate. An 'intention to treat' analysis should be carried out which includes the outcomes of all randomized subjects, including those who were lost to follow-up during the study.

Systematic reviews and meta-analyses

Secondary research aims to summarize and draw conclusions from all the known primary studies on a particular topic (i.e. those which report results at first hand). The main advantage of these studies is the resulting increase in the combined sample size. A problem of secondary research is the presence of publication bias, i.e. small negative results are less likely to be published. Therefore, ideally, one should attempt a comprehensive search strategy that includes not only published results but also those reported in abstracts, personal communications and the like.

Meta-analyses are a type of secondary research tool which integrate the numerical data from more than one study and then statistically re-analyse these pooled data. In comparison, a systematic review simply summarizes (sometimes quantitatively) the results of primary studies using a pre-defined methodology. When pooling or comparing data from different studies, a researcher should check that the comparison is indeed valid by testing for heterogeneity between studies. Individual studies can vary in methodological quality of the research, and there are concerns about giving equal weighting to studies of different qualities.

Epidemiology and evaluation

Randomized versus non-randomized evidence

Evidence-based medicine has grown out of the application of statistical and epidemiological concepts to clinical medicine. Doctors have been using evidence upon which to base their clinical practice for many years, but if there is anything

'new' about evidence-based medicine it is in the suggestion that the production and synthesis of evidence should be done in a more explicit and quantitative way.

One consequence of this movement has been the increasing emphasis placed upon RCTs as providing the best evidence for clinical effectiveness. Clinical anecdote and experience is now largely discounted as a basis for clinical decision making, unless there is no evidence from other sources. Using observational designs, whether case–control or cohort, to investigate clinical effectiveness is of course fraught with the difficulties of identifying and adjusting for confounders. Sadly, the problem of confounding is rarely acknowledged in non-randomized studies of clinical effectiveness but there are circumstances under which non-randomized evidence is of potential value (Black, 1996).

It is also of importance to recognize the limitations of RCTs in guiding clinical practice. Though randomization should eliminate confounding, the internal validity of an RCT can also be affected by chance, the possibility of measurement bias and losses to follow-up. Of more concern to health service researchers is the external validity, the difficulty in generalizing the results from an RCT to real-life clinical situations. This has led to the development of the pragmatic RCT. Anyone familiar with the arguments over the findings of RCTs [e.g. correspondence on NIMH Depression trial (Elkin *et al.*, 1989)] will regard the idea that RCTs are 'gold standards' as somewhat naïve. There are still serious difficulties in interpretation even after well-conducted studies.

RCTs often have a number of limitations in informing clinical practice. Many clinical trials have quite restrictive inclusion criteria. For example, trials of antidepressants almost always exclude those who are at risk of suicide even though they are the group about whom most clinicians would like good evidence on clinical effectiveness.

Pragmatic randomized controlled trials

Schwartz and Lellouch (1967) are usually credited with contrasting explanatory and pragmatic attitudes in clinical trials. Explanatory trials are aimed at providing evidence of efficacy, or to answer theoretical questions about treatments; "can they work?" For that reason, it might be reasonable to analyse data only on those subjects who received the course of treatment rather than adopting an intention to treat analysis. Pragmatic trials, on the other hand, are concerned with providing evidence for the effectiveness of treatments under real service conditions: "Do they work?" Table 5.2 lists some of the questions one can ask when criticizing pragmatic trials. One of the important principles is to ensure that the trial is addressing a dilemma faced by clinicians or health managers. It is also important to realize that the costs of treatments have to take account of use of other health and social services, and personal costs.

Research, guidelines and audit

There are always difficulties in generalizing the results from single trials and there is always the possibility that the results of small trials, particularly the well-known ones, are a result of random error. Systematic reviews of research studies should be the backbone of providing advice to clinicians about treatment. These can therefore be used to provide guidelines for best practice. Audit is therefore about determining the extent to which guidelines are adhered to. There has been much talk also about measuring outcomes in routine clinical practice in the context of auditing services. This practice would produce unrandomized evidence usually with a poor understanding of potential confounders. In our view, this is unlikely to be of much use to clinicians in deciding upon what treatments to use. If the research evidence is thought to be inadequate, it is best to advocate carrying out pragmatic clinical trials that are relevant to practice in that locality.

Psychiatry and public health

Preventive strategies and public health

Geoffrey Rose (Rose, 1992) made the distinction between high risk and population-based strategies

Table 5.2 *Questions to ask in critically appraising pragmatic randomized controlled trials*

1. Aims
    Does the trial address a clinically important dilemma?
    Are the subjects in the trial those patients in which the treatment would normally be considered in clinical practice?
    Is the intervention a realistic reflection of likely good practice in the Health Service?
    Is it a 'Rolls Royce' service provided in a centre of excellence that would be difficult to sustain elsewhere?

2. Design
    What was the method of randomization and how did the investigators ensure that it was adhered to?
    Who was blind to the randomized allocation—patient, physician, the research assistant measuring outcomes, the investigator who analysed the data? How was blindness ensured and was it assessed?
    Did the experimenters include an assessment of 'quality of life'?
    Is there an economic assessment that measures health and social service costs not directly concerned with the treatment?

3. Analysis
    Was there an imbalance between the randomized groups in any important prognostic variables?
    How is missing data analysed? Is an intention to treat strategy used or are other statistical methods used?
    Have the investigators performed multiple statistical tests on a variety of outcomes?
    Was the main outcome specified before the trial was started? Is the power calculation from the research proposal described?
    If a negative result, how large are the confidence intervals? Have the investigators ruled out the possibility of an important treatment effect?

for preventing disease. The high risk approach identifies individuals at high risk, and any intervention is directed purely at them. An example might be the usual medical approach towards hypertension in which GPs screen and treat the hypertensive. The population-based approach aims to reduce the frequency of risk factors in the whole population, for example by encouraging everyone to exercise more and eat less salt in order to reduce blood pressure and the incidence of cardiovascular diseases. Unfortunately, our knowledge of the aetiology of psychiatric disorder is such that we are not yet in a position to adopt preventive strategies.

High risk strategies fit better with the medical model and restrict any intervention to those whom would benefit most. However, Rose has shown repeatedly that there are many circumstances where high risk strategies have rather modest effects in reducing the rates of disease because they exclude the large numbers of people at moderate risk. This point can be illustrated using data from the Epidemiologic Catchment Area Program study in the USA (Broadhead *et al.*, 1990; Table 5.3) In this study, the authors examined the association between disability days (e.g. days off work) and major depression, dysthymia and two categories representing those with neurotic symptoms that fell below the threshold for DSM-III diagnoses. Those with major depression had higher rates of disability days. However, in aggregate, there was more disability as a result of those with the less severe disorders.

Conclusions

The epidemiological approach is an essential element of planning services, evaluating interventions, investigating aetiology and devising and evaluating preventive strategies. It can be considered as one of the basic sciences underpinning health service research and the future of community psychiatry.

Acknowledgements

P.B.J gratefully acknowledges support from the Stanley Foundation.

References

Black, N. (1996) Why we need observational studies to evaluate the effectiveness of health care. *British Medical Journal*, 312, 1215–1218.

Broadhead, W.E., Blazer, D., George L. *et al.* (1990) Depression, disability days and days lost from work. *Journal of the American Medical Association*, 264, 2524–2528.

Brown, G.W. and Harris, T. (1978) *Social Origins of Depression*. London: Tavistock.

Elkin, I., Shea, T., Watkins, J.T. *et al.* (1989) National Institute of Mental Health Treatment of Depression Collaborative Research Program: general effectiveness of treatments. *Archives of General Psychiatry*, 46, 971–983.

Table 5.3 *Disability, depression and symptoms not fulfilling DSM-III criteria*

	Major depression	Minor depression (with mood disorder)	Minor depression (without mood disorder)	No symptoms
Sample size	49	178	696	1997
Mean disability days (SD)	11.0 (29.0)	6.1 (21.4)	4.0 (16.3)	2.0 (10.7)
Excess disability days	474	712	1356	Baseline

From Broadhead *et al.* (1990).

Evidence-Based Medicine Working Group (1992) Evidence-based medicine. A new approach to teaching the practice of medicine. *Journal of the American Medical Association*, 268, 2420–2425.

Lewis, G., David, A., Andreasson, S. *et al.* (1992) Schizophrenia and city life. *Lancet,* 340, 137–140.

O'Callaghan, E., Gibson, T., Colohan, H.A. *et al.* (1992) Risk of schizophrenia in adults born after obstetric complications and their association with early onset of illness: a controlled study. *British Medical Journal,* 305, 1256–1259.

Rose, G. (1992) *The Strategy of Preventive Medicine.* Oxford: Oxford University Press.

Sainsbury, P. (1955) *Suicide in London.* London: Chapman and Hall.

Schwartz, D. and Lellouch, J. (1967) Explanatory and pragmatic attitudes in therapeutic trials. *Journal of Chronic Diseases,* 20, 637–648.

Snow, J. (1936) *On the Mode of Communication of Cholera.* New York: The Commonwealth Fund.

6 | *Methods for evaluating community treatments*

Peter Tyrer

Introduction

New treatments are constantly being introduced to all forms of psychiatry and, for most of these, the setting in which the treatment is administered is not of special importance. Thus the introduction of a new and effective drug for a mental disorder will require similar testing in hospital, community or other settings and does not require special description here. However, all treatments given in the community have a common problem associated with them, compliance, or what is now termed more appropriately 'concordance' or 'adherence' (Mullen, 1997). Because treatment in the community rarely can be supervised satisfactorily, a great deal depends on the motivation of individual patients to continue whatever intervention is being given without the need to be monitored closely. Increasingly, therefore, the evaluation of community treatment is going to involve (i) some check on whether the treatment is being given appropriately and (ii) if not, whether additional treatments are able to be introduced to improve concordance and adherence. New treatments to improve compliance have now been introduced for the major psychoses and shown to be effective (Kemp *et al.*, 1996, 1998; Perry *et al.*, 1999) and these approaches are likely to impinge increasingly on those working in the community and be amongst the areas of competence being evaluated for such workers (described in Chapter 21).

The word 'evaluation' is now being used increasingly to describe any type of description of an intervention, and increasingly it is being used inappropriately with regard to community treatments. The word 'evaluate' is a mathematical expression originally used to give a numerical value to something which previously had no such value. It is still used in this sense in related expressions such as 'evaluable', but increasingly it has been broadened in use to describe any form of assessment, whether or not it is quantified accurately.

Three key questions

Before discussing different forms of evaluation of community treatment, it is necessary to establish what type of evaluation is proposed in any one instance. One of three main questions normally is being asked in such evaluations and it is important not to blur these because doing so creates confusion. The three questions are:

- Is the treatment efficacious? (i.e. is it better than a standard or control treatment)
- Does the treatment work in practice? (i.e. is in effective)
- Is the treatment cost-effective?

Is the treatment efficacious?

There is no point in any treatment being introduced to clinical practice in medicine unless it is an improvement on no treatment. The first prerequisite of any putative treatment is, therefore, to develop its efficacy. The circumstances in which such efficacy is shown has been the subject of considerable dispute over the past few years. Since the pioneering paper by Schwarz and Lellouch in 1967 (see below), a distinction has been made between explanatory and pragmatic trials of treatment effectiveness. Most, if not all, treatments in community psychiatry are determined by pragmatic trials as the circumstances in which treatments are given in ordinary practice may be very different from those which demonstrate the efficacy of a treatment. Such comparisons can be carried out in any setting but may not necessarily be appropriate to ordinary practice. For example, some years ago, Soloff and colleagues demonstrated that haloperidol in relatively low dosage (~7 mg a day) was superior to both antidepressants and placebo tablets in patients with borderline personality disorder treated in a penitentiary. There were no drop-outs from care because all the patients were in a locked environment and, not surprisingly, all patients took their medication as prescribed (Soloff *et al.*, 1986). The prerequisite of efficacy had been established, but this is no guarantee that in ordinary clinical usage the treatment would be appropriate for the general population of people with borderline personality disorder. In fact, subsequent studies in more typical samples have not shown the same degree of superiority for antipsychotic drugs (Cornelius *et al.*, 1993; Soloff, 1994).

Is the treatment effective in practice?

In a pragmatic trial, the circumstances in which the treatment would be used in ordinary clinical practice are being tested and these may be very different from those appertaining in an explanatory trial. Pragmatic trials are more relevant to community mental health services and are also favoured by those supporting evidence-based medicine, a subject which is now at the heart of clinical governance in the UK (Scally and Donaldson, 1998). A distinction is sometimes made between the words 'effective' and 'efficacious' in this context. If the treatment is superior to a control treatment, it can be said to show 'efficacy', but it is only when it has been tested in ordinary circumstances of clinical practice and shown to be superior to other treatments that it can be regarded as 'effective'. This might stretch interpretation of the English language too far. 'Effective' refers to the ability of a treatment to bring

about a desired effect, and this is virtually the same as 'efficacious', something 'that produces, or is certain to produce, the intended effect (i.e. effective)' (*Shorter Oxford English Dictionary*, 1973). The definition of a good service need not therefore be strictly determined by the results of a randomized controlled trial, and although such trials should never be regarded as redundant or unnecessary, evaluation can be reinforced greatly by a range of other sources of information (for a review, see Thornicroft and Tansella, 1999, pp. 101–105).

Cost

It is no longer satisfactory merely to demonstrate the effectiveness of a treatment. If the cost of this is so much greater than that of existing treatments, and the gain only a small advance, it is difficult to justify its introduction except on a very limited scale. It is fortunate that most treatments in community psychiatry are relatively cheap compared with the high cost of in-patient services. A substantial part of cost-effectiveness of community treatments is the demonstration that in-patient care is reduced as a consequence of introducing the treatment. Even if the reduction in in-patient care is only modest, in most cases it would be more than sufficient to make the cost of treatment less than the alternative (Knapp and Beecham, 1990).

Stages of evaluation

The evaluation of complex health interventions, which includes community treatments, can be viewed as a graded process occurring in a set of phases (Campbell *et al.*, 2000), somewhat similar to the phases that have now become common parlance in the evaluation of new drugs.

(Phase 0)—pre-clinical or theoretical phase

At the first stage of evaluation, it is legitimate to think broadly about an issue and decide whether it is an important subject to examine and research, and then to think about the methods that might be employed. Thus, for example, in the later 1980s there was concern about the failure of many patients who formerly would be resident in psychiatric hospitals to keep appointments with their psychiatric services and who therefore disappeared from the network of care. This could be recorded in simple quantitative data or could merely be an impression (reinforced by public inquiries of major incidents, usually involving homicide). Thus, for example, this type of speculation could lead naturally to the suggestion that systems to produce closer supervision of psychiatric patients might lead to fewer drop-outs from care, and this could be a prelude to formal testing of the hypothesis in a fully controlled trial. In this particular instance, the findings of such trials show that the number of drop-outs from care is reduced (Tyrer *et al.*, 1995; Marshall *et al.*, 1997). Similarly, the first description of a new specific intervention such as counselling in general practice can consist of a description of its specific input and apparent impact on outcome in a way that could only be described as speculative since there could be so many confounding factors that could result in the findings apart from the specific intervention concerned. It is only later that the value of the intervention can be measured. In the case of counselling, this first stage might have been carried out more diligently as subsequent work has been handicapped by ignorance as to what exactly is the specific input that distinguishes counselling from other interventions (Corney, 1992).

Phase 1—modelling

In this phase, the effects of a new intervention or treatment are described and, to some extent, measured before and after its introduction and an idea of its likely effect size obtained. This goes beyond simple description and gives some idea of the impact of the new intervention. However, most open studies exaggerate the degree of change created by the new intervention and, invariably, further studies show that its impact is considerably less. Nevertheless, these studies serve a valuable purpose in demonstrating that the intervention is

(i) feasible in clinical practice, (ii) is more likely to have a positive impact than a negative one and (iii) gives some idea of its relative advantages and disadvantages. Other improvements that can be made in such studies include (i) reduction in numbers of other treatments that are given so confounding is less, (ii) formal assessment using rating scales at the beginning and end of the treatment period so that change is measured more precisely, (iii) better selection of patients for treatment and (iv) formal pre–post designs that reduce other forms of variance a little.

Phase 2—exploratory trial

In this phase, the information gathered in phase 1 is used to develop the ideal form of intervention and to choose the best study design for a formal comparison. This often involves testing further the feasibility of delivery of the intervention and its acceptability to providers and patients. It may also be helpful to work with user groups at this stage in order to develop a strong case for the trial within the community of patients likely to be treated.

Also included in this phase are a range of interventions that fall short of the requirements of the randomized controlled trial in that randomization of the population does not take place but other measures are introduced to make the groups as similar as possible at baseline. The problems of randomization are prominent when community services are being compared (an der Heiden, 1996; Thornicroft *et al.*, 1998) and are discussed in more detail in Chapters 5 and 7.

Phase 3—randomized controlled trials

In the last stage of comparison, the new treatment is compared with a standard treatment under the rigorous conditions of a randomized controlled trial. Whilst this has always been the 'gold standard' whereby any new treatment is to be judged, it is important not to be carried away by the scientific arguments for using such trials (which are incontrovertible) without considering alternatives which may be more appropriate *at that particular time in the development of the treatment.*

Randomized controlled trials are still relatively new to medicine and particularly to psychiatry, and the first major studies [of the treatment of schizophrenia in the USA (Casey *et al.*, 1960) and of depression in the UK (Clinical Psychiatry Committee, Medical Research Council, 1965] are still within my experience in psychiatry.

Attitudes towards the randomized controlled trial have changed markedly in the last 10 years because of the distinction made between pragmatic and explanatory trials of interventions (Schwartz and Lellouch, 1967). Before this time, all was invested in the explanatory trial, a tightly organized and controlled trial of highly selected individuals who were homogeneous for the condition being treated and who were likely to complete the course of treatment. The findings of these studies were then generalized to routine clinical practice. Schwartz and Lellouch pointed out that this approach was not valid. The explanatory trial was "aimed at understanding whether a difference existed between two treatments" whereas the pragmatic trial "aimed at decision by answering the question 'which of the two treatments should we prefer?'" (Schwartz and Lellouch, 1967). It is this question that is at the heart of any service evaluation and it is asked at a later stage than the explanatory trial.

Johnson (1998) has pointed out recently that, despite long use of the randomized controlled trial in psychiatry, it continues to be used inefficiently and often wrongly. There are greater problems with psychiatric disorders (and with psychiatric patients) than in other medical conditions and these include (i) problems of achieving reliable diagnoses, (ii) the difficulties of maintaining blind assessments, (iii) the common practice of simultaneously giving many treatments and (iv) the difficulties in selecting control groups, particularly for psychosocial treatments. However, these do not excuse the generally laxity of design and poor presentation and interpretation of findings. Johnson recommends that those involved in carrying out clinical trials of treatment interventions in psychiatry should follow seven principles when choosing a suitable design: (i) choose no more than two outcome variables; (ii) concentrate on obtaining follow-up information on all randomized patients

on a few occasions rather than many; (iii) use a multi-centre design wherever possible; (iv) ensure that the entry criteria are as broad as possible so that the results are likely to be generalizable; (v) forget power calculations and aim to recruit at least 100 patients for analysis in each treatment group; (vi) develop the strategy for analysis *before* the trial database is 'unblinded' to reveal treatments; and (vii) use recently introduced statistical modelling techniques to enable analysis of all available data rather than restrict this to those with full follow-up information (Everitt, 1995).

Individual randomization may not always be appropriate in mental health service evaluation. For example, if an intervention is directed towards a team intervention, cluster randomization frequently is used and this will affect the numbers needed to show benefit (these are usually larger than when individual randomization is made) (Kerry and Bland, 1998) and may pose important ethical issues (Edwards *et al.*, 1999). Randomized incomplete block designs have also been used when full randomized studies are not deemed to be possible.

Because it is rarely possible to blind both patients and investigators in trials of community mental health services, there is great potential for bias. Attempts to minimize bias need to be made explicit, and one way of ensuring this is to make the investigating (research) team independent of the service providers. The characteristics of those who refuse to participate or who drop-out at an early stage of evaluation are likely to differ from those who participate throughout, and should be recorded.

The sample size necessary for a trial is dependent on the power calculation which relies on estimating the difference between the effects of two or more interventions and the likely variance of the data. This may be possible if an exploratory trial has been carried out using the same design, but in most instances there is a great deal of guesswork in making such estimations. In practice, many investigators work backwards. They estimate how many patients they are likely to have available for treatment and then work out the power calculations to fit these figures. This was not the purpose for which power calculations were introduced, and the recommendation of Johnson (1998) that investigators should aim for a minimum of 100 patients in each arm of the trial is a better solution.

Phase 4—dissemination and implementation

This final phase is sometimes neglected by researchers who feel their work has been done when they complete their main trials. The growth of research and development in health service research has achieved greater prominence because of the failure to implement advances quickly enough; this was the main impetus behind the development of the Cochrane Collaboration. Part of this phase is equivalent to post-marketing surveillance after the introduction of a new drug, and it is fair to add that health service interventions have been slow to introduce this adequately. However, it has a role in the establishment of audit.

Audit is often undervalued by experienced research workers who are used to working with good resources and no time pressures. However, audit is the best way of ensuring that the benefits of research advance are not only disseminated to clinical practice but are also maintained. In clinical practice, good audit ensures quality control so that sound practice is maintained.

Patient preference

Although randomized trials provide the best evidence of efficacy for treatments such as a comparison of new drugs in which patient preference is a very minor factor, the situation is different for many psychosocial treatments or those in which drugs and other treatments are being compared. In a consumer society, the issue of patient preference with respect to treatment is coming more to the fore. This is particularly true in community settings. One common example is the prescription of antipsychotic drugs in schizophrenia. Although the evidence for the efficacy of these drugs in schizophrenia is overwhelming, there is still a large minority of patients who prefer to take other

forms of treatment, particularly 'alternative therapies', of unproven and doubtful value. In my personal experience, the strong personal belief of such patients that these treatments are the only valid ones does have an influence on response to treatment which goes far beyond the simple placebo effect for the preferred treatment and the nocebo effect (Tyrer, 1991) of the rejected one. The nocebo effect (i.e. the expectation that a treatment will harm) is now as prevalent as the placebo effect in clinical practice. Fifty years ago, new treatments were mainly 'wonder drugs' that led to marvel, amazement and the expectation of improvement. Now we have a more sophisticated and informed population that is likely to look up all the adverse effects on the Internet before agreeing to start treatment.

There is also the possibility that there are important interactions between an individual's preferences and the effects of treatment, yet, in the standard randomized controlled trial, these are not detected. If these are important, the results of the randomized controlled trial may be attributed wrongly to the specific content of the intervention alone (McPherson *et al.*, 1997). As a consequence of this, there is increasing interest in non-experimental methods in the assessment of efficacy of treatments (Wennberg, 1988) and in different research designs that take account of patient (or indeed, other people's such as clinicians) preferences. Brewin and Bradley (1989) proposed a partially randomized patient-centred design for psychosocial treatments in which patients who had strong preferences for a particular treatment were allocated to it whereas those who had no particular preference were allocated randomly in the usual way. The problem with this approach is that it breaks one of the fundamental principles of the randomized controlled trial, ensuring equivalent populations for all factors apart from the treatments under consideration. If, as has been shown to be the case, patients who have strong preferences differ from others in their level of education and other potentially important factors (Feine *et al.*, 1998), then their results cannot be compared satisfactorily with others.

This does not mean that patient preference trials are inappropriate, but it is probably preferable to avoid contaminating the randomized controlled trial by attempting to combine randomization and patient preference in one design. If a patient preference trial is carried out independently of a randomized controlled trial, then the results can be compared and policy decisions made after taking account of both sets of findings (Wennberg *et al.*, 1993).

Choice of evaluation for different treatments

Although circumstances vary greatly, it is possible to list the most appropriate forms of evaluation for different treatments (Table 6.1). For most drug treatments, it is preferable to concentrate on randomized controlled trials as the main method of evaluation as, despite their difficulties in community settings, the ability to make treatments more or less double-blind is a major advantage. However, when multiple drug treatments are being evaluated, it is almost impossible to obtain adequate numbers of patients to test hypotheses adequately, and in these circumstances it is better to carry out audit studies and introduce standards to reduce the extent of polypharmacy (Wressell *et al.*, 1990).

For psychosocial interventions, the choice is not so straightforward; the difficulties in ensuring blind assessment (or even masked assessment when a small amount of information sometimes is leaked) are often very great. For treatments such as psychotherapy, patient preference should be taken into account more and be linked to single-blind trials, whereas for more clearly defined therapies such as cognitive and behaviour therapy, it is appropriate to concentrate on good single-blind trials with tightly defined outcomes.

In the settings of ordinary community practice, many treatments are given simultaneously, both pharmacological and non-pharmacological. It has to be admitted that the process of evaluation here is not satisfactory and no sleight of hand in the form of complex assessment procedures and designs can conceal this. At the same time, it is quite clear that the answers to therapy in these settings are much more important than for most single treatments. It is reasonable to attempt such evaluations only if the investigators are prepared to combine data from several interventions in analysing data. Thus drug and psychological treatments could be combined separately prior to

Table 6.1 *Common psychiatric treatments and their evaluation in community psychiatry*

Treatment	Problems of community evaluation	Most common form of evaluation
Single drug therapy	Adherence	Randomized controlled trial
Multiple drug therapy	Adherence	Audit
Psychodynamic therapy	Choice of outcomes	Preference and randomized controlled single-blind trials
Behaviour therapy	Choice of outcomes	Single-blind trials
Cognitive therapy	Treatment fidelity	Single-blind trials
Mixed drug and psychological therapies	Choice of control populations	Trials of complex design with insufficient numbers but with opportunities for combining data

analysis and interactions examined. Ideally, studies should be multi-centre ones in which sufficient numbers can be generated to test several hypotheses, but for many involved in such research the special circumstances of their own community settings seem to make them reluctant to pool resources in this way. As a consequence, we have a large number of small-scale studies carried out in different settings with silly differences in methodology which prevent data from being combined or meta-analysis from being carried out successfully. Organizations such as ENMESH (European Network for Mental Health Service Evaluation) could play an important part in fostering a common basis for evaluation that could aid such multi-centre studies.

Outcome measures

Although it would be wrong to think that community mental health practice leads to a different set of outcome than other forms of treatment, there is a recurring set of themes involved in community care which has to be borne in mind in order to process an evaluation. These themes will be discussed in order of importance. This is also relevant in view of the tendency of evaluations of community treatment to attempt to measure large numbers of outcomes on the grounds that all can contribute to the overall effect of a treatment policy.

Cost

Although at various times during the move towards community care, emphasis has been placed on improving the quality of life for patients, de-stigmatizing the mentally ill and promoting the dignity of self-sufficiency, the major reason why community care has been promoted in psychiatry is that it is considerably cheaper than hospital care. This is illustrated in Figure 6.1 in which the relative cost of providing care for a population of psychotic patients was recorded over 1 year. The figures show that, even when community care is focused specifically upon in the practice, its costs are dwarfed completely by the costs

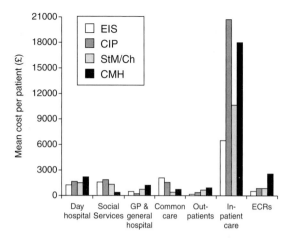

Figure 6.1 *Comparison of costs of randomly allocated community-oriented and hospital-orientated care over 1 year for 144 patients with recurrent psychotic disorder, illustrating the much greater expense of hospital in-patient care compared with community services. (Derived from Tyrer et al., 1998.) EIS = early intervention service (community team); ECR = extra-contractual referral (in-patient care away from parent hospital); CIP = community intervention project (community team); St M/Ch = St Mary's/St Charles Hospital (hospital team); CMH = Central Middlesex Hospital (hospital team).*

of in-patient care. Thus the best resourced team in the study (Early Intervention Service; EIS) shown in Figure 6.1 still accounted for a much smaller proportion of the total budget than in-patient care despite accounting for a large fraction of the cost of community care in the study. The slogan 'a week in hospital is worth a year in the community' is essentially true even when considerable input is given to the community services.

In all countries of the world, we now have to accept that medical services are rationed to some extent and any treatment in the community that is more expensive than other treatments, even if it is more effective, has a hard task in getting preference. In practice, most treatments in community psychiatry do not demonstrate such clear-cut advantages over the best of existing treatments, and the most frequent scenario is that a number of treatments produce equivalent clinical findings but the one that does it most cheaply is the one that is recommended for adoption. In many cases, the treatment might appear to be more expensive than the comparison ones but if it saves money by reducing admissions to hospital it would turn out to be cheaper overall. Thus, for example, the atypical neuroleptic drugs are much more expensive than the standard antipsychotic drugs, but the case has been made for their adoption in clinical practice because, overall, they save money (Guest *et al.*, 1996; Aitcheson and Kerwin, 1997).

Although cost is an obvious target for outcome measurement, it is fraught with difficulties in analysis. Almost invariably, costs show a grossly skewed distribution with few outliers costing a very large amount of money and many others costing very little if intervention had been minimal. In terms of analysis, non-parametric statistics are appropriate and yet these data do not deal with real figures. Mean costs constitute real resources whereas median costs are hypothetical even though they are more appropriate for statistical analyses. One of the consequences of this is that most analyses of costs tend to be carried out poorly (Barber and Thompson, 1998), and much more rigour is needed in the analysis of data. In our personal work, we found the statistical technique called the 'bootstrap method' (Efron and Tibshirani, 1993) to be an appropriate way of dealing with cost data, and this allows arithmetic means to be used in analysis despite skewing of the data (Evans *et al.*, 1999).

Generalizability

Good evaluations of treatment lead to findings that can be used widely across a range of settings. In standard research trial methodology, this is achieved by broad entry criteria to studies so that the population treated is representative of all those at risk and drop-out rates are kept as low as possible so that the intervention can be analysed within this representative population.

The issue that commonly leads to different findings in community studies is that of treatment fidelity. It is tested most often in studies of

psychological treatments that can be defined formally, such as cognitive therapy, but it could equally well be addressed in all forms of treatment, including drug therapy. With respect to drug therapy, treatment fidelity is concerned primarily with compliance, adherence or concordance. Although this is true of all forms of treatment, it is the essential element in drug treatment since the consumption of the medication constitutes the essential part of treatment fidelity. Pharmacokinetic differences may lead to the drug being less effective in some people compared with others, but these are in no way under the voluntary control of the patient or therapist. In community comparisons of drug treatment, it is very difficult to be certain of adherence to treatment, since simple measures such as counting of tablets after each course of treatment does not guarantee that those which have been taken have been consumed by the patient, and the detection of drugs which can be tested in the urine or in other body fluids do not guarantee that the drug concerned has been taken in regular dosage over the total course of treatment.

What seems to be most important in ensuring compliance is education and knowledge. The more a patient knows about the reasons for a treatment and the consequences of not taking it, the more likely they are to comply with a treatment regime. One of the reasons why cognitive and behavioural approaches have been so valuable in recent years is that they essentially involve a collaborative approach with the patient which involves an explanation as to why treatment is necessary and which the patient has to adopt if treatment is to proceed successfully (Kemp *et al.*, 1996, 1998; Perry *et al.*, 1999).

For psychological treatments, the variance in treatment fidelity may be much greater. If we regard the basic unit of community treatment as the community mental health team, it is clear that there is a wide range of experience and knowledge across the range of treatments available, and most team members will not be capable of giving psychological treatment competently without training and periodic refresher courses. The standard way of determining treatment fidelity in psychosocial interventions is to tape-record interviews and, ideally, have them rated blind by an independent assessor. Although this is a perfectly reasonable procedure to adopt, it is important to realize that it may interfere with the therapeutic session, may not always be representative of all parts of treatment since the therapist and patient know they are being monitored and it is not usually representative of ordinary practice. It merely tests whether patient and therapist are *capable* of carrying out treatment in a proper manner; it does not confirm that this treatment is being given consistently in this way. Such measures also beg the question, "what do we do with the results when treatment fidelity is not satisfactory?" In ordinary practice, there is, as yet, no standard way of ensuring that patients are treated by competent therapists (e.g. Kingdon *et al.*, 1996).

Summary

The methodology of evaluation of community treatments is still a young area of science. However, we have moved far from following in the paths of John Conolly at Hanwell and Edward Charlesworth at Lincoln 150 years ago when they removed constraint and encouraged rehabilitation as the first stage of community treatment. These initiatives had face validity in that they illustrated that patients with mental illness could have a much better quality of life when the right intervention was given. We have become much better informed in the last few years and have moved a long way from the stage of what Thornicroft and Tansella term 'naïve community mental health' in which the chant of the animals in Orwell's *Animal Farm* 'four legs good, two legs bad' could be paraphrased as 'community treatment good, hospital treatment bad'. As Thornicroft and Tansella (1999, p. 266) suggest, we should now "recognise the value of facilities both at hospital and at community sites, as part of a well-integrated mental health system of care", and, if we are to hone and develop these to their maximum effect, we need to use the range of methodologies described here. There is also an urgent need to develop new approaches that are not as time-consuming, expensive and limited in scope as the randomized

controlled trial. It is likely that progress will be made more effectively by integrating qualitative and quantitative approaches in this regard. Above all, we need to be pragmatic and flexible in the use of the methodologies and not allow them to become masters rather than servants.

References

Aitcheson, K.J. and Kerwin, R.W. (1997) Cost-effectiveness of clozapine. *British Journal of Psychiatry*, 171, 125–130.

An der Heiden, W. (1996) Experimental and quasi-experimental design in evaluative research. In: Knudsen H.C. and Thornicroft, G. (eds), *Mental Health Service Evaluation*. Cambridge: Cambridge University Press, pp. 143–155.

Barber, J. and Thompson, S.G. (1998) Analysis and interpretation of cost data in randomised controlled trials: review of published studies. *British Medical Journal*, 317, 1195–1200.

Brewin, C.R. and Bradley, C. (1989) Patient preferences and randomised clinical trials. *British Medical Journal*, 299, 313–315.

Campbell, M., Fitzpatrick, R., Haines, A., Sandercock, P., Spiegelhalter, D. and Tyrer, P. (2000) A framework for the design and evaluation of complex interventions to improve health. *British Medical Journal*, in press.

Casey, J.F., Lasky, J.J., Klett, C.J. and Hollister, L.E. (1960) Treatment of schizophrenic reactions with phenothiazine derivatives. *American Journal of Psychiatry*, 117, 97–105.

Clinical Psychiatry Committee, Medical Research Council (1965) Clinical trial of the treatment of depressive illness. *British Medical Journal*, i, 881–886.

Cornelius, J.R., Soloff, P.H., George, A., Ulrich, R.F. and Perel, J.M. (1993) Haloperidol vs. phenelzine in continuation therapy of borderline disorder. *Psychopharmacology Bulletin*, 29, 333–337.

Corney, R. (1992) The effectiveness of counselling in general practice. *International Review of Psychiatry*, 4, 331–338.

Edwards, S., Braunholtz, D., Stevens, A. and Lilford, R. (1999) Ethical issues in the design and conduct of cluster RCTs. *British Medical Journal*, 318, 1407–1409.

Efron, B. and Tibshirani, R. J. (1993) *An Introduction to the Bootstrap*. London: Chapman and Hall.

Evans, K., Tyrer, P., Catalan, J., Schmidt, U., Davidson, K., Dent, J. *et al.* (1999) Manual-assisted cognitive-behaviour therapy (MACT): a randomised controlled trial of a brief intervention with bibliotherapy in the treatment of recurrent deliberate self-harm. *Psychological Medicine*, 29, 19–25.

Everitt, B.S. (1995) The analysis of repeated measures: a practical review with examples. *The Statistician*, 44, 113–135.

Feine, J.S., Awad, M.A. and Lund, J.P. (1998) The impact of patient preference on the design and interpretation of clinical trials. *Community Dental and Oral Epidemiology*, 26, 70–74.

Guest, J.S., Hart, W.N., Cookson, R.S. and Lindstrom, E. (1996) Pharmaco-economic evaluation of long-term treatment with risperidone for patients with chronic schizophrenia. *British Journal of Medical Economics*, 10, 59–67.

Johnson, T. (1998) Clinical trials in psychiatry: background and statistical perspective. *Statistical Methods in Medical Research*, 7, 209–234.

Kemp, R., Hayward, P., Applewhaite, G., Everitt, B. and David, A. (1996) Compliance therapy in psychotic patients: randomised controlled trial. *British Medical Journal*, 312, 345–349.

Kemp, R., Kirov, G., Applewhaite, G., Everitt, B., Hayward, P. and David, A. (1998) Randomised controlled trial of compliance therapy: 18 month follow-up. *British Journal of Psychiatry*, 172, 413–419.

Kerry, S.M. and Bland, J.M. (1998) Analysis of a trial randomised in clusters. *British Medical Journal*, 316, 54.

Kingdon, D., Tyrer, P., Seivewright, N., Ferguson, B. and Murphy, S. (1996) The Nottingham Study of Neurotic Disorder: influence of cognitive therapists on outcome. *British Journal of Psychiatry*, 169, 93–97.

Knapp, M. and Beecham, J. (1990) Costing mental health services. *Psychological Medicine*, 20, 893–908.

Little, W., Fowler, H.W. and Coulson, J. Revised and edited by Onions, C.T. (1973) *Shorter Oxford English Dictionary*. Oxford: Oxford University Press.

Marshall, M., Gray, A., Lockwood, A. and Green, R. (1997) Case management for severe mental disorders. In: Adams, C.E., Duggan, L., de Jesus Mari, J. and White, P. (eds), *Schizophrenia Module of the Cochrane Database of Systematic Reviews*. Oxford: Cochrane Collaboration.

McPherson, K., Britton, A.R. and Wennberg, J.E. (1997) Are randomised controlled trials controlled? Patient preferences and unblind trials. *Journal of the Royal Society of Medicine*, 90, 652–656.

Mullen, P.D. (1997) Compliance becomes concordance. *British Medical Journal*, 314, 691–692.

Perry, A., Tarrier, N., Morriss, R., McCarthy, E. and Limb, K. (1999) Randomised controlled trial of efficacy of teaching patients with bipolar disorder to identify early symptoms of relapse and obtain treatment. *British Medical Journal*, 318, 149–153.

Scally, G. and Donaldson, L.J. (1998) The NHS's 50th anniversary: clinical governance and the drive for quality improvement in the new NHS in England. *British Medical Journal*, 317, 61–65.

Schwartz, D. and Lellouch, J. (1967) Explanatory and pragmatic attitudes in therapeutic trials. *Journal of Chronic Diseases*, 20, 637–648.

Soloff, P.H. (1994) Is there any drug treatment of choice for the borderline patient? *Acta Psychiatrica Scandinavica*, 379 (Suppl.), 50–55.

Soloff, P.H., George, A., Nathan, R.S., Schulz, P.M., Ulrich, R.F. and Perel, J.M. (1986) Progress in pharmacotherapy of personality disorders: a double blind study of amitriptyline, haloperidol and placebo. *Archives of General Psychiatry*, 43, 691–697.

Thornicroft, G. and Tansella, M. (1999) *The Mental Health Matrix: A Manual to Improve Services*. Cambridge: Cambridge University Press.

Thornicroft, G., Strathdee, G., Phelan, M., Holloway, F., Wykes, T., Dunn, G. *et al.* (1998) Rationale and design: the PRiSM Psychosis Study. *British Journal of Psychiatry*, 173, 363–370.

Tyrer, P. (1991) The nocebo effect—poorly known but getting stronger. In: Dukes, M.N.G. and Aronson, J.K. (eds), *Side Effects of Drugs Annual 15*. Amsterdam: Elsevier, pp. 19–25.

Tyrer, P., Morgan, J., Van Horn, E., Jayakody, M., Evans, K., Brummell, R. *et al.* (1995) A randomised controlled study of close monitoring of vulnerable psychiatric patients. *Lancet*, 345, 756–759.

Tyrer, P., Evans, K., Gandhi, N., Lamont, A., Harrison-Read, P. and Johnson, T. (1998) Randomised controlled trial of two models of care for discharged psychotic patients. *British Medical Journal*, 316, 106–109.

Wennberg, J.E. (1988) Non-experimental methods in the assessment of efficacy. *Medical Decision Making*, 8, 175–176.

Wennberg, J.E., Barry, M.J., Fowler, F.J., and Mulley, A. (1993) Outcomes research, PORTs, and health care reform. *Annals of the New York Academy of Sciences*, 703, 52–62

Wressell, S.E., Tyrer, S.P. and Berney, T.P. (1990) Reduction in antipsychotic drug dosage in mentally handicapped patients. A hospital study. *British Journal of Psychiatry*, 157, 101–106.

7 | *Methods for evaluating community mental health services*

Wolfram an der Heiden

Introduction

When considering methods for the evaluation of community mental health care, one has to take into account that typical evaluation projects are characterized by the following features (Wottawa, 1996):

- there may be a feedback loop between the results of the study and changes in the clinical and social context of the study, so that the context changes over time, and sometimes will change during the course of the study;
- since the study aim usually is the optimization of patient benefit, the dependent variables chosen in evaluation studies should directly or indirectly reflect patient benefit.

There is a considerable difference between evaluation studies and basic scientific research. Because the results of evaluation may be incorporated in service planning decisions, researchers often are confronted with specific expectations by planners, politicians and managers. This is of concern since the method usually applied in basic research to protect against bias—control studies and cross-validation—is often not a real option for most evaluation questions. As Milne (1987) noted, "... as we learn more about how best to measure client change, we tend to change the measures: we decide that we need 'better' ways of evaluating their response to therapy. This may enhance the next evaluation, but it simultaneously

reduces our capacity to relate a series of programme changes to one another, since we are comparing different programmes using different measures, so creating problems of interpretation. In a similar way the growing experience of the practitioner may dictate 'better' experimental designs. These are equally capable of annulling comparisons over time" (p. 43).

One response to this dilemma would be to carry out evaluation studies with special emphasis on methodological soundness. Because of the non-repeatability of many real-life evaluative studies, it is necessary to raise the standards of research design, of sampling procedures and the measures used. However, one is faced with the following challenges (Wottawa, 1996):

- research designs in the real world are usually weaker than designs in experimental basic research;
- the formation of true probability samples or comparable control groups often is not possible; and
- blindness often is not achievable, and the people included in an investigation normally have a clear idea of what they think the result should be.

As a consequence, methodological efforts in evaluation studies may be seen as 'walking a tightrope' between what seems to be useful, and possible with regard to resources, and what is desirable. The interests of the different stakeholders involved are also significant influences.

For Dunn *et al.*, the 1981 enterprise of evaluation is an 'ill-structured problem', because it may show one or more of the following characteristics:

(i) Unknown decision-makers: the persons, groups or agencies who will affect and be affected by the results are unknown.

(ii) Unidentifiable alternatives: the range of appropriate approaches to understanding and improving programmes cannot be identified.

(iii) Unspecifiable criteria: criteria for choosing among alternative programmes or competing approaches are not specified.

(iv) Inestimable probabilities: the probability that some decision-maker(s) will utilize information from the study results cannot be estimated.

The enterprise of evaluation

The diversity within evaluation is extraordinary (Suchman, 1967), despite the fact that the use of scientific methods and techniques is regarded as indispensable. 'Programme evaluation' lies in between evaluation and rigorous scientific investigation (e.g. randomized controlled trials, RCTs) (J.H. Abramson, 1979; Wittmann, 1985). The distinction between 'hard' scientific methods on the one hand and 'weaker' methods on the other hand points to the problems that have dominated the discussion about methods in evaluative research for the last two decades, and which may be defined by the terms 'qualitative' versus 'quantitative' evaluation (Cook and Reichardt, 1979b; Patton, 1980; Sechrest and Sidani, 1995; Shadish, 1995).

The elements of evaluative research

According to Attkisson *et al.* (1978), the enterprise of evaluation:

• is based on systematic data collection and analysis;

• involves a process of making reasonable judgements about programme inputs, effectiveness, efficiency and adequacy;

• is designed for use in programme management, external accountability and future planning;

• measures the amount of change that occurs; and

• focuses especially on accessibility, awareness, availability, comprehensiveness, continuity, integration and cost of services.

In *input evaluation*, the analysis is centred around the activities that take place in a programme or service and the related resources (Suchman, 1967; Milne, 1987). The assumption is that increased input correlates with increased efficiency. In *process evaluation*, utilization data, for example the number of clients served and the range of services provided over time, are used as descriptive measures of service activity. When there is an emphasis on the cost of attaining programme goals and on developing less expensive alternatives, it is called *efficiency evaluation*. *Client satisfaction evaluation* looks at services from a consumer point of view. According to Lebow (1982a), this form of evaluation is the result of the movement to a more consumer-oriented society and an increased financing of treatment services by government and third party payers. When the focus is on the impact of services on clients health or functioning, it is called *outcome evaluation*.

Another differentiation is that by Lebow (1982b), who distinguishes between:

• an organizational model: a focus on the management of a facility assessing the appropriateness and viability of the organizational structure, the scope of the operation, the efficiency of the management, the quantity of services provided and the relationship of services to community need and demand;

• a care process model: the quality of services is compared against a standard practice;

• a consumer evaluation model: a focus on the consumer's opinion about services;

• a community impact model: examining the effects of the intervention on the wider local community; and

- the efficacy model: a service's ability to change client outcomes.

One of the challenges for evaluation research is to investigate the associations between inputs, processes and outcomes. Data on staffing, equipment and facilities ('input') and on their utilization ('process') are required comparisons of costs and outcomes of different service interventions. "These differences stand in the way of implementing the design and they must be reduced as much as possible by developing clear understandings and consensual agreements on objectives, procedures, and standards ..." (Riecken and Boruch, 1974, p. 158).

According to the focus of the study and the organizational context, there are a host of methodological choices (Patton, 1980):

(i) Measurement options: what kinds of data should be collected and what kinds of measures should be used?

(ii) Design options: how much manipulation or control should be exerted in the settings under study? Options vary from controlled experiments to naturalistic field studies with a considerable variation in between.

(iii) Personal involvement options: what kinds of interpersonal contacts, if any, should the researchers have with the subjects under study?

(iv) Analysis options: to what extent should the study be open to whatever emerges (inductive analysis) and to what extent should prior hypotheses be examined (deductive analysis)?

Depending on the questions, different data and research designs are needed. Table 7.1 shows the diversity of available methods.

Process evaluation in psychiatric services

The variables used in evaluative research need to be selected on the basis of how relevant they are to the objectives of the study. T. Abramson (1979) separates three types of variables that should be considered for inclusion:

(i) 'universal' variables: variables that should always be considered because of their relevance in any study of groups and populations; for example sex, age, ethnic group, marital status, social class, place of residence;

(ii) measures of time: these are especially important in longitudinal studies, for example for the definition of treatment episodes or observation periods,

(iii) variables which delineate the study population or populations; the demographic characteristics, for example, may indicate the extent to which generalizations could be made from the findings.

Many evaluative studies rely exclusively on data of these three types, without any additional data about the individuals affected by the study. This development has been favoured by the introduction of computerized information systems at the organizational level as the principal tool for planning and managing, and which allow the possibility of using routinely collected data for evaluation purposes. Process evaluation comprises all the processes by which inputs are translated into outcomes (Attkisson and Broskowski, 1978) and it often comprises process monitoring alone. An evaluator, for example, may examine demographic characteristics of the clients served in order to assess accessibility, or the referral of clients from one level of care to another.

In the field of mental health care, information systems exist at different levels, from primary level information systems (hospital records or files) to linked uniform reporting systems. In its most elaborate form, this system constitutes a comprehensive population-based case register. A case register is a patient-centred longitudinal record of contacts with a defined set of psychiatric services, originating from a defined population (ten Horn, 1983), and is patient related instead of event related. Each patient is assigned a unique identifier to prevent him or her from being counted more than once. Registers can be used to trace a patient through different services over time. In

Table 7.1 *Domains of evaluation: examples for criteria, data sources and methodological tools*

Domains of evaluation	Criteria and data sources	Methodological tools
Input measurement	Amount and distribution of resources (staffing, equipment, facilities, financing, staff–patient interaction, use of equipment, etc.)	Management information systems; explicit structural and process standards; service availability, etc.
Performance measurement	Outcome and effectiveness (acceptance of services offered, changes in incidence/ prevalence of problems/disorders, acceptability of services, availability and accessibility)	Assessment of patients' status and functioning, client satisfaction, enumeration of cultural, geographical, organizational obstacles to accessibility
Adequacy measurement (output/need)	Input and process relative to community needs/demand and analysis of management information systems	Developing of methods for needs-resources assessment, review
Efficiency measurement (outcomes/ input)	How inputs are organized to achieve performance/adequacy (comparison of services with respect to performance measures, costs)	Costs per unit, cost–outcome and cost-effectiveness analysis for different target groups
Process measurement (outcomes mediated via inputs)	Processes by which inputs are translated into outcomes (specification of service and client characteristics associated with different outcome; causal relationship between input and outcome; secure external validity; ruling out alternative explanations)	Descriptive, quasi-experimental and experimental methods, replication of studies and cross-validation of results

From Attkisson and Broskowski (1978; abridged version).

addition, a case register is population based, which makes it possible to calculate rates or to include information from other registers covering the same area. A standardized, prospective, cumulative and population-based collection of patient-centred data, with the possibility of making record linkages covering different services and time periods, provides some of the essential prerequisites for the evaluation of community mental health services.

During the last three decades, new policies in psychiatric care in many European countries have been the subject of case register analyses (e.g. Wing and Hailey, 1972; Hailey 1973, 1974; Wing and Fryers, 1976; Häfner and Klug, 1980, 1982; Giel and ten Horn, 1982; Dupont, 1983; Gibbons *et al.*, 1984; Giel, 1986; ten Horn *et al.*, 1986; Munk-Jorgensen, 1986; Fryers and Wooff, 1989; Tansella, 1991). A comparison of results, however, has turned out to be difficult due to differences in the structure and method of the registers. In addition, because an essential characteristic of psychiatric case registers is their service orientation, information is obtained exclusively from affiliated services. Even those registers which claim to cover a wider range of services often neglect out-patient care or even omit it completely.

As a whole, process evaluation is usually restricted to the description of service use over time. As Wing (1986) stated, administrative indices of this kind can be used to monitor trends, but " ... they cannot allocate value to the policies or practices that are responsible for those trends occurring" (p. 38). The direction of causes and effects cannot be specified without further investigation.

Outcome evaluation of psychiatric services

Outcome evaluation is often considered the 'core' of evaluative research. It focuses on the effects of treatments or services. In outcome evaluation, the primary goal is " ... to determine the extent to which an activity is associated with the occurrence of results" (Suchman, 1966, p. 72), which means

that a cause–effect relationship between treatment and outcome is identified. When the study of cause is the primary purpose of outcome evaluation, it is acknowledged that an experimental design provides the strongest inferences. Experimental conditions and designs are used when the evaluator wants to introduce as much control as possible and to reduce variation in extraneous variables.

The basic tools for excluding alternative explanations are control and randomization. As for control, Cook and Campbell (1979a) make a distinction between the ability to control the situation in which an experiment is being conducted, the ability to determine which units receive a particular treatment in a particular time, and the ability to identify and measure a particular threat to valid inference so that it can be used in data analysis to rule out the threat. Control of the experimental situation requires the exclusion of the influences of extraneous variables—concerning the period between outset and completion of the study and therefore taking effect after randomization—by isolation, elimination or stabilization. Treatment control is exercized through randomization.

The function of randomization is twofold (Kluiter and Wiersma, 1996): (i) in order to secure the applicability of statistical techniques of comparison, all subjects recruited must have the same chance of being placed in either the experimental or the control group; and (ii) by random assignment of subjects to experimental and control conditions, we will ensure that at the start of the experiment the different groups are similar with respect to each known or unknown characteristic (e.g. living conditions, treatment history, age, sex) that may exert an influence on the outcome variable additional to that of the independent variable(s) of interest. The groups differ systematically only on those variables controlled for by the design (service use).

In the classical clinical experiment, the experimental conditions typically are given by competing methods of therapy (e.g. different drugs), and the units of investigation are individual patients. In contrast, the evaluation of mental health care systems aims at investigating different forms of treatment or services, for example in-patient versus extra-mural care. In principle, the objectives addressed in the evaluation of psychiatric services are the very same as in the controlled clinical trial. The so-called 'patient care trial', according to Spitzer and colleagues (1975) one of the two variants for the evaluation of mental health care systems, differs from the clinical trial solely by the additional inclusion of non-clinical outcome measures, as for example use of medical and social services, administrative problems, 'burden on the family', length of stay in hospital and absence from work.

The potential of the RCT design is so highly valued that for some evaluators there is no justifiable alternative to RCT methods. Newcombe (1988) recommended that the RCT should be adopted as the norm in all evaluative studies of mental health care. This attitude is also reflected in the reviews by Test and Stein (1978), May and Simpson (1984) and Braun *et al.* (1981) who confine themselves to 'prospective experiments' or 'controlled experimental designs'.

However, when looking into existing studies in more detail, we came to realize that we will rarely find an outcome evaluation of psychiatric care systems that meets the criteria of a controlled clinical trial. The reasons for this are manifold, reflecting issues of both feasibility and desirability (Smith, 1980).

Although the experimental design seems applicable, many confounders cannot be excluded

It often seems unethical to withhold treatment from individuals due to random selection, so that some of the most needy fail to receive the best available services. As a consequence, trials in health care evaluation often rely upon volunteers willing to accept randomization. As Taylor and Thornicroft (1996) point out, most of the so-called randomized controlled trials in mental health care evaluation are marred by obstacles to the random allocation of patients to different treatment conditions, resulting in some artificially composed samples. They summarize the problems

that are common when trying to apply the RCT method in health services research:

- Challenges to achieve random allocation
- Non-application of intention to treat analysis
- Limitations imposed by patient consent and motivation
- Incomplete blindness
- The natue of the experimental condition
- The nature of the control condition
- Compromise to internal and external validity
- Difficulties in measuring outcomes.

One of the greatest threats to internal validity is attrition. Some individuals refuse to participate in their randomly assigned groups because some services are more attractive than others and individuals differentially drop out of the trail. This is especially a problem when (i) drop-outs differ systematically from subjects remaining to provide providing information and when (ii) this relationship differs between the treatment and control groups (Foster and Bickman, 1996).

The majority of therapeutic and rehabilitation inputs are set up to promote medium- to long-term recovery, while the experiment is best suited to short-term interventions. Kish (1959) made the point that many events that occur during the time span between outset and outcome measure, or as a function of time, escape from control. Evaluations within the experimental framework may not be based on realistic assumptions about the nature of a service and the way in which treatment is delivered.

There seems to be an increasing concern among researchers as to whether outcome-focused evaluations, treating services as 'black boxes', are appropriate (Dobson and Cook, 1980). A common assumption underlying many evaluations of services and interventions is that clients uniformly receive the services available. However, the treatment of interest is often non-standardized within a service and tailored to the specific needs of individual subjects. As Schulberg and Bromet (1981) noted, mental health services increasingly are designed to meet the particular needs of given patients on the premise that different problems are best resolved by different services, ". . . i.e. the service should fit the patient rather than the patient fitting the service" (p. 932). As a consequence, the way in which a treatment is delivered in a service may differ from one person to another and treatments are planned for varying duration. In addition, therapy and rehabilitation measures not only attempt to reduce or even eliminate the effects of an illness, they often aim at developing abilities compensating for such effects as well as at the prevention of primary and secondary disabilities.

Under these kinds of intervention, an exact specification of what treatments clients did or did not receive is difficult. Many services to be evaluated have broad aims with multiple treatments and several anticipated outcomes, while experimental designs require the selection of a limited number of variables, thus resulting in 'underspecification' of the programme being evaluated: the narrow range of experimentally assessed impacts will not represent the broad influence of the service adequately (Smith, 1980). Randomized studies, focusing on main effects, often ignore the fact that people react differently to a given treatment.

If services are not described clearly, it is likely that evaluation results will be distorted due to the failure to consider the nature of a service. Scanlon *et al.* (1977; quoted from Dobson and Cook, 1980) characterized this situation in terms of 'type 3 error'. While a type 1 error means rejecting a hypothesis where it should be accepted and a type 2 error means accepting a hypothesis when it should be rejected, evaluators commonly make two types of errors in undertaking evaluations: a type 3 error is to try to measure something that is not meaningfully measurable, while a type 4 error is measuring something that is of no interest to managers or to policy makers.

Experimental studies are expensive

The logic of scientific argumentation in confirmatory data analysis requires that the construction of hypotheses, and the selection of the central methods for testing the hypotheses should precede data collection (Cohen, 1982). The evaluator must have a clear idea of the interactional model

he wants to test. In reality, evaluative research data are used regularly for both the development of models and the estimation of parameters, thus inflating type 1 error. The restriction to purely confirmatory testing makes the experimental design an expensive enterprise.

The results of experimental studies have little validity in routine clinical settings

The role of context or setting frequently is an important factor in evaluating a community mental health service. However, experimental methods try to control such factors rather than attempting to understand their influence. Filstead (1979) wrote: "It is quite common to obtain results which do not fit with what was expected. Engaging in speculation about rival explanations becomes frustrating because of the lack of contextual understanding which often surrounds the assessment. What could have caused such puzzling results? Was the instrument OK? Did the questions asked tap the area under study? Did the subjects perceive these questions in a different manner from what was anticipated? Did events internal or external occur (. . .) which could have affected the evaluation? The list of questions goes on and on. But the thrust of these questions is the same: Is there any qualitative data that can provide the framework for comprehending this evaluation within the larger context within which it occurred? . . . the qualitative methods provide the context of meanings in which the quantitative findings can be understood" (p. 44).

While the last point in essence touches on the paradigmatic controversy concerning the appropriateness of qualitative versus quantitative methods in evaluative research, even from a natural science point of view there is a series of reasons preventing an investigation of the efficacy of psychiatric services meeting the ideal of a controlled clinical trial. In such cases, where the essential features of the experimental design are met only in part, the term 'quasi-experimental design' or 'observational study' is used (Cook and Campbell, 1979a). As a rule, quasi-experiments show less standardization, less control and isolation, and test longer lasting, more complex interventions. However, the key factor is that the groups under observation are not assigned randomly to different treatment conditions. In most cases, the evaluator must be satisfied with the role of a neutral observer. The objectives of such design variants, in principle, are the same as in an experiment: identification of cause–effect structures through the exclusion of rival explanations. However, because of lack of essential control mechanisms, there are more alternative explanations for given data structures.

Quasi-experimental designs may be classified into three basic types (Fife-Schaw, 1995). (i) Non-equivalent control group design: no control group, or a control group without random assignment. Most of the so-called 'experiments' in mental health care evaluation belong to this design type, including model programmes and model services (Pasamanick *et al.*, 1967; Mosher *et al.*, 1975; Stein *et al.*, 1975). (ii) Time-series design: only one experimental group, assessed several times before and after treatment to identify a temporal development, in the dependent variable. (iii) Time-series design combined with the non-equivalent control group design.

The non-equivalent control group design—according to Cook and Campbell (1979a) including design types with single measurements in subjects' after service use ('one-group post test-only design' and 'post-test-only design with non-equivalent control group'), as well as the 'one-group pre-post test design'—belongs to the most frequently used designs in mental health services evaluation. Here again, three groups may be separated. (i) According to the occurrence or frequency of an event relevant to the assessment of treatment outcome (dependent variable Y), the patients under study are grouped *a posteriori* into two or more subgroups. The subgroups are then compared with respect to differences in previous use of services (independent variable X). Nuehring *et al.* (1980), for example, compared patients with and without readmissions to hospital over an observation period of 6 months with respect to continuity of previous out-patient treatment (see also Christensen, 1974; Franklin *et al.*, 1975). (ii) Observation of patients over an extended period of time with respect to use of services. The total group will be subdivided *a posteriori* into subgroups according to service use, which are compared in terms of outcome. McCranie and Mizell (1978) compared readmission rates of three patient groups who differed in their frequency of contacts with an aftercare clinic (see also Anthony and Buell, 1973; Kirk, 1976; Solomon *et al.*, 1984; Middelboe *et al.*, 1996). (iii) Comparison of an 'experimental' group with one or more 'a priori' defined non-equivalent control groups (Claghorn and Kinross-Wright, 1971; Beard *et al.*, 1978; Dincin and Witheridge, 1982). Studies with 'true' random allocation to different services or treatment conditions are rare (Wiersma *et al.*, 1995; Lehman *et al.*, 1997).

An evaluation study normally requires specifically trained personnel, and in practice this is time-consuming and expensive. When calling to mind the inputs that are required for the organization, data collection, preparation and analysis, and the limitations attending the attempt to transfer laboratory conditions to real life, one must ask the question: does the benefit justify the input? What benefit does one expect from an experimental design?

The difficulties in carrying out evaluation studies according to the RCT paradigm are evident. At the same time, the evaluation of the efficacy of new forms of psychiatric care or services often cannot be carried using routinely collected data. The renunciation of the RCT paradigm to secure internal validity as far as possible seems to be justifiable when control is possible only at the expense of reduced external validity. As internal and external validity are reciprocal, one can secure either one or the other. The reduction in the degree of control over bias will be balanced by generalizability to other situations (Gadenne, 1976). This is a central dilemma challenging the evaluation of mental health services.

References

Abramson, J.H. (1979) *Survey Methods in Community Medicine*. New York: Churchill Livingstone.

Abramson, T. (1979) Issues and models in vocational education evaluation. In: Abramson, T., Kehr-Tittle, C. and Cohen, L. (eds), *Handbook of Vocational Educational Evaluation*. Beverly Hills, CA: Sage, pp. 133–160.

Anthony, W.A. and Buell, G.J. (1973) Psychiatric aftercare effectiveness as a function of patient demographic characteristics. *Journal of Consulting and Clinical Psychology*, 41, 116–119.

Attkisson, C.C. and Broskowski, A. (1978) Evaluation and the emerging human service concept. In: Attkisson, C.C., Hargreaves, W.A., Horowitz, M.J. and Sorensen, J.E. (eds), *Evaluation of Human Service Programs*. New York: Academic Press.

Beard, J.H., Malamud, T.J. and Rossman, E. (1978) Psychiatric rehabilitation and long-term rehospitalization rates: the findings of two research studies. *Schizophrenia Bulletin*, 4, 622–635.

Braun, P., Kochansky, G., Shapiro, R.W., Greenberg, S., Gudeman, J.E., Johnson, S. and Shore, M.F. (1981) Overview: deinstitutionalization of psychiatric patients, a critical review of outcome studies. *American Journal of Psychiatry*, 138, 736–749.

Christensen, J.K. (1974) A 5-year follow-up study of male schizophrenics: evaluation of factors influencing success and failure in the community. *Acta Psychiatrica Scandinavica*, 50, 60–72.

Claghorn, J.L. and Kinross-Wright, J. (1971) Reduction in hospitalization of schizophrenics. *American Journal of Psychiatry*, 128, 344–347.

Cohen, P. (1982) To be or not to be. Control and balancing of type I and type II errors. *Evaluation and Program Planning*, 5, 147–254.

Cook, T.D. and Campbell, D.T. (1979a) *Quasi-experimentation. Design and Analysis Issues for Field Settings*. Boston: Houghton Mifflin Co.

Cook, T.D. and Reichardt, C.S. (1979b) *Qualitative and Quantitative Methods in Evaluation Research*. Beverly Hills: Sage.

Dincin, J. and Witheridge, T.F. (1982) Psychiatric rehabilitation as a deterrent to recidivism. *Hospital and Community Psychiatry*, 33, 645–650.

Dobson, L.D. and Cook, T.J. (1980) Avoiding type III error in program evaluation. Results from a field experiment. *Evaluation and Program Planning*, 3, 269–276.

Dunn, W.N., Mitroff, I.I. and Deutsch, S.J. (1981) The obsolescence of evaluation research. *Evaluation and Program Planning*, 4, 207–218.

Fife-Schaw, C. (1995) Quasi-experimental designs. In: Breakwell, G.M., Hammond, S. and Fife-Schaw, C. (eds), *Research Methods in Psychology*. London: Sage, pp. 85–98.

Filstead, W.J. (1979) Qualitative methods: a needed perspective in evaluative research. In: Cook, T.D. and Reichardt, C.S. (eds), *Qualitative and Quantitative Methods in Evaluation Research*. Beverly Hills: Sage, pp. 33–48.

Foster, E.M. and Bickman, L. (1996) An evaluator's guide to detecting attrition problems. *Evaluation Review*, 20, 695–723.

Franklin, J.L., Kittredge, L.D. and Thrasher, J.H. (1975) A survey of factors related to mental hospital readmissions. *Hospital and Community Psychiatry*, 26, 749–751.

Gadenne, V. (1976) *Die Gültigkeit psychologischer Untersuchungen*. Stuttgart: Kohlhammer.

Kirk, S.A. (1976) Effectiveness of community services for discharged mental hospital patients. *American Journal of Orthopsychiatry*, 46, 646–659.

Kish, L. (1959) Some statistical problems in research design. *American Sociological Review*, 24, 328–338.

Kluiter, H. and Wiersma, D. (1996) Randomised controlled trials of programmes. In: Knudsen, H.C. and Thornicroft, G. (eds) *Mental Health Service Evaluation*. Cambridge: Cambridge University Press, pp. 259–280.

Lebow, J. (1982a) Consumer satisfaction with mental health treatment. *Psychological Bulletin*, 91, 244–259.

Lebow, J. (1982b) Models for evaluating services at community mental health centers. *Hospital and Community Psychiatry*, 33, 1010–1014.

Lehman, A.F., Dixon, L.B., Kernan, E., DeForge, B.R. and Postrado, L.T. (1997) A randomized trial of assertive community treatment for homeless persons with severe mental illness. *Archives of General Psychiatry*, 54, 1038–1043.

May, P.R.A. and Simpson, G.M. (1984) Schizophrenic: Beurkilung des Behenllungserfolger. In Freedman, A.M. Kaplan, H.I., Sadock, B.J. and Peters, U.H. (eds.), *Psychiatrie in Praxis und Klinik, Band 1: Schizophrenic, affective Ehrenkungen, Verlust und Trener*. Stuttgert: Thienne, pp. 203–259.

McCranie, E.W. and Mizell, T.A. (1978) Aftercare for psychiatric patients: does it prevent rehospitalization? *Hospital and Community Psychiatry*, 29, 584–587.

Middelboe, T., Nordentoft, M., Knudsen, H.C. and Jessen-Petersen, B. (1996) Small group homes for the long-term mentally ill. Clinical and social characteristics of the residents. *Nordic Journal of Psychiatry*, 50, 297–303.

Milne, D. (1987) Evaluating mental health practice: an introduction. In: Milne, D. (ed.), *Evaluating Mental Health Practice—Methods and Applications*. London: Croom Helm, pp. 1–22.

Mosher, L.R., Menn, A.Z. and Matthews, S.M. (1975) Soteria: evaluation of a home-based treatment for schizophrenia. *American Journal of Orthopsychiatry*, 45, 455–467.

Newcombe, R.G. (1988) Evaluation of treatment effectiveness in psychiatric research. *British Journal of Psychiatry*, 152, 696–697.

Nuehring, E.M., Thayer, J.H. and Ladner, R.A. (1980) On the factors predicting rehospitalization among two state mental hospital patient populations. *Administration in Mental Health*, 7, 247–270.

Pasamanick, B., Scarpitti, F. and Dinitz, S. (1967) *Schizophrenics in the Community: An Experimental Study in the Prevention of Hospitalization*. New York: Appleton Century Crofts.

Patton, M.Q. (1980) Making methods choices. *Evaluation and Program Planning*, 3, 219–228.

Riecken, H.R. and Boruch, R.F. (1974) *Social Experimentation*. New York: Academic Press.

Schulberg, H.C. and Bromet, E.J. (1981) Strategies for evaluating the outcome of community services for the chronically mentally ill. *American Journal of Psychiatry*, 138, 930–935.

Sechrest, L. and Sidani, S. (1995) Quantitative and qualitative methods: is there an alternative? *Evaluation and Program Planning*, 18, 77–87.

Shadish, W.R. (1995) Philosophy of science and the quantitative-qualitative debates: thirteen common errors. *Evaluation and Program Planning*, 18, 63–75.

Smith, N.L. (1980) The feasibility and desirability of experimental methods in evaluation. *Evaluation and Program Planning*, 3, 251–256.

Solomon, P., Davis, J.M. and Gordon, B. (1984) Discharged state hospital patients' characteristics and use of aftercare: effect on community tenure. *American Journal of Psychiatry*, 141, 1566–1570.

Spitzer, W.O., Feinstein, A.R. and Sackett, D.L. (1975) What is a health care trial? *Journal of the American Medical Association*, 233, 161–163.

Stein, L.I., Test, M.A. and Marx, A.J. (1975) Alternative to the hospital: a controlled study. *American Journal of Psychiatry*, 132, 517–522.

Suchman, E.A. (1966) A model for research and evaluation on rehabilitation. In: Sussmann, P. (ed.), *Sociology and Rehabilitation*. Washington, DC: American Sociological Association, pp. 52–70.

Suchman, E.A. (1967) *Evaluative Research. Principles and Practice in Public Health Service and Social Action Programs*. New York: Russell Sage Foundatation.

Taylor, R. and Thornicroft, G. (1996) Uses and limits of randomised controlled trials in mental health service research. In: Thornicroft, G. and Tansella, M. (eds) *Mental Health Outcome Measures*. New York: Springer, pp. 143–151.

ten Horn, G.H.M.M. (1983) *Psychiatric Case Registers. Report on a Working Group. Mannheim, May 1983*. Copenhagen: WHO.

Test, M.A. and Stein, L.I. (1978) Community treatment of the chronic patient: research overview. *Schizophrenia Bulletin*, 4, 350–364.

Wiersma, D., Kluiter, H., Nienhuis, F.J., Ruphan, M. and Giel, R. (1995) Costs and benefits of hospital and day treatment with community care of affective and schizophrenic disorders. *British Journal of Psychiatry*, (Suppl.), 52–59.

Wing, J.K. (1986) The cycle of planning and evaluation. In: Wilkinson, G. and Freeman, H. (eds), *The Provision of Mental Health Services in Britain: The Way Ahead*. Oxford: Gaskell, Royal College of Psychiatrists, pp. 35–48.

Wittmann, W.W. (1985) *Evaluationsforschung*. Heidelberg: Springer

Wottawa, H. (1996) Methoden der Evaluations forschung. In: Erdfelder, E., Mausfeld, R., Meiser, T. and Rudinger, G. (eds), *Handbuch Quantitative Methoden*. Weinheim: Psychologie Verlags Union, pp. 551–566.

8 | *The application of epidemiology to mental disorders*

Glyn H. Lewis, Hollie V. Thomas, Mary Cannon and Peter B. Jones

Introduction

In Chapter 5, we presented the main tools used by epidemiologists to measure the occurrence and aetiology of disease in populations. In this chapter, we summarize the results of epidemiological studies when applied to mental disorders.

Epidemiology of neurosis

Diagnostic boundaries

There is a long-running controversy over the nature and relevance of diagnoses in studies of common mental disorder. Studies have tended to concentrate on either depression or treated psychiatric disorder in the community as a single category. Much of the literature has concentrated on investigating depression, though evidence that depression and anxiety disorders have different risk factors is relatively sparse (Eaton and Ritter, 1988). There is also evidence that depression and generalized anxiety disorder have the same genetic vulnerability (Kendler *et al.*, 1993). The main difference between the mental health of individuals can be explained in terms of a single dimension, but there are also likely to be factors that increase the risk of, for example, depression over and above the risk of common mental disorder.

Descriptive epidemiology

In community surveys, the majority of the population have at least one neurotic symptom at any one time. For example, in the British Health and Lifestyle survey (Cox *et al.*, 1987), 70% of the population reported at least one of the symptoms on the General Health Questionnaire (GHQ; Goldberg, and Williams, 1988). In that sense, the abnormal individuals are those without neurotic symptoms. Fatigue was the most common symptom in the OPCS National Survey of Psychiatric Morbidity conducted in Great Britain, and is present in about 27% of the population (Jenkins *et al.*, 1997). Irritability and worry are also more common than depression and anxiety.

In the OPCS National Survey of Psychiatric Morbidity, about 15% of the population had a neurotic psychiatric disorder in the week before interview. The threshold in this study indicates a degree of symptomatology that would generate concern in a primary care physician. Of those studied in the multi-national WHO study of common mental disorders in primary care, 21% fulfilled one or more ICD-10 diagnosis, mostly neurotic conditions (Ormel *et al.*, 1994). Table 8.1 shows the prevalence of the main neurotic disorders from three population-based studies and the WHO study of primary care. There are quite marked differences in prevalence between the surveys. These result from using different diagnostic criteria, different assessments for psychiatric disorder and geographical and temporal variation.

Gender

Neurotic disorders of whatever type are more common in women in community surveys, although it is usually stated that there are two exceptions, social phobias and obsessive–compulsive disorder.

Table 8.1 *Prevalence (%) of neurotic disorders from three population surveys and a primary care study*

Period prevalence	ECA, USA[a] 1 month	OPCS, UK[b] 1 week	NCS, USA[c] 12 months	WHO, PHC[d] 12 months
Depression	2.4	1.7	10.3	10.5
Phobias—total	6.7	1.8		
Agoraphobia	7.6[e]		2.8	1.5
Social phobia	3.2[e]		7.9	
Specific phobia	15.1[e]		8.8	
Panic disorder	0.5	0.8	2.3	1.1
Obsessive–compulsive disorder	1.3	1.3		
Generalized anxiety disorder	1.3	2.9	3.1	7.9
Mixed anxiety–depression		7.1		
Diagnostic criteria	DSM-III	ICD-10	DSM-III-R	ICD-10

[a]Robins and Regier (1991) ECA five USA sites.
[b]Jenkins *et al.* (1997) OPCS National Survey of Psychiatric Morbidity.
[c]Kessler *et al.* (1994) US National Comorbidity Survey.
[d]Ormel *et al.* (1994) WHO Primary Care study.
[e]Lifetime prevalence.

There are also some studies where the gender difference is less marked than those done in the UK and USA (Jenkins, 1985).

There are a number of possible explanations for neurosis being more common in women than in men. Many of the studies are cross-sectional and so the excess prevalence may result from either a higher incidence in women or a longer duration of illness, though longitudinal studies have usually confirmed a higher incidence. The difference between the sexes may result because women are more likely to divulge details of their emotional life or be more aware of them. One other possibility is some underlying inherited or acquired characteristic, for example related to endocrine differences or differences in upbringing. Alternatively, differences between the sexes may result from differences in environmental factors in

development, for example sexual abuse is more common in female than male children.

One of the most likely explanations for the gender difference concerns the different social roles occupied by men and women. Women are more likely to be in low status jobs and are also more likely to have too many roles. For example, most women continue to provide child care and home keeping while out at work. Studies that investigate relatively homogenous groups of men and women, for example civil servants of the same grade, find that there is no gender difference in psychiatric disorder (Jenkins, 1985).

Socio-economic status

There are some contradictory results concerning whether neurotic disorders are more common in those with lower socio-economic status (SES). It is likely that these can be accounted for by the varying ways of measuring or conceptualizing SES. There are three aspects of SES that are measured commonly: occupational status, such as Registrar General Social Class as used in the UK; educational attainment; and standard of living. In a recent study, it has been argued that a poor standard of living does show a consistent independent relationship with an increased prevalence of common mental disorder (Lewis *et al.*, 1998). It is likely that this is mediated by delaying recovery from episodes of depression. This is also probably true of the association between unemployment and psychiatric disorder (Weich and Lewis 1998).

Geographical variation

Geographical variations in the rates of disease can help provide clues to aetiology and are also useful in planning services. There have been many reports that neurotic psychiatric disorders are more common in urban areas, at least in western societies (Blazer *et al.*, 1985; Lewis and Booth, 1994). The reasons for this are not understood, though Brown and colleagues found that stressful life events were more common in South London than in North Uist in the Outer Hebrides, Scotland (Brown *et al.*, 1977).

Disability

Major depression and other neurotic disorders are associated with profound morbidity and social impairment, equal to or in excess of that seen in many chronic physical illnesses (Wells *et al.*, 1989). There is considerable impact on industry of neurotic disorder as well as direct costs on the health service (Croft-Jefferys and Wilkinson, 1989; Smith *et al.*, 1995). However, for psychiatrists, psychotic disorders are more important and they are more disabling for the individual. For the community as a whole, depression and anxiety disorders are sufficiently common that they lead to a considerable aggregate burden. This falls mostly on primary care. If one takes account of morbidity as well as mortality, then by the year 2020 unipolar depression will account for >5% of

the Disability Adjusted Life Years lost to ill-health (Murray and Lopez, 1997), second only to ischaemic heart disease.

Epidemiology of needs assessment

It is important to remember that the epidemiological assessment of neurotic symptoms is different from an assessment of needs. It is relatively difficult to make assessments of need in this area as more knowledge is needed about the relationship between the epidemiological criteria for defining a case and the criteria for defining who would benefit from particular interventions. One study has attempted to relate the criteria used in admission to antidepressant trials to the assessment used in the OPCS National Survey in the UK. They concluded that up to 6% of the population might have a neurotic disorder that is severe enough to benefit from antidepressant medication. However, such figures have a number of limitations and need to be interpreted with caution.

Aetiology of common mental disorder

In the long term, preventive strategies for neurotic disorder will need to be based upon sound epidemiological findings concerning the environmental causes of the conditions. At the moment, a public health approach towards preventing these conditions is premature, but an important priority for research must be to understand more about the aetiology of these conditions and translate the findings into practical preventive strategies.

The literature on the aetiology of common mental disorder is voluminous, and the suggestions of important aetiological factors correspondingly large. Three main areas have been studied: childhood experience; adult experience; and current stressors and personality. A genetic contribution has also been established, but its nature is as yet unknown.

Childhood experience

Parental loss and separation The seminal studies of Brown and Harris (1978) suggested that loss of a mother before 11 years of age increased the risk of adult depression. Subsequent studies have produced contradictory findings (Parker *et al.*, 1992). Separation or loss of a parent rarely occurs in isolation and any association with neurotic disorder may be confounded by other variables. For example, childhood parental loss is often followed by socio-economic disadvantage and inconsistent or inadequate parenting by alternative care-givers. Parker's work from Australia has also linked style of parenting during childhood to later depression, but also, albeit to a lesser extent, anxiety (Parker *et al.*, 1979).

Other early experiences There recently has been considerable interest in the possibility that child sexual abuse increases the risk of neurotic disorder in adulthood. Community-based studies find that adults with a variety of neurotic diagnoses report increased rates of early traumatic sexual encounters (Angst and Vollrath, 1991; Brown *et al.*, 1993). Disentangling the links between abuse and adult disorder is not easy, since child sexual abuse does not happen randomly, and is associated with other adversity, including poverty, parental discord, inadequate parenting and physical abuse. However, child sexual abuse was associated independently with the prevalence of adult psychiatric disorder in a community survey from New Zealand (Mullen *et al.*, 1993).

Although childhood experiences are important in the aetiology of adult neurosis, there is no simple relationship between childhood and adult neurotic disorder. Most emotionally disordered children do not become neurotic adults, and most neurotic disorders develop in adult life (Rutter, 1985). However, there is a striking continuity between depression as a child and depression as an adult (Harrington *et al.*, 1990).

Adolescent experiences In general, the literature on the social aetiology of neurosis concentrates on childhood predictors of adult disorder, and adult experiences. Mental health in childhood is also addressed frequently, but the change from childhood to adulthood has received less attention. Specific issues such as unemployment (Banks and Jackson, 1982) and acute life events have been addressed (Goodyer *et al.*, 1987). A recent

community-based study showed that 17% of girls living at home showed evidence of psychiatric disorder; independent risk factors were maternal distress and the quality of the parental marriage (Monck *et al.*, 1994).

Adult experiences and current stressors

Life events The relationship between life events and neurotic disorder has been reviewed extensively elsewhere. This body of work has provided some of the most convincing evidence for establishing psychosocial environmental stresses as an important cause of depression. In particular, George Brown's work has been influential in arguing that the social context of life events and the meaning attached to them by the individual is also an important determinant of the likelihood of developing depression.

One of the limitations of the life event approach is that it seems to have a limited relevance to public health. Life events, such as bereavement, are an inevitable part of the human condition. Though other life events such as redundancy could, in principle, be influenced by economic policy, it is more likely that the context of the life event is more amenable to policy changes than the occurrence of life events themselves. Future research should include the role of the context of life events, for example poor housing, financial problems or inadequate child care, in the hope of drawing conclusions that potentially could influence government policy or give more insight into the social and psychological mechanisms leading to depression.

Social support and social networks One consistent finding is an association between poor social support and neurotic disorder. Brown and Harris (1978) found that women who lacked an intimate or confiding relationship had an increased risk of depression (in the presence of a life event). Scott Henderson and colleagues (Henderson *et al.*, 1981) in Australia went on to find a more general association between neurotic disorder and lack of satisfaction with the social network. In the Epidemiological Catchment Area (ECA) programme, all anxiety disorders were more common among the separated or divorced, whilst in New Zealand females who were widowed, separated or divorced were more likely to have neurotic disorder than those currently married (Romans *et al.*, 1993).

There are two areas of controversy in this area. The first is the rather technical point of whether social support interacts with life events in increasing the risk of depression. In other words, is there a stronger association between life events and depression in the presence of poor social support? This issue depends upon the nature of the statistical model that is being used by the researchers (Alloway and Bebbington, 1987). Of more importance, however, is the question of whether the association with poor social support is causal or results from either a personality attribute or measurement bias resulting from depression. Henderson has argued for the latter, while Brown maintains the former position.

Unemployment Unemployment is associated with higher rates of neurosis (Jenkins *et al.*, 1997). Warr (1987) has conducted some elegant studies showing that men made unemployed are at increased risk of developing neurotic disorder and their mental health improves when they return to work. The situation for women is more complicated because of the expectation of work within the home.

Physical illness Physical and psychiatric illnesses are associated by more than chance alone. In general, there is a threefold increase in psychological disorder in people with medical illness. The relationship between physical and psychological illness is complex. Psychological disorder may result from illness or chronic disability. Sometimes, physical and psychological illness may have a common aetiology, for example diseases of the central nervous system are more likely to have a co-existent psychiatric disorder. There may also be a Berksonian, or referral bias that leads to the association seen in health care settings. However, the most common reason for the association between physical and psychological illness is somatization, illness behaviour and its effect on symptoms reporting.

Personality

It is widely assumed that personality characteristics are an important risk factor for developing neurotic disorder. Eysenck's neuroticism scale is claimed to be such a dimension, those scoring high on neuroticism having an increased risk of developing neurotic illness (Eysenck and Eysenck, 1964). However, there is a considerable overlap between the questions asked by neuroticism scales and the actual symptoms of neurotic disorder. A number of studies (Coppen and Metcalfe, 1965; Kendell *et al.*, 1968; Hirschfeld, 1983) have found that neuroticism scale scores are closely correlated with measures of neurotic disorder and change with recovery from depression. Duncan-Jones *et al.* (1990) have also argued, with evidence from statistical models, that the neuroticism scale is effectively measuring the same thing as the average level of neurotic psychiatric disorder measured by the GHQ. Nevertheless, the idea of a general liability to develop neurotic symptoms, with a genetic contribution, is probably an important part of the aetiology of neurotic disorder.

An alternative and perhaps complementary approach is based upon theories of personality developed by social learning theorists. For example, Warr's (1987) studies on unemployment have found that 'commitment to work' is related to poor mental health during unemployment and good mental health in employment. Work commitment was assessed by a short and simple scale incorporating attitudinal questions such as "If you had won a million pounds, would you still want to work?" This series of studies provide a model for studying personal attributes and their relationship with mental illness, and show an interaction between personality and the impact of a life event. They also illustrate the link between an individual's attitudes and societal norms, in this instance the social and economic importance of the 'work ethic'.

Epidemiology of psychosis

Diagnostic preamble

As for neurosis, the question as to what is a case is fundamental to counting, treating or establishing cause. The debate surrounding the definition of diagnostic categories within psychosis has been fierce (Clare, 1980). Over the century since our modern concepts of schizophrenia and bipolar affective disorder were first described, opinion has varied considerably as to how best to define them and, indeed, whether they existed at all. This is esoteric stuff for the clinician and service planner faced with the imperative of people with delusions, hallucinations, thought disorder, negative features, severe depression or mania.

The disturbance and disability involving individuals, carers and community seem a long way from academic arguments about operational criteria. Current research is focusing once more on diagnostic boundaries, but is more inclusive within the psychoses. Ultimately, a classification based upon causes or mechanisms may be a goal. For the moment, many services are making routine diagnoses and management returns using standard operational criteria such as those defined in the 10th revision of the International Classification of Disease (World Health Organization, 1994). This is favoured by European psychiatrists and is similar to its American stepsister DSM-IV (American Psychiatric Association, 1994). Both these systems have undergone a 'narrowing' in their definitions of schizophrenia and other psychotic syndromes from previous, to present versions. Together with a more general recent history of the schizophrenia concept, these are considered by Cannon and Jones (1996).

From the point of view of a community psychiatric service, the majority of people with psychosis will have syndromes adequately described by schizophrenia or non-affective psychosis. These will outnumber those with affective psychoses, i.e. bipolar disorder and psychotic depression, by about fivefold, although the needs of this group may be high (see below). There will be smaller group with other psychotic syndromes, including those related to drugs.

In some quarters, the pendulum has swung towards talk of 'severe mental illness' (SMI), a catch-all term, too loose for epidemiology. The term is of some use to service planning where many requirements are common across diagnoses, and where there is heterogeneity of needs within any one diagnosis. *Post-hoc* attempts to define this term have invoked composite notions of diagnosis, severity, disability and duration. As mentioned above, the majority of this 'SMI' comprises schizophrenia.

The advantage of the term is that it puts the concept of needs to the fore. The danger is that aspects of care specific to individual diagnoses may be forgotten. This is particularly the case for those people with neurotic syndromes that may be severe, disabling and long-lasting. A person with severe obsessive–compulsive disorder may benefit from common aspects of a service designed for the majority of people with SMI who have schizophrenia. However, they also need distinct therapy that will be left untried if diagnostic accuracy and precision are neglected. Similarly, 'blue skies' research concerning causes and mechanisms, referred to earlier in chapter 5, may be impossible if there are no boundaries, although some research is relevant to a wider group. In this chapter, we have been using recent operational concepts when we refer to schizophrenia.

Descriptive epidemiology

The low incidence (10–40 cases per 100 000 per year) and relatively low lifetime prevalence (0.5–1%) of schizophrenia in the population have led to a reliance on case–control study designs in research. Chronic patients recruited from hospital wards are compared with volunteer controls from the community, and consequent problems of bias and confounding have led to many contradictory findings that are not replicated. Cannon and Jones (1996) have pointed out that, for a time, schizophrenia looked as if it would prove to be the undoing of epidemiologists, just as it had once been the 'graveyard of neuropathologists' (Plum, 1972). Over the past two decades, however, the application of advances in cohort and case–control methodology to psychiatric epidemiology has led increasingly to more robust results (Lewis and Pelosi, 1990).

Incidence and time trends

Examination of incidence rates may be potentially more informative than prevalence of schizophrenia. The latter can be influenced by many factors such as changes in treatment and changes in mortality rate; both are affected by changes in the age and sex structure of the population (see below). Ideally, incidence studies should be based on community incidence samples but, as this is difficult to achieve, case registers and hospital admission data commonly are used.

Eagles and Whalley (1985) first reported a decline in the diagnosis of schizophrenia among first admissions in Scotland between 1969 and 1978. There have since been 14 further papers examining this issue in England (Der *et al.*, 1990; De Alarcon *et al.*, 1990; Castle *et al.*, 1991; Bamrah *et al.*, 1991; Harrison *et al.*, 1991), Scotland (Eagles *et al.*, 1988; Geddes *et al.*, 1993; Kendell *et al.*, 1993), Denmark (Munk-Jorgensen, 1986; Munk-Jorgensen and Mortensen, 1992), New Zealand (Joyce, 1987), Canada (Nicole *et al.*, 1992), Ireland (Waddington and Youssef, 1994) the USA (Stoll *et al.*, 1993) and The Netherlands (Oldehinkel and Giel, 1995). Those based on national statistics have found a large (40–50%) decline in first-admission rates for schizophrenia during the 1970s and the 1980s (Joyce, 1987; Bamrah *et al.*, 1991; Castle *et al.*, 1991; Munk-Jorgensen and Mortensen, 1992). Findings based on case register data have been less consistent and, indeed, two such studies from Camberwell (Castle *et al.*, 1991) and Salford (Bamrah *et al.*, 1991) in the UK actually found a slight increase in the incidence of schizophrenia during the same period. Others have reported a decrease in first-admission rates for schizophrenia among females only (Kendell *et al.*, 1993; Waddington and Youssef, 1994; Oldehinkel and Giel, 1995).

The major question is whether the decrease noted in first-admission rates corresponds to an actual decrease in the incidence of the condition. Many factors influence this apparent 'administrative decline' in schizophrenia. The introduction of more restrictive diagnostic criteria for schizophrenia may cause a shift to diagnoses such as 'borderline states' (Munk-Jorgensen, 1986) or affective psychosis (Stoll *et al.*, 1993; Oldehinkel and Giel, 1995). The move to community care over the past two decades could have affected hospital admission rates (Nicole *et al.*, 1992). Clinicians' attitudes have changed and they are now more reluctant to make a diagnosis of schizophrenia on the first hospital admission (Munk-Jorgensen, 1986), and this could lead to a spurious fall in incidence rates over the last few years of the period under observation. Private health insurance companies' policies regarding schizophrenia may be partly responsible for this effect (Stoll *et al.*, 1993). Changes in the age, sex and ethnic structure of the population over the period under study have not been taken into account in most studies. The two areas of the UK that have shown an increased incidence of schizophrenia, Camberwell and Salford, are both areas with a high proportion of immigrants (Bamrah *et al.*, 1991; Castle *et al.*, 1991). Unfortunately, schizophrenia has such a low incidence that it may be impossible to disentangle all these effects and reach any firm conclusions regarding changes in incidence in the developed world in recent decades (Jablensky, 1995).

Geographical variation

In 1978, a large multi-centre study of schizophrenia was initiated by WHO, the Ten-Country Study, to provide information about the incidence, course and outcome of schizophrenia in different cultures (Jablensky *et al.*, 1992). Two case definitions of schizophrenia were used: a broad, clinical definition comprising ICD-9 schizophrenia and paranoid psychoses; and a narrow, restrictive definition including only cases classified as 'nuclear' schizophrenia using the CATEGO computer program (Wing *et al.*, 1974). For narrowly defined schizophrenia, rates ranged only between seven and 14/100 000 per year. The parsimonious conclusion is that rates for narrowly defined schizophrenia are the same in all centres. However, confidence intervals for these estimates were wide and there may not have been sufficient statistical power to detect differences.

The incidence rates for broadly defined schizophrenia do seem to vary between countries (range between 16 and 42/100,000), and the rates for centres in the developing world were about twice as high as those in the developed world. However, the variation in incidence rates for schizophrenia worldwide is very small compared with illnesses such as ischaemic heart disease or cancer which are known to have major environmental risk factors.

Prevalence

The lifetime prevalence of schizophrenia in the western world seems to lie somewhere between 0.4 and 1.4%, and may have decreased over the past decade. Two major prevalence studies of psychiatric illness carried out in the USA indicate a decrease in prevalence of schizophrenia over one decade. The ECA (Keith *et al.*, 1991) surveyed 17803 persons between 1980 and 1984 and found a lifetime prevalence of schizophrenia of 1.4%. The National Comorbidity Survey (NCS; Kessler *et al.*, 1994) interviewed 8098 people between 1990 and 1992 and found that lifetime prevalence for the summary category of non-affective psychosis was 0.7%. This discrepancy may be related to issues of sampling, interview methodology or actual change over time, and remains to be clarified by future reports.

The OPCS Psychiatric Morbidity Survey (Meltzer *et al.*, 1995; Mason and Wilkinson, 1996; Jenkins *et al.*, 1997) indicated that four per 1000 people of working age living in private households had experienced psychosis in the previous 6 months. This prevalence is lower than that found in the NCS, but 37% of those who screened positive for psychosis refused a second diagnostic interview, so the true prevalence may have been higher. Also, some people with psychosis will have been in residential care and therefore outside the scope of this part of the survey.

A number of other studies have been undertaken in the UK and Ireland to define the prevalence of a more tightly defined schizophrenia syndrome. These have been summarized by Jeffreys *et al.* (1997) and are shown in Table 8.2, adapted and updated. The results show a fairly tight range, with studies yielding prevalence estimates of between 4.8 and 11.3 cases per 1000 after correction for the age of the population. Such age correction is useful given the fact that schizophrenia is a disorder of adult life, rather than of the extremes of age.

The more recent studies indicate that the prevalence may be higher in urban than in rural populations. This has already been alluded to in terms of incidence, but a similar finding is of key importance for service planning, and for understanding the factors associated with causation and determinants of outcome.

Age and sex distribution

Total lifetime risk for schizophrenia appears to be just about equal in both sexes (Keith *et al.*, 1991; Jablensky *et al.*, 1992) but the details of the relationship with the life-course differ for men and women. Schizophrenia can occur at any age (Castle and Murray, 1993; Asarnow and Asarnow, 1994; van Os *et al.*, 1995) but onset commonly is in early adulthood. The mean age of onset for males is 3–4 years earlier than for females, irrespective of whether 'onset' of schizophrenia is defined as first sign of mental disorder, first psychotic symptom or first hospital admission (Häfner *et al.*, 1993). The peak age of onset for males is between 15 and 30 years, while females have a slower and more even rate of onset, with a peak between the ages of 20 and 35 years and a second smaller peak after the age of 45. No satisfactory explanation yet exists for this sex difference.

Social class

An association between schizophrenia and low social class was confirmed by the ECA prevalence study which showed that schizophrenic patients in the USA were 10 times more likely to be in the lowest socio-economic group than the highest. Evidence from birth cohorts in Britain (Done *et al.*, 1994; Jones *et al.*, 1994) and Finland (Aro *et al.*, 1995) show that this relationship is not causal, as schizophrenic patients at birth have the same socio-economic distribution as the general population. What is remarkable is the steep decline in social status that accompanies the illness and is evident even before the clinical onset (Jones *et al.*, 1993). This decline is far greater than that experienced by patients with severe affective disorder. Recent evidence (Croudace *et al.*, 2000)

Table 8.2 *Prevalence studies of schizophrenia in the UK and Ireland*

Study (type of study)	Place	Schizophrenia prevalence per 1000		
		Total population	Age correction (15 plus)	Age correction (Weinberg)
Wing (1976)[a] (CR, U: point)	Camberwell	2.0		
Wing (1976)[a] (CR, U: point)	Salford	2.8		
Freeman and Alpert (1986) (CR, U: 1 year)	Salford		6.8	
McCreadie (1982) (K, R: point)	Nithsdale	2.4 (1.7)		
Walsh (1986)[a] (CR, U: point)	Dublin, Ireland	1.7	2.5	
Walsh (1986)[a] (CR, R: point)	Three Counties, Ireland	4.9	7.1	
Youssef *et al.* (1991) (K, R: 1 year)	Co. Cavan, Ireland	[3.3]	[4.6]	[6.4]
Pantelis (1997)[b] (K, U: point)	S. Camden[c]	7.3 (4.7) [4.9]	8.3 (5.3) [5.6]	11.3 (7.2) [7.6]
Harvey (1996) (K, U: point)	N. Camden[c]	4.7	5.3	7.3
Jeffreys *et al.* (1997) (K, U: point)	Hampstead	5.1 (2.9) [3.0]	5.9 (3.4) [3.5]	8.0 (4.7) [4.8]
Thornicroft *et al.* (1998) (K, U: 1 year; all psychosis)	South London	7.7 All psychosis		

CR, case register; K, key informant; U, urban; R, rural.
[a]Data available in Torrey (1987).
[b]Data available in Harvey (1996).
[c]Camden data based on population estimates near census.
Figures in ( ) refer to patients with Feighner diagnosis of schizophrenia.
Figures in [ ] refers to patients with DSM-III-R diagnosis of schizophrenia.

suggests a non-linear gradient between summary scores of deprivation and occurrence of psychosis in the UK. This study demonstrated a dispropor-tionate amount of incidence and administrative prevalence (admissions) in the most deprived areas.

Marital status

People with schizophrenia are unlikely to be married and they have low fertility. Married patients have a better clinical and social outcome than single patients (Jablensky *et al.*, 1992). Marriage may, of course, merely reflect better pre-morbid social adjustment and later age at onset, both independent predictors of good outcome. However, the prevalence of schizophrenia among separated or divorced people in the USA (2.9%) is similar to that among single people (2.1%), suggesting that marriage may confer an independent protective effect (Keith *et al.*, 1991). An interaction between marital status and gender was found in the 1-year follow-up of the ECA study (Tien and Eaton, 1992). Single women were 14 times more likely to develop schizophrenia than married women, but single men were almost 50 times more likely to develop schizophrenia than their married counterparts. The role of marital status as a risk indicator or modifier for schizophrenia requires further study. However, it is clear that the basic characteristics of a population will predict some of the requirements of a community psychiatric service, in terms of its provision for those with psychosis.

Ethnicity and migrant status

Gender, age and social characteristics of a community all, therefore, have a bearing on service requirements. However, migration and ethnic group are the two least understood and emotive factors that have a massive effect on the services that must be provided and that may hold keys to understanding the genesis of psychosis.

To date, no single *indigenous* ethnic group appears to have a significantly higher occurrence of schizophrenia than any other, although some 'pockets' of high prevalence may exist in isolated areas such as North Sweden (Böök *et al.*, 1978). The west of Ireland (Torrey, 1980, 1987) and the Istrian peninsula in Croatia (Crocetti *et al.*, 1971) previously had been identified as 'high-risk' cultures, but the higher incidence and prevalence rates originally found among these peoples are now thought to be due to bias (Eaton, 1991). The

ECA study (Keith *et al.*, 1992) found a higher prevalence for schizophrenia among black people than among white people in the USA (2.1% versus 1.4%). However, controlled for age, gender, marital status and, most importantly, socio-economic group, the difference disappeared.

Schizophrenia in immigrants

The report of a 10-fold increase in the incidence of schizophrenia among the African-Caribbean population in Nottingham (Harrison *et al.*, 1988) is yet to be explained. It has been replicated convincingly in other centres in the UK (Wessley *et al.*, 1991; Thomas *et al.*, 1993; King *et al.*, 1994; van Os *et al.*, 1994), again in Nottingham (Harrison *et al.*, 1997), and in The Netherlands (Selten and Sijben, 1994). In these replications, the incidence ratio has been rather lower (3–4) when the denominator has been adjusted for possible under-reporting in census data (King *et al.*, 1994; van Os *et al.*, 1996). An increased incidence ratio for schizophrenia has also been found among African and Asian (King *et al.*, 1994) immigrants in the UK, indicating that the effect is not confined solely to a single ethnic minority; not all studies concur on this.

The hospital admission rate for schizophrenia among migrants is higher in their host country than in their country of origin (Burke, 1974; Hickling, 1991; Odegaard, 1932), implicating factors occurring principally after migration. The risk of schizophrenia is greater for second-generation migrants than first-generation migrants (McGovern and Cope, 1987), arguing against selective migration of pre-schizophrenic individuals. Both first- and second-generation migrants are exposed to psychosocial stresses, but these may have differential effects on generations exposed to different socio-economic climates or other epigenetic events (Sugarman and Craufurd, 1994). The fact that immigrants from poor countries tend to show higher rates of schizophrenia than immigrants from affluent countries implicates factors associated with improved living conditions, industrialization or urbanization. There is as yet little evidence to support more 'biological' explanations (Eagles, 1991; Warner, 1995).

The evidence for a unique epidemic of schizophrenia among certain immigrant groups is not conclusive, but is intriguing. Possible confounders such as low socio-economic and marital status may reduce the incidence ratio even further. Ethnicity probably represents a 'proxy' variable for a variety of social and perhaps biological factors. Once these are controlled, there may be little or no residual effect of ethnicity, but we would gain information about other, perhaps preventable, risk factors. The most parsimonious conclusion would be that schizophrenia in immigrants is caused by the same factors that cause schizophrenia in other groups but that these factors are more common (and therefore more conspicuous) following migration. There are two alternatives: there may be specific causes in immigrants that do not occur in other populations, or there may be effect modification with ubiquitous factors causing schizophrenia in only some groups. These possibilities currently are the subject of investigation in the Medical Research Council ÆSOP study.

Course and outcome

The definition of schizophrenia or other psychoses is of importance here, as some have an element of chronicity built in to them. Outcome studies are usually based on hospital treatment samples and so may not be representative (Ram *et al.*, 1992); indeed, the true natural course of schizophrenia nowadays is always masked by treatment. The results of outcome studies are difficult to summarize because the definitions of outcome and methods of assessment used are so varied. However, all show marked heterogeneity in course and outcome (Ram *et al.*, 1992). At the extremes of outcome, about a fifth of patients seem to recover after a single episode of psychosis (Leff *et al.*, 1992; Tohen *et al.*, 1992; Geddes *et al.*, 1994), while about the same proportion, perhaps a little less, develop a chronic unremitting psychosis and never fully recover (Shepherd *et al.*, 1989; Jablensky *et al.*, 1992; Leff *et al.*, 1992). Clinical outcome at 5 years can be summarized by the rule of thirds, with approximately 35% of patients in the poor outcome category (Shepherd *et al.*, 1989; Leff *et al.*, 1992); 36% in the good outcome category (Bleuler, 1978; Hegarty *et al.*, 1994) and the remainder with intermediate outcome. Prognosis does not appear to worsen after 5 years (Bleuler, 1978; Jablensky, 1995; Mason *et al.*, 1996).

Predictors of course and outcome

Mutable factors represent important targets for psychiatric services. High levels of 'expressed emotion' among close relatives, i.e. criticism, hostility and overinvolvement (Brown *et al.*, 1972; Leff *et al.*, 1983), predict early relapse. Substance abuse (Jablensky *et al.*, 1992; Linzen *et al.*, 1994) also predicts poor prognosis.

Delay in receiving treatment results in poorer outcome (Johnstone *et al.*, 1986; Wyatt, 1991; Loebel *et al.*, 1992). This intriguing finding might be due to reverse causality, with poorer prognosis itself resulting in delayed treatment. However, it is possible that a more biological process is involved where untreated positive symptoms alter the 'hard-wiring' in the brain. Alternatively, or in addition, secondary disabilities and the ongoing psychological impact of psychosis are both likely to affect outcome.

Immutable factors: patients from developing countries have a better outcome than patients from developed countries (Jablensky *et al.*, 1992). It is not yet known which aspects of non-western 'culture' are responsible for this effect. Possible social factors include lower levels of 'expressed emotion' (Leff *et al.*, 1990), stronger social support networks or lack of 'stigma'. Ethnicity does not appear to be associated strongly with outcome (Harrison *et al.*, 1999). Other favourable prognostic factors are good pre-morbid social adjustment, female gender, being married and later age at onset (Jablensky *et al.*, 1992), but these factors are unlikely to act independently (Eaton, 1991). Acute onset of illness and the experience of negative life events prior to illness are also related to better outcome (Leff *et al.*, 1992; van Os *et al.*, 1994).

Aetiology

Genetic and epigenetic events are involved in causation, and it appears that events over the life-course may interact to form complete causal

Table 8.3 *'Best-estimate' effect sizes of various genetic and environmental risk factors for schizophrenia (expressed as odds ratios or relative risks)*

Category of risk factor	Specific risk factors	'Best-estimate' of effect size[a]
Genetic[b]	Monozygotic twin of schizophrenic patient	46
	Child of two schizophrenic parents	40
	Dizygotic twin of schizophrenic patient	14
	Child or sibling of schzophrenic patient	10
	Parent of schizophrenic patient	5
Developmental[c]	Delayed milestones	3
	Speech problems	3
	Cerebral ventricular enlargement	2
Post-natal environment[c]	Immigrant/ethnic minority status	3
	Chronic cannabis consumption	2
	Solitariness as child	2
Pre- and perinatal environment[c]	Birth complications	2
	Severe undernutrition (1st trimester)	2
	Maternal influenza (2nd trimester)	2
	Born in city	1.4
	Born in winter/early spring	1.2

[a] Rounded to nearest whole number >1.
[b] Relative risk.
[c] Odds ratio.
Adapted from Cannon and Jones (1996).

constellations. The aetiology of the psychoses is complex and not yet understood. Table 8.3, adapted from Cannon and Jones (1996), summarizes some of the factors that have been implicated. The examination of relative risks can give clues to causation.

Table 8.3 shows that only genetic risk factors come anywhere near the effect size expected for a strong causal agent. However, we cannot ignore the existence of so many pre- and post-natal risk factors with small effect sizes. These environmental risk factors of small effect could be 'proxy' measures for an unrecognized major environmental causal agent, or may act additively with each other, or with chance events. They could also indicate the existence of gene–environment interactions.

One key point is the emergence of the whole life-course as a period during which genetic or epigenetic events may increase the risk for psychosis (Jones, 1999), the effects not being specific for schizophrenia (Jones and Tarrant, 1999). Moreover, the effects of early events may be apparent, albeit in subtle ways, many years before psychosis emerges. This developmental reformulation has had a considerable effect on biological views of the causes and mechanisms of schizophrenia, although most would now concede that psychosocial stress and other precipitants ought to be included in any complete causal model. Biological or organic factors (including genetics) may account for the majority of liability for predisposition (vulnerability or diathesis), with psychosocial factors being important for precipitation or triggering in what is essentially a 'stress-diathesis' model (Zubin and Spring, 1977). This dichotomy in timing of effects whereby biological effects (including genetics) act early and psychosocial effects are triggers is unlikely to be valid. Certainly, only complex models drawing from genetic and epigenetic factors, and across the life-course are likely to explain the main epidemiological variations for psychosis such as sex differences in incidence, and migrant group effects.

Are prediction and primary prevention feasible?

Another important issue for community psychiatry that arises from new, developmental views of the aetiology of psychosis is the prospect of prediction and primary prevention (Jones, 1999). Theoretical attempts are being made (Davidson *et al.*, 1999). However, useful prediction is not yet feasible because the predictive power of any models in current cohort studies is so low, and there is no science of pre-psychotic interventions. The problem with low power of models is due to the combination of modest relative risks, involving fairly common characteristics and, thankfully, a relatively rare outcome. With lifetime odds in the general population of 99% for not getting schizophrenia, it is a much safer proposition to identify who will not get the disorder, than it is those who will. Improving prediction by adding more variables to a model may not be helpful in a real-life setting; data on cognition and family history are candidates but would have to be available on a routine basis.

Current evidence does allow some comments to be made. Prediction in high-risk samples, where the likelihood of disorder is an order of magnitude higher than in the general population, is much more feasible. Those known to be at genetic high risk, or in clinics taking referrals for possible psychosis are examples (Jackson and McGorry, 1999; see http://yarra.vicnet.net.au/~eppic). If there were a feasible intervention, the number needed to treat in order to prevent one case of schizophrenia may be in the realm of acceptability once side effects (including stigma and fear) are

taken into account (Jones and Croudace, 1999). Such an equation, however, is radically different for different interventions; drugs psychotherapy, for instance.

Dose–response relationships between possible causes and risk of schizophrenia give rise to some exciting possibilities. Those being described for psychosis are similar in nature to those between smoking and lung cancer, blood pressure and cerebrovascular disease. The majority of cases arise from the majority of the population at medium risk. High-risk individuals are rare and account for only a small proportion of the disorder. Rose (1989) pointed out that, in these situations, the most efficient interventions are not those aimed at the few cases arising from the high-risk population. Rather, they are aimed at the majority at medium risk from which most cases would arise. Thus, the exciting public health implications of the new epidemiology of psychosis (Jones and Cannon, 1998) are very similar to those for common mental disorder, though the true impact of the latter is likely to be greater.

However, there is a problem for all outcomes. Most people in this majority will not become ill, certainly they will not get schizophrenia. Most people have to suffer an intervention unnecessarily. Rose called this the prevention paradox. However, there is another paradox; this is where the lack of specificity between developmental deviance and later schizophrenia may even turn out to be an advantage. Other outcomes after developmental problems encompass a church broader than just affective disorder. They include conduct disorder and sociopathic personality disorder, criminality, poor educational achievement and a penumbra of other outcomes. If widespread interventions aimed at children and adolescents were relatively inefficient at preventing schizophrenia but also impinged upon the incidence of more common, deleterious outcomes, then the population may benefit. If such interventions were generally beneficial with no 'side effects' (better education, for instance), then the prevention paradox is low. The data suggest that this kind of situation would be a stark contrast to a hypothetical programme using current antipsychotic drugs in children at high risk for schizophrenia but not yet psychotic. Thus, in terms of prediction and prevention of schizophrenia, the scope for community psychiatry may lie way beyond secondary and tertiary prevention, or the 'fire-fighting' that drives it today.

Conclusions

The epidemiological approach is an essential element when applied to planning services, evaluating interventions, investigating aetiology and devising and evaluating preventive strategies.

Acknowledgement

P.B.J. gratefully acknowledges support from the Stanley Foundation.

References

Alloway, R. and Bebbington, P. (1987) The buffer theory of social support—a review of the literature. *Psychological Medicine*, 17, 91–108.

American Psychiatric Association (1994) *Diagnostic and Statistical Manual*, 4th edn. Washington, DC: American Psychiatric Association.

Angst, J. and Vollrath, M. (1991) The natural history of anxiety disorders. *Acta Psychiatrica Scandinavica*, 84, 446–452.

Aro, S., Aro, H. and Kesmäki, I. (1995) Socio-economic mobility among patients with schizophrenia or major affective disorder: a 17-year retrospective follow-up. *British Journal of Psychiatry*, 166, 759–767.

Asarnow, R.F. and Asarnow, J.R. (1994) Childhood onset schizophrenia. *Schizophrenia Bulletin*, 20, 591–597.

Bamrah, J.S., Freeman, H.L. and Goldberg, D.P. (1991) Epidemiology of schizophrenia in Salford 1974–1984. Changes in an urban community over ten years. *British Journal of Psychiatry*, 159, 802–810.

Banks, M.H. and Jackson, P.R. (1982) Unemployment and risk of minor psychiatric disorder in young people: cross-sectional and longitudinal evidence. *Psychological Medicine*, 12, 789–798.

Blazer, D., George, L.K., Landerman, R. *et al.* (1985) Psychiatric disorders: a rural/urban comparison. *Archives of General Psychiatry*, 42, 651–656.

Bleuler, M. (1978) *The Schizophrenic Disorders: Long-term Patient and Family Studies*. New Haven, CT: Yale University Press.

Böök, J.A., Wetterberg, L. and Modrzewska, K (1978) Schizophrenia in a North Swedish geographical isolate 1900–1977: epidemiology, genetics and biochemistry. *Clinical Genetics*, 14, 373–394.

Brown, G.W. and Harris, T. (1978) *Social Origins of Depression*. London: Tavistock.

Brown, G.W., Birley, J.L.T. and Wing, J.K. (1972) Influence of family life on the course of schizophrenic disorders. *British Journal of Psychiatry*, 121, 241–258.

Brown, G.W., Davidson, S., Harris, T. *et al.* (1977) Psychiatric disorder in London and North Uist. *Social Science and Medicine*, 11, 367–377.

Brown, G., Harris, T. and Eames, M. (1993) Aetiology of anxiety and depressive disorders in an inner-city population. II. Comorbidity and adversity. *Psychological Medicine*, 23, 155–165.

Burke, A.W. (1974). First admission rates and planning in Jamaica. *Social Psychiatry*, 15, 17–19.

Cannon, M. and Jones, P.B. (1996) Neuro-epidemiology reviews: schizophrenia. *Journal of Neurology, Neurosurgery and Psychiatry*, 61, 604–613.

Castle, D., Wessley, S., Der, G. and Murray, R.M. (1991) The incidence of operationally-defined schizophrenia in Camberwell 1965–84. *British Journal of Psychiatry*, 159, 790–794.

Clare, A. (1980) *Psychiatry in Dissent. Controversial Issues in Thought and Practice*, 2nd edn. London: Tavistock, pp. 120–168.

Coppen, A. and Metcalfe, M. (1965) Effect of a depressive illness on MPI scores. *British Journal of Psychiatry*, 111, 236–239.

Cox, B.D., Blaxter, M., Buckle, A.L.J. *et al.* (1987) *The Health and Lifestyle Survey*. Cambridge: Health Promotion Research Trust.

Crocetti, G.J., Lemkau, P.V., Kulcar, Z. and Kesic, B. (1971) Selected aspects of the epidemiology of psychoses in Croatia, Yugoslavia. II. The cluster sample and the results of the pilot survey. *American Journal of Epidemiology*, 94, 126–134.

Croft-Jefferys, C. and Wilkinson, G. (1989) Estimated costs of neurotic disorder in UK general practice. *Psychological Medicine*, 19, 549–558.

Croudace, T.J., Kayne, R., Jones, P.B. and Harrison, G.L. (2000) Non-linear relationship between an index of social deprivation, psychiatric admission prevalence and the incidence of psychosis. *Psychological Medicine*, in press.

Davidson, M., Reichenberg, A., Rabinowitz, J., Weiser, M., Kaplan, Z. and Mark, M. (1999) Behavioural and intellectual markers for schizophrenia in apparently healthy male adolescents. *American Journal of Psychiatry*, 156, 1328–1335.

De Alarcon, J., Seagroatt, V. and Goldacre, M. (1990) Trends in schizophrenia. *Lancet*, 335: 852–853.

Der, G., Gupta, S. and Murray, R.M. (1990) Is schizophrenia disappearing? *Lancet*, 335, 513–516.

Done, D.J., Crow, T.J., Johnstone, E.C. and Sacker, A. (1994) Childhood antecedents of schizophrenia and affective illness: social adjustment at ages 7 and 11. *British Medical Journal,* 309, 699–703.

Duncan-Jones, P., Fergusson, D.M., Ormel, J. *et al.* (1990) A model of stability and change in minor psychiatric symptoms: results from three longitudinal studies. *Psychological Medicine Monograph*, Supplement 18.

Eagles, J.M. (1991) The relationship between schizophrenia and immigration. Are there alternative hypotheses? *British Journal of Psychiatry*, 159, 783–789.

Eagles, J.M. and Whalley, L.J. (1985) Decline in the diagnosis of schizophrenia among first admissions to the Scottish mental hospitals from 1969–78. *British Journal of Psychiatry*, 146, 151–154.

Eagles, J.M., Hunter, D. and McCance, C. (1988) Decline in the diagnosis of schizophrenia among first contacts with psychiatric services in North East Scotland, 1969–84. *British Journal of Psychiatry*, 152, 793–798.

Eaton, W.W. (1991) Update on the epidemiology of schizophrenia. *Epidemiologic Reviews*, 13, 320–328.

Eaton, W.W. and Ritter, C. (1988) Distinguishing anxiety and depression using field survey data. *Psychological Medicine*, 18, 155–166.

Eysenck, H.J. and Eysenck, S.B.G. (1964) *Manual of the Eysenck Personality Inventory*. London: University of London Press.

Freeman, H. and Alpert, M. (1986) Prevalence of schizophrenia in an urban population. *British Journal of Psychiatry*, 149, 603–611.

Geddes, J.R., Black, R.J., Whalley, L.J. *et al.* (1993). Persistence of the decline in the diagnosis of schizophrenia among first admissions to Scottish hospitals from 1969–1988. *British Journal of Psychiatry*, 163, 620–626.

Geddes, J., Mercer, G., Frith, C.D. *et al.* (1994) Prediction of outcome following a first episode of schizophrenia: a follow-up study of Northwick Park first episode study subjects. *British Journal of Psychiatry*, 165, 664–668.

Goldberg, D.P. and Williams, P. (1988) *The User's Guide to the General Health Questionnaire*. Windsor: NFER-NELSON.

Goodyer, I., Kolvin, I. and Gatzanis, S. (1987) The impact of recent undesirable life events on psychiatric disorder in childhood and adolescence. *British Journal of Psychiatry*, 151, 179–184.

Häfner, H., Maurer, K., Loeffler, W. and Reicher-Rossler, A. (1993) The influence of age and sex on the onset and early course of schizophrenia. *British Journal of Psychiatry*, 162, 80–86.

Harrington, R., Fudge, H., Rutter, M., Pickles, A. and Hill, J. (1990) Adult outcomes of childhood and adolescent depression. I. Psychiatric status. *Archives of General Psychiatry*, 47, 465–473.

Harrison, G., Owens, D., Holton, A., Neilson, D. and Boot, D. (1988) A prospective study of severe mental disorder in Afro-Caribbean patients. *Psychological Medicine*, 18, 643–657.

Harrison, G., Cooper, J.E. and Gancarczyk, R. (1991) Changes in the administrative incidence of schizophrenia. *British Journal of Psychiatry*, 159, 811–816.

Harrison, G., Glazebrook, C., Brewin, J. *et al.* (1997) Increased incidence of psychotic disorders in African Caribbean migrants to the U.K. *Psychological Medicine*, 27, 799–806.

Harrison, G., Amin, S., Singh, S.P., Croudace, T. and Jones, P. (1999) Outcome of psychosis in people of African Caribbean family origin. *British Journal of Psychiatry*, 175, 43–49.

Harvey, C.A. (1996) The Camden Schizophrenia Survey, 1: the psychiatric behavioural and social characteristics of the severely mentally ill in an inner London health district. *British Journal of Psychiatry*, 168, 410–417.

Harvey, C.A., Pantelis, C., Taylor, J. *et al.* (1996) The Camden Schizophrenia Surveys, II: high prevalence of schizophrenia in an inner London borough and its relationship to sociodemographic factors. *British Journal of Psychiatry*, 168, 418–426.

Hegarty, J.D., Baldessarini, R.J., Tohen, M., Waterman, C. and Oepen, G. (1994) One hundred years of schizophrenia: a meta-analysis of the outcome literature. *American Journal of Psychiatry*, 151, 1409–1416.

Henderson, A.S., Byrne, D.G. and Duncan-Jones, P. (1981) *Neurosis and the Social Environment*. Sydney: Academic Press.

Hickling, F.W. (1991) Psychiatric hospital admission rates in Jamaica, 1971 and 1988. *British Journal of Psychiatry*, 159, 817–821.

Hirschfeld, R.M.A., Klerman, G.L., Clayton, P.J., Keller, M.B., Mcdonald-Scott, P. and Larkin, B. (1983) Assessing personality: effects of the depressive state on trait measurement. *American Journal of Psychiatry*, 140, 695–699.

Jablensky, A., Sartorius, N., Ernberg, G. *et al.* (1992) Schizophrenia: manifestations, incidence and course in different cultures. A World Health Organisation Ten-Country Study. *Psychological Medicine Monograph*, Supplement 20.

Jablensky, A. (1995) Schizophrenia: recent epidemiologic issues. *Epidemiologic Reviews*, 17, 10–20.

Jeffreys, S.E., Harvey, C.A., McNaught, A.S., Quayle, A.S., King, M.B. and Bird, A.S. (1997) The Hampstead Schizophrenia Survey 1991. I: prevalence and service use comparisons in an inner London health authority, 1986–1991. *British Journal of Psychiatry*, 170, 301–306.

Jenkins, R. (1985) Sex differences in minor psychiatric disorder. *Psychological Medicine Monographs*, Supplement 7.

Jenkins, R., Lewis, G., Bebbington, P. *et al.* (1997) The National Psychiatric Morbidity Surveys of Great Britain: initial findings from the Household Survey. *Psychological Medicine*, 27, 775–790.

Johnstone, E.C., Crow, T.J., Johnson, A.L. and MacMillan, J.F. (1986) The Northwick Park study of first episode schizophrenia. 1. Presentation of the illness and problems relating to admission. *British Journal of Psychiatry*, 148,115–120.

Jones, P.B. (1999) Longitudinal approaches to the search for the causes of schizophrenia: past, present and future. In: Gattaz, W.F. and Hafner, H. (eds), *Search for the Causes of Schizophrenia Vol. IV Balance of the Century*. Darmstadt: Steinkopff (Springer), pp. 91–119.

Jones, P.B. and Cannon, M. (1998) The new epidemiology of schizophrenia: common methods for genetics and the environment. *Psychiatric Clinics of North America*, 21, 1–25.

Jones, P.B. and Croudace, T. (2000) Predicting schizophrenia from teachers' reports of behaviour. Results from a general population birth cohort. In: Mednick, S.A. and McGlashan, T. (eds), *Early Intervention in Psychiatric Disorders*. NATO ARW, in press.

Jones, P.B. and Tarrant, C.J. (1999) Specificity of developmental precursors to schizophrenia and affective disorders. *Schizophrenia Research*, 39, 121–125.

Jones, P.B., Bebbington, P., Foerster, A., Lewis, S.W., Murray, R.M., Russell, A., Sham, P.C., Toone, B.K. and Wilkins, S. (1993) Premorbid social underachievement in schizophrenia. Results from the Camberwell Collaborative Psychosis Study. *British Journal of Psychiatry*, 162, 65–71.

Jones, P., Rodgers, B., Murray, R. and Marmot, M. (1994) Childhood developmental risk factors for schizophrenia in the 1946 national birth cohort. *Lancet*, 344, 1398–1402.

Joyce, P.R. (1987) Changing trends in first admissions and readmissions for mania and schizophrenia in New Zealand. *Australian and New Zealand Journal of Psychiatry*, 21, 82–86.

Keith, S.J., Regier, D.A. and Rae, D.S. (1991) Schizophrenic disorders. In: Robins, L.N. and Regier, D.A. (eds), *Psychiatric Disorders in America: the Epidemiologic Catchment Area Study*. New York: The Free Press, pp. 33–52.

Kendell, R., Discipio, W. and Eysenck. (1968) Personality inventory scores of patients with depressive illness. *British Journal of Psychiatry*, 11, 767–770.

Kendell, R.E., Malcolm, D.E. and Adams, W. (1993) The problem of detecting changes in the incidence of schizophrenia. *British Journal of Psychiatry*, 162, 212–218.

Kendler, K.S., Kessler, R.C., Neale, M.C. *et al.* (1993) The prediction of major depression in women: toward an integrated etiologic model. *American Journal of Psychiatry*, 150, 1139–1148.

Kessler, R.C., McGonagle, K.A., Zhao, S. *et al.* (1994) Lifetime and 12-month prevalence of DSM-III-R psychiatric disorders in the United States: results from the National Comorbidity Survey. *Archives of General Psychiatry*, 52, 8–19.

King, M., Coker, E., Leavey, G., Hoare, A. and Johnson-Sabine, E. (1994) Incidence of psychotic illness in London: a comparison of ethnic groups. *British Medical Journal*, 309, 1115–1119.

Leff, J., Kuipers, L., Berkowitz, R., Vaughan, C. and Sturgeon, D. (1983) Life events, relative's expressed emotion and maintenance neuroleptics in schizophrenic relapse. *Psychological Medicine*, 13, 799–800.

Leff, J., Wig , N.N., Bedi, H. *et al.* (1990) Relatives expressed emotion and the course of schizophrenia in Chandigargh: a two-year follow-up study of a first contact sample. *British Journal of Psychiatry*, 156, 351–356.

Leff, J., Sartorius, N., Jablensky, A., Korten, A. and Ernberg, G. (1992) The International Pilot Study of Schizophrenia: five-year follow-up findings. *Psychological Medicine*, 22, 131–145.

Lewis, G. and Booth, M. (1994) Are cities bad for your mental health? *Psychological Medicine*, 24, 913–916.

Lewis, G. and Pelosi, A. (1990) The case–control study in psychiatry. *British Journal of Psychiatry*, 157, 197–207.

Lewis, G., Bebbington, P., Brugha, T. *et al.* (1998) Socio-economic status, standard of living and neurotic disorder. *Lancet*, 352, 605–609.

Linzen, D.H., Dingemans, P.M. and Lenior, M.E. (1994) Cannabis abuse and the course of recent-onset schizophrenic disorders. *Archives of General Psychiatry*, 51, 273–279.

Loebel, A.D., Lieberman, J.A., Alvir, J.M.J. *et al.* (1992) Duration of psychosis and outcome in first-episode schizophrenia. *American Journal of Psychiatry*, 149, 1183–1188.

Mason, P. and Wilkinson, G. (1996) The prevalence of psychiatric morbidity. OPCS survey of psychiatric morbidity in Great Britain. *British Journal of Psychiatry*, 168, 1–3.

McCreadie, R.M. (1982) The Nithsdale schizophrenia survey: 1. Psychiatric and social handicaps. *British Journal of Psychiatry*, 140, 582–586.

McGovern, D. and Cope, R.V. (1987). First psychiatric admission rate of first and second generation Afro-Caribbeans. *Social Psychiatry*, 22, 139–149.

Meltzer, H., Gill, B, Petticrew, M. and Hinds, K. (1995) *Economic Activity and Social Functioning of Adults with Psychiatric Disorders*. London: OPCS.

Monck, E., Graham, P., Richman, N. and Dobbs, R. (1994) Adolescent girls II; background factors in anxiety and depressive states. *British Journal of Psychiatry*, 165, 770–780.

Mullen, P., Martin, J., Anderson, J., Romans, S. and Herbison, G. (1993) Child sexual abuse and mental health in adult life. *British Journal of Psychiatry*, 163, 721–732.

Munk-Jorgensen P. (1986) Decreasing first-admission rates of schizophrenia among males in Denmark from 1970 to 1984. *Acta Psychiatrica Scandanavica*, 73, 645–650.

Munk-Jorgensen, P. and Mortensen, P.B. (1992) Incidence and other aspects of the epidemiology of schizophrenia in Denmark, 1971–87. *British Journal of Psychiatry*, 161, 489–495.

Murray, C.J. and Lopez, A.D. (1997) Alternative projections of mortality and disability by cause 1990–2020: Global Burden of Disease Study. *Lancet*, 349, 1498–1504.

Nicole, L., Lesage, A. and Lalonde, P. (1992). Lower incidence and increased male:female ratio in schizophrenia. *British Journal of Psychiatry*, 161, 557–556.

Odegaard, O. (1932). Emigration and insanity. *Acta Psychiatrica Scandinavica Supplement* 4.

Office of Population Censuses and Surveys. *The Prevalence of Psychiatric Morbidity Among Adults aged 16–64 Living in Private Households in Great Britain*. London: OPCS.

Oldehinkel, A.J. and Giel, R. (1995) Time trends in the care-based incidence of schizophrenia. *British Journal of Psychiatry*, 167, 777–778.

Ormel, J., von Korff, M., Ustun, B. *et al.* (1994) Common mental disorders and disability across cultures: results from the WHO collaborative study on psychological problems in general health care. *Journal of the American Medical Association*, 272, 1741–1748.

Pantelis, C., Jeffreys, S.E., Harvey, CA., Quayle, A.S., King, M.B. and Bird, A.S. (1997) The Hampstead Schizophrenia Survey 1991. II: Incidence and migration in inner London.

Parker, G.B., Barrett, E.A., and Hickie, I. B. (1992) From nurture to network: examining links between perceptions of parenting in childhood and social bonds in adulthood. *American Journal of Psychiatry*, 149, 877–885.

Parker, G., Tupling, H. and Brown, L.B. (1979) A parental bonding instrument. *British Journal of Medical Psychology*, 52, 1–10.

Plum, F. (1972) Prospects for research on schizophrenia. 3. Neuropsychology. Neuropathological findings. *Neurosciences Research Program Bulletin*, 10, 384–388.

Ram, R., Bromet , E.J., Eaton, W.W., Pato, C. and Schwartz, J.E. (1992) The natural course of schizophrenia: a review of first admission studies. *Schizophrenia Bulletin*, 18, 185–207.

Robins, L. and Regier, D. (eds) (1991) *Psychiatric Disorders in America: The Epidemiological Catchment Area Study*. New York: The Free Press.

Romans. S., Walton, V., McNoe, B., Herbison, G. and Mullen, P. (1993) Otago Women's Health Survey: 30-month follow-up. I: onset patterns of non-psychotic psychiatric disorder. *British Journal of Psychiatry*, 163, 733–738.

Rose, G. (1989) The mental health of populations. In: Williams, P. and Rawnsley, K. (eds), *The Scope of Epidemiological Psychiatry*. London: Routledge, pp. 77–85.

Rutter, M.L. (1985) Resilience in the face of adversity: protective factors and resistance to psychiatric disorder. *British Journal of Psychiatry*, 147, 598–611.

Selten. J.P. and Sijben, N. (1994) First admission rate for schizophrenia in immigrants to The Netherlands: the Dutch National Register. *Social Psychiatry and Psychiatric Epidemiology*, 29, 71–72.

Shepherd, M., Watt, D., Falloon, I. and Smeeton N. (1989) The natural history of schizophrenia: a five-year follow-up study of outcome and prediction in a representative sample of schizophrenics. *Psychological Medicine Monograph*, Supplement 15.

Smith, K., Shah, A.J., Wright, K. and Lewis, G. (1995) The prevalence and costs of psychiatric disorders and learning disabilities. *British Journal of Psychiatry*, 166, 9–18.

Stoll, A.L, Tohen, M., Baldessarini, R.J. *et al.* (1993) Shifts in diagnostic frequencies of schizophrenia and major affective disorders at six North American psychiatric hospitals, 1972–88. *American Journal of Psychiatry*, 150, 1668–1673.

Sugarman, P.A. and Craufurd, D. (1994) Schizophrenia in the Afro-Caribbean community. *British Journal of Psychiatry*, 164, 474–480.

Thomas, C.S., Stone, K., Osborn, M., Thomas, P.F. and Fisher, M. (1993) Psychiatric morbidity and compulsory admission among UK-born Europeans, Afro-Caribbeans and Asians in central Manchester. *British Journal of Psychiatry*, 163, 91–99.

Thornicroft, G., Strathdee, G., Phelan, M., Holloway, F., Dunn, G., McCrone, P., Leese, M., Johnson, S. and Szmukler, G. (1998) PriSM Psychosis Study I. Rationale and design. *British Journal of Psychiatry*, 173, 363–370.

Tien, A.Y. and Eaton, W.W. (1992) Psychopathological precursors and sociodemographic risk factors for the schizophrenia spectrum. *Archives of General Psychiatry*, 49, 37–46.

Tohen, M., Stoll, A.L., Strakowski, S.M. *et al.* (1992) The McLean first-episode psychosis project: six-month recovery and recurrence outcome. *Schizophrenia Bulletin*, 18, 273–282.

Torrey, E.F. (1980) *Schizophrenia and Civilisation*. New York: Jason Aronson.

Torrey, E.F (1987) Prevalence studies in schizophrenia. *British Journal of Psychiatry*, 150, 598–608.

van Os, J., Fahy, T., Bebbington, P. *et al.* (1994) The influence of life events on the subsequent course and outcome of psychotic illness. A prospective study of the Camberwell Collaborative Psychosis Study. *Psychological Medicine*, 24, 503–513.

van Os, J., Castle, D.J., Der, G., and Murray, R. M. (1996) Psychotic illness in ethnic minorities: clarification from the 1991 census. *Psychological Medicine*, 26, 203–208.

van Os J., Howard., R., Takei, N. and Murray, R. (1995) Increasing age is a risk factor for psychosis in the elderly. *Social Psychiatry and Psychiatric Epidemiology*, 30, 161–164.

Waddington, J.L. and Youssef, H.A. (1994) Evidence for gender-specific decline in the rate of schizophrenia in a rural population over a fifty-year period. *British Journal of Psychiatry*, 164, 171–176.

Warner, R.. (1995) Time trends in schizophrenia: changes in obstetric risk factors with industrialization. *Schizophrenia Bulletin*, 21, 483–500.

Warr, P. (1987) *Work, Unemployment and Mental Health*. Oxford: Oxford Science Publications.

Weich, S. and Lewis, G. (1998) Poverty, unemployment and the common mental disorders: a population based cohort study. *British Medical Journal*, 317, 115–119.

Wells, K.B., Stewart, A., Hays, R.D. *et al.* (1989) The functioning and well-being of depressed patients: results from the medical outcomes study. *Journal of the American Medical Association*, 262, 914–919.

Wessley, S., Castle, D., Der, G. and Murray, R. (1991) Schizophrenia and Afro-Caribbeans. A case–control study. *British Journal of Psychiatry*, 159, 795–801.

Wing, J.K and Fryers, T. (1976) *Statistics from the Camberwell and Salford Psychiatric Registers, 1964–1974*. London: Institute of Psychiatry.

Wing, J.K., Cooper, J.E. and Sartorius, N. (1974) *The Measurement and Classification of Psychiatric Symptoms*. Cambridge: Cambridge University Press.

World Health Organisation (1994) *The ICD-10 Classification of Mental and Behavioural Disorders: Diagnostic Criteria for Research*. Geneva: WHO.

Wyatt, R..J. (1991) Neuroleptics and the natural course of schizophrenia. *Schizophrenia Bulletin*, 17, 325–351.

Youssef, H.A., Kinsella, A. and Waddington, J.L (1991) Evidence for geographical variations in prevalence of schizophrenia in rural Ireland. *Archives of General Psychiatry*, 48, 254–258.

Zubin, J. and Spring, B. (1977) Vulnerability—a new view of schizophrenia. *Journal of Abnormal Psychology*, 86, 103–126.

9 | *Mental disorder and disability in the population*

Rachel Jenkins and Bruce Singh

Introduction

The association of a range of psychiatric disorders with consequent functional disability has been demonstrated in a series of epidemiological studies in the community (Jenkins *et al.*, 1998), in primary care (Ustun and Sartorius, 1995) and in out-patient mental health settings in a wide variety of developed and low income countries. These studies have been conducted over the past two decades and have illustrated that a considerable burden of disability accompanies the presence of the range of common disorders—a fact that was already well known for the psychoses (Lehman, 1996). However, the measurement of disability is only a relatively recent phenomenon in psychiatric assessment compared with the large amount of work conducted on symptom rating scales and diagnostic instruments (Thompson, 1989).

The importance of quantifying disability is twofold: it gives an idea of the burden that psychiatric disorders cause for individuals and their communities and it provides a baseline measure to evaluate the outcomes of interventions. Comprehensive evaluation of new treatments needs to provide data on disability or quality of life outcomes and cost implications, as well as the clinical outcomes based on the presence or severity of the psychiatric disorder (McDowell and Newell, 1987; Thornicroft and Tansella, 1996).

One of the first proxy measures of health were mortality data. Mortality is unambiguous and, because death may be recordable by law, the data are generally complete. However, recorded mortality is a good indicator of actual mortality; it is not a good indicator of health and it is only a very partial indicator of morbidity. The selection of an indicator has important consequences. Indicators are chosen to reflect issues of public concern. Thus mortality, whilst it might have been appropriate for an era of infectious diseases, becomes less adequate in an era of chronic disease. Rising health expectations of the past centuries have led to a shift away from viewing health in terms of survival, to defining it more in terms of freedom from disease. In this transition, there has also been an increased appreciation of the value, not only of the observations of health professionals, but also of the legitimacy of subjective judgements by individual patients.

The WHO framework

The World Health Organization (WHO, 1980) developed a framework to describe the consequences of disease in 1980 when it published the International Classification of Impairments, Disabilities and Handicaps (ICIDH), to disentangle the potential confusion that can result when disease and its consequences are confused.

The classification came from an awareness that studies have shown that, in the health services sector, diagnosis alone does not predict service needs, length of hospitalization, level of care or outcomes. It was also known that diagnosis alone is not a good predictor of receipt of disability benefits, work performance, return to work potential or the likelihood of social integration. So a classification system based on diagnosis alone does not provide us with sufficient information for planning and management purposes. However, when everyday functioning is taken into account, the predictive power and understanding of needs and outcomes are increased.

The original WHO classification of disability referred to three dimensions of the consequences of disease, namely impairment, disability and handicap, with the following definitions, shown in Table 9.1.

The sequence, which is not necessarily unidirectional, is defined as follows.

- Awareness of symptoms and signs manifesting as a result of dysfunction at the organ level (impairments).
- Objective alterations of behaviour or performance at the level of the individual (disabilities).
- Involvement with society resulting in disadvantages at the level of environmental and social interaction (handicaps).

The WHO currently is in the process of revising the ICIDH for a second edition, which should be available in the year 2001. It is doing this because it believes that the classification requires revision in the light of the changes in health care and a new social understanding of social disability. One significant change will involve a new terminology; *activity* will be used instead of disability and *participation* rather than handicap.

The ICIDH2 has been constructed to reflect a specific model of *disablement*, the bio- psychosocial model. In this model, human functioning and disablement are viewed as outcomes of an interaction between a person's physical or mental condition and the social and physical environment. The so-called medical model of disablement locates disablement entirely within the person, views medical interventions as the only possible response to disablement and has such a narrow model long criticized and rejected by experts. Yet there are appropriate medical responses to some aspects of disablement, so the underlying message of the medical model cannot be wholly abandoned, rather the model needs to be synthesized with the social model.

In the new classification, the definition of *impairment* remains the same; however, *activity* is now used in the broader sense to capture everything that a person does at any level of complexity from simple activities to complex skills and behaviours. They include simple or basic physical functions of the person as a whole (e.g. grasping, moving a leg or seeing); basic and complex mental functions, e.g. remembering past events; and collections of physical and mental activities at varying levels of complexity, e.g. driving a car or interacting with people in social settings. Activity limitation (formerly disability) is a difficulty in the performance, accomplishment or completion of an activity at the level of the person. Difficulty encompasses all of the ways in which doing an activity may be affected, doing it with pain, doing it too slowly, not at the right time and place, and doing it awkwardly or otherwise not in the manner expected. It may range from a slight to a severe deviation in terms of the quality or quantity of doing the activity. The term disability is related to the word ability that is an aptitude or skill. The former classification focused mainly on activities related to the performance of individuals in daily life. The main criticism was that society did not distinguish between the individual's disability and the disabling imposed by society on a person because of society's limitations (e.g. by not being able to provide education for the blind).

Table 9.1 *WHO classification of impairment, disability and handicap*

An *impairment* is any loss or abnormality of a psychological, physiological or anatomical structure or function

A *disability* is any restriction or lack resulting from an impairment of ability to perform an activity in the manner within the range considered normal for a human being

A *handicap* is a disadvantage for a given individual resulting from an impairment or disability that limits or prevents the fulfilment of a role that is normal for age, sex, social and cultural dimensions for that individual.

Participation (formerly handicap) is the interaction of impairments and disabilities with contextual factors that are features of the social and physical environment and personal factors. Participation consists of all areas or aspects of human life, including the full experience of being involved in a practice, custom or social behaviour. Dimensions of participation include personal maintenance, mobility, exchange of information and social relationships. Participation restriction is a disadvantage for a person with an impairment or disability that is created or worsened by features of the environment. The disadvantage may take many forms, e.g. the creation of additional disablement as a result of stigma associated with the mental condition.

The evolution of disability measures

The development of disability scales parallels the sequences specified in the ICIDH. From early impairment scales (covering physical capacities such as balance and movement), attention shifted towards measuring disability (e.g. self-care activities) and later to handicap (inability to work or fulfil social roles).

The earliest measures were those which assessed activities of daily living (ADL) and were concerned with severe levels of disability relevant mainly to institutionalized patients and the elderly. During the 1970s, this concept was expanded to the instrumental activities of daily living (IADL), namely shopping, cooking and managing money, as care started to move out into the community. This move also led to extension of the scale and to cover indices of social function. Finally, multi-dimensional scales evolved which covered physical, social and emotional function or so-called general health measurements.

Disability and quality of life

The second major conceptual framework for non-fatal health outcomes falls under the concept of health-related quality of life. Health-related quality of life includes at least four broad concepts: opportunity, health perceptions, functional status and impairment (Patrick and Ericsson, 1993). Unfortunately, the same vocabulary as in the ICIDH is used in different ways in the health-related quality of life field. Within each of these concepts, various domains have been identified; for example the domains of social or cultural disadvantage, and resilience. Functional status can include the domains of social function, psychological function and physical function. Each of these three domains can in turn be divided into subdomains such as affect, integration, contact, intimacy and fitness. Impairment includes domains such as symptoms, signs, tissue alterations or diagnosis.

As can be seen, there is conceptual confusion, which arises from the fact that different investigators started to develop instruments independently of each other and without a coherent framework. The first instruments were developed by clinicians and clinical psychologists, and focused on the measurement of quality of life before and after various therapeutic interventions. Later, several of these instruments were adapted by epidemiologists, psychologists and sociologists for use in cross-sectional surveys of the general population. There is thus no one overreaching conceptualization of quality of life. Instruments used to measure it have a multi-dimensional approach. At the minimum, most would agree that the domains of physical functioning, psychological well-being, social and role functioning and health perceptions should be included. Some concepts of quality of life include the additional domains of opportunities and resources to pursue and achieve life goals, which have particular relevance to people with disabilities (McDowall and Newall, 1987).

Unlike the ICIDH, where the distinction between disability and handicap lies in the consequences for the individual, the health-related quality of life approach does not draw such a sharp distinction. Rather, the impact on the individual is one of many domains making up the health-related quality of life. Furthermore, a clear distinction is not made between living in a particular health state and the valuation of time spent in that health state. Some domains such as satisfaction with health are obviously a mixture of perceived health status and the valuation of that health status by the individual.

Disability and psychiatric conditions

Disability ratings have now been created for a large number of psychiatric conditions. These include depression and anxiety (Jenkins *et al.*, 1998), panic disorder (Sheehan *et al.*, 1996), obsessive–compulsive disorder (OCD; Gudex, 1996) and schizophrenia (Van-Nieuwenhuizen *et al.*, 1997). As might be expected, they demonstrate that the majority of mental disorders are associated with significant disability. However, as in the case of physical conditions, diagnosis does not necessarily correlate with level of disability. Because few studies have used comparable measures across conditions, empirical data on relative levels of disability among mental conditions and between mental disorders and physical conditions are lacking. Studies such as one which demonstrated that depressed patients suffered as much disability as those with heart disease do reinforce the growing awareness of the consequences of psychiatric illness (Pyne *et al.*, 1997).

Considerable confusion has arisen by virtue of the widespread use of the term 'serious mental illness' synonymous with psychosis, and minor psychiatric morbidity synonymous with the previous term 'neurosis', referring to the spectrum of anxiety and depressive disorders. The use of terms such as serious versus minor often is mistakenly assumed to imply that the one is associated with significant disability and the other not. Yet the majority of clinicians are aware that within the term minor psychiatric morbidity are conditions such as depression, OCD and panic disorder, which can be devastating to an individual's level of functioning.

It is this difficulty in linking diagnosis to disability which has been at the heart of the problems in developing a reliable case mix classification for mental disorder similar to the Diagnosis Related Groups used for funding many physical health conditions. Diagnosis alone has not been found to be a good predictor of health service use, but needs to be combined with other variables such as disability, severity, chronicity and important socio-demographic information such as martial status and housing status, before health service use can be predicted with any accuracy.

Disability and the global burden of disease

The concept of quality of life has been utilized by economists to develop a measure to allow health status to be measured in various circumstances across conditions. It is based on the proposition that health as an output of health services is a function of both quantity of health, of mortality and morbidity. The Quality Adjusted Life Year (QALY) allows individuals to trade-off quantity of life against quality of life, arguing that, for example, according to people's preferences, 10 years living with a chronic condition is equivalent to 8 years of full health. The quality adjustment for the condition would thus be 0.8 and consequently if a cure was available it would result in improvement in quality of life of 0.2 QALYs per annum. The development of QALYs, with their incorporation of a large subjective and value-laden decision into the measure, can be considered an advance in that it led to the explicit recognition that such value judgements had validity in measuring health outcomes.

The QALY has been modified by the World Bank to translate into the so-called Disability Adjusted Life Years or DALY. This has been used to calculate the burden of different diseases. Unlike the QALY, however, the assumptions, which led to the weights, are standardized and made explicit in the publication of *The Global Burden of Disease*.

The DALY has a uniform method of estimating disability and estimating preference for different health states. This statistic summates the morbidity and the mortality resulting from identifiable diseases into a single numerical measure. The full impact of mortality is taken into account by considering the age at which it occurs. The number of years of potential life lost by that death are calculated by subtracting the age at which it occurred from the expectation of life remaining at that age. To give the same weight to premature death in poor and rich countries, the figure for life expectancy chosen is the one for low mortality countries. Moreover, the calculation recognizes that years of life do not have the same value to individuals throughout the life span, i.e. most persons value a year in young adulthood as worth several times more than a year in late life. To measure disability resulting from disease, each surviving year is discounted against the severity of the disability and the expected duration of the disability. The disadvantage from a given handicap is assigned a position on a scale from 0 for complete health to 1 for death by expert consensus, for example blindness is rated at a severity of 0.6 whereas disease of the female reproductive tract is rated at a severity of 0.22. Thus, DALYs take into account the age when a specific disease is acquired, the potential years of life lost, the relative value of those years and the years compromised by persisting handicap.

In the chapter of *The Global Burden of Disease* entitled 'Rethinking DALYs', Murray describes in detail how the disability weights for the conditions are calculated (Murray and Lopez, 1996). He makes the point that in order to compare the time lived in various health states with years of life loss due to premature mortality, it is necessary to develop a set of weights for time spent in different health states. An important issue is to define what exactly it is intended to value (e.g. one can value time spent being blind, time spent with a reading disability or time spent unable to work because of blindness). The methods available to measure preferences include visual analogue scale, magnitude estimation, standard gamble, time trade-off and person trade-off.

A second important issue in making preferences for time lived with different non-fatal outcomes is the choice of respondents, or in other words *whose values* should be measured. At least four groups often are distinguished: those living in the

given health state; family of individuals in that health state; the general public; and health care providers. The person trade-off method forced individuals to undertake interpersonal comparisons of utility between groups of individuals with different conditions with the assumption that its resulting weight is intended to influence the allocation of resources between groups. As with time preference, individuals may have different preferences for trade-off between quantity of life for one set of individuals, and quality of life for another set of individuals. Murray also makes the point that deliberation is important, what he calls 'reflective equilibrium', where individuals are faced with the policy consequences of their valued choices and given the opportunity to reflect. He quotes Madison who argued that a representative democracy would be preferable to a direct democracy because some judgements require deliberation, reflection on the implications of choice and sufficient time to arrive at an informed judgement. Since the general public would not have adequate time and opportunity for such deliberation, Madison argued for indirect representative democracy as preferable to direct democracy. Murray eventually decided on the person trade-off protocol, and used a deliberative process to ensure that the consequences of the decisions were fed back to participants. Two forms of person trade-off were used. In the first form, participants are asked to trade-off life extension of individuals in a given health state. Thus participants were asked questions such as "Would you as decision maker prefer to purchase through a health intervention, one year of life for 100 perfectly healthy individuals or 200 blind individuals." In the second form of the person trade-off, participants trade-off between raising the quality of life of those in a reduced state of health to perfect health for 1 year, versus extending life for healthy individuals for 1 year. In both forms, preference weights for the health state under consideration are achieved.

Murray used 22 indicator conditions, which individuals participating had to consider were affecting people for a full 12 months of relevance to mental disorders (Murray and Lopez, 1996). Amongst the 22 were the psychiatric condition of active psychosis, Downs's syndrome and mild mental retardation, dementia and unipolar major depression. The relevant descriptions were;

- active psychosis—'an individual with paranoid delusions, auditory hallucinations and disorganized speech';
- mild mental retardation—'IQ level between 55 and 70';
- Down's syndrome—'the average individual with Downs syndrome';
- unipolar major depression—'the loss of interest or pleasure in nearly all activities, the depressed individual has change in appetite or weight, sleep and psychomotor activity, decreased energy, feeling of worthlessness or guilt, difficulty thinking, concentrating or making decisions';
- dementia—'an individual with multiple cognitive defects including memory impairment, aphasia and apraxia'.

The weights, which were finally achieved by this method and utilized in further calculations, are given in Table 9.2.

In calculating the DALYs for unipolar major depression, the DALYs from depression were combined with the DALYs from suicide. Using these methods, neuropsychiatric conditions contributed 10.5% of the global burden of disease, 22% in the developed world and 9% in the developing world. As can be seen in Table 9.3, the reasons for psychiatric DALYs worldwide being so high is that psychiatric conditions are amongst the leading causes of disability in the world even though their contribution to mortality although significant is not so visible.

Epidemiological surveys

Psychiatric epidemiological studies are now in their third generation (Tsuang *et al.*, 1996). The *first-generation* studies described by Tsuang and his colleagues took place between the turn of the century and the Second World War. Investigation tended to rely on key informants and records to supply information to enable them to identify cases. When interviewers were used (six studies), the median for all types of disorder was only 3.6% compared with a prevalence of 20% in the second-generation studies. This difference can be explained by an expansion of the concept of psychiatric disorders as a result of the mental health

Table 9.2 *Weights for relative time spent in different health states*

Disability class	Severity weights	Indicator conditions
1	0.00–0.02	Vitiligo on face, weight-for-height <2 SDs
2	0.02–0.12	Watery diarrhoea, severe sore throat, severe anaemia
3	0.12–0.24	Radius fracture in a stiff cast, infertility, erectile dysfunction, rheumatoid arthritis, angina
4	0.24–0.36	Below-the-knee amputation, deafness
5	0.36–0.50	Rectovaginal fistula, mild mental retardation, Down syndrome
6	0.50–0.70	Unipolar major depression, blindess, paraplegia
7	0.70–1.00	Active psychosis, dementia, severe migraine, quadriplegia

From Murray and Lopez (1996).

Table 9.3 *The top 10 causes of the world's disability adjusted life years (DALY)*

	Total (millions)	Percentage of total
All causes	427.7	
1. Unipolar major depression	50.8	10.7
2. Iron-deficiency anaemia	22.0	4.7
3. Falls	22.0	4.6
4. Alcohol use	15.8	3.3
5. Chronic obstructive pulmonary disease	14.7	3.1
6. Bipolar disorder	14.1	3.0
7. Congenital anomalies	13.5	2.9
8. Osteoarthritis	13.3	2.8
9. Schizophrenia	12.1	2.6
10. Obsessive–compulsive disorders	10.2	2.2

From Murray and Lopez (1996).

profession experience with psychiatric screening for serious and subsequent psychiatric casualties. *Second-generation* studies, also described by Tsuang and his colleagues from the Second World War to 1970, relied on direct interviews. Either a single psychiatrist conducted interviews or interviews were conducted by others. Case identification depended on psychiatrists' evaluation of protocols. They were supplemented by studies where lay interviewers administered instruments, which had been developed as aids to service screening in the Second World War. The results of all these studies were expressed not as diagnostic types but as ratings of caseness or impairment

Third-generation studies build on progress made in systematizing and refining diagnostic system. The basis of these studies was semistructured interviews conducted by key interviews achieving high reliability in large samples. One example of these is the DIS, which was used in the Epidemiological Catchment Area (ECA) programme in the USA (Robins and Regier, 1991),

and the Composite International Diagnostic Instrument (CIDI) developed by the WHO (Witchen and Eassau, 1993). The majority of these surveys, however, incorporated no measure of disability, although the WHO Disability Assessment Schedule was developed specifically to be administered with it.

The generation of the DALYs mentioned above depended on epidemiological surveys which had been conducted in various parts of the world and from which the data were generated. It is important to note that the weight for depression was calculated for someone who would be considered to have a moderately severe case of depression for 1 year. Prevalence rates in community surveys subsume people whose depression is relatively brief as well as those whose depression is chronic and may last for several years if untreated. We do not have sufficient information to know whether a person with moderate depression for 1 year is a reasonable average to take for the whole population. Nonetheless, a message from *The Global*

Burden of Disease is that psychiatric disorders are considerable causes of worldwide morbidity and are likely to increase over the next 20 years.

Epidemiological surveys measuring disability

In this section, three recent community surveys which used disability measures will be described. In each survey, the methodology is outlined, and then the results are presented firstly for the prevalence of psychiatric disorder and then for levels of disability resulting from disorder.

WHO study of mental illness in general health care

In 1995, the WHO published the results of a major survey of mental illness in general health care (Ustun and Sartorius, 1995) which screened over 25 000 patients in primary care in 14 countries. The methodology used multiple methods to assess patients in that they were self-rated, interviewer rated and physician rated for psychological illness, functional disability and physical health as shown in Table 9.4.

The sample originally was screened, 1500 at each site, with the General Health Questionnaire 12, of whom 400 were selected for a baseline diagnostic assessment, and then all with current disorder and 20% of a random sample were followed-up 3 months later. The CIDI was used to achieve psychiatric diagnoses, and a brief disability questionnaire composed of six self-report disability items taken from the medical outcomes survey short form SF36 was used to assess limitations of function. In addition, questions concerning daily functioning, motivation for work and personal efficiency and deterioration in social relationships were added. Interviewer ratings of disability in work role from the Social Disability Schedule were included to provide a disability measure that did not depend on self-assessment. In this assessment, the global score was based on interviewer ratings of adjustment to daily routine, energy input at performance, contact with people

Table 9.4 *Study of mental ilness in general health care*

Point prevalence of current ICD-10 disorders	%
Current depression	10.4
Generalized anxiety disorder	7.9
Neurasthenia	5.4
Harmful use of alcohol	3.3
Alcohol dependence	2.7
Somatization disorder	2.7
Dysthymia	2.1
Panic disorder	1.1
Agoraphobia with panic	1.0
Hypochondriasis	0.8
Agoraphobia without panic	0.5
Any CIDI diagnosis	24.0
Two or more mental disorders	9.5

at work and other relevant daily activities. The assessment permitted the interviewer to take local norms regarding work role performance into account. Subjects were also asked to report the number of days in the prior month that they were unable to carry out fully their usual daily activities. The overall result of this study was that 24% of consecutive attenders have current mental disorders reaching ICD-10 criteria for well-defined psychiatric disorder (see Table 9.5).

For all diagnostic categories, the proportion of patients with moderate or severe disability was approximately 3–5 times higher relative to patients without a psychiatric disorder. This pattern was similar across all measures of disability. However, these increased disability rates among patients with psychiatric illness may be biased by psychiatric co-morbidity as almost half of the

Table 9.5 Impact of psychopathology on disability—WHO study

Current ICD-10 diagnosis (patients with psychiatric co-morbidity are excluded)	Moderate or severe Occupational role dysfunction (%)	Self-reported physical disability (%)
Psychiatrically well patients	7	12
ICD Depressive Episode	39	46
ICD Panic Disorder	53	34
ICD Agoraphobia	14	47
ICD Neurasthenia	37	48
ICD Hypochondriasis	42	45
ICD Generalized Anxiety	26	53
ICD Alcohol Dependence	20	18
ICD Somatization Disorder	21	42

Disability by current ICD-10 diagnosis pooled across centres.

patients with at least one psychiatric disorder had a disorder from at least one other cluster. The clusters were depressive episode; agoraphobia, panic and anxiety disorders; somatization, hypochondriasis and somatoform pain; and alcohol dependence.

When disability levels among patients with only one psychiatric disorder were examined, self-reported disability dropped; however, it was still higher than for those without. When a logistic regression was used to look at the relative contribution of physical and psychiatric ill-health to the disability, it was shown that both have a substantial independent effect, but occupational disability appears to be more sensitive to mental illness than to physical illness. It was interesting that there were substantial differences here between centres, suggesting that the contributions of illness to disability vary in different cultures (see Figure 9.1).

This consistent relationship of psychological and disability and negative health perceptions across a wide range of countries and cultures underscores the worldwide public health significance of the common forms of psychological illness experienced by primary care patients. The significance of these disorders appears to extend beyond the considerable personal suffering that they induce.

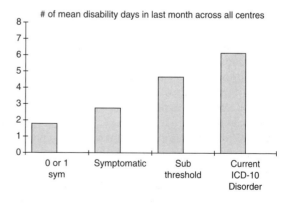

Figure 9.1 Disability in mental disorders

The Australian national survey of mental health and well-being

The Australian survey was conducted in two parts as a national survey of common mental disorders and an additional study looking particularly at the psychoses. The 1997 National Survey of Mental Health and Wellbeing of Adults (ABS, 1997) was conducted from May to August 1997 from a representative sample of persons living in private dwellings across Australia. Approximately 13 000 dwellings were selected and approximately 10 600 people aged 18 years and over participated in the survey; a response rate of 78%. The survey was designed to look for psychiatric disorders using the CIDI, particularly looking for the spectrum of anxiety disorders, affective disorders, and alcohol and substance abuse disorders.

Disability was measured using the Brief Disability Questionnaire (BDQ) which is a standard questionnaire containing eight questions which measured general levels of disability. This constitutes an 8-item scale (Belloc *et al.*, 1971) which emphasizes physical aspects of disability. Respondents are asked whether they are limited because of health problems in a number of activities such as running or sports, climbing stairs or walking long distances. They are also asked whether they have cut down or stopped activities at decreased motivation or personal efficiency or deterioration in their social relationships. The items in the BDQ refer to the 4 weeks prior to the interview. The medical outcomes study method of scoring scale from 0 to 16 was used, a high score indicating that the respondent has been limited in their activities by health problems. Also used were the SF12 (Ware *et al.*, 1996) which is a standard international instrument containing 12 questions, which provide a generic measure of health status. It may be considered as a measure of disability because it addresses limitations due to physical and mental health. It measures eight concepts: physical functioning; role limitation due to physical health problems; bodily pain; general energy; vitality; social functioning; role limitations due to emotional problems; and mental health, psychological distress and psychological well-being. For this survey, most items refer to the 4 weeks prior

to the interview. From these items, the physical component summary (PCS) and the mental component summary (MCS) are derived. As expected, the PCS focuses mainly on limitations in physical role functioning, whilst the MCS focuses mainly on role limitations due to emotional problems. Both scales are transformed to have a mean of 50 and a standard deviation of 10, a lower score indicating a greater level of disability.

The overall results of the study demonstrate that 18% of the sample had a mental disorder at some time during the 12 months prior to the survey, with the prevalence gradually decreasing with age. Young adults aged 18–24 years have the highest prevalence, mental disorder (27%) declining steadily to 6.1% for those aged 65 years and over. Men and women had similar overall prevalence rates; however, from age 35 years, women were more likely to have a mental disorder than men. For people with mental disorder, co-morbidity was common, for example nearly one in three who had an anxiety disorder also had an affective disorder, while one in five also had a substance abuse disorder. Those with mental disorders were more likely to report physical symptoms than those without (see Table 9.6).

The results of the disability survey showed that most people (66%) were disability free as measured by the BDQ, 13% had mild, 15% moderate and 6.5% severe disability. Of those with a mental disorder, 44% had mild, moderate or severe disability and averaged 3 days out of role in the 4 weeks prior to interview compared with 1 day for those with no mental disorder.

Persons with physical conditions scored lower on the PCS but higher on the MCS, while the pattern was reversed for those with mental disorders (combinations of disorders had an accumulative effect on disability) and this co-morbid group were among the lowest scorers on the SCF12 measures and reported the highest number of days out of role at an average of 5.6 days out of the 4 weeks prior to interview. Anxiety and affective disorders of any group generally had a more disabling impact that substance abuse disorders. Overall, those with anxiety disorders were most troubled by physical aspects of disability while those with affective disorders fared worse in terms of the

Table 9.6 *Prevalence of disorders in Australian National Survey*[a]

	Males ×1000	%	Females ×1000	%	Total ×1000	%
Physical conditions	2396.0	36.2	2823.7	41.3	5219.6	38.8
Mental disorders						
Anxiety disorders						
Panic disorder	36.7	0.6	133.8	2.0	170.5	1.3
Agoraphobia	49.2	0.7	101.9	1.5	151.1	1.1
Social phobia	161.4	2.4	207.3	3.0		
Generalized anxiety disorder	156.8	2.4	256.0	3.7	412.8	3.1
Obsessive–compulsive disorder	19.3	0.3	29.2	0.4	48.6	0.4
Post-traumatic stress disorder	153.3	2.3	285.8	4.2	439.2	3.3
Total anxiety disorders	470.4	7.1	829.6	12.1	1299.9	9.7
Affective disorders						
Depression	227.6	3.4	465.3	6.8	629.9	5.1
Dysthymia	63.4	1.0	88.3	1.3	151.7	1.1
Total affective disorders[b]	275.3	4.2	.3	7.4	778.6	5.8
Substance use disorders						
Alcohol harmful use	285.4	4.3	123.8	1.8	409.2	3.0
Alcohol dependence	339.8	5.1	126.9	1.9	466.7	3.5
Drug use disorders[c]	206.9	3.1	89.2	1.3	296.0	2.2
Total substance use disorders	734.3	11.1	307.5	4.5	1041.8	7.7
Total mental disorders	1151.6	17.4	1231.5	18.0	2383.1	17.7
No mental disorders or physical conditions	3531.8	53.3	3351.6	49.0	6883.4	51.1
Total[d]	6627.1	100.0	6837.7	100.0	13464.8	100.0

[a]During the 12 months prior to interview.
[b]Includes other affective disorders such as mania, hypomania and bipolar affective disorder.
[c]Includes harmful use and dependence.
[d]A person may have more than one mental disorder with or without a physical condition. The components when added may therefore be larger than the total.

mental component in days out of role (see Tables 9.7 and 9.8).

The Australian Low Prevalence Study, which complemented the National Survey, provided detailed clinical and social data on 1000 people with psychotic disorders around Australia. This included those in both in-patient and out-patient care and those currently not in contact. The instrument used was the Diagnostic Interview for Psychosis (DIP) which includes items from the WHO DAS disability assessment schedule (WHO, 1988).

Table 9.7 Co-morbidity of disorders[a] by disability status[b] in the Australian survey

	None	Mild	Moderate	Severe	Total	Total (×1000)
Physical conditions only	45.4	17.2	25.3	12.1	100.0	4198.3
Mental disorders only						
Anxiety only	71.7	9.4	14.2	*4.7	100.0	386.3
Affective only	78.4	*7.3	10.4	*3.8	100.0	191.7
Substance use only	75.8	12.0	10.9	*1.3	100.0	479.7
Combination of mental disorders only[c]	55.0	22.9	14.0	8.1	100.0	304.1
Total mental disorders only	70.4	13.0	12.5	4.1	100.0	1361.8
Mental disorders and physical conditions						
Anxiety and physical only	29.4	18.4	33.2	19.0	100.0	348.7
Affective and physical only	34.7	*16.0	28.3	21.0	100.0	114.2
Substance use and physical only	65.0	14.5	14.0	*6.6	100.0	238.6
Combination of mental disorders and physical conditions[c]	25.6	18.7	31.1	24.7	100.0	319.8
Total mental disorders and physical conditions	37.1	17.3	27.5	18.1	100.0	1021.3
Total mental disorders	56.1	14.9	18.9	10.1	100.0	2383.1
Total mental disorders or physical conditions	49.3	16.4	23.0	11.4	100.0	6581.4
No mental disorders or physical conditions	81.8	9.6	6.7	1.9	100.0	6883.4
Total	65.9	12.9	14.7	6.5	100.0	13464.8

[a]During the 12 months prior to interview.
[b]During the 4 weeks prior to interview, according to the Brief Disability Questionnaire (BDQ).
[c]Combinations of mental disorders from more than one of the major groupings (anxiety, affective and substance use).
*High Standard error.

In the study, social impairment in daily life was high in that 50% had impaired participation in household tasks and 45% impaired interpersonal relationships (40% having no intimate relationships, 36% no sexual relationship and 12% no friends).

Based on global ratings of disability, 23% had major impairments in all areas while 64% had social and occupational impairment; 87% of the sample had no carer available.

The OPCS surveys of psychiatric morbidity in Great Britain

The Office of Population Census and Surveys (OPCS) Surveys of Psychiatric Morbidity in Great Britain were commissioned by the Department of Health to provide up to date information about the prevalence of psychiatric problems among adults in Great Britain, as well as associated social disability. Four separate surveys were carried out

Table 9.8 *Average days out of role[a] by co-morbidity of disorders[b] in the Australian survey*

	Males	Females	Total
Physical conditions only	2.4	2.4	2.4
Mental disorders only			
Anxiety only	1.8	2.2	2.1
Affective only	3.5	2.3	2.7
Substance use only	1.3	0.8	1.1
Combination of mental disorders only[c]	3.1	3.9	3.6
Total mental disorders only	1.9	2.4	2.2
Mental disorders and physical conditions			
Anxiety and physical only	4.2	3.5	3.7
Affective and physical only	7.2	6.0	6.3
Substance use and physical only	1.6	2.4	1.8
Combination of mental disorders and physical conditions[c]	5.3	5.7	5.6
Total mental disorders and physical conditions	3.7	4.5	4.1
Total mental disorders	2.6	3.4	3.0
Total mental disorders or physical conditions	2.5	2.7	2.6
No mental disorders or physical conditions	0.9	1.1	1.0
Total	1.7	1.9	1.8

[a]During the 4 weeks prior to interview.
[b]During the 12 months prior to interview.
[c]Combinations of mental disorders from more than one of the major groupings (anxiety, affective, and substance use).

in the 1993–1994 period. The major survey was a private household survey of 10 000 adults aged 16–64 years living in the community; a supplementary sample of 350 with psychosis, 1200 people living in institutions and 1100 homeless people were also surveyed. The household survey demonstrated that one in six adults had suffered some type of neurotic disorder in the week before the survey interview, half of which were mixed anxiety–depression (see Table 9.9), 0.4% had a psychosis, 4.7% reported alcohol abuse and 2.2% drug abuse.

In order to measure daily functioning, all subjects were asked about their economic activity and were placed into one of eight categories: working; looking for work; intending to look for work but prevented by temporary ill-health; going to school or college; permanently unable to work; retired; looking after the home or family; or other. Disability was assessed by evaluating activities of daily living. Seven areas of functioning were covered by the survey: personal care; using transport; medical care; household activities; practical activities; dealing with paperwork; and managing money. Respondents were asked whether they had difficulty with each task.

The results of the disability and economic activity were that adults with neurotic health problems

Table 9.9 *Prevalence of psychiatric disorders per 1000 population in adults aged 16–64 years, in Great Britain 1993 in OPCS survey*

	Women	Men	All adults
Rate per thousand in past week (SE)			
Mixed anxiety and depressive disorder	94 (5)	54 (4)	77 (3)
Generalized anxiety disorder	34 (3)	28 (2)	31 (2)
Depressive episode	25 (2)	17 (2)	21 (1)
Phobias	14 (2)	7 (1)	11 (1)
Obsessive–compulsive disorder	15 (2)	9 (2)	12 (1)
Panic disorder	9 (1)	8 (2)	8 (1)
Any neurotic disorder	195 (7)	123 (5)	160 (5)
Rate per thousand in past 12 months (SE)			
Functional psychosis	4 (1)	4 (1)	4 (1)
Alcohol dependence	21 (2)	75 (5)	47 (3)
Drug dependence	14 (2)	29 (3)	22 (2)

Table 9.10 *Difficulties in activities of daily living (ADL) in household samples*

Subject group	% with any ADL difficulties	Base
Suicidal thoughts in past week	50	80
Psychosis in past year	40	44
Neurosis in past week	32	1557
None of the above	12	8184

were 4–5 times more likely than the rest of the sample to be permanently unable to work; those with two or more neurotic disorders who had been working for at least 1 year had on average 28 days a year off sick compared with 8 days a year for those with one neurotic disorder. Among the sample with any neurotic disorder who were unemployed and seeking work, 70% had been unemployed for a year or more, i.e. approximately

7% of all people with neurotic disorder. Compared with the general population, adults with neurosis were twice as likely to be receiving income support and 4–5 times more likely to be on invalidity benefit. As far as activities of daily living amongst adults reporting no physical health problem, 35% of those with two neurotic disorders had at least one ADL difficulty, practically twice the proportion of those with one neurotic disorder. People with phobia, depressive episode phobia and OCD had the highest proportions with any ADL difficulty, 55, 45 and 42%, respectively. Between 10 and 20% of adults with generalized anxiety disorder, depressive episode phobia or OCD experienced difficulty with handling money or dealing with paperwork. Only four in 10 adults with a psychotic disorder were working compared with nearly six in 10 with neurotic disorder, and seven in 10 of those unaffected by a mental disorder (see Tables 9.10 and 9.11).

Conclusion

Psychiatric disorders are associated with relatively high levels of disability. The distribution of dis-

Table 9.11 *Mean number of 'days off work due to ill-health' in past year by type of disorder*

	Mixed anxiety and depressive disorder	Generalized anxiety disorder	Depressive episode	Phobias	OCD	Panic	Any neurotic disorder
Proportion employed for 1 year or more	47%	30%	32%	20%	31%	34%	38%
Base = no. with disorder	750	439	220	180	157	93	1557
Mean no. of days off work in past year	7	15	25	16	23	10	10
Base = no. of people employed for 1 year or more	351	130	71	36	48	32	599

ability in mental disorders is as important in understanding the impact of mental disorder as a population as is the distribution of symptomatology. Hitherto, the focus of psychiatric epidemiologists has been to study symptomatology and its relationship with socio-demographic variables. Three recent major surveys of psychiatric morbidity have now extended this focus into an exploration of levels of concomitant disability.

All three surveys have revealed strikingly similar findings with regard to prevalence and the relationship of disorders to functioning. Two of these were major community surveys both involving approximately 10 000 people aged 16–65 years in the UK and Australia. The other involved 25 000 patients presenting to primary care practitioners in 14 countries. The surveys found that:

- psychiatric disorders of the 'neurotic' type are of high prevalence in the community and in patients presenting to GPs
- they are associated with a significant degree of disability
- co-morbid psychiatric disorder, if present, further decreases functioning.

These findings have major implications for health services—the high level of disability accompanying the common mental disorders emphasizes the need to support primary care (via basic training and continuing education) in its role of assessing and managing the bulk of these conditions, and particular help may be needed to address co-morbidity. Since the disability is comprised largely of difficulties in social functioning, there is a need to incorporate social aspects of care into the primary care level. The even higher levels of disability accompanying the psychoses reinforce the emphasis which should be given to occupational rehabilitation as well as to social rehabilitation in this group of clients.

References

Australian Bureau of Statistics (1997) *Mental Health and Well Being. Profile of Adults.* Canberra: Australian Bureau of Statistics.

Belloc, N.B., Breslow, L. and Hochstim, R.J. (1971) Measurement of physical health in a general population. *American Journal of Epidemiology*, 93, 328–376.

Gudex, C. (1996) Measuring patient benefit in mental illness. *European Psychiatry*, 11, 155–158.

Jenkins, R., Bebbington, P., Brugha, T.S., Farrell, M., Lewis, G. and Meltzer, H. (1998) British Psychiatric Morbidity Survey. *British Journal of Psychiatry*, 173, 4–7.

Lehman, A.F. (1996) Measures of quality of life among persons with severe and persistent mental disorders. *Social Psychiatry and Psychiatric Epidemiology*, 31, 78–88.

McDowell, I. and Newall, C. (1987) *Measuring Health. A Guide to Rating Scales and Questionnaires.* Oxford: Oxford University Press.

Murray, C.J.L. and Lopez, A.D. (1996) *The Global Burden of Disease.* Geneva: WHO.

Patrick, D.L. and Erickson, P. (1993) *Health Status and Policy: Allocating Resources to Health Care.* New York: Oxford University Press.

Pyne, J., Patterson, T.L., Kaplan, R.M., Gillin, J.C., Koch, W.L. and Grant, I. (1997) Assessment of the quality of life of patients with major depression. *Psychiatric Services*, 48, 224–229.

Robins, L.N., Rejier, D.A. (eds) (1991) *Psychiatric Disorders in America.* New York: Toronto: Free Press: Collier Macmillan

Sheehan, D.V., Harnett-Sheehan, K. and Raj, B.A. (1996) The measurement of disability. *International Clinical Psychopharmacology*, 11, 89–95

Thompson, C. (1989) *The Instruments of Psychiatric Research.* Chichester: Wiley

Thornicroft, G. and Tansella, M. (1996) *Mental Health Outcome Measures.* New York Springer-Verlag.

Tsuang, M.T., Tuhen, M. and Zahner, G.E.P. (1995) *Textbook of Psychiatric Epidemiology.* New York: Wiley.

Ustun, T.B. and Sartorius, N. (1995) *Mental Illness in General Health Care.* Chichester: Wiley.

Van-Nieuwenhuizen., C., Schene, A.H., Boevink, W.A. and Wolf, J.R.L.M. (1997) Measuring the quality of life of clients with severe mental illness: a review of instruments. *Psychiatric Rehabilitation Journal*, 20, 33–34.

Ware, J.T., Kosinski, M., Keller, S.D. (1996) A 12-Item Short-Form Health Survey. *Medical Care*, 34, 220–233.

WHO (1980) *International Classification of Impairment Disability and Handicap.* Geneva: WHO.

World Health Organisation (1988) *Psychiatric Disability Schedule.* Geneva: WHO

Wittchen, H.U. and Eassau, C.A. (1993) An overview of the Composite International Diagnostic Interview (CIDI). *International Journal of Methods in Psychiatric Research*, 3, 79–85.

10 | *The needs of people with mental disorders*

Mike Slade and Gyles Glover

Introduction

The term 'need' has become increasingly influential in European psychiatric practice. In Britain, government policy recently has restated the importance of needs assessment underpinning the planning, development and evaluation of mental health services (NHS Executive, 1998). At the individual level, all mental health and social care should be provided on the basis of need. At the population level, funding allocation is intended to match the needs of the population, so that whether or not overall resources are adequate, efficiency and equity are achieved.

This chapter will provide a conceptual overview of the meaning of the term 'need', at both the individual and population level. The context of health politics in Britain will then be described, followed by a description of available approaches to needs assessment. Finally, issues in using needs assessment information will be considered.

Needs at the individual level

At the individual level, the concept of need has been grounded in various theories. Maslow (1954) put forward a theory of motivation in terms of a hierarchy of needs: physiological; safety; belongingness and love; esteem; and self-actualization. Different types of need have been identified by Bradshaw (1972): felt (experienced); expressed (experienced and communicated); normative (judgement of professionals); and comparative (based on comparison with the position of other individuals or reference groups). This takes account of the different perceptions of need that can exist. Within health care, the concept of need has been used to inform service provision. It is taken to mean the ability to benefit in some way from health care (Stevens and Gabbay, 1991), and thus distinguished from demand (what the person asks for) and supply (services given). For example, the MRC Needs for Care Assessment Schedule (NCA) is premised on the assumption that need is "a normative concept which is to be defined by experts" (Bebbington, 1992, p. 107).

Some assessments of need focus on strengths, with a need indicating an area of potential development, while others focus on deficits, in which needs are for treatment. Holloway (1994) calls these the 'implicit' and 'psychiatric' models of mental disorder, and highlights key issues such as the legitimacy of professional knowledge, the proper location of the user's perspective and the primacy of the person's stated wishes. He suggests that the different ideological models create difficulties in communication between psychiatrists and community staff. A disparity exists in practice, as shown by a Joseph Rowntree Foundation study of how social services practitioners assess need, which found that instinct-guided assessments and moral judgements were common (Ellis, 1993).

The model of need which is used will impact on individual clinical practice. For example, what response is appropriate when patient and clinician disagree about either the problem or the proposed solution? This happens frequently, for reasons ranging from patient antipathy towards mental health practitioners to clinician preference for one treatment modality (e.g. psychological therapy or pharmacotherapy) over another. One approach is to give primacy to the staff view, another to give primacy to the patient's view, and a third to attempt to negotiate. Each approach will lead to a different pattern of therapeutic interactions.

Population needs

In the attempt to move from considering the needs of mentally ill individuals to establishing overall community needs, these complexities are compounded in three ways. Firstly, the needs of a wider range of individuals must be considered. These include immediate carers, people such as neighbours, and local authority staff, for example in housing and environmental health. Secondly, the translation of counts of treatment-amenable problems or service needs into institutional or staff provision requirements raises questions about service design models. What sort of agency should provide particular services, in what type of setting and how much user choice in service style should be supported by public funding authorities? Finally, since reasonable requests for assistance are likely to outstrip available resources, the practical questions which emerge relate to relative rather than absolute need. Thus we need to determine not only the existence and scale of needs, but also their importance in comparison with each other.

The overall level of needs for mental health services varies between places, reflecting differences in the prevalence of disorders. The nature of need has also changed over recent decades, reflecting developments in therapeutic capabilities, particularly in the provision of psychological therapies, changes in the extent to which severely mentally ill peoples' service needs have been moulded by institutionalization, and also possibly secular trends in the incidence of schizophrenia (Der et al., 1990).

Administrative and political context

In England, changes in administrative arrangements have influenced the tone of writing in this area. The inception of the National Health Service in 1949 removed responsibility for most types of mental health care from county authorities. Initially, 14 regional level health care authorities with a strategic rather than managerial remit assumed this function in collaboration with the central government department. Not until the advent of the market structure in 1991 did a single authority at reasonably local level once again acquire both the administrative and financial responsibility for providing health care to mentally ill people from geographically defined areas (Secretaries of State, 1989). While parallel responsibility for social care provision has rested throughout this period with local government, which has always had clear geographic domains, the boundary between health and social care has shifted considerably as care for chronically mentally ill people has moved from asylums to community-based services.

Studies from the 1960s to the 1980s reflect the methodological developments made possible by the development of case registers, and by improvements in mental hospital statistics within the Health Service (e.g. Tooth and Brooke, 1961; Wing, 1989) While these studies elegantly develop the conceptual framework, they seem to lack a clear target for their conclusions. In contrast, literature of the 1990s provides practical advice to the new health care purchasing authorities, with a recognition that, notwithstanding the imprecision of available evidence, contracts must be signed and budgets spent (e.g. Conway et al., 1994; Wing, 1994; Johnson et al., 1996).

Measures to assess individual need

Brewin (1992) categorizes definitions of need within mental health care into three types: (i) a lack of health; (ii) a lack of access to services or institutions; and (iii) a lack of action by lay or professional mental health workers. Existing needs assessment tools used in mental health services will be reviewed using these three categories.

Needs for improved health

The Community Care Act states that needs are "the requirements of individuals to enable them to achieve, maintain or restore an acceptable level of social independence or quality of life" (Department of Health Social Services Inspectorate, 1991, p. 10). This definition equates need with social disablement, which occurs when a person experiences lowered psychological, social and physical functioning in comparison with the norms of society (Wing, 1986). Indeed, involvement with psychiatric services generally occurs only when psychiatric illness is compounded by problems in social functioning (Wykes and Hurry, 1991). Three categories of social functioning measures have been identified: social attainment measures, social role performance measures and instrumental behaviour measures (Wykes and Hurry, 1991).

Social attainments are achievements in the major life roles, such as marriage and employment. They have the advantage of being easily measurable with relatively high reliability, and so are particularly suited to large-scale, nomothetic studies and epidemiological research. For example, at a population level, significantly higher admission rates are associated with being unmarried, living alone, social deprivation and drug misuse (Jarman, 1992), and there is a large negative correlation between recovery from schizophrenia and unemployment (Warner, 1985). However, it is difficult to establish whether variables being measured are in a causal or correlative relationship. Further shortcomings of this approach are reviewed by Wykes and Hurry (1991).

Social role performance measures relate to how well a person is coping in their major roles of work, relationships, home and self-care. They give a more in-depth assessment of a person's performance than social attainment measures, and cover a wide range of subdivided areas, such as instrumental and affective tasks (Weissman, 1975). It can be difficult to take account of the person's social and cultural background, although this has been attempted by using consensual professional judgement, e.g. the SSIAM (Gurland *et al.*, 1972), or by using normative scales (e.g. Cochrane and Stopes-Roe, 1977). Definitions of what constitutes pathological lack of function are culture specific, although some scales have attempted to produce culture-free thresholds—87% of a general population sample had no major difficulties in role areas assessed using the MRC Social Role Performance Schedule, which the authors suggest is evidence that difficulties being measured transcend cultural boundaries (Hurry and Sturt, 1981).

The Camberwell Assessment of Need (CAN) addresses this issue by separate staff and service user assessments (Phelan *et al.*, 1995), and is intended specifically to meet the requirements of the National Health Service and Community Care Act (1990). Clinical, research and brief versions of the CAN have been developed, all suitable for making a comprehensive assessment of the health and social needs of adults with severe mental illness. Forensic, older adult and learning disability versions have been developed, and translations have been made into 13 other languages. The CAN is suitable for routine clinical use, and has been used extensively as an outcome measure in intervention studies (Slade *et al.*, 1999).

Instrumental measures record social behaviour, and are more suited to a detailed assessment of individual psychiatric patients, some of whom may not fulfil many life roles. A detailed description of behaviour allows consideration of cultural factors when analysing the data. The Clifton Assessment Procedures for the Elderly (CAPE) scale entails cognitive assessment and a behaviour rating scale, which is combined to give a measure of dependency (Pattie and Gilleard, 1976). The Social Behaviour Scale (SBS) assesses 21 types of behaviour, each of which are deemed to be prerequisites for independent social functioning (Wykes and Sturt, 1986). REHAB assesses both general and deviant behaviour (Baker and Hall, 1988). Both SBS and REHAB are derived from the Ward Behavior Rating Scale (Wing, 1961). Instrumental measures do not take account of the context in which behaviour takes place—the person with hygiene problems who does not have access to pleasant washing facilities. They are often designed for use with very disabled people, and so rely on staff reports which may not take account of the person's perceptions of their needs.

Social functioning measures have been used for some time to identify and quantify levels of need in a psychiatric population (Mann and Cree, 1976). For instance, the SBS has been used to assess care needs in a study of long-term psychiatric patients under the Camberwell community services (Wykes *et al.*, 1985). However, there is as yet no consensus on what social functioning scales should measure, so that they tend to be an enumeration of symptoms. For example, categories in the SBS include 'panic attacks and phobias' and 'overactivity and restlessness' (Wykes and Sturt, 1986). Whilst undoubtedly all important areas to consider, they can lead to a client's psychiatric symptomatology being assessed, rather than their needs.

Needs for services

The second category of needs assessment schedules suggested by Brewin incorporates those measuring access to psychiatric services. Underlying these measures is the assumption that an unmet need indicates a lack of access to some form of psychiatric service. This category is used for informing the development of mental health services. It is less appropriate at an individual level, since it assesses needs through the filter of existing psychiatric services.

The Mini Finland Health Survey equated unmet need with an inadequate level of service response for the severity of problem (Lehtinen *et al.*, 1990). Need of care was assessed using self-reports, benefit information, the 36-item General Health Questionnaire (GHQ) and the short version of the Present State Examination. Sixty percent of people in need were not receiving any treatment, and self-perceived need was reported by 7.3% whereas clinically assessed need was found in 17.4% of subjects. No attempt was made to discriminate types of need.

The National Institute of Mental Health Epidemiologic Catchment Area programme collected data on psychiatric disorder prevalence (Regier *et al.*, 1984), using the Diagnostic Interview Schedule (DIS) (Robins *et al.*, 1981), supplemented by questionnaires covering socioeconomic factors, physical health, psychotropic medication, life events and social support networks. A lower estimate of need in the (USA) population was made at 7.1%, with an upper bound of 34.5%. Although only considering emotional problems, no account was taken of cultural factors in seeking help from medical professionals.

The Community Placement Questionnaire (CPQ) is designed to inform placing of long-term residents of psychiatric hospitals which are scheduled for closure (Clifford *et al.*, 1991). Three types of data are recorded: basic epidemiological data, factors affecting placement (social skills, problem behaviours, social contact) and community placement possibilities (daytime activities, accommodation). The CPQ is a planning tool, and the sacrifice of precision for utility is acknowledged. However, the design accords with Hall's principles for ward rating scales: reliability; validity; rational scale selection; specification of the observation period; and the provision of norms for defined patient groups (Hall, 1980).

Various difficulties arise in using any assessment of need for services to infer an individual user's needs. Most of the existing scales are designed for use with long-term patients, prior to resettlement. This limits their utility for the psychiatric population, and they tend to rely on staff reports. The data being collected typically are not sensitive to change, as would be desirable in assessing the needs of an individual. Scales also tend to consider institutional services rather than individual needs, oriented as they are to large-scale planning rather than individual assessment. Finally, assessments are used for informing the provision of broad service categories, and therefore may not assess individual needs in a discriminating manner.

Needs for action

The final category of needs assessment schedules measure the need for action by professional or lay mental health workers. The MRC NCA defines need as present when the person's functioning falls below a specified level *due to a potentially remediable cause* (Brewin *et al.*, 1987). This reduces the extent to which assessment is needs-led, since intervention effectiveness rather than need is being assessed. More recent formulations of the schedule have introduced a new category of 'no meetable need' (Mangen and Brewin, 1991). Modified versions of the NCA have been used with diabetics (Brewin *et al.*, 1991) and relatives (MacCarthy *et al.*, 1989), and in cross-cultural studies (LeSage *et al.*, 1991).

There are difficulties in assessing when there is an available intervention which would be at least partly effective—deciding that a treatment has not worked is seldom easy. There is also a cultural bias in stating what constitutes a problematic level of functioning requiring intervention. However, as Bebbington notes, "the inevitable value judgements inherent in the procedure have the virtue of being public and consequently accessible to argument" (Bebbington, 1992, p. 106).

Measures to assess population need

Measures to assess population-based need can be classified by the data and by the analytical approaches they use. Three types of data commonly are used. The most readily accessible documents the use of current mental health services. While this can be criticized as reflecting only current service provision, its ready availability and nationwide coverage mean that it is used extensively, particularly for the development of needs indices, described below. The failure of simple service activity statistics to indicate the adequacy of the services described can be tackled by asking simple additional questions, an approach which has been used with telling political effect by the Research Unit of the Royal College of Psychiatrists. Using a simple battery of questions, repeated at intervals, about the signs of excess pressure on in-patient mental health services in London, they produced evidence which did much to keep London's mental health services high on the political agenda (Audini *et al.*, 1995).

Secondly, direct surveys of population-based morbidity, using epidemiological instruments, undertaken on a small or a large scale, offer a perspective independent of service activity. Major national studies have been undertaken in the USA (Regier *et al.*, 1984) and the UK (Jenkins *et al.*, 1997a). These give precise estimations of the overall prevalence of the more common mental disorders. From a needs assessment perspective, one of the more interesting aspect of these studies is their evidence about the limited extent to which individuals with treatable mental health problems make use of services which could help them (Shapiro *et al.*, 1984; Brugha, 1995).

Simple population-based samples are very inefficient in estimating the prevalence of relatively rare conditions such as schizophrenia. Studies thus tend to use two-stage procedures, with a relatively brief initial screening process applied to a large number of people followed by in-depth interviews for a selected few. 'Booster' samples, perhaps including all the known psychiatric patients for the areas surveyed, may be sought through mental health services (Jenkins *et al.*, 1997b). Population surveys depend on the identification of randomly sampled individuals. Some types of mental health problem, notably substance misuse, commonly are associated with socially marginal lifestyles, making it likely that sufferers will be under-represented systematically by traditional population sampling approaches. More sophisticated sampling approaches, such as capture–recapture methods, have been used for these situations (Hay and McKeganey, 1996).

The third type of data relate to the views of local people. Local needs assessment studies entail a structured approach to eliciting the views of service users, their carers, interested voluntary sector organizations and all statutory agencies with responsibilities in the area. Smith (1998) has described how this type of study can be integrated into the overall planning process.

A range of analytical approaches has been employed. Beyond the realm of direct descriptive statistics with local survey data, these seek to explore variations in need either over time or between places. In the 1960s and early 1970s, developing awareness of the fall in asylum populations sparked debate about how to predict the future course and eventual end point of this decline (Tooth and Brooke, 1961). Recent work has attempted to quantify the impact of this shift in service design on requirements for acute admission facilities.

More recently, in England, government initiatives have tried to base the allocation of money between areas on the morbidity as well as the size of their populations. This has led to studies modelling this variation. The first widely used index (Jarman, 1983) was developed on the basis of consensus between GPs about patient characteristics associated with high use of primary care services. While developed for wider purposes, this was shown to relate reasonably closely to variations in psychiatric admission. Later indices have been established by statistical modelling exercises seeking to quantify the relationship between social variables measured in censuses and either service use (Thornicroft, 1991; Carr-Hill *et al.*, 1994; Glover *et al.*, 1998) or population-based epidemiological findings. The variation between places in the prevalence of the less severe types of mental illness commonly dealt with in primary care is less that that for problems usually managed by specialist mental health services, which again is much less than that observed for forensic services. Thus models developed for one level of care should not be used to estimate patterns of need for other levels.

In practice, no single approach to assessing the needs of a population will suffice. Needs assessment at this level requires the integration of many perspectives. The Kings Fund review of London's mental health services (Johnson *et al.*, 1997) illustrates how a detailed perspective can be assembled from many fragments of evidence, each of which would be inadequate in isolation.

Issues in needs assessment

Whose views should be assessed?

There is now considerable evidence that staff and patient assessments of need differ (MacCarthy *et al.*, 1986; Slade *et al.*, 1996, 1998). In Britain, the National Health Service and Community Care Act (1990) requires that *"all users ... should be encouraged to participate to the limit of their capacity. ... Where it is impossible to reconcile*

*different perceptions, these **differences should be acknowledged and recorded**"* (Department of Health SSI, 1991a, pp. 51 and 53). The user group MIND (The National Association for Mental Health) advocate a policy framework based on *"the actual wishes and needs of people who use the service"* (Sayce, 1990). It is therefore important for scientific, political and ethical reasons to overcome the power differential between staff and patients, and to facilitate active patient involvement. The involvement of informal carers is also encouraged, although not yet required. In the future, it may be that other people contribute to the assessment, such as a community member to comment on the risk of violence by the person to others in society. It is therefore not possible to have a single assessment of need, since each person assessed will have their own perceptions.

Who should assess need?

The person undertaking an assessment will have their own agenda. Practitioners are influenced by their training, and will be more skilled at (and, given their choice of profession, often more interested in) some areas of need than others. For example, a study investigating how mental health professionals in Australia, England and India prioritize needs found that professional subgroups demonstrated a tendency to rate according to emphasis in training (Slade, 1996). Thus five times as many occupational therapists rated benefits as a priority area for help as any other profession, social workers gave the highest priority of any profession to daytime activities, and clinical psychologists rated accommodation needs relatively low. The implication is that the results of an assessment of need will differ according to who is doing the assessment.

Can individual needs be aggregated to population levels?

While it is theoretically feasible to undertake routine standardized needs assessments on all patients within a service, this approach alone has three drawbacks. Firstly, the prevailing culture of clinical practice does not encourage the routine use of standardized assessment (Bilbrey and Bilbrey, 1995; Walter *et al.*, 1996; Stein, 1999). This is not seen universally as a valued clinical activity, and experience from studies which involve the routine collection of simple outcome measures suggests that there may be substantial professional resistance to widespread use of routine outcome measures. Secondly, there is not yet a sufficiently developed information infrastructure to support the national collection, management and analysis of such data. Thirdly, even if individual needs assessments were aggregated nationally, the diversity of views (patient, staff, carer, tax-payer) would make a shared interpretation of the data problematic.

Why is the assessment being carried out?

As described, assessment can be at the individual or population level. At the individual level, the purpose of assessing need can vary. The goal for the (potential) service user may be to communicate clearly their perceptions of their difficulties. The mental health professional is concerned with assessing whether the person's unmet needs are sufficiently serious to merit interventions by services. For informal carers, assessment is an opportunity both to act as advocates for the mentally ill person and to access support and respite services for themselves. A further goal of assessment is to address the social and political concern with safety both to the public and to the mentally ill person.

Population level assessment can be at the sector or district level, to assess whether the pattern of services being provided locally is the best use of available resources. It can also be at a national level, to determine whether adequate resources are being provided to meet the needs of mentally ill people. Population assessments ideally involve aggregating information from individual assessments, but the disparity in current needs assessment methodologies precludes this approach. Proxy measures (e.g. bed usage, day care facilities) are therefore used to infer the level of need in the population. For example, El-Guebaly and

colleagues (1993) equate meeting needs with reducing the shortage of psychiatrists.

In practice, the principal outcome of population-based needs assessment, resource allocation, is not a neat business. Any study to identify an equitable new allocation pattern creates winners and losers. Since the results only indicate relative levels of need, losers inevitably argue that their current absolute level of resourcing is already inadequate. Essentially political decisions are thus introduced about how quickly resources should be reassigned to achieve the new idea of 'equity', and whether the shift should be achieved by actual transfer or by differential growth. Shifts of revenue resources are much easier than shifts of capital, but moving the former out of step with the latter may lead to inefficiencies.

At the same time, special resources (as always) are likely to be made available to encourage implementation of currently promising service innovations. This process may push the overall distribution of funds away from the point of equity. It is rare for this dimension to be considered formally in the allocation of special allowances.

At a local level, service innovations which are indicated by needs assessment work can seldom all be implemented at once. Needs studies tend to identify a range of pressing gaps in services, only some of which can be funded in the short term. Thus questions of the relative importance of needs identified arise. Of the methodologies identified above, only local consensus surveys can shed any light on this essentially value-based question. Issues of timeliness, political necessity, expedience, synergy and leadership are all also likely to influence which of the many possible service developments eventually is implemented.

Using individual needs assessments to inform future interventions

Needs assessment can be used to inform decisions about future interventions. For example, if day centre attendance has had a beneficial impact on the person's reported satisfaction with life, increased their life experiences and reduced their level of need, then it is probably an appropriate intervention to continue. However, more often, there is a mixed picture, and in these cases particular outcomes need to be prioritized. This requires knowledge about the natural course of the mental illness (Ruggeri and Tansella, 1995), and the same factors confound the necessary epidemiological research, since untreated conditions are rarely encountered. Diagnosis is known to be a poor predictor of service utilization (McCrone and Strathdee, 1994). Schizophrenia is the most researched major mental disorder, with various factors implicated in outcome, including symptom severity, stressful events, living and working conditions and social support (McGlashan, 1991; Jablensky *et al.*, 1992). The inter-relationship of these factors is important but unclear. If we knew, for example, that a good social network caused (rather than was associated with) lower relapse rates, then the need for an increased social network could be prioritized over some other needs. Given the lack of clarity about which factors give a better outcome, the decision about which needs of a person should be prioritized and by what interventions cannot be fully informed.

This is not simply an academic debate, since these choices are made in day to day clinical work. It is common that there is no single set of interventions which maximizes all outcome criteria, so some interventions are given at the expense of others. For example, patients who refuse neuroleptic medication (i.e. are unsatisfied with the quality of their care) because of the associated side effects (i.e. its deleterious effect on their satisfaction with life) can, under certain circumstances, be compelled to accept it. The rationale for this typically will be that that their disability or the burden on their care-giver will be reduced. Implicit in this rationale is the assumption that minimizing disability and care-giver burden is, in some circumstances, more important than life experiences (e.g. compulsory hospitalization) and satisfaction. Mental health professionals are aware of these issues, and consider all outcome criteria as important. However, the choice of one intervention will preclude others, so should be as informed as possible. There is a need for more epidemiological information about the inter-relationship of vari-

ous outcome criteria, and which are the most helpful prognostic indicators.

Although best practice is not clear, good practice has evolved and should be disseminated. For example, the CAN involves assessing the perceptions of both mental health service staff and users separately (Phelan *et al.*, 1995), thus facilitating an active, collaborative process of negotiation in identifying and prioritizing needs. The establishment of a standard approach to needs assessment would allow data to be aggregated nationally, so that the level and targeting of resources can be debated more rationally.

Conclusion

In summary, assessment of need can involve compromises between desirable and attainable information, and value-based judgements about how and what to measure. However, it is a politically, ethically and scientifically important concept, and so assessment should be as rigorous and comprehensive as possible. For both individual and population level needs assessment, this means that assessment should cover a wide range of health and social domains, should take account of different perspectives (e.g. patient, staff) and should be a separate process from treatment and resourcing decisions.

In the longer term, a more sophisticated understanding of exactly what is being measured is required, along with a consensus about what information is to be collected. This will allows information collected locally to be aggregated to a national level, and information collected nationally to be applied locally.

References

Audini, B., Crowe, M., Feldman, J., Higgitt, A., Kent, A., Lelliot, P. *et al.* (1995) Monitoring inner London mental illness services. *Psychiatric Bulletin*, 19, 276–280.

Baker, R. and Hall, J. (1988) REHAB: a new assessment instrument for chronic psychiatric patients. *Schizophrenia Bulletin*, 14, 97–111.

Bebbington, P. (1992) Assessing the need for psychiatric treatment at the district level: the role of surveys. In: Thornicroft, G., Brewin, C. and Wing, J. (eds), *Measuring Mental Health Needs*. London: Royal College of Psychiatrists, pp. 99–117.

Bilbrey, J. and Bilbrey, P. (1995) Judging, trusting and utilizing outcomes data: a survey of behavioral healthcare payors. *Behavioral Healthcare Tomorrow*, 4, 62–65.

Bradshaw, J. (1972) A taxonomy of social need. In: McLachlan, G. (ed.), *Problems and Progress in Medical Care: Essays on Current Research* (7th series). London: Oxford University Press, pp. 69–82.

Brewin, C. (1992) Measuring individual needs for care and services. In: Thornicroft, G., Brewin, C. and Wing, J. (eds), *Measuring Mental Health Needs*. London: Royal College of Psychiatrists.

Brewin, C., Wing, J., Mangen, S., Brugha, T. and MacCarthy, B. (1987) Principles and practice of measuring needs in the long-term mentally ill: the MRC Needs for Care Assessment. *Psychological Medicine*, 17, 971–981.

Brewin, C., Bradley, C. and Home, P. (1991) Measuring needs in patients with diabetes. In Bradley, C., Home, P. and Christie, M. (eds.), *The Technology of Diabetes Care*. Reading: Harwood, pp. 142–155.

Brugha, T.S. (1995) Depression undertreatment: lost cohorts, lost opportunities? *Psychological Medicine*, 25, 3–6.

Carr-Hill, R.A., Hardman, G., Martin, S., Peacock, S., Sheldon, T.A. and Smith, P. (1994) *A Formula for Distributing NHS Revenues Based on Small Area Use of Hospital Beds*. York: Centre for Health Economics, University of York.

Clifford, P., Charman, A., Webb, Y., Craig, T. and Cowan, D. (1991) Planning for community care: the Community Placement Questionnaire. *British Journal of Clinical Psychology*, 30, 193–211.

Cochrane, R. and Stopes-Roe, M. (1977) Psychological and social adjustment of Asian immigrants to Britain: a community survey. *Social Psychiatry*, 12, 195–206.

Conway, M., Melzer, D., Shepherd, G. and Troop, P. (1994) *A Companion to Purchasing Adult Mental Health Services*. Oxford: Anglia and Oxford Regional Health Authority.

Department of Health Social Services Inspectorate (1991) *Care Management and Assessment: Practitioners' Guide*. London: HMSO.

Der, G., Gupta, S. and Murray, R. (1990) Is schizophrenia disappearing? *Lancet*, 35, 86–88.

El-Guebaly, N., Kingstone, E., Rae-Grant, Q. and Fyfe, I. (1993) The geographical distribution of psychiatrists in Canada: unmet needs and remedial strategies. *Canadian Journal of Psychiatry*, 38, 212–216.

Ellis, K. (1993) *Squaring the Circle: User and Carer Participation in Needs Assessment*. York: Joseph Rowntree Foundation.

Glover, G.R., Robin, E., Emami, J. and Arabsheibani, G.R. (1998) A needs index for mental health care. *Social Psychiatry and Psychiatric Epidemiology*, 33, 89–96.

Goldberg, D. (1972) *The Detection of Psychiatric Symptoms by Questionnaire. Maudsley Monograph 21*. London: Oxford University Press.

Gurland, B., Yorkstone, N., Stone, A. and Frank, J. (1972) The Structured and Scaled Interview to Assess Maladjustment (SSIAM) 1. Description, rationale and development. *Archives of General Psychiatry*, 27, 264–267.

Hall, J. (1980) Ward rating scales for long-stay patients: a review. *Psychological Medicine*, 10, 277–288.

Hay, G. and Mckeganey, N. (1996) Estimating the prevalence of drug misuse in Dundee, Scotland: an application of capture–recapture methods. *Journal of Epidemiology and Community Health*, 50, 469–472.

Holloway, F. (1993) Need in community psychiatry: a consensus is required. *Psychiatric Bulletin*, 18, 321–323.

Hurry, J. and Sturt, E. (1981) Social performance in a population sample: relation to psychiatric symptoms. In Wing, J., Bebbington, P. and Robbins, L. (eds), *What is a Case*. London: Grant McIntyre, pp. 202–213.

Jablensky, A., Sartorius, N., Ernberg, G., Anker, M., Cooper, J. and Day, R. (1992) *Schizophrenia: Manifestations, Incidence and Course in Different Cultures. A World Health Organisation Ten-country Study. Psychological Medicine Monograph* Supplement 20. Cambridge: Cambridge University Press.

Jarman, B. (1983) Identification of underprivileged areas. *British Medical Journal— Clinical Research*, 286, 1705–1709.

Jarman, B., Hirsch, S., White, P. and Driscoll, R. (1992) Predicting psychiatric admission rates. *British Medical Journal*, 304, 1146–1151.

Jenkins, R., Lewis, G., Bebbington, P., Brugha, T., Farrell, M., Gill, B. *et al.* (1997a) The National Psychiatric Morbidity surveys of Great Britain—initial findings from the household survey. *Psychological Medicine*, 27, 775–789.

Jenkins, R., Bebbington, P., Brugha, T., Farrell, M., Gill, B., Lewis, G. *et al.* (1997b) The National Psychiatric Morbidity surveys of Great Britain—strategy and methods. *Psychological Medicine*, 27, 765–774.

Johnson, S., Thornicroft, G. and Strathdee, G. (1996) Assessing population needs. In: Thornicroft, G. and Strathdee, G. (eds), *Commissioning Mental Health Services*. London: HMSO, pp. 37–52.

Johnson, S., Ramsay, R., Thornicroft, G., Brooks, L., Lelliot, P., Peck, E. *et al.* (1997) *London's Mental Health. The Report of the Kings Fund Commission.* London: Kings Fund Publishing.

Karnofsky, D., Abelmann, W. and Craver, L. (1948) The use of nitrogen mushrooms in the palliative treatment of carcinoma. *Cancer*, 1, 634–656.

Lehtinen, V., Joukamaa, M., Jyrkinen, E., Lahtela, K., Raitasala, R., Maatela, J. and Aromaa, A. (1990) Need for mental health services of the adult population in Finland: results from the Mini Finland Health Survey. *Acta Psychiatrica Scandinavica*, 81, 426–431.

LeSage, A., Mignolli, G. and Faccincani, C. (1991) Standardised assessment of the needs for care in a cohort of patients with schizophrenic psychoses. *Psychological Medicine* 19 (Suppl.), 426–431.

MacCarthy, B., Benson, J. and Brewin, C. (1986) Task motivation and problem appraisal in long-term psychiatric patients. *Psychological Medicine*, 16, 431–438.

MacCarthy, B., LeSage, A., Brewin, C., Brugha , T., Mangen, S. and Wing, J. (1989) Needs for care among relatives of long-term users of day care. *Psychological Medicine*, 19, 725–736.

Mangen, S. and Brewin, C. (1991) The measurement of need. In: Bebbington, P. (ed.), *Social Psychiatry: Theory, Methodology, and Practice*. New Brunswick, NJ: Transaction Press, pp. 163–181.

Mann, S. and Cree, W. (1976) 'New' long-stay psychiatric patients: a national sample of fifteen mental hospitals in England and Wales 1972/3. *Psychological Medicine*, 6, 603–616.

Maslow, A. (1954) *Motivation and Personality*. New York: Harper and Row.

McCrone, P. and Strathdee, G. (1994) Needs not diagnosis: towards a more rational approach to community mental health resourcing in Britain. *International Journal of Social Psychiatry*, 40, 79–86.

McGlashan, T. (1991) Selective review of recent North American long-term follow-up studies of schizophrenia. In: Mirin, S., Grosset, J. and Grob, J. (eds), *Psychiatric Treatment: Advances in Outcome Research*. Washington, DC: American Psychiatric Press, pp. 121–134.

NHS Executive (1998) *Modernising Mental Health Services: Safe, Sound and Supportive*. London: HMSO

Pattie, A. and Gilleard, C. (1976) The Clifton Assessment Schedule—further validation of a psychogeriatric assessment schedule. *British Journal of Psychiatry*, 129, 68–72.

Phelan, M., Slade, M., Thornicroft, G., Dunn, G., Holloway, F., Wykes, T., Strathdee, G., Loftus, L., McCrone, P. and Hayward, P. (1995) The Camberwell Assessment of Need (CAN): the validity and reliability of an instrument to assess the needs of people with severe mental illness. *British Journal of Psychiatry*, 167, 589–595.

Regier, D., Myers, J., Kramer, M., Robins, L., Blazer, D., Hough, R., Eaton, W. and Locke, B. (1984) The NIMH Epidemiologic Catchment Area Program: historical context, major objectives and study population characteristics. *Archives of General Psychiatry*, 41, 934–941.

Robins, L., Helzer, J., Croughan, J. and Ratcliff, K. (1981) National Institute of Mental Health Diagnostic Interview Schedule: its history, characteristics and validity. *Archives of General Psychiatry*, 38, 381–389.

Ruggeri, M. and Tansella, M. (1995) Evaluating outcome in mental health care. *Current Opinion in Psychiatry*, 8, 116–121.

Sayce, L. (1990) *Waiting for Community Care: Implications of Government Policy for 1991*. London: MIND publications.

Secretaries of State (1989) *Working for Patients*. Cm 555. London: HMSO.

Shapiro, S., Skinner, E.A., Kessler, L.G., Von Korff, M., German, P.S. *et al.* (1984) Utilization of health and mental health services. Three Epidemiologic Catchment Area sites. *Archives of General Psychiatry*, 41, 971–978.

Slade, M. (1996) Assessing the needs of the severely mentally ill: cultural and professional differences. *International Journal of Social Psychiatry*, 42, 1–9.

Slade, M., Phelan, M., Thornicroft, G. and Parkman, S. (1996) The Camberwell Assessment of Need (CAN): comparison of assessments by staff and patients of the needs of the severely mentally ill. *Social Psychiatry and Psychiatric Epidemiology*, 31, 109–113.

Slade, M., Phelan, M. and Thornicroft, G. (1998) A comparison of needs assessed by staff and an epidemiologically representative sample of patients with psychosis, *Psychological Medicine*, 28, 543–550.

Slade, M., Loftus, L., Phelan, M., Thornicroft, G. and Wykes, T. (1999) *The Camberwell Assessment of Need*. London: Gaskell.

Smith, H. (1998) Needs assessment in mental health services: the DISC framework. *Journal of Public Health Medicine*, 20, 154–160.

Stein, G.S. (1999) Usefulness of the Health of the Nation Outcome Scale. *British Journal of Psychiatry*, 174, 375–377.

Stevens, A. and Gabbay, J. (1991) Needs assessment needs assessment. *Health Trends*, 23, 20–23.

Thornicroft, G. (1991) Social deprivation and rates of treated mental disorder. Developing statistical models to predict psychiatric service utilisation. *British Journal of Psychiatry*, 158, 475–484.

Tooth, G.C. and Brooke, E.M. (1961) Trends in the mental hospital population and their effect on future planning. *Lancet*, i, 710

Walter, G., Kirkby, K., Marks, I. *et al.* (1996) Outcome measurement sharing experiences in Australia. *Australasian Psychiatry*, 4, 316–318.

Warner, R. (1985) *Recovery from Schizophrenia. Psychiatric and Political Economy.* London: Routledge and Kegan Paul.

Weissman, M. (1975) The assessment of social adjustment by patient self-report. *Archives of General Psychiatry*, 32, 357–365.

Wing, J. (1961) *A Simple and Reliable Subclassification of Chronic Schizophrenia.* Cambridge: Cambridge University Press.

Wing, J. (1986) The cycle of planning and evaluation. In: Wing, J. (ed.), *Long-term Community Care: Experience in a London Borough. Psychological Medicine Monograph* Supplement No. 2, 41–55.

Wing J. (1989) Health Services Planning and Research. *Contributions from Psychiatric Case Registers.* London: Royal College of Psychiatrists, Gaskell imprint.

Wing, J.K. (1994) Mental illness. In: Stevens, A. and Raftery, J. (eds), *Health Care Needs Assessment*, Vol. 2. Oxford: Ratcliffe Medical Press, pp. 202–304.

Wykes, T. and Hurry, J. (1991) Social behaviour and psychiatric disorders. In: Bebbington, P. (ed.), *Social Psychiatry: Theory, Methodology, and Practice.* New Brunswick, NJ: Transaction Press, pp. 183–208.

Wykes, T. and Sturt, E. (1986) The measurement of social behaviour in psychiatric patients: an assessment of the reliability and validity of the SBS Schedule. *British Journal of Psychiatry*, 148, 1–11.

Wykes, T., Sturt, E. and Creer, C. (1985) The assessment of patients' needs for community care. *Social Psychiatry*, 20, 76–85.

11 | *The costs of mental disorder*

Martin Knapp

The relevance of economics

The impacts of mental illness are wide-ranging, often long lasting and sometimes profound. They are felt not only by those people who are ill, but also by their families, neighbours and the wider society. Some of those impacts can be seen as 'economic', having effects associated with personal income, the ability to work, productive contributions to the national economy or the utilization of treatment and support services. These economic impacts are often considerable, as we show in this chapter. Indeed, because increasing attention has been focused upon them by health care decision makers, politicians, the general public and others, their true scale is beginning to be appreciated more widely. However, we need to keep the economic perspectives and issues in context. They should not, for example, be elevated to a position where they dominate the personal and family pain and impaired quality of life so often associated with mental illness.

What are the sources of interest in these economic impacts? One is this very recognition that the costs of mental disorders are likely to be substantial, falling on those who are ill, their families and the national economy. A second is that the professional, pharmaceutical and other resources needed to treat these disorders are not sufficient to meet all assessed needs: scarcity is endemic. In the face of scarcity, choices have to be made between alternative uses of the same resource or service, which raises questions about comparative costs and effects.

Another factor generating interest in the economics of mental illness is the seemingly high cost of some new treatment modalities. The selective serotonin re-uptake inhibitors (SSRIs) for depression, atypical antipsychotics and cholinesterase inhibitors for Alzheimer's disease are all marketed at much higher prices than the older treatments they potentially could replace. Not surprisingly, many people feel there is an urgent need to determine whether the newer treatments are cost-effective.

In the context of these growing interests, the aim of this chapter is to look at the main economic consequences of mental illness. We initially organize the discussion around the main dimensions of economic impact: service utilization, lost employment, family and care-giver consequences, and so on. We then discuss how these impacts might be costed, although we should emphasize that it does not always make sense to try to express each of them in monetary terms. We also summarize estimates of the overall costs of some particular psychiatric disorders. This summary is more illustrative than comprehensive. The final section discusses the relevance of these estimates. This chapter will not, however, discuss the cost-effectiveness of particular care arrangements, service configurations or treatment modalities.

Economic impacts

What are the main economic impacts of mental illness, and how large are they? Some impacts are identified readily in principle and measured readily in practice. For instance, there is usually a close association between mental illness and the use of specialist psychiatric services, and the latter could be measured in terms of either the frequency and intensity of receipt or their costs. Other effects may be largely hidden from view or difficult to express in tangible terms. One example would be the effects of depression on performance at work, widely believed to be quite substantial but rarely quantified. Another would be the impact of some mental health problems on patients' families. In the discussion that follows, we identify and assess the likely importance of the main economic impacts. Potentially, each of them—whether readily identified or obscured, and whether easily quantified or not—can be seen as a cost. The methods used to arrive at cost measures are described in a later section.

Health service utilization

The most immediately and frequently measured economic consequences of mental illness are the costs of the health services, both specialist and generic, used by individuals. Working from the 1992/93 programme budgets of the National Health Service (NHS) in England and Wales, expenditure has been disaggregated by diagnostic group (NHS Executive, 1996). Table 11.1 summarizes the estimates for the main psychiatric diagnostic groups (discussed further in Patel and Knapp 1998).

The general approach in these calculations was to allocate total expenditure to the immediate (diagnostic) cause, based mainly on Hospital Episode Statistics. The resultant expenditure burden will often be lower than estimated in other studies—particularly cost-of-illness estimates—which (usually) also include costs of associated secondary diseases (cf. Andrews *et al.*, 1998). The estimates in Table 11.1 obviously could not include secondary effects without substantial double counting. Missed diagnoses of mental illness, or mental health symptoms taken as secondary to other symptoms for classification purposes, would result in underestimated costs. (Another reason for underestimation was that 15% of total expenditure could not be allocated to diagnostic categories.)

Notwithstanding these caveats, the expenditure figures in Table 11.1 make interesting reading. For instance, 22% of total national expenditure on in-patient services is accounted for by mental illness (and >5% by schizophrenia alone), compared with less than 4% of primary care expenditure and only 5% of the drugs budget. (The latter should be set in context, however, because they pre-date the recent 'revolution' in psychotropic medications.) The high in-patient proportions

have given further encouragement to the search for alternative, community-based care arrangements.

An illuminating perspective on the expenditure implications of different illnesses comes from Meerding *et al.* (1998). They used comprehensive data from most health care sectors in The Netherlands in 1994 to compute costs by ICD-9 code. Costs were based on prevalence but included only direct (service) costs. Across all ages, mental disorders accounted for 23.2% of total expenditure (learning disability 8.1%, dementia 5.6%, depression and anxiety 2.3%, schizophrenia 1.4%, alcohol and drug problems 0.8% and other mental disorders 5.0%). Meerding and colleagues also reported that one or both of the two most costly diagnostic groups in each of the five age bands used to categorize the population were mental disorders. (These expenditure figures include long-term care, including old people's homes, so that the denominator for these percentage calculations would be larger than for countries adopting a tighter definition of health care spending.)

Other formally delivered services

Health service providers cannot meet all of the needs of people with mental health problems. Indeed, they may be able to address only a fraction. Many seriously or chronically ill people consequently need support from a range of non-health professionals and organizations:

• Former long-stay psychiatric in-patients who moved to community care settings when two North London hospitals were closed used an enormously diverse collection of services, including social care, general and special housing, education, criminal justice, supported employment and welfare advice (Hallam *et al.*, 1995).

• Children with behavioural problems may require psychiatric treatment, but they are likely already to be in receipt of special educational inputs, and they may also be supported by social work agencies (Burns *et al.*, 1995; Health Advisory Service, 1995; John *et al.*, 1995).

Table 11.1 *Programme budget costs of mental health problems, England, 1992–1993, and percentage of total NHS expenditure (all ICD)*

Disease group and ICD-9 codes	Hospital in-patient[a] £m	%	Hospital out-patient £m	%	Primary care £m	%	Pharmaceutical £m	%	Community health £m	%	Social services £m	%
Dementia (290)	424	3.49	5	0.23	21	0.59	–	–	52	1.8	348	6.5
Other organic psychoses (291–294)	49	0.40	3	0.13	10	0.29	–	–	–	0.0	59	1.1
Schizophrenia (295)	652	5.37	1	0.04	2	0.05	32[b]	1.06	26	0.9	96	1.8
Other non-organic psychoses (296–299)	294	2.42	12	0.53	16	0.45	–	–	–	0.0	–	–
Neuroses (300)	75	0.62	29	2.13	39	1.09	96[c]	3.13	139	4.8	150	2.8
Alcohol and drug misuse (303–305)	51	0.42	11	0.50	3	0.09	5	0.17	160	5.5	75	1.4
Other neuroses (301, 302, 306–316)	230	1.89	73	3.18	37	1.06	26[d]	0.84	–	0.0	11	0.2
Learning disability (317–319)	839	6.91	6	0.26	–	0.00	–	–	212	7.3	745	
All mental health	2614	21.5	160	6.97	128	3.62	159	5.20	589	20.3	1484	27.7

Source: NHS Executive (1996).
[a]Includes residential provision (e.g. hostels) funded by NHS.
[b]Schizophrenia and other non-organic psychoses excluding depression.
[c]Depression (includes dementia, other organic psychoses, neuroses).
[d]Excluding depression.
[e]Other organic and non-organic psychoses combined.

- In many countries, responsibility for co-ordi-nating or financing continuing care for older people with dementia sits outside the health service (OECD, 1996).

- Psychiatric problems are particularly prevalent among the homeless and prison populations yet, for these groups, health care provision is often very limited or non-existent.

- Voluntary (non-profit) and private sector orga-nizations may play significant roles in mental health care, not just as providers but as fund-ing bodies, patient advocates and lobbyists for change (Knapp *et al.*, 1997).

Multi-agency care systems are the norm, not the exception. To overlook their roles in supporting and treating people with mental health problems is to risk a host of problems for service delivery and co-ordination, with obvious implications for patient quality of life, service effectiveness and system efficiency. Inter-agency boundary prob-lems and the perverse incentives they can engen-der lie at the root of many of the difficulties faced by mental health care systems (Kavanagh and Knapp, 1995).

Lost employment and reduced productivity

A large part of the global economic impact of mental illness stems from the difficulties that patients encounter in finding and keeping paid employment, and in contributing productively when they are able to work. The UK Psychiatric Morbidity Surveys found that only 20% of peo-ple with psychoses were in paid employment (Foster *et al.*, 1996). About a third of all sickness absence from work has been attributed to com-mon mental disorders (Jenkins, 1985). Employees with affective disorders have lower productivity in the workplace. The effects of mental illness may start even earlier: adults with social phobia, the onset of which is usually in the teenage years, are more likely than people without psychiatric mor-bidity *never* to have sought employment (Patel *et al.*, 2000). Note, however, that the causal con-nection linking mental illness and employment difficulties may run in the opposite direction: for

example, in the general population, unemploy-ment and poverty increase the duration (but not the likelihood of onset) of anxiety and affective disorders (Weich and Lewis, 1998).

These employment difficulties could have a number of corollaries. Someone whose illness pre-vents them working, or achieving their full poten-tial, may become both economically and socially marginalized ('socially excluded'). If they are com-pensated through social welfare payments from the state, there will be a cost to tax-payers. If the econ-omy is running close to full employment, there could be productivity losses. Whilst these effects overlap, and double counting should be avoided, they are clearly considerable and widespread.

Family and care-giver impacts

Some of the costs of services and some of the bur-den of lost employment could clearly fall on the families of people with mental health problems. Creed *et al.* (1997), for example, measured what families spent transporting their relatives to out-patient and day activity settings. In public sector or social insurance health care systems, however, where families generally have to make few out-of-pocket payments for services, a much greater con-sideration will be the care-giver role (Schene *et al.*, 1996). The effects are by no means all negative (Szmukler, 1996), but estimates of the time that families devote to the care-giver role are substan-tial, and there are often also major implications for health and quality of life.

- One five-country European study reported that family care-givers for adults with schizophrenia spent on average between 6 and 9 hours per day providing support (the average varied across sites; Magliano *et al.*, 1998). The most common 'burdens' reported were constraints on social activities, negative effects on family life and feelings of loss.

- A study of 408 families in the USA with a men-tally ill family member (80% with schizophre-nia) showed that care-giving absorbed most of their spare time (67 hours per month), with knock-on employment and financial difficulties (McGuire, 1991).

- An American study found that people with dementia needed almost 4 hours of care per day from the primary care-giver (Stommel *et al.*, 1994). An Italian study found an even higher average of 45 hours a week of unpaid personal care for Alzheimer's sufferers (Cavallo and Fattore, 1997).

- Interviews with 10 families with a conduct-disordered child being treated at the Maudsley Hospital revealed that a third of the total cost of more than £15 000 per year was carried by parents through lost earnings, damage to the home and the additional burden of housework (Knapp *et al.*, 1999).

- Families where there is a parent with a mental illness have increased risks of obstetric complications, divorce/separation, employment problems, poor educational attainment and school problems, needing specialist health and social care services and needing informal care (Göpfert *et al.*, 1995).

Mortality

Mortality among people with schizophrenia is 1.6 times greater than would be expected in a general population of similar age and gender, and the risk of suicide is nine times greater. Among people with major depression, the equivalent risks are 1.4 and 21 times higher than in a general population. Suicide risk is even greater for people with eating disorders (33 times higher) and substance abusers (86 times higher for those taking a combination of legal and illegal drugs). These estimates come from a substantial meta-analysis of 20 studies, covering 36 000 people from nine countries (Harris and Barraclough, 1998). Above-average mortality rates have cost consequences associated with lost productivity, although this is a minor consideration compared with the huge personal and social losses of premature death.

Crime and public safety

In the UK and in some other countries, there is heightened public concern about violent incidents involving psychiatric patients who are insufficiently supported or supervised. However, as Taylor and Gunn stress, "Most people with a mental disorder offer no risk to others" (1999, p. 13), and they present compelling evidence from a number of countries to counter the oft-expressed view that community-based care is to blame for homicides committed by people with mental health problems. Moreover, proportionately fewer homicides today are committed by people with mental disorders than was previously the case: for the UK, they find a 3% annual decline in the proportionate contribution between 1957 and 1995.

Societal concern about violent incidents, homicides and suicides—whether well-founded or not—can be seen as a cost (colloquially and in economic terms), albeit one that is hard to measure. The follow-on costs to the criminal justice system are more straightforward to assess. Estimated contacts with criminal justice agencies in the USA by people with schizophrenia amounted to $464 million (Rice and Miller, 1996). A study of heavy drug users in the UK found that the costs of criminal behaviour (costs to victims and to the criminal justice system) were almost four times as large as the costs of drug dependency treatments and other health service utilization (Healey *et al.*, 1998).

Transfer payments

Social security or welfare payments are transfers from one part of society (tax-payers) to another (benefit recipients), and economists therefore exclude them from calculations of the aggregate costs of an illness. They are 'transfer payments' and may double-count other costs. Nevertheless, to tax-payers, these welfare payments can represent a sizeable drain on fiscal resources. In England in the mid-1990s, welfare payments to people with mental health problems may have amounted to more than £7 billion (Patel and Knapp 1998).

Long-term consequences

Almost all of the economic impacts discussed above could have long-term consequences, whilst the figures given in this section merely represent snapshots at a point in time. Particular concern has been expressed about the enduring effects of many disorders of childhood and adolescence, where the longer term (adulthood) effects can often be much larger than those experienced in childhood (Knapp, 1997a).

Costing the impacts

The impacts described above are felt in a variety of areas, and can be measured in a variety of ways. For some purposes, it is helpful to try to transform these diverse impacts into a single, cost-based measure of the consequences of mental illness. This would give us a better overall understanding of the relative magnitude of an illness compared with the burdens associated with other illnesses. It also has the signal virtue of drawing attention to what could be a large and wide-ranging impact. The danger is that such a cost measure might oversimplify the complexity of the real world, and might also introduce further measurement error into what is already generally only a rough approximation of impact.

Cost-of-illness or burden-of-disease studies, as these global conflation exercises are often called, may or may not offer useful guides to decision makers about the best use of resources: another drawback is that they do not say anything about efficiency or equity attainment. In fact, cost-of-illness (COI) estimates can even be somewhat misleading because the extent of service use will be a function not only of the severity and duration of a disorder but also of the availability of hospital, residential and community-based services. The heterogeneous nature of these latter, supply side factors can make it difficult to derive a standard global account. Despite these difficulties of interpretation, there are quite well developed methods for this kind of exercise (Rice and Miller, 1996).

COI estimates are either constructed 'top-down' by disaggregating national or regional budgets by diagnostic group or they can be built 'bottom-up' based on prevalence or incidence figures. Prevalence-based COIs calculate the direct and indirect economic burden of illness according to the current time period in which the illness takes place—usually a year. Incidence-based COIs

represent the full lifetime costs of an illness from its onset. The majority of COI studies are prevalence based. The 'bottom-up' approach would follow a standard series of questions.

- What is the prevalence or incidence of a particular disorder?
- What services do people with the disorder use in the cross-section (prevalence estimate) or at different stages of their lives (incidence estimate)?
- What is the unit cost of each of these services?
- What other costs (not related directly to services) need to be included in the calculation, such as family burden or lost employment?
- Finally, how representative are these total costs?

Most COI studies aim to include a wide range of impacts, and do so from a broad societal perspective (i.e. not restricting the analysis to, say, health care expenditures). In this way, they generally aim to reflect the full social costs of the disorder.

Ideally, all resource impacts would be *opportunity costs*, that is the values forgone by not using these resources in their next best employment. The costs of services such as hospital in-patient days, out-patient visits, specialist-supported accommodation, and so on could be based on expenditure figures, probably after minor adjustment (Knapp, 1993; Netten *et al.*, 1998). The costs of lost employment, crime (property loss or victimization), care-giver support and other impacts for which there is no ready 'market-based' monetary measure are more difficult to estimate. There are some methodological disputes about what is legitimate to include in some of these non-service costs, and about how they are to be valued (Koopmanschap *et al.*, 1995; Drummond *et al.*, 1997; Johanneson and Karlsson, 1997). There is insufficient space to discuss these methodological issues here, but it should be noted that apparently modest differences in approach can sometimes produce quite wide discrepancies in overall cost estimates (Wyatt *et al.*, 1995).

The scale of the impacts

With such a wide range of possible impacts of the kind discussed above, it is not surprising that there have been few successful attempts to measure the complete costs of mental disorders. The most useful, and usually the most comprehensive aggregate measures have been constructed from national epidemiological surveys which have not only sought to estimate prevalence of particular disorders but have also asked questions about service utilization patterns, living circumstances and employment experiences. Most attention has been focused on either the more common mental disorders or those with sizeable individual-level impacts. There are still quite limited data about some diagnostic groups; for instance there are no reliable aggregate estimates for any of the disorders in childhood or adolescence.

The Epidemiologic Catchment Area (ECA) survey conducted by the National Institute of Mental Health in the USA allowed Rice *et al.* (1990) to use a prevalence approach to estimate total direct and indirect costs for all mental illnesses. They calculated an aggregate cost of $148 billion (at 1990 prices) for all diagnostic groups together, distinguishing direct and indirect costs. The latter were based on the human capital approach, the value of labour at market prices forgone as a direct result of illness, using average incomes. Regression analysis predictions were used to standardize income effects by taking into consideration other socio-economic variables. This partly explains the relatively low morbidity cost compared with findings from some other studies.

The calculations by Rice and colleagues covered most of the elements expected of a comprehensive COI estimate. They included the utilization of health care and other services, the value of reduced or lost productivity due to morbidity, the costs of premature mortality, victim costs of crime and criminal justice system expenditures, and the value of time spent by family care-givers supporting their relatives. Anxiety disorders were the highest cost group within Rice's calculations ($47 billion per annum nationally), but schizophrenia ($33 billion), affective disorders ($30 billion) and other disorders ($38 billion) were also clearly having major economic impacts.

COI estimates for specific mental health problems illustrate the components of the overall economic impact. It would be tedious to attempt to summarize all such estimates, but there are relevant findings to highlight.

Schizophrenia

In Rice's calculations, the direct (service) costs of schizophrenia in the USA in 1990 amounted to $17 billion, reflecting the high costs of institutionalization as well as the large number of ambulatory visits per person. This was approximately 2.5% of total national health care expenditure. Mental health organizations and nursing homes made up the bulk of direct costs (68%). Indirect costs were $12 billion, whereas other estimates for schizophrenia suggest that indirect costs might be 3–4 times higher than direct costs (e.g. Andrews *et al.*, 1985; Davies and Drummond, 1994). Crime, social welfare administration, imprisonment and family care-giver costs together amounted to $3.2 billion.

A recent calculation for England and Wales suggested annual figures of £810 million for direct costs (2.8% of all NHS expenditure) and £2.6 billion for both direct and indirect costs (Knapp, 1997b). These figures underestimated the value of care-giver time and did not look at the intangible consequences of the illness for quality of life. An earlier UK calculation showed that 97% of the direct costs were incurred by less than 50% of schizophrenia sufferers (Davies and Drummond, 1994).

One other national study shows how the economic impact of schizophrenia is closely tied to the structure of the health care system. In three areas of Spain (Burlada, Cantabria and Barcelona), patients were selected on the basis of first-time contacts with any psychiatric service, and costs were calculated for the third year after onset. The direct costs of care were substantially lower than figures reported for other western European countries, probably due to lower availability of services and the larger roles played by families. Comparing across the three areas, costs were higher in the areas that had the better developed community mental health systems.

Affective disorders

Depression is much more prevalent than schizophrenia, but has generally been found to have lower aggregate health care costs. Depression has a greater economic impact through its effects on work performance. Different studies have produced markedly different estimates for these employment/productivity costs of affective disorders, reflecting differences in methodology. This can clearly be seen from the two most widely quoted USA studies. Based on the ECA, Rice *et al.* (1990) suggest that lost work days due to affective disorders cost the US economy $2.2 billion in 1990, whilst mortality (also reckoned in terms of lost productivity) cost another $7.7 billion. In total, these were equivalent to just over half the total health care costs of treating people with these disorders ($19.8 billion). Greenberg *et al.* (1993) reported lower health care costs for the same year ($12.4 billion). However, their estimated costs for work days lost ($11.7 billion), reduced productivity whilst at work ($12.1 billion) and mortality ($7.5 billion) were much larger. By Greenberg's reckoning, the employment-related impacts were 2.5 times larger than the health care costs.

For England and Wales, Kind and Sorensen (1993) measured the total health service costs of affective psychoses and depressive disorders to be £416 million in 1986 (at 1991 price levels), based on data collected in the Royal College of General Practitioners (1986) morbidity survey. Estimates of service utilization were approximate. Their figures for the costs of lost work days were £3 billion, which does not include any estimate for mortality (although they suggest that 90 000 life years are lost due to affective disorders).

Anxiety disorders

There have been few economic studies of anxiety disorders, but one feature common to the best of them is that the costs of lost work days due to morbidity dwarf all other costs. This is vividly demonstrated by the ECA-based figures of Rice *et al.* (1990) which indicate that lost work days and reduced work performance cost the US economy $34 billion in 1990. This represented just over half the total of such morbidity costs for all mental illnesses together, and 73% of the aggregate costs of anxiety disorders. Smaller scale studies for particular disorders confirm this pattern (e.g. Edlund and Swann, 1987, on panic disorder; Patel *et al.*, 2000, on social phobia).

Dementia

One American estimate pitched the full cost of Alzheimer's disease at around $67 billion, 31% of which were direct care costs (formal services), 49% unpaid care-giver costs and 20% the value of lost productivity due to illness and premature mortality (Ernst and Hay, 1994). Equivalent exercises for other countries reach similar conclusions regarding the considerable proportional size of family or care-giver contributions, generally between 1.4 and 3 times the costs of formal care services (Knapp *et al.*, 1998). Among the aggregate figures suggested for the national costs of Alzheimer's disease are 8.9 billion lire for Italy (Cavallo and Fattore, 1994) and £1 billion for England (Gray and Fenn, 1993), although both now look like sizeable underestimates.

For dementia more generally, Kavanagh *et al.* (1995) looked at the component and total costs for England in 1992/93 (totalling £5 billion, including community living costs). They then used their sample-based national data to project the cost consequences of a number of alternative policy scenarios (such as greater emphasis on home-based care, greater availability of respite services and quality improvements in residential care settings). There are strong associations between the degree of cognitive impairment, service use patterns and costs (Kavanagh and Knapp, 1999). Consequently, treatment interventions or preventative measures that can delay the rate of cognitive decline have the potential to reduce quite considerably the costs of supporting people with dementia, especially if the admission to nursing home or in-patient care can be postponed.

Interpreting the figures

This chapter has focused on the main economic consequences of mental illness. Aggregate COI figures of the kind summarized in the previous section clearly show the enormous impact of mental health problems on national economies. Within these totals, there are a number of substantial contributory factors, particularly those discussed earlier. Some have immediately obvious economic implications (such as services used and work days lost), whilst others have not (such as mortality and family care-giver support).

There are many important messages coming from these figures. Some of these messages are picked up in later chapters, and their individual and community impacts discussed more fully. Among those that certainly warrant further consideration are the following.

- Most obviously, mental health problems require interventions from mental health services. What is not always so obvious is the high proportion of national health care expenditures that are allocated to the treatment of mental illnesses. As these proportions or totals are more widely appreciated, so too does pressure grow to find more cost-effective arrangements for treatment and support.

- In-patient services account for a large part of total expenditure, particularly for illnesses such as schizophrenia, and prompt the search for community-based care alternatives. However, we must remember that high costs do not necessarily mean low cost-effectiveness, and there have been concerns that the balance between in-patient and community care may have shifted too far or too fast.

- In contrast, a small component of health service costs is expenditure on drugs. This sometimes appears to be overlooked in discussions about newer (and more expensive) generations of pharmaceutical treatments. It is essential, of course, to examine carefully the cost-effectiveness of *any* new treatment modality, but some reactions to the higher prices of new drugs (and indeed, of new forms of

psychological treatment) sometimes appear to be driven by quite narrow cost considerations.

- There are many service cost implications of mental illness beyond those conventionally labelled 'mental health', including those to non-health services. Decision making should be cognisant of these, not merely for completeness but because a partial view of the consequences of a particular decision could set in train a series of unwanted events to the detriment of patient quality of life and system efficiency.

- Many economic impacts—perhaps the larger ones—are hidden from view. They too need to be brought into the reckoning, particularly because many of them may reflect major impacts of mental illness on sufferers and their families. Examples are the effects of ill-health on the ability to find employment and the intangible effects on families and other care-givers.

Finally, we should remember that the *real* impact of mental illness is felt at the individual level, through the suffering and stigma of those people with an illness or their close relatives. The ease with which it is possible to quote aggregate figures for the cost of a particular disorder must not distract attention away from these very personal impacts.

References

Andrews, G., Hall, W., Goldstein, G. *et al.* (1985) The economic costs of schizophrenia. *Archives of General Psychiatry*, 42, 537–543.

Andrews, G., Sanderson, K. and Beard, J. (1998) Burden of disease: methods of calculating disability from mental disorder. *British Journal of Psychiatry*, 173, 123–131.

Burns, B.J., Costello, E.J., Angold, A., Stangl, D., Farmer, E.M.Z. and Erkanli, A. (1995) Children's mental health service use across sectors. *Health Affairs*, 14, 147–159.

Cavallo, M.C. and Fattore, G. (1997) The economic and social burden of Alzheimer's disease on families in the Lombardy region. *Alzheimer's Disease and Associated Disorders*, 11(4), 184–90.

Creed, F., Mbaya, P., Lancashire, S., Tomenson, B., Williams, B. and Holme, S. (1997) Cost effectiveness of day and inpatient psychiatric treatment. Results of a randomised controlled trial. *British Medical Journal*, 314, 1381–1385.

Davies, L.M. and Drummond, M.F. (1994) Economics and schizophrenia: the real cost. *British Journal of Psychiatry*, 165 (Supplement 25), 18–21.

Drummond, M.F., O'Brien, B., Stoddart, G.L. and Torrance, G.W. (1997) *Methods for the Economic Evaluation of Health Care Programmes*, 2nd edn. Oxford: Oxford Medical Publications.

Edlund, M.J. and Swann, A.C. (1987) The economic and social costs of panic disorder. *Hospital and Community Psychiatry*, 38, 1277–1279.

Foster, K., Meltzer, H., Gill, B. and Hinds, K. (1996) *Adults with a Psychotic Disorder Living in the Community*. OPCS Survey of Psychiatric Morbidity Report 8. London: HMSO.

Göpfert, M., Webster, J. and Seemen, M.V. (eds) (1995) *Disturbed Mentally Ill Parents and Their Children*. Cambridge: Cambridge University Press.

Gray, A.M. and Fenn, P. (1993) Alzheimer's disease: the burden of illness in England. *Health Trends*, 25, 31–37.

Greenberg, P.E., Stiglin, L.E., Finkelstein, S.N. *et al.* (1993) The economic burden of depression in 1990. *Journal of Clinical Psychiatry*, 54, 405–418.

Hallam, A., Knapp, M.R.J., Beecham, J.K. and Fenyo, A. (1995) Eight years of psychiatric provision: an economic evaluation. In: Knapp, M.R.J. (ed.), *The Economic Evaluation of Mental Health Care*. Aldershot, UK: Arena, pp. 103–124.

Harris, E.C. and Barraclough, B. (1998) Excess mortality of mental disorder. *British Journal of Psychiatry*, 173, 11–53.

Healey, A., Knapp, M.R.J., Astin, J., Gossop, M., Marsden, J., Stewart, D., Lehmann, P. and Godfrey, C. (1998) Economic burden of drug dependency: social costs incurred by drug users at intake to the National Treatment Outcome Research Study. *British Journal of Psychiatry*, 173, 160–165.

Health Advisory Service (1995) *Child and Adolescent Mental Health Services: Together We Stand*. London: HMSO.

Jenkins, R. (1985) Minor psychiatric disorder in employed young men and women and its contribution to sickness absence. *British Journal of Industrial Medicine*, 42, 147–154.

Johanneson, M. and Karlsson, G. (1997) The friction cost method: a comment. *Journal of Health Economics*, 16, 249–255.

John, L.H., Offord, D.R., Boyle, M.H. and Racine, Y.A. (1995) Factors predicting use of mental health and social services by children 6–16 years old. *American Journal of Orthopsychiatry*, 65, 76–86.

Kavanagh, S.M. and Knapp, M.R.J. (1995) Market rationales, rationing and rationality: mental health care in the UK. *Health Affairs*, 14, 260–268.

Kavanagh, S.M. and Knapp, M.R.J. (1999) Cognitive disability and direct care costs for elderly people. *British Journal of Psychiatry*, 174, 539–546.

Kavanagh, S.M., Schneider, J., Knapp, M.R.J., Beecham, J.K. and Netten, A.P. (1995) Elderly people with dementia: costs, effectiveness and balance of care. In: Knapp, M.R.J. (ed.), *The Economic Evaluation of Mental Health Care*. Aldershot, UK: Arena, pp. 125–156.

Kind, P. and Sorensen, J. (1993) The costs of depression. *International Clinical Psychopharmacology*, 7, 191–195.

Knapp, M.R.J. (1993) Background theory. In: Netten, A. and Beecham, J.K. (eds), *Costing Community Care: Theory and Practice*. Aldershot, UK: Ashgate, pp. 9–23.

Knapp, M.R.J. (1997a) Economic evaluation and interventions for children and adolescents with mental health problems. *Journal of Child Psychology and Psychiatry*, 38, 3–26.

Knapp, M.R.J. (1997b) Cost of schizophrenia. *British Journal of Schizophrenia*, 171, 509–518.

Knapp, M.R.J., Beecham, J.K. and Hallam, A.J. (1997) The mixed economy of reprovision. In: Leff, J. (ed.), *Community Care: Illusion or Reality?* Chichester: John Wiley & Sons, pp. 37–47.

Knapp, M.R.J., Wilkinson, D. and Wigglesworth, R. (1998) The economic consequences of Alzheimer's disease in the context of new drug developments. *International Journal of Geriatric Psychiatry*, 13, 531–543.

Knapp, M.R.J., Scott, S. and Davies, J. (1999) The cost of antisocial behaviour in younger children. *Clinical Child Psychology and Psychiatry*, 4(4), 457–473.

Koopmanschap, M.A., Rutten, F.F.H., van Ineveld, B.M. and van Roijen, L. (1995) The friction cost method for measuring indirect costs of disease. *Journal of Health Economics*, 14, 171–189.

Magliano, L., Fadden, G., Madianos, M., Caldas de Almeida, J.M., Held, T., Guarneri, M., Marasco, C., Tosini, P. and Maj, M. (1998) Burden on the families of patients with schizophrenia. *Social Psychiatry and Psychiatric Epidemiology*, 33, 405–412.

McGuire, T. (1991) Measuring the economic costs of schizophrenia. *Schizophrenia Bulletin*, 17, 375–378.

National Health Service Executive (1996) *Burdens of Disease*. London: Department of Health.

Netten, A., Dennett, J.H. and Knight, J. (1998) *Unit Costs of Health and Social Care 1998*. University of Kent at Canterbury: Personal Social Services Research Unit.

OECD (1996) *Caring for Frail Elderly People*. Social Policy Studies 19. Paris: OECD.

Patel, A. and Knapp, M.R.J. (1998) Costs of mental illness in England. *Mental Health Research Review*, 5, 4–10.

Patel, A., Knapp, M.R.J., Henderson, J. and Baldwin, D. (2001) The economic consequences of social phobia, *Journal of Affective Disorders*, forthcoming.

Rice, D.P. and Miller, L.S. (1996) The economic burden of schizophrenia: conceptual and methodological issues, and cost estimates. In: Moscarelli, M., Rupp, A. and Sartorius, N. (eds), *Schizophrenia*. London: Wiley, pp. 321–334.

Rice, D., Kelman, S., Miller, L.S. *et al.* (1990) *The Economic Costs of Alcohol and Drug Abuse and Mental Illness: 1985*. Publication No. (ADM) 90-1694. Rockville, MD: Alcohol, Drug Abuse and Mental Health Administration.

Schene, A.H., Tessler, R.C. and Gamache, G.M. (1996) Caregiving in severe mental illness: conceptualisation and measurement. In: Knudsen, H.C. and Thornicroft, G. (eds), *Mental Health Service Evaluation*. Cambridge: Cambridge University Press. pp. 296–316.

Stommel, M., Collins, C.E. and Given, B.A. (1994) The costs of family contributions to the care of persons with dementia. *Gerontologist*, 34, 199–205.

Szmukler, G. (1996) From family 'burden' to caregiving. *Psychiatric Bulletin*, 20, 449–451.

Taylor, P.J. and Gunn, J. (1999) Homicides by people with mental illness: myth and reality. *British Journal of Psychiatry*, 174, 9–14.

Weich, S. and Lewis, G. (1998) Poverty, unemployment, and common mental disorders: population based cohort study. *British Medical Journal*, 317, 115–119.

Wyatt, R.J., Henter, I., Leary, M.C. and Taylor, E. (1995) An economic evaluation of schizophrenia—1991. *Social Psychiatry and Psychiatric Epidemiology*, 30, 196–205.

12 | *The impact of mental disorders on families and carers*

Harriet P. Lefley

Introduction

Severe mental disorders such as schizophrenia or major affective disorders have an impact on the lives of other persons who are attached by love or kinship and are personally invested in the patient's well-being. These other individuals are of interest to community psychiatrists not only because of their interactions with patients, but because their own emotional or even physical health status may be affected by the burdens imposed by the mental illness of a loved one (Greenberg *et al.*, 1993; Schene *et al.*, 1998). For the most part, these persons are family members, although they may be significant others such as unmarried partners or devoted friends. Some individuals, not related by kinship, may have developed affectionate bonds with patients through years of administering long-term care.

The research and self-report literature on the impact of mental illness, however, is restricted almost exclusively to families. These are the people who knew the patient in his or her premorbid state and have shared the confusions, disruptions and emotional ravages of the illness. In most cases, a caring family continues to be the most stable resource for patients throughout a lifetime of stressors, shifting resources and changing clinical services. Even when they do not live with the patient, concerned family members find services for their ill relative, provide social, financial and emotional support, and serve as a last resort when the system fails (Clark and Drake, 1993). Families are thus the encompassing group about whom we speak.

In English-speaking countries outside of the USA, family members who provide ongoing support and are committed to the welfare of both child and adult patients are typically called 'carers'. The more common terms in the USA, however, are 'care-givers' or 'care-takers'. Elsewhere I have commented that the latter are functional words, seemingly anchored to tasks and responsibilities rather than to emotional investment (Lefley, 1998a). 'Carers', on the other hand, suggests individuals whose own happiness is entwined with the well-being of people who are dear to them.

The semantic distinction is meaningful with respect to the relationship of patients and family members, and to the mindset of the mental health professionals with whom they interact. The concept of caring families, of family love, has had little currency in the clinical literature. Since the literature has been preoccupied with pathogenic or toxic relationships, the idea that many families love their psychotic relatives is sometimes a revelation to even the most empathic professionals (Lefley, 1998a). Yet caring underlies families' assumption of responsibility for care-giving, and the quality and stability of family support. Caring also informs the confusions, ambivalences and conflicted emotions found in families throughout the world who are trying to cope with the incomprehensible behaviours of mental illness.

For families, the impact of mental illness is multiply determined. Apart from the shared grief of unfulfilled life expectations, there are various categorical sources of stress that affect family members of persons with major psychiatric disabilities. At one level are behavioural disturbances and their disruptive effects on family life. This is the thrust of the family burden research, which will be discussed further in this chapter. There is also iatrogenic stress, the residual of now discredited theories that often resulted in mistreatment of families by professionals, denied information to families and generated inappropriate and sometimes damaging treatment models (McFarlane and Lukens, 1994). Although this mistreatment has abated in recent years, exclusionary confidentiality barriers and totally inadequate family education continue to be problems in most mental health systems, whether in the USA (Dixon et al., 1999), Europe (Bergmark, 1994) or Australia (Bland, 1994).

Perhaps the most important source of stress is society itself, ranging from the generalized social stigma of mental illness to inadequate funding for research and services. In all societies, political and economic forces affect the structure of mental health systems and the adequacy of services for the mentally ill. Decision-making bodies far from the centres of service delivery determine resources available to families for coping with crises and accessing long-term care. A society's legal decisions affect the rights of individuals who may be floridly psychotic to reject involuntary treatment, and the criminalization of mental illness through incarceration of sufferers in jails rather than hospitals (Lamb and Weinberger, 1998). These have become issues of great concern to family carers (Lefley, 1997a).

In this chapter, accordingly, we explore the impact of mental illness on families in several domains. Research on the family's experience generally has focused on the burden of coping with the reality problems and psychological distress incurred by the illness. Studies of the factorial structure and dimensions of family burden currently are being enriched by a self-report literature that puts a human face on the graphs and tables of empirical research (e.g. Backlar, 1994). In addition to research on some clinical correlates of burden, we discuss the family's experience as a function of the illness trajectory and the family life cycle; effects on siblings and children; and issues specific to parents and spouses.

The social issues focus on the adequacy of mental health services and barriers to treatment. Crisis management, dealing with violence and involuntary treatment, and attempts to find alternatives to homelessness and jail are constant dilemmas for family carers. There are now some empirical examples from other countries, cross-cultural comparisons that indicate how societal resources for aftercare and employment may affect families' well-being and their ability to sustain an ongoing care-giving relationship (Warner et al., 1998).

Services for families include psychoeducational interventions, family education, family support groups and linkages with advocacy groups. Some issues of family and consumer movements, their areas of concordance as well as conflict, are discussed in terms of their relevance to carer and patient well-being. Mental health systems offer increasing promise to patients in the combination of the new atypical neuroleptics with sophisticated techniques of psychiatric rehabilitation. Currently, there are moves toward incorporating as standard practice empirically validated services such as assertive community treatment and family psychoeducation. There is increasing attention on training former patients as case managers and peer counsellors. For families, ongoing support, education, respite and advocacy decrease the burdensome impact of mental illness. However, many more societal initiatives are necessary to lower the negative impact of mental illness on families and patients alike, and to implement promising trends in both biological and psychosocial spheres. Affiliative initiatives with professionals through joint political advocacy for services and research, enhanced by mutual support groups or appropriate psychotherapy, can increase family members' feelings of self-efficacy and control over their lives.

Dimensions of family burden

The vast literature on families of persons with mental illness typically has focused on the impact of the family on the patient. In the flow of theory and research, whether postulating or discrediting paradigms that implicated families in the aetiology or systemic maintenance of major psychotic disorders (McFarlane and Lukens, 1994), or demonstrating the relationship of high expressed emotion to relapse (Kavanagh, 1992; Bebbington and Kuipers, 1994), the direction of effect has been largely unilateral.

The family burden literature was the first to assess the effects of mental illness on the family. These effects typically have been characterized as objective burden (the multiple tasks associated with taking care of the patient) and subjective burden, a concept initially anchored to these tasks in terms of their personal costs. Subjective burden has been expanded into an overall assessment of the emotional distress engendered by the illness. Schene *et al.* (1994) identified 21 instruments developed to measure care-giver burden in severe mental illness. Comprehensive reviews of the research may be found in Maurin and Barmann Boyd (1990) and Lefley (1996), among others.

Years of experience in working with families of persons with severe mental illness suggest that the research instruments often fail to capture the extent and the psychological parameters of either objective or subjective burden. Examples of objective burden include: (i) the restrictive effects on carers' lives of adult patients' continuing dependency and inability to fulfil expected role functions; (ii) disruptions of household routines; (iii) carers' investments of time and energy in help-seeking and in negotiating the mental health, social welfare and legal systems; (iv) carers' confusing and often humiliating interactions with service providers; (v) deprivation of needs of other family members, sometimes with long-term psychological sequelae; (vi) social isolation of the family and impaired relations with the outside world; (vii) difficulties in obtaining timely crisis intervention or hospitalization; (viii) difficulties in finding acceptable residential facilities outside of the home; and (ix) financial costs of the illness, which in some cases have impoverished families without commensurate benefit to the patient.

Subjective burden includes the emotional costs associated with each component of objective burden. However, this concept also encompasses carers' mourning for the premorbid personality and for the failed aspirations of someone they love. There are also feelings of stigmatization, frustrations due to inability to make or fulfil personal plans, and worries of ageing parents about the future of a disabled child who will surely outlive

them. Economic strain, isolation, burnout and need for respite are common. Negative effects of the illness on other family members, on siblings and young children, is an ongoing concern and may result in a need for ancillary interventions and a new generation of psychotherapy bills (see Marsh, 1998).

Behaviour management issues create ongoing tensions. Carers may have to contend with abusive or assaultative behaviours, socially offensive or embarrassing situations in public places; mood swings and unpredictability; conflicts over money; or negative symptoms of amotivation or anhedonia. Conflicts arise about excessive smoking, poor personal hygiene, damage to household property or sleep reversal patterns that may keep the household awake. Patients' rejection of medications is a major area of contention, particularly when there is a known pattern of relapse.

Although these behaviours are characteristic of many family situations, they are not universal and their effects within individual families are a function of many factors. The notion of family burden as a common correlate or sequela of mental illness has been criticized as pejorative, and the distinctions between objective and subjective burden ill-defined. For these reasons, Szmukler (1996) has suggested rejecting the term 'burden' and instead operationalizing the dimensions of care-giving, which may have some positive as well as negative aspects. Conceptualizing care-giving within a 'stress–appraisal–coping' theoretical framework, Szmukler *et al.* (1996a) developed *The Experience of Caregiving Inventory* as a vehicle for determining how the 'burdens' of care-giving may be appraised and dealt with by individual families. Concordant with the findings on other instruments (Schene *et al.*, 1994), they found that the experience of care-giving is multi-dimensional, but that the 'mastery' factor may be useful as a global measure of coping.

A qualitative study explored themes of the family's experience in narrative accounts of care-givers. Themes included dealing with unpredictable or difficult behaviours, mixed feelings about the professional treatment system, need for care-giver support, societal stigmatization and particularly fears about the future. In stories that tried to make sense out of the disruptions incurred by the illness, however, the authors identified two types of narrative structure. *Stories of restoration or reparation* tried to turn the illness into a meaningful event by developing a *platform* that located the illness within their map of the world. These care-givers were able to reconstruct their personal identity in terms of a moral quest and a life worth living. In *chaotic or frozen narratives*, the illness remained a series of random events. These carers could not construe any patterned whole out of scattered events. "Carers seemed unable to break loose from a roundabout, repetitive way of telling ... inhibiting the movement from disruption to *platform* to reconstruction" (Stern, 1999, p. 359).

This study was based on a small sample, and the relationship between narrative structure and the themes regarding external stressors was unclear. The care-giving inventory developed by Szmukler *et al.* (1996a) was intended to assess the degree to which care-givers' perceived stress and coping styles might predict their psychological well-being or morbidity without the concept of objective burden. The phenomenology of care-giving, however, is subject to the trait–state dilemma, i.e. perceptual and coping styles may be stable or they may vary according to situational factors. A study of 480 families of persons with chronic psychosis in The Netherlands found four care-giving domains: tension, supervision, worrying and urging (Schene *et al.*, 1998). The investigators found that these domains were positively related to three variables: the patient's symptomatology, contact between the relative and the patient's mental health professional (greater contact implying more of a care-giving role, and hence more tension, supervision and urging) and the hours of actual contact with the patient (contact of <1 hour a week meant more worrying but less distress). When patients live with their families, distress may be evoked by greater responsibility and tension and fewer hours of respite for carers..

Cultural differences

The greater contact inherent in co-residence may be associated with greater or lower perceived family burden. On the one hand, the tension suggested in the research by Schene *et al.* (1998) is concordant with findings that some patients are likely to be more troublesome and even violent with family members with whom they live (Straznickas *et al.*, 1993). On the other hand, cross-racial/ethnic comparisons, as well as international studies, suggest that in more traditional cultures, co-residence may be associated with more tolerance, less depression and lower reported burden (see Lefley, 1998a,b).

Co-residence appears to be a function of cultural norms, social support and the availability of outside residential facilities. Research by Warner *et al.* (1998) indicated that 70% of schizophrenic patients being treated in the mental health system in Bologna, Italy were living with their families versus 17% in Boulder, Colorado, a city that arguably has a greater array of housing alternatives. In most studies, co-residence in the USA ranges from 40 to 75%, with the figures varying by ethnicity (Lefley, 1996). One study found that approximately 60% of African-American and 75% of Hispanic-American families lived with their mentally ill family member, versus 32% of Anglo- or European-American families (Guarnaccia and Parra, 1996). Yet a body of research has found that in contrast to Anglo-/European-American care-givers, Hispanic- and African-American family care-givers report significantly less subjective burden in terms of the impact of mental illness on their own physical and mental health (Lefley, 1997b).

In cross-ethnic research on families of psychiatric patients, racial and ethnic differences have also been found in causal attributions, prognostic expectations, kinship roles of primary care-givers, hospitalization and service utilization patterns and, as indicated, in perceived psychological distress (Lefley, 1996). Across cultural and ethnic groups, however, patients' current symptomatology shows the strongest relationship with care-giving patterns and family burden. This is in good accord with the findings of Schene *et al.* (1998) in Holland, and with the American research findings on both developmentally and mentally disabled adults. Throughout the literature, patients' level of behavioural disturbance is the most clear predictor of perceived carer burden and psychological distress (Lefley, 1997b)

Clinical dimensions of carers' response

In recent years, there have been a few attempts to explore gratifications in care-giving as a contrast to family burden (e.g. Greenberg *et al.*, 1994). These studies typically focus on companionship and practical help offered by mentally ill adults to ageing parents, but the figures are very low. Most studies continue to focus on the emotional costs of mental illness to family members. Adverse emotional reactions on clinical scales have been found in 75% of family members confronting first-episode schizophrenia (Scottish Schizophrenia Research Group, 1985). For longer duration mental illness, research on a clinic sample of care-givers in England indicated that both objective and subjective measures on a family burden scale were significantly correlated with anxiety, insomnia and depression scores on clinical scales (Oldridge and Hughes, 1992). In an Australian study, Winefield and Harvey (1993) found that care-givers of persons with mental illness showed high levels of psychological distress when compared with norms on various standardized instruments of adjustment. Significantly, levels of care-giver distress were predicted by the level of behavioural disturbance of the mentally ill relative after controlling for multiple related variables.

A study of mental health professionals with mentally ill family members found that 67% reported that at least one family member was seriously affected psychologically by the experience of their relative's illness, and 38% reported an adverse effect on physical health. As an example of stressful life events during a 1-year period, 75% of the sample reported multiple emergency calls and over 73% had needed to hospitalize their relative at least once (Lefley, 1987). Research on maternal care-givers by Greenberg *et al.* (1993) found that subjective burdens related to worry and stigma were significant predictors of poor physical health after controlling for multiple variables related to health status.

Grieving and loss

Despite the conventional picture of young adults with schizophrenia or major affective disorder as having been withdrawn loners in their premorbid lives, many are remembered as popular, competent and bright with promise (Backlar, 1994). Parents and siblings who knew the premorbid personality suffer the experience of dual loss. They mourn the loss of the person who was, and the person who might have been. Marsh (1998) reports that in her survey of mothers of mentally ill adults, 75% reported chronic mourning. The feelings of many parents are summed up in the words of one mother, who had experienced the death of one child and the mental illness of another. She said, "I've lost a child to death. This is worse because death is final . . . I have to continue to see him suffer. To see a handsome, young, bright life destroyed" (Marsh, 1998, p. 221).

Ambiguous loss is a term that Boss (1999) applies to the disappearance of a beloved personality without the closure of death. Relatives experience unresolved or frozen grief. This is well manifested in research by Atkinson (1994). The study compared grief among three groups of parents of adults who at a mean age of 21–22 years had suffered either schizophrenia, head injury with organic personality disorder or death. Parents of young adults with schizophrenia had more ongoing grieving than the others. The other parents had a greater initial grief reaction, because the child had died or was expected to die through head injury, but in both cases the grieving diminished over time. In contrast, parents of schizophrenic children had low initial levels of grieving that rose over time. The authors concluded that once the diagnosis is established, parental loss of a child through schizophrenia leads to a pattern of chronic mourning.

Marsh (1998) reports that siblings who have known a previously high functioning brother or sister experience the multiple losses of love, comfort, entertainment, companionship, admiration and protection. "To me, it was a death. The person whom I knew . . . had died, and I didn't know this person who was living in the house any more." (p. 272). If siblings were young children at the onset of illness, they may grieve for the loss of a normal childhood and family life or the loss of a potential mentor, an older brother or sister. Siblings may also experience the loss of the attention and mentoring of their parents who are consumed by grief, or the loss of other well siblings who may respond to the family tragedy with anger or disengagement

Surveys of offspring of mentally ill parents indicate mourning for the loss of protection and guidance, the loss of remembered beauty and strength. Children or adolescents may mourn for a family that can no longer meet their needs. They may share the grief of the well parent, and yet be unable to compensate for the loss of a beloved mate. In recording the childhood memories and later reactions to the loss of a parent to mental illness, Marsh (1998, p. 294) suggests that "During their adulthood, the early losses of offspring may have an amorphous jurisdiction over their lives."

Spouses, similarly, may mourn the loss of the person they once knew but still love. They may also grieve for companionship and intimacy, for their own changes in lifestyle and unfulfilled dreams, and for the suffering of their partner and children. It should be noted, however, that in comparison with other familial relationships, spouses are likely to be more high functioning and potentially capable of retaining their competencies and productive roles in life, particularly with the new medications. Regardless of the burdens imposed by mental illness, a patient's ability to maintain an intact personality and a capacity for relating does much to prevent or counteract grief and mourning in family members.

The family life cycle and role relationships

Many commentators have pointed out the need for practitioners to view their patients within a life cycle perspective. Stromwall and Robinson (1998) sketch the typical stages of the family life cycle in terms of normally expected developmental tasks and the disruptive impact of a major psychiatric disorder such as schizophrenia. At a developmental stage in late adolescence or early adulthood that usually entails separation from the family of origin, parents must now be involved with adult children who cannot develop age-appropriate peer, partnership and work relationships.

For many years, unmarried dependent adults may share households with ageing parents who, lacking acceptable community alternatives, feel unable to relinquish the care-giving role. The resultant drain on the parents' physical and emotional health, and their dashed expectations of freedom in their older years, co-mingle with anxieties about who will replace their care-giving after they are gone (Lefley and Hatfield, 1999).

The sequelae of deinstitutionalization also mean that psychiatrically disabled adults now living in the community are engaging in more conjugal relationships and parenting roles. Although this is a salutary development for many persons with mental illness, these new roles bring many problems and adjustments. Among patients able to form partnerships, a new partner with schizophrenia or bipolar disorder may have difficulty devoting energy and maintaining commitments to the dyad. In families with young children, the partner with serious mental illness may have difficulty relating to or caring for a child. The well partner must assume responsibility for all adult roles in the household, and a young child's needs may not be optimally met. Young marriages are particularly fragile because the well partner with dual and sometimes conflicting responsibilities is unable to rely on a supportive mate. Mental illness often means the loss of companionship and intimacy that might otherwise have carried the couple through difficult life situations.

In families with adolescents, a mentally ill parent needs care and support from the spouse and children, and often the adolescent child must take on adult roles. In families with adult children, the psychiatrically disabled parent needs continuing support and the adult offspring may be reluctant to introduce friends or potential mates due to stigma. Across the life cycle, children, adolescents and adults, regardless of kinship roles, frequently are unwilling to bring friends home and are likely to seek friendships and mentors outside of the family because of their fear of embarrassing behaviours.

Lefley (1996) has also detailed aspects of the illness trajectory and its effects at different points in the life cycle of both the family and the patient. Family interactions are greatly affected by the role expectations of adults with major mental disorders, and the appraisal of symptoms by both patients and family members. Conflicts may be exacerbated by the cyclical patterns of many disorders, the remission and exacerbation of symptoms and attendant capacities for functioning. This is one of the most common complaints of family members: they do not know what to expect in the way of functioning nor how to assess patients' responsibility for their own behaviours.

Patient violence

One of the most critical issues for parents of adult patients is the dual impact of their children's inability to fulfil age-appropriate productive roles, and the patients' projection of rage because of their own dependency. Many of these families are locked in unresolved independence–dependency conflicts of adolescence. Patients may assert their own autonomy while resenting limit-setting or demands for performance. This is a situation that can lead to over-reaction on the part of family members, and sometimes to aggressive or assaultative behaviour of patients.

Among patients admitted to psychiatric hospitals who had physically assaulted someone, studies in the USA showed that family members were the targets from 50 to 65% of the time, particularly if they were living in the same household (Lefley, 1996). In a major study of assaultative hospitalized patients, Estroff *et al.* (1994) reported that financial dependence was associated with violent threats and acts. Interestingly, respondents who were violent perceived their significant others as threatening but did not perceive themselves as threatening in return. "The respondents who were violent felt malice and danger from significant others and perceived and experienced hostility in their interpersonal networks" (p. 677).

The study by Estroff *et al.* found that violence was directed most frequently toward mothers living with the patient. Straznickas *et al.* (1993) found that patients who attacked parents, children and siblings were most likely to live with their victims in the same household. They found that primary care-givers were more at risk because of their frequent contact. "Our results suggest that attempts by caretakers to place limits on patients often precede assaults. Also, psychotic symptoms such as paranoid delusions involving the family caregiver are common in patient assaults on family members in violent acts, as is concurrent drug or alcohol abuse by the patient" (p. 387).

The research suggests that violence may be triggered by normative expectations and limit-setting, or by any perceived encroachments on patients' autonomy. It also suggests that patients' financial dependence, and carers' power in money management, may be a factor in eliciting rage. The perception of threatening intent from carers is likely to be delusional, yet threat may be implicit in the patient's perception of control by others. Battles over money, expectations of performance and issues of control create hostile tension between carers and patients. There is now a well-known body of research that suggests that a patient's sensitivity to critical hostility in the family environment may be instrumental in triggering relapse.

Expressed emotion (EE)

Although the family burden research is related most directly to the subject of this chapter, a focus on families' effects on patients continues through the ongoing research on expressed emotion (EE). By now, multiple studies have found that high EE in families, operationalized as a specific level of hostile criticism or emotional overinvolvement verbally expressed by at least one family member, is predictive of a greater tendency to relapse in schizophrenia (Kavanagh, 1992; Bebbington and Kuipers, 1994). The focus on high EE in the literature has obscured the fact that despite cross-cultural variability, in most of the world families of persons with schizophrenia tend to show low EE (Kavanagh, 1992; Bentsen, 1998). Initially described by Leff and Vaughn (1985) as calm, empathic, accepting and respectful, low EE families appear to defy the stereotypes of schizophrenogenesis, and indeed most EE researchers deny any aetiological implications. Rather, as EE pioneer George Brown (1985) pointed out, high EE behaviours are within the range of ordinary family transactions and normative responses to stress, but they may have an unduly negative impact on persons with the sensitivities and psychophysiological deficits of schizophrenia.

The direction of effect and interactional aspects of familial EE have been constant themes. Scazufca and Kuipers (1996) found that high EE relatives, both critical and overinvolved, had twice as high burden of care scores as low EE relatives (P = 0.0002). Numerous other studies have found high EE characteristics linked with both objective and subjective burden of care, as well as reactive to patients' negative behaviours (Bentsen, 1998). One study of patient–family interactions found that schizophrenic patients in high EE families displayed four times as many odd or disruptive behaviours as did patients in low EE families (Rosenfarb et al., 1995). Warner (1999) has also presented research indicating that households with more criticism and intrusiveness tend to be those of patients whose personality attributes make them more difficult to live with. He thinks the research evidence suggests that one way that some families adapt to difficult behaviours is to become unusually low key and permissive. Many persons with schizophrenia do well under these conditions. It may be pointed out, however, that if permissiveness is excessive and precludes limit-setting, this may be a potentially maladaptive form of low EE.

Schene et al. (1998) have postulated that the connection between EE and care-giver burden, the latter encompassing patients' disturbing behaviours, may also be explained by attributional differences in families. An example is the finding by Barrowclough et al. (1996) that care-givers' attributions, their cognitive appraisals of the illness and of patients' accountability for their behaviours, are related both to EE and care-givers' level of distress. "An intriguing question ... concerns the causal pathway between the patient's symptomatology/functioning, caregiving, family-member distress, and the further interactions with concepts like expressed emotion ... future studies will need to examine the reciprocity between these different concepts." (Schene et al., 1998, p. 616).

Overall, then, it seems that family transactions are informed by objective and subjective family burden, including patients' disturbing behaviours. We seem to see a feedback loop of stressors that evoke negative responses in carers, and these in turn may negatively affect the patient and thereby reinforce the stress. This cycle may be broken by basic family education together with other appropriate help, which may range from psychotherapy to involvement of families in advocacy in order to provide external resources for carer relief.

Help for carers

Help for carers comes from both clinical and non-clinical interventions, and from the therapeutic and practical effects of self-help and advocacy. The question that is still unresolved, and of great interest to community psychiatrists, is whether the helping intervention should be evaluated in terms of the well-being of the patient or that of the family. The two outcome measures obviously are inter-related and perhaps interdependent, but until recent years little attention was paid to the well-being of the family except as an auxiliary to patient care.

Psychoeducational interventions are the most empirically validated family interventions, in terms of deterring patient relapse and rehospitalization (Dixon and Lehman, 1995). In contrast to older family therapy models with their notions of systemic dysfunction, psychoeducational models eschewed presumptions of family pathology. Instead, they taught a biologically based stress-vulnerability model of schizophrenia (and later bipolar disorder), with an eye to reducing complexity and overstimulation in the social environment and improving functional skills. In so doing, psychoeducators gave families that which they had long desired but had seldom received from clinicians: information, understanding and support; behaviour management and communication techniques; and problem-solving strategies.

Psychoeducational interventions essentially developed as research projects in Great Britain, ultimately spreading to the USA and subsequently to numerous other countries in the world, including rural China (see Leff *et al.*, 1985; Falloon *et al.*, 1984; Anderson *et al.*, 1986; Birchwood *et al.*, 1992; Xiong *et al.*, 1994; McFarlane *et al.*, 1995). Unfortunately, despite the fact that these are among the most carefully studied and validated psychosocial treatments for major mental illnesses, few mental health facilities offer educational services to families on any consistent basis. As noted by Dixon *et al.* (1999) in surveying services for a national sample of over 15 000 patients with schizophrenia in the USA, when it comes to educating families there is a wide gap between best practices and standard practice..

Various models of family psychoeducation have been developed by clinicians, ranging from individual behavioural family management (Mueser *et al.*, 1994) to multi-family groups, that have proven superior in long-range outcome to single family treatment (McFarlane *et al.*, 1995). Other interventions have been developed that are primarily educational, focusing on families' needs rather than on patient outcomes. Solomon (1998) notes that "Family education is a non-clinical intervention that has a strengths approach as its empirical base, with stress reduction, improved coping and adaptation as its targeted outcomes. In contrast to psychoeducation, which was designed to meet the needs of the ill relative, family education was developed primarily to meet the needs of families. These programmes comes from an adult learning and health promotion orientation" (p. 8).

Although there have been numerous studies of the effects of psychoeducation, there are few studies of interventions aimed at alleviating families' distress. Partly this is because many psychoeducational interventions were developed as funded research projects, with carefully developed designs, adequate length of family and patient participation (typically many months) and clear but limited patient outcome measures—typically relapse or rehospitalization.

Studies of interventions that alleviate families' distress are hampered by the ambiguity of dependent variables and also by the heterogeneity of samples and investment of time. Most reviews of family interventions have reported positive effects on relatives' burden and distress, although findings are not always significant or consistent with positive patient outcome (Kazarian and Vanderheyden, 1992; Solomon, 1996). In Chapter 40 of the present volume, Margaret Leggatt notes that there are studies that do not meet the 'gold standard' for randomized controlled trials but that nevertheless suggest positive outcomes for family members in various dimensions, such as more confidence and adaptability, reduced self-blaming and a greater capacity for advocacy.

Johnson (1994) reviewed six studies of family interventions that did not include the member with mental illness and that focused on relief of family burden. Three studies reported positive effects, and three reported no significant effects. Szmukler *et al.* (1996b) conducted a controlled trial of six weekly home-based counselling sessions for principal care-givers with the patient absent. The control group received a 1-hour educational session. Relatives in the intervention group reported better understanding of the patient and a more positive relationship, including a sense of the carer's contributing to the patient's well-being. There were no group differences in negative aspects of care-giving or coping style. The authors concluded that their findings are congruent with other studies of short-term family interventions, indicating that "it is easier to influence understanding of, and attitudes toward the patient than caregiver distress or coping" (p. 154).

Do short educational programmes significantly increase knowledge or satisfaction with services? Merinder *et al.* (1999) conducted a randomized study of the effectiveness of an eight-session psychoeducational programme for patients with schizophrenia and their relatives in two community mental health centres in Denmark. They found significant increases in knowledge of schizophrenia among both patients and relatives and in their satisfaction with relatives' involvement in care. However, the authors noted that these improvements were not sufficient to influence important variables such as relapse, compliance, psychopathology, insight or psychosocial functioning.

Cuipers (1999) conducted a meta-analysis of 16 studies of family interventions in which at least one outcome measure involved relatives' burden of care. The measure had to refer to an element that could be interpreted as subjective burden (e.g. psychological distress) or objective burden (e.g. family–patient relations, social support), and had to report at least pre-test and post-test data. The analysis found that family interventions can have considerable effects on relatives' psychological distress, the relationship between the patient and family, and family functioning. Taken together, the 16 studies yielded only moderate effect sizes at post-test and small effect sizes at follow-up. Large effects were found in a subset of six studies but, of these, the majority had 13 or more sessions.

Cuipers concluded that interventions with less than 10 sessions have no important effects on relatives' burden. However, the number of sessions could not explain completely the differences between effective and less effective interventions. The author suggested that length of total time rather than the number of sessions may be a factor, as well as diagnosis. "It is possible that greater effects can be expected from interventions aimed at partners or relatives of patients with other illnesses than schizophrenia" (pp. 282–283). Since most successful psychoeducation was initiated with families of schizophrenic patients, this is an important consideration. It is possible that the behaviours and disruptions of schizophrenia are such that more than psychoeducation is needed to alleviate family burden.

Nevertheless, there are more and more calls to include patient and family education as a component of standard practice. It currently is recommended in the *Journal of Clinical Psychiatry*'s expert consensus treatment guidelines for schizophrenia (McEvoy *et al.*, 1999) with a comprehensive content guide for patients and families. In the USA, the Therapeutic Education Association (TEA), comprised of mental health professionals who have developed models of patient and family education for the major psychiatric disorders, was organized about 6 years ago. The TEA meets annually as an allied organization of the American Psychiatric Association's Institute on Psychiatric Services. Numerous models of family education deal with both generic and specific issues, the latter attentive to discrete informational needs associated with the age of patients and care-givers, diagnosis, functional level, stage of illness, family life cycle, and the like. Some of these models were developed by clinicians with mentally ill relatives within the American family movement, The National Alliance for the Mentally Ill (NAMI). In recent years, however, NAMI has developed its own Family-to-Family Educational Program, an intensive 12-week programme based on a 'trauma and recovery model' of mental illness (Burland, 1998).

Therapeutic aspects of support and advocacy groups

In addition to clinical interventions, the growth of family movements has generated invaluable sources of help for patients' relatives. Family organizations typically combine mutual support groups; education about mental illness for both internal and public consumption; anti-stigma initiatives and campaigns; and, wherever possible, fundraising and legislative advocacy for improved services and research. In Chapter 40 of this book, Margaret Leggatt describes the rise and functions of family organizations worldwide.

The superiority of the multi-family group model, as discovered by McFarlane *et al.* (1995), replicates the experiences of multiple members of the family organizations. In their mutual support groups, they have found an empathic understanding of shared experiences, resource information, exchange of coping strategies and a social network for families who have suffered stigma and social isolation. The multi-family group tends to normalize reactions of grief and guilt, and sometimes offers concrete aid for members' relatives in terms of social support and job-finding. Members offer each other help in negotiating the mental health, welfare and even criminal justice systems. McFarlane *et al.* (1995) attribute to the group experience an enhanced problem-solving capability, an antidote to overinvolvement, a cross-parenting capacity and techniques for crisis intervention.

These variables are quite evident in a support group that I have led for many years for families of psychiatric patients at a large urban medical centre. Members helped a socially isolated widow, whose only relative was her schizophrenic son, deal with her terminal cancer over a 2-year period. As her sole support system, group members accompanied Mrs N to physicians, took her to a competent attorney to make a will and special needs trust for her disabled heir, arranged her funeral, and still provide social support for her son. They continue to visit him and invite him to their homes. This type of support goes far beyond psychoeducation and family education, since it provides both a therapeutic milieu and a practical capability for meeting experiential crises. In essence, the support group can become a surrogate family for isolated patients and their relatives.

Many participants in family support groups feel they want to advance beyond their own situation to advocate for the whole population of persons with mental illness. In this case, joining and becoming active in advocacy groups begins to fulfil a socially useful and personally therapeutic function. As suggested in the chapter on carer organizations, families' affiliation with professionals on both the case-centred and societal levels enable formerly powerless people to take an active role in controlling their own destinies.

Resolving the family dilemma: toward a collaborative model of care

In evaluating how best to help carers, it is important to recognize that the major stressor for families is probably the reconciliation of conflicting realities. Families face the dilemma of dealing with difficult behaviours in the home while trying to ensure greater societal acceptance and lessened stigma in the world outside the home. They must acknowledge and deal with the violence of a small subset of patients while trying to convince society that the mentally ill are no more violent than other members of society, that they are more victims than victimizers.

In many countries, new patient organizations have had salutary effects in the counselling, mutual support, role-modelling and hope offered by high-functioning consumers to peers, and in developing patient-operated enterprises. Yet families must vie with those members who, typically identifying themselves as ex-patients or survivors, demand for all persons with mental illness the right to refuse medications and other psychiatric services, regardless of levels of dysfunction or self-neglect. Carers of individuals manifesting life-threatening decompensation and severely impaired judgement must contend with a system that makes it difficult to obtain mandatory treatment (see Lefley, 1997a). Whether cast as anti-civil libertarians, or as controlling and paternalistic, families are critically viewed as combating autonomy and self-determination while they feel they are literally fighting to save the life of a person whose continued well-being is entwined with their own.

Above all, families of individuals who are severely impaired must balance the need to live their own lives with the need to do everything they can to help their relatives. Functionally, this means that they must protect themselves from being overwhelmed by the demands of care-giving without feeling they have abandoned someone they love. In most cases of severe disability, this means families must look to mental health systems for care-giving in order to avoid too stressful an impact of mental illness on their own lives and those of vulnerable members such as children.

With ongoing deinstitutionalization, we are now in an era of ageing patients and parental carers approaching their geriatric years. Research suggests that almost all carers worry about their relatives' future "when I am gone", about adequate housing, medication oversight, money management, social outlets and quality of life. Yet few carers know how to make provisions for the financial or social welfare of loved ones (Lefley and

Hatfield, 1999). Fewer still know how to ensure continuity of care for relatives who may stop taking medications, drop out of treatment, perhaps lose their housing and become homeless. This is left up to mental health systems that in many cases are poorly organized for follow-up services to long-term patients. The field badly needs data and projections of what happens to psychiatrically disabled adults when carers die, the replacement resources available, and studies of family disruptions due to carers' death and patient transitions after periods of mourning and loss.

Families can continue to provide emotional and financial support to patients, but they must also do legislative advocacy to ensure the availability of high quality resources for treatment and independent living outside the home. For a better quality of life for themselves, they must also deal with their own paternalistic tendencies and reinforce the message of the consumer movements for greater autonomy and self-determination.

The interests of the carer and consumer movements coincide in terms of more autonomy and independence for the patient. Community psychiatrists and other mental health professionals can help in this process by offering education and support to families, by providing resources for multi-family groups and by promoting their patients' participation in available self-help groups and consumer-operated enterprises. It is increasingly evident that collaborative efforts of the three constituencies—clinicians, carers and patients—are important for long-range rehabilitation at the individual case level, and for joint advocacy at the societal level to ensure adequate resources for independent living in the community. In any part of the world, organized families add a powerful stimulus to adequate funding for mental health services, basic and applied research, and the continued support and development of the psychiatric professions.

References

Anderson C.M., Reiss D.J. and Hogarty, G.E. (1986) *Schizophrenia and the Family*. New York: Guilford Press.

Atkinson, S.D. (1994) Grieving and loss in parents with a schizophrenic child. *American Journal of Psychiatry*, 151, 1137–1139.

Backlar, P. (1994) *The Family Face of Schizophrenia*. New York: Tarcher/Putnam.

Barrowclough, C., Tarrier, N. and Johnston, M. (1996) Distress, expressed emotion, and attributions of relatives of schizophrenic patients. *Schizophrenia Bulletin*, 22, 691–702.

Bebbington, P. and Kuipers, L.(1994) The predictive utility of expressed emotion in schizophrenia: an aggregate analysis. *Psychological Medicine*, 24, 707–718.

Bentsen, H. (1998) *Predictors of Expressed Emotion in Relatives of Patients with Schizophrenia or Related Psychoses*. Oslo, Norway: University of Oslo Faculty of Medicine.

Bergmark, T. (1994) Models of family support in Sweden: from mistreatment to understanding. *New Directions for Mental Health Services*, 62, 71–77.

Birchwood, M., Smith, J. and Cochrane, R. (1992) Specific and non-specific effects of educational interventions for families living with schizophrenia: a comparison of three methods. *British Journal of Psychiatry*, 160, 806–814.

Bland, R. (1994) Supportive approaches to families in Australia: drawing conclusions from practice. *New Directions for Mental Health Services*, 62, 61–69.

Boss, P. (1999) *Ambiguous Loss*. Cambridge, MA: Harvard University Press.

Brown, G. (1985) The discovery of expressed emotion: induction or deduction? In: Leff, J. and Vaughn, C. (eds), *Expressed Emotion in Families*. New York: Guilford Press, pp. 7–25.

Burland, J.(1998) Family-to-family: a trauma and recovery model of family education. *New Directions for Mental Health Services*, 77, 33–41.

Clark, R.E. and Drake, R.E. (1994) Expenditures of time and money of families of people with severe mental illness and substance abuse disorders. *Community Mental Health Journal*, 30, 145–163.

Cuijpers, P. (1999) The effects of family interventions on relatives' burden: a meta-analysis. *Journal of Mental Health*, 8, 275–285.

Dixon, L.B. and Lehman, A.F. (1995) Family interventions for schizophrenia. *Schizophrenia Bulletin*, 21, 631–643.

Dixon, L., Lyles, A., Scott, J., Lehman, A., Postrado., L., Goldman H. *et al.* (1999) Services to families of adults with schizophrenia: from treatment recommendations to dissemination. *Psychiatric Services*, 50, 233–238.

Estroff, S.E., Zimmer, C., Lachicotte, W.S. and Benoit, J. (1994) The influence of social networks and social support on violence by persons with serious mental illness. *Hospital and Community Psychiatry*, 45, 669–679.

Falloon, I.R.H., Boyd, J.L. and McGill, C.W. (1984) *Family Management of Schizophrenia*. Baltimore: Johns Hopkins University.

Greenberg, J., Greenley, .R., McKee, D., Brown, R. and Griffin-Francell, C. (1993) Mothers caring for an adult child with schizophrenia: the effects of subjective burden on maternal health. *Family Relations*, 42, 205–211.

Greenberg, J., Greenley, J.R. and Benedict, P. (1994) Contributions of persons with serious mental illness to their families. *Hospital and Community Psychiatry*, 45, 475–480.

Guarnaccia. P.J. and Parra, P. (1996) Ethnicity, social status, and families' experiences of caring for a mentally ill family member. *Community Mental Health Journal*, 32, 243–260.

Johnson, D.L. (1994) Current issues in family research: can the burden of mental illness be relieved? In: Lefley, H.P. and Wasow, M. (eds), *Helping Families Cope with Mental Illness*. Newark, NJ: Harwood Academic, pp. 309–328.

Kavanagh, D. (1992) Recent developments in expressed emotion and schizophrenia. *British Journal of Psychiatry*, 160, 601–620.

Kazarian, S.S. and Vanderheyden, D.A. (1992) Family education of relatives of people with psychiatric disability: a review. *Psychosocial Rehabilitation Journal*, 15, 67–84.

Lamb, H.R. and Weinberger, L.E. (1998) Persons with severe mental illness in jails and prisons: a review. *Psychiatric Services*, 49, 483–492.

Leff, J.P., Kuipers, L., Berkowitz R. and Sturgeon, D. (1985) A controlled trial of social intervention in families of schizophrenia patients: two year follow-up. *British Journal of Psychiatry*, 146, 594–600.

Leff, J.P. and Vaughn, C. (1985) *Expressed Emotion in Families*. New York: Guilford Press.

Lefley, H.P. (1987) Impact of mental illness in families of mental health professionals. *Journal of Nervous and Mental Disease*, 175, 613–619.

Lefley, H.P. (1996) *Family Caregiving in Mental Illness*. Thousand Oaks, CA: Sage.

Lefley, H.P. (1997a) Mandatory treatment from the family's perspective. *New Directions for Mental Health Services*, 75, 7–16.

Lefley, H.P. (1997b) Synthesising the family caregiving studies: implications for service planning, social policy, and further research. *Family Relations*, 46, 443–450.

Lefley, H.P. (1998a) Families, culture and mental illness: constructing new realities. *Psychiatry*, 61, 335–355.

Lefley, H.P. (1998b) The family experience in cultural context: implications for further research and practice. *New Directions for Mental Health Services*, 77, 97–106.

Lefley, H.P. and Hatfield, A.B. (1999) Helping parental caregivers and mental health consumers cope with parental aging and loss. *Psychiatric Services*, 50, 369–375.

Marsh, D.T. (1998) *Serious Mental Illness and the Family: The Practitioner's Guide*. New York: Wiley.

Maurin, J.T. and Barmann Boyd, C. (1990) Burden of mental illness on the family: a critical review. *Archives of Psychiatric Nursing*, 4, 99–107.

McEvoy, J.P., Scheifler, P.L. and Frances, A. (eds) (1999) The expert consensus guidelines series. Treatment of schizophrenia 1999. *Journal of Clinical Psychiatry*, 60 (Suppl. 11), 4–80.

McFarlane, W. and Lukens, E. (1994) Systems theory revisited; research on family expressed emotion and communication deviance. In: Lefley, H.P. and Wasow, M. (eds), *Helping Families Cope with Mental Illness*. Newark, NJ: Harwood Academic, pp. 70–103.

McFarlane, W.R., Lukens, E., Link, B., Dushay, R., Deakins, S.A., Newmark, M. *et al.* (1995) Multiple-family groups and psychoeducation in the treatment of schizophrenia. *Archives of General Psychiatry*, 52, 679–687.

Merinder, L.B., Viuff, A.G., Laugesen, H.D., Clemmensen, K., Misfelt, S. and Espensen, B. (1999) Patient and relative education in community psychiatry: a randomized controlled trial regarding its effectiveness. *Social Psychiatry and Psychiatric Epidemiology*, 34, 287–294.

Mueser K.T., Glynn, S.M. and Liberman, R.P. (1994) Behavioral family management for serious psychiatric illness. *New Directions for Mental Health Services*, 62, 37–50.

Oldridge, M.L. and Hughes, I.C.T. (1992) Psychological well-being in families with a member suffering from schizophrenia. *British Journal of Psychiatry*, 161, 249–251.

Rosenfarb, I.S., Goldstein, M.J., Mintz, J. and Neuchterlein, K.H. (1995) Expressed emotion and subclinical psychopathology observable within the transactions between schizophrenic patients and their family members. *Journal of Abnormal Psychology*, 104, 259–267.

Scazufca, M. and Kuipers, E. (1996) Links between expressed emotion and burden of care in relatives of patients with schizophrenia. *British Journal of Psychiatry*, 168, 580–587.

Schene A.H., Tessler, R.C. and Gamache, G.M. (1994) Instruments measuring family or caregiver burden in severe mental illness. *Social Psychiatry and Psychiatric Epidemiology*, 29, 228–240.

Schene, A.H, van Wijngaarden, B. and Koeter, M.W.J. (1998) Family caregiving in schizophrenia: domains and distress. *Schizophrenia Bulletin*, 24, 609–618.

Scottish Schizophrenia Research Group (1985) First episode schizophrenia: IV. Psychiatric and social impact on the family. *British Journal of Psychiatry*, 150, 340–344.

Solomon, P. (1996) Moving from psychoeducation to family education for families of adults with serious mental illness. *Psychiatric Services*, 47, 1364–1370.

Solomon, P. (1998) The cultural context of interventions for family members with a seriously mentally ill relative. *New Directions for Mental Health Services*, 77, 5–16.

Stern, S., Doolan, M., Staples, E., Szmukler, G. I. and Eisler, I. (1999) Disruption and reconstruction: narrative insights into the experience of family members caring for a relative diagnosed with serious mental illness. *Family Process*, 38, 353–369.

Straznickas, K.A., McNiel, D.E. and Binder, R.L. (1993) Violence toward family caregivers by mentally ill relatives. *Hospital and Community Psychiatry*, 44, 385–387.

Stromwall, L.K. and Robinson, E.A.R. (1998) When a family member has a schizophrenic disorder: practice issues across the family life cycle. *American Journal of Orthopsychiatry*, 68, 580–589.

Szmukler, G. (1996) From family 'burden' to caregiving. *Psychiatric Bulletin*, 20, 449–451.

Szmukler, G. I., Burgess, P., Herrman, H., Benson, A., Colusa, S. and Bloch, S. (1996a) Caring for relatives with serious mental illness: the development of the Experience of Caregiving Inventory. *Social Psychiatry and Psychiatric Epidemiology*, 31, 137–148.

Szmukler, G. I., Herrman, H., Colusa, S., Benson, A. and Bloch, S. (1996b) A controlled trial of a counselling intervention for caregivers of relatives with schizophrenia. *Social Psychiatry and Psychiatric Epidemiology*, 31, 149–155.

Warner, R. (1999) Environmental interventions in schizophrenia: I. The individual and the domestic level. *New Directions in Mental Health Services*, 83, 61–70.

Warner, R., de Girolamo, G., Belelli, B., Bologna, C., Fioritti, A. and Rosini, G. (1998) The quality of life of people with schizophrenia in Boulder, Colorado and Bologna, Italy. *Schizophrenia Bulletin*, 24, 559–568.

Winefield, H.R. and Harvey, E.J. (1993) Determinants of psychological distress in relatives of people with chronic schizophrenia. *Schizophrenia Bulletin*, 19, 619–635.

Xiong, W., Phillips, M.R., Hu, X., Wang, R., Dai, Q., Kleinman, J. and Kleinman, A. (1994). Family-based interventions for schizophrenic patients in China: A randomized controlled trial. *British Journal of Psychiatry*, 165, 239–247.

13 | *The principles underlying community care*

Michele Tansella and Graham Thornicroft

Introduction

In this chapter, we examine the principles which underlie community care. We start by defining terms, and proceed from the stage of conceptualizing and planning services to discuss their delivery and evaluation. We argue that an ethical basis for mental health services is a necessary complement to the evidence-based approach, and that the interaction between these two perspectives is particularly important. In this respect, we consider it helpful to think of three stages: (i) the identification of *fundamental principles*; (ii) the identification of *applied principles*; and (iii) the translation of applied principles into standardized input, process and outcome measures, to be used for improving the planning, delivery and evaluation of mental health services, considered as a continuing cyclic activity (Thornicroft and Tansella, 1999a).

In concluding this chapter, we will argue that the physical manifestation of services is the embodiment of the principles (both fundamental and applied) held as important at each prior stage in their development. Using this form of 'intellectual archaeology' (i.e. the interpolation of the principles which appear to have been predominant in planning services from the shape which they ultimately assumed), we argue that principles are *inputs* into mental health service, at both the national and local catchment area level (Thornicroft and Tansella, 1999b). These types of input, moreover, are as important in shaping services as are other inputs such as financial investment and the mental health legislative framework. We therefore turn first to the principles which inform the conceptual basis of community care.

Principles underlying the concepts and scope of community care

Turning first to the meaning of 'principle', Table 13.1 shows the definitions of 'principle', defined in the *Concise Oxford Dictionary* as 'a fundamental truth or law as the basis of reasoning or action', etymologically originating in *principium* meaning 'source' or 'foundation'. We refer in this chapter to the principles underlying community care, and choose not to use the term 'values' for this purpose. This is first because the meaning of 'values' overlaps to a large degree with that of 'principles', and secondly because an element of avoidable confusion is added by the term 'values' since this can refer either (i) to the broader sense of worth which is accorded to something, that is to say what is deemed important, or (ii) to a more specific usage, which means utility or the ability to serve a particular purpose (*Concise Oxford Dictionary*, 1993).

The meaning of 'community'

Moving now to the meaning of 'community', Table 13.2 shows five definitions, selected from the *Concise Oxford Dictionary*. The first two of these ('*all the people living in a specific locality*', '*a specific locality, including its inhabitants*'), include both the people in a particular area and that locality itself. The third definition ('*body of people having a religion, a profession, etc., in common*') is consistent with a public health perspective which considers disaggregated subgroups of the total population (e.g. immigrants or people

Table 13.1 *The definition of principle*

Principle *n.*

1a fundamental truth or law as the basis of reasoning or action (*arguing from first principles; moral principles*).

2a a personal code of conduct (*a person of high principle*). b (in pl.) such rules of conduct (*has no principles*).

3a general law in physics etc. (*the uncertainty principle*).

4a law of nature forming the basis for the construction or working of a machine etc.

5a fundamental source; a primary element (*held water to be the first principle of all things*).

6   Chem. A constituent of a substance, esp. one giving rise to some quality, etc.

Etymology ME f. OF *principe* f. L *principium* source, (in pl.) foundations

From the *Concise Oxford Dictionary* (1993).

Table 13.2 *The definition of 'community'*

Community

1 all the people living in a specific locality

2 a specific locality, including its inhabitants.

3 body of people having a religion, a profession, etc., in common (*the immigrant community*).

4 fellowship of interests etc.; similarity (*community of intellect*).

5 the public.

From the *Concise Oxford Dictionary* (1993).

who are homeless), who may be at higher risk for particular mental disorders, or whose needs for services are distinct. The fourth and fifth definitions of 'community' refer to the *fellowship of interests* and to the *general public*, respectively. This wider community of citizens can be seen to delegate responsibility for the care of mentally ill people to the mental health services: in effect, an unwritten contract exists in which the public agree to fund and support (or fail to oppose) those services which contract to provide treatment.

Intriguingly, the word 'community' becomes increasingly complex upon closer inspection. The sense conveyed by the term 'community care', for example, presumes that a functioning social entity exists in a local area. This positive aura for the term may relate to a 'remembered community', which is a symbolic, idealized concept, but which in fact may never have existed (Banton *et al.*, 1985). This notional 'remembered community' has four characteristics: a small and manageable size; the interpenetration of communication and experience of its members; a shared sense of membership or belonging; and participation in a common cause. In any particular local area, some or all of these characteristics may be absent, and indeed this somewhat naïve sense of 'community' has already been supplanted by a more pragmatic approach in the field of 'community' psychiatry, as well as in the wider context of community health and social services.

Re-appraising the meaning of 'common'

The etymological root of 'community' originates in the Latin 'communitas' meaning '*common*'. As Table 13.3 shows, the *Concise Oxford Dictionary* offers five definitions of 'common', all of which may be relevant to the central themes of this chapter (see also Thornicroft and Tansella, 1999b). The *first definition* is 'occurring often', and there are the following implications for the commonness of the mental disorders. Their widespread occurrence means that they will have a very substantial impact on every community and in every type of society. Further, the nature of each local community and each social environment is known

Table 13.3 *The definitions of 'common'*

Common (*adjective*)

1 occurring often (*a common mistake*).

2 ordinary; of ordinary qualities; without special rank or position (*no common mind*; *common soldier*; *the common people*).

3 shared by, coming from, or done by, more than one (*common knowledge*; *by common consent*; *our common benefit*)

4 belonging to, open to, or affecting, the whole community or the public (*common land*).

5 derogatory, inferior (*a common little man*).

Adapted from the *Concise Oxford Dictionary* (1993).

to be closely related to the relative risk of mental illness and the likelihood that an illness will become chronic. Equally, since mental disorders are so widely distributed, it is reasonable to plan responses to these disorders based upon the assumption that many core services should be decentralized commensurately.

The *second meaning* of common is **ordinary**, which may refer to the need to provide routine care, support and treatment in everyday 'real world' clinical settings, and to address the ordinary, practical problems that patients cannot solve alone. A similar concept can apply to the *third meaning* of 'common': '**shared by, coming from, or done by, more than one**' which can also refer to an aspect of community-based services, namely the multi-disciplinary teamwork. A *fourth meaning* of 'common' is '**belonging to, open to, or affecting, the whole community or the public**'. This meaning is also important because it may be linked to one aspect of community-based mental health services, namely their easy access by the whole local community or by all members of the public.

Defining 'community care' and 'community mental health'

Having discussed the meanings of 'community' and its etymological roots, how then should '*community care*' be defined? The term 'community care' was first officially used in Britain, for example, in 1957 (Report on the Royal Commission on Mental Illness and Mental Deficiency), and its historical development has been traced by Bulmer (1987), who has offered four interpretations. It may mean: (i) care outside large institutions; (ii) professional services provided outside hospitals; (iii) care by the community; or (iv) normalization or ordinary living. Later usages include: (v) care in one's own home and (vi) the full range of social care services. Taking into account these roots of 'community', how can *community mental health services* best be defined? Taking these previous contributions into account, we have proposed the following definition:

"A *community-based mental health service* is one which provides a full range of effective mental health care to a defined population, and which is dedicated to treating and helping people with mental disorders, in proportion to their suffering or distress, in collaboration with other local agencies." (Thornicroft and Tansella, 1999b).

The wider context to research in mental health services is the recent explosion of interest in evidence-based medicine (EBM). This reflects the maturation of systematic reviews and other meta-analytical techniques to provide methodologically sound overviews of the strength of scientific evidence in all areas of biomedical research. The origins of EBM lie with the birth of randomized clinical trials and the increasing recognition of the importance of scientific evidence to guide the delivery of health care interventions (Cochrane, 1972; Kassirer, 1993). The EBM approach is, in our view, necessary but not sufficient to inform decisions about priorities and the allocation of resources in the planning and delivery of mental health care. Even when relevant evidence exists, it will nevertheless still need to be interpreted in relation to either explicit or implicit *fundamental principles*, which attach varying degrees of value to the specific results of research. We shall refer later to those principles which have greater salience when applied to the operation of mental health services. The distinction which we denote between *fundamental and applied principles* (which are not different in kind) is useful only in so far as they have explanatory power to assist our understanding of the ethical base of mental health services.

Fundamental principles underlying community care

Within the field of mental health, there is a particular need for an agreed statement of fundamental principles. Many service users lack confidence in professional practice and provision, and find the experience of receiving services alienating, discriminatory and oppressive. Legitimate professional differences of perspective can undermine collaborative partnerships in providing services. The public may lack confidence in the policies being pursued, and may not wish to include people with mental health problems within their local communities. A common *value-base* is an essential step forward in overcoming these obstacles.

Any statement of principles for mental health services may need to command the confidence of service users, their relatives and carers, the range of professionals involved, politicians and the public. It can draw upon social and clinical models of the care and treatment of people who experience mental health problems and social disability. The statement of principles could also adopt a framework for protecting the basic human and civil rights of individuals, and of the public as a whole. It may be able to make clear the responsibilities of all parties, and support the standards of conduct and good practice which will further these aims. These principles do not replace the need for clear, specific and practical guidance, but they can be the necessary building blocks for establishing consensus on how to improve services.

The National Service Framework for Mental Health in England (Department of Health, 1999)

recently has given examples of such fundamental principles, which are summarized in Table 13.4. This national mental health plan proposes that people with mental health problems, and their carers, who require help can expect that the services offering care and treatment show *openness and honesty* in providing information about the results of assessment, and about the range of services which are available. Contacts with every type of care should show that the people working in the services offer users and carers *respect and courtesy*. Care and treatment should be provided *equitably*, should be *proportional* to the changing needs of individuals, and should be provided in the least restrictive way. Resources for services should be distributed according to criteria which are clear, specified and which have widespread acceptance as being fair. In addition, services should be *open to learning and change*, for example as a result of comments or complaints from users of the service, or from the results of internal audit, when service providers act as learning organizations. In fact, as we shall argue below, some of these points are applied rather than fundamental principles.

Table 13.4 *Fundamental principles for planning services for people with mental health problems*

People with mental health problems can expect that services providing their care and treatment will:

show openness and honesty

demonstrate respect and offer courtesy

be allocated fairly and provided equitably

be proportional to their needs

be open to learning and change

From the National Service Framework for Mental Health in England (Department of Health, 1999).

Principles as applied to community care

To propose this selection of ethical principles, we have reviewed the literature and drawn upon our own clinical and research experience to identify those which we consider to be the most relevant to mental health service research, and which are mutually independent. In relation to biomedical ethics as a whole, the approach of 'principalism' has been best set out in the 'Principles of Biomedical Ethics', in which four principles are described as the basis for medical ethics: respect for autonomy; non-maleficence; beneficence; and justice (Downie and Calman, 1987; Beauchamp and Childress, 1994; Holm, 1995). In more particular relation to quality at the service level, Maxwell (1984) has recognized that quality of care cannot be reduced to a single measure, and has described six dimensions: access to services; relevance to need; effectiveness; equity; social acceptability; and finally efficiency and economy. Building upon this, we have selected nine principles: autonomy; continuity; effectiveness; accessibility; comprehensiveness; equity; accountability; coordination; and efficiency (which, from their initials, could be termed 'the three ACEs').

While some degree of overlap still remains, we regard these particular nine principles as largely conceptually distinct, and as exerting the most impact upon mental health services in economically developed countries.

Autonomy

Autonomy has been defined as 'personal freedom', or the 'doctrine of the self-determination of the will'. This is not a characteristic of a health service, but rather a product of what the service does. It refers to the capability of the service to preserve and promote independence by positive experiences, and to reinforce the strengths or healthy aspects of each patient, especially the most severely disabled, while controlling symptoms (Hall, 1992; Jinnett-Sack, 1993). There is a balance between this principle and continuity of care, in that overintrusive or overfrequent follow-up

effectively can interrupt the processes of recovery and rehabilitation. Autonomy is closely associated with another of our key principles: accessibility. The ability to exercise autonomy through choice is negated unless a real choice is possible between actual alternatives that are both available and seen to be relevant by patients.

We define *autonomy* as 'a patient characteristic consisting of the ability to make independent decisions and choices, despite the presence of symptoms or disabilities. Autonomy should be promoted by effective treatment and care'.

Continuity

Continuity has been defined as 'a continuous or connected whole', or 'coherence'. These definitions are pertinent to our purpose here in that they stress the ongoing need by many patients for reliable sources of treatment and social support. Johnson *et al.* (1997) distinguished the longitudinal and cross-sectional dimensions of continuity of care. *Longitudinal continuity* refers to the ability of services to offer an uninterrupted series of contacts over a period of time. *Cross-sectional continuity* includes continuity between different service providers.

The implementation of this principle may also be a way of increasing efficiency, for example the avoidance of multiple or overlapping interventions can reduce costs and adverse effects. At the same time, there are disadvantages from a too compulsive stress upon continuity, which can encourage patients to develop an unhealthy degree of dependence on a particular service, which in turn may foster a chronic sick role (Dickenson, 1997). For these reasons, we consider that for long-term illnesses an appropriate balance is needed to provide *variable continuity*.

We define *continuity* as 'the ability of the relevant services to offer interventions, at the patient or at the local level, and (i) which refers to the coherence of interventions over a shorter time period, both within and between teams [*cross-sectional continuity*], or (ii) which are an uninterrupted series of contacts over a longer time period [*longitudinal continuity*]'.

Effectiveness

The Cochrane database defines effectiveness as 'The extent to which a specific intervention, when used under ordinary clinical circumstances, does what it is intended to do.' (Cochrane Database of Systematic Reviews, 1996). In this sense, effectiveness applies to routine clinical settings, as compared with 'efficacy' which means how far a specific intervention achieves its intentions under ideal, experimental conditions, such as those which are required for randomized controlled trials (Adams *et al.*, 1996; see also Chapter 6).

As one moves from the individual patient level to the treatment programme level, the amount of evidence from controlled studies decreases rapidly, as does its quality, and the primary issue becomes one of effectiveness rather than efficacy. To make research useful in practice, we need to move from efficacy to effectiveness, that is to extend research from selected patient groups to more representative patient samples taken from ordinary clinical settings.

We define *effectiveness* at the individual patient level as 'the proven, intended benefits of treatments provided in real-life situations, and at the treatment programme level as the proven, intended benefits of services provided in real-life situations'.

Accessibility

Accessibility can be understood as *'capable of being entered or reached'* or *'get-at-able'*. This relates directly to the central point, which is that patients should be able to reach and 'get at' services where and when they are needed. Accessibility remains a complex concept. It is used in relation to geographical distance or to travel times from patients' homes to health services sites, to delays in how long it takes for patients to be assessed or treated, and to selective barriers or filters which reduce the uptake of services by all patients (such as stigma) or for some subgroups of the population (such as ethnic minorities).

There may be disadvantages associated with too much accessibility. If specialist services or hospitals are too easily available, then patients may have a low threshold to consult when in difficulty, may by-pass primary care services where these exist, and may expect specialist attention when suffering from relatively minor, brief and self-remitting conditions. Such contacts may divert time and resources away from more severely disabled patients, and access may be delivered at the expense of equity. Secondly, if accessibility is too high, then efficiency may reduce as minor disorders are seen in the more expensive specialist services. Accessibility therefore cannot be unlimited, and services may need to encourage self-limited use by patients, for example in relation to night-time emergency services.

We define *accessibility* as 'a service characteristic, experienced by patients and their carers, which enables them to receive care where and when it is needed'.

Comprehensiveness

A central dilemma for health services is the balance between offering more intensive care to fewer patients or less intensive care to more. The degree of comprehensiveness of a service therefore raises the key question: comprehensive for whom? Taking mental health as an example, psychiatric disorders will affect about a quarter of the general adult population in any year, and since the capacity of the specialist mental health services, even in most economically developed countries, means that they can provide a service usually to between 2 and 6% of the adult population, these services will *necessarily* be limited to only a minority of those suffering from mental illnesses. The question then becomes one of quality *or* quantity. Services which selectively treat first the more severely mentally ill, such as in Britain, will provide a relatively poor service for the majority of patients who have neurotic illnesses. Many of these cases remain untreated if they are not recognized by primary care staff. This lack of treatment, in turn, may increase the risk of chronicity and of developing subsequent disabilities and handicaps. Similarly, in other areas of medicine, services given to people with lesser degrees of severity may replace those given to those with more severe forms of illness.

We define **comprehensiveness** as 'a service characteristic with two dimensions. By *horizontal comprehensiveness*, we mean how far a service extends across the whole range of severity of mental illnesses, and across a wide range of patient characteristics. By *vertical comprehensiveness*, we mean the availability of the basic components of care, and their use by prioritized groups of patients'.

Equity

Commonly defined as aspect of 'fairness', the application of the principle of equity implies that the distribution of money for health services should be made according to criteria which are specified, transparent and which have widespread acceptance as being fair. There is a need to adapt and apply such rational and explicit approaches to resource allocation in settings where historical and inequitable patterns may predominate (Chodoff, 1981; Mooney, 1986; Westrin *et al.*, 1992; see also Chapters 14 and 44).

In our view, there is a useful distinction between explicit and implicit equity in allocating resources to health services. Implicit methods often are based on decisions taken by restricted groups of people which are not transparent, since the criteria used are not in the public domain. These decisions may be defined as equitable by using *post-hoc* independent procedures. We believe that the basis upon which resources are allocated should be a process of needs assessment, although in this respect is it notable that Hunter in Chapter 14 advocates the advantages of 'muddling through elegantly', and warns against the dangers of being too transparent (Beecham *et al.*, 1995).

We define **equity** as 'the fair distribution of resources. The rationale used to prioritize between competing needs, and the methods used to calculate the allocation of resources, should be made explicit'.

Accountability

At the individual patient level, the principle of accountability refers to the element of responsibility within the relationship between staff and individual patients, a relationship that needs to be based upon confidence and trust. Each patient has a legitimate expectation that the clinician will offer treatment based upon a 'duty of care', and will do this in accordance with accepted standards of professional practice. For example, one aspect of direct accountability to the patient is that clinical information remains confidential. This type of direct patient accountability may be challenged by requests from family members (or others), who express the need for services also to be accountable to them. At the treatment programme level, a wider set of considerations apply, and health services operate in a way which offers *dual accountability*; both to the patient and to the wider society. In practice, health services are held accountable by the public to act in a way that maintains public confidence in their viability.

We define **accountability** as 'a function which consists of complex, dynamic relationships between mental health services and patients, their families and the wider public, who all have legitimate expectations of how the service should act responsibly'.

Co-ordination

We can distinguish between cross-sectional and longitudinal types of co-ordination. The first refers to the co-ordination of information and services within an episode of care (both within and between services). The latter refers to the inter-relationships between staff and between agencies over a longer period of treatment, often spanning several episodes.

We define **co-ordination** as 'a service characteristic which is manifested by coherent treatment plans for individual patients. Each plan should have clear goals and include interventions which are needed and effective: no more and no less. By **cross-sectional co-ordination**, we mean the co-ordination of information and services within an episode of care. By **longitudinal co-ordination**, we mean the inter-linkages between staff and between agencies over a longer period of treatment'.

Efficiency

There will never be 'enough' resources allocated for health services in the eyes of patients, their carers or staff. If we accept this scarcity as the basic condition, our starting point is therefore the narrower question of allocation. The pursuit of efficiency can mean, therefore, reducing the costs for a given level of effectiveness (outcome), or improving the level of effectiveness or the volume and quality of outcomes achieved from fixed budgets (Knapp, 1995).

Three types of economic efficiency have been defined by Drummond and O'Brien (1997). *Technical efficiency* is 'achieving maximum physical output from resource use' (without considering the costs implications). *Productive efficiency* means 'achieving maximization of output for a given cost'. *Allocative efficiency* is defined as 'achieving maximization of the value attached to the output for a given cost'. In terms of the patient level, Cochrane (1972) described inefficiency in two senses: the use of ineffective therapies and the use of effective therapies at the wrong time.

We define *efficiency* as 'a service characteristic, which minimizes the inputs needed to achieve a given level of outcomes, or which maximizes the outcomes for a given level of inputs'.

Two illustrations serve to show how such applied principles can be used for the development of mental health policy. First, a joint European Commission/World Health Organization meeting on the balance between mental health promotion and mental health service provision, held in Brussels in April 1999, included eight of the nine components of the three ACEs in its final communiqué summarizing the core relevant principles (WHO/EC, 1999). Secondly, the National Service Framework for Mental Health in England (Department of Health, 1999) has itemized a series of applied principles which should inform the development of mental health services for adults of working age (Table 13.5).

A conceptual framework for mental health services

Having discussed fundamental and applied principles, we move next to consider a framework within which these principles can be set in

Table 13.5 *Applied principles of the National Service Framework for Mental Health in England (Department of Health, 1999)*

People with mental health problems can expect that services will:

meaningfully involve users and their carers in planning and delivery of care

deliver high quality treatment and care which is known to be effective and acceptable

be well suited to those who use them and non-discriminatory

be accessible so that help is available when and where it is needed

promote their safety and that of their carers, staff and the wider public

offer choices which promote independence

be well co-ordinated between all staff and agencies

empower and support their staff

deliver continuity of care for as long as this is needed

be properly accountable to the public, users and carers

context. For planning, delivering and evaluating mental health services, there is a clear need for an overall conceptual framework. We have proposed such a framework (the matrix model) which uses two dimensions, the *geographical* (country, local and patients levels, identified by the numbers 1, 2 and 3) and the *temporal* (input, process and outcome phases, referred to by the letters A, B and C) (Tansella and Thornicroft, 1998). Using these two dimensions, a 3x3 matrix with nine cells is constructed to bring into focus critical issues for mental health services, and the overall scheme is illustrated in Table 13.6.

As Table 13.7 shows, these principles are most relevant at different levels of the matrix model.

Table 13.6 Overview of the matrix model

Geographical dimension	Temporal dimension		
	(A) Input phase	(B) Process phase	(C) Outcome phase
(1) Country/regional level	1A	1B	1C
(2) Local level (catchment area)	2A	2B	2C
(3) Patient level	3A	3B	3C

Table 13.7 Principles for community mental health services: 'the three ACEs' in relation to the three geographical levels of the matrix model

	Principle	Geographical level of the matrix model		
		Patient	Local	Country
1st ACE	1 Autonomy	x		
	2 Continuity	x	x	
	3 Effectiveness	x	x	
2nd ACE	4 Accessibility		x	
	5 Comprehensiveness		x	
	6 Equity		x	
3rd ACE	7 Accountability		x	x
	8 Co-ordination		x	x
	9 Efficiency		x	x

While the first ACE (autonomy, continuity and effectiveness) applies to the patient level, in comparison, the second and third ACEs apply only at higher levels. Autonomy is directly relevant only at the patient level; nevertheless, if data from this level are aggregated, information about the application of this principle can be used to describe outcomes at the local or regional levels.

As outlined in the Introduction, following the identification of the fundamental and applied principles, the next stage in elaborating a well-articulated relationship between an ethically based and an evidence-based approach to mental health services is to operationalize these nine principles through *scale construction and standardization*. Once developed, such scales may be implemented in research studies, to provide a multi-dimensional assessment of mental health service inputs, processes and outcomes.

Conclusions

In concluding this chapter, we wish to emphasize the *practical* usefulness of principles (both fundamental and applied) in relation to mental health services. Although they could be considered as abstractions without direct impact on the real world, in fact we argue that they are the foundations upon which all the practical manifestations of mental health services and treatments are built. Although such fundamentals are necessarily present, in fact they are usually covert rather than overt, and are therefore less open to scrutiny and debate. For example, in the common situation where over 75% of the mental health service budget is spent on in-patient beds, this does not occur by chance alone, but may reflect the fact that decisions continue to made which attach higher principle to providing *continuity* of care, along with *vertical comprehensiveness*, to those relatively few patients who are in hospital, than to ensure the *autonomy* of these patients, or the *accessibility* to assessment and treatment for the larger number of patients outside hospital who may benefit from specialist care.

We identify five main practical uses for principles in relation to mental health services.

(i) *Principles may be used in the absence of evidence*, for example in establishing a service where no strong evidence base exists, such as one for the treatment of people with antisocial personality disorders. The Italian psychiatric reform offers a second illustration of the impact of principles in the absence of *scientific* evidence, because these radical changes were enacted when a widely based platform of political, mass media, lay and professional beliefs moved policy towards deinstitutionalization on the humanitarian and ideological grounds that community-based treatment offering greater *accountability* and *accessibility*, while aiming to promote the *autonomy* of service users, would offer conditions better than those found at that time within the large and neglected psychiatric institutions.

(ii) The situation where *principles may be used instead of evidence* (evidence exists but is discounted), for example on political or financial grounds. To illustrate this, it may be impossible to open a new community-based mental health facility in a climate where there is widespread and strongly felt local opposition to such a proposal, or when financial constraints limit or prohibit any new services, even when research evidence would support such a service development.

(iii) *Principles may be used in conjunction with available evidence*. This can be: (a) to attach relative value to the results of research or (b) to adjudicate where the research evidence is unclear or conflicting. An example of the first situation is in the choice of medication for psychotic disorders, where the evidence is that the newer, atypical neuroleptic drugs produce fewer adverse effects, but at much greater purchasing price. In the short term, therefore, the evidence will not be sufficient alone to answer the question of whether this category of drugs should the first-line treatment of choice. A principle needs to be attached to the relief of suffering (from having fewer adverse effects) and this benefit then weighed against the additional costs of the atypical neuroleptic drugs, compared with their traditional counterparts, for a purchasing decision to be made.

(iv) *Principles may be used to produce new outcome measures*, as we have outlined in the previous section. It is notable that so far the domains of measures for mental health services have included the translation of only three principles into measures, to be used in accordance with the EBM paradigm: effectiveness of treatments, efficiency and continuity of care. The latter has been initiated recently (Sytema *et al.*, 1997; Saarento *et al.*, 1998; Sytema and Burgess, 1999), and there is as yet no consensus on how continuity can be operationalized in a standardized manner.

(iv) *Principles may orient decisions on directions for research funding* and future scientific developments. For example, the activities of scientific funding bodies and international grant committees are not immune to the wider social and political atmosphere of the times, which will reflect the fundamental values which have commanded a common currency at those particular times and places.

References

Adams, C., Freemantle, N. and Lewis, G. (1996) Meta-analysis. In: Knudsen, H.C. and Thornicroft, G. (eds), *Mental Health Service Evaluation*. Cambridge: Cambridge University Press, pp. 176–196.

Banton, R., Clifford, P., Frosch, S., Lousada, J. and Rosenthall, J. (1985) *The Politics of Mental Health*. London: Macmillan.

Beauchamp, T.L. and Childress, J.F. (1994) *Principles of Biomedical Ethics*, 4th edn. New York: Oxford University Press.

Bulmer, M. (1987) *The Social Basis of Community Care*. London: Allen and Unwin.

Calman, K.C. (1994) The ethics of allocation of scarce health care resources: a view of randomized controlled trials of health care. *Millbank Quarterly*, 71, 411–437.

Chodoff, P. (1981) The responsibility of the psychiatrist to his society. In: Bloch,S. and Chodoff, P. (eds), *Psychiatric Ethics*. Oxford: Oxford University Press, pp. 306–321.

Cochrane, A.L. (1972) *Effectiveness and Efficiency. Random Reflections on Health Services*. London: Nuffield Provincial Hospitals Trust.

Cochrane Database of Systematic Reviews (1996) Adams, C., Anderson, J. and Mari, J. (eds), Available in *The Cochrane Library* (database on disk and CDROM). The Cochrane Collaboration; Issue 3. Oxford: Update Software; 1996. Updated quarterly. Available from: BMJ Publishing Group: London.

Dickenson, D. (1997) Ethical issues in long-term psychiatric management. *Journal of Medical Ethics*, 23, 300–304.

Department of Health (1999) *The National Service Framework for Mental Health. Modern Standards and Service Models*. London: Department of Health.

Downie, R.S. and Calman, K.C. (1987) *Healthy Respect. Ethics in Healthcare*. London; Faber and Faber.

Drummond, M. and O'Brien, B. (1997) *Methods for the Economic Evaluation of Heath Care Programmes*, 2nd edn. Oxford: Oxford University Press.

Hall, S.A. (1992) Should public health respect autonomy? *Journal of Medical Ethics*, 18, 197–201.

Holm, S. (1995) Not just autonomy. The principles of American biomedical ethics. *Journal of Medical Ethics*, 21, 332–338.

Jinnett-Sack, S. (1993) Autonomy in the company of others. In: Grubb, A. (ed.), *Choices and Decisions in Healthcare*. London: Wiley, pp. 97–136.

Johnson, S., Prossor, D., Bindman, J. and Szmukler, G. (1997) Continuity of care for the severely mentally ill: concepts and measures. *Social Psychiatry and Psychiatric Epidemiology*, 32, 137–142.

Kassirer, J.P. (1993) Clinical trials and meta-analysis. What do they do for us? *New England Journal of Medicine*, 327, 273–274.

Knapp, M. (1995) Community mental health services: towards an understanding of cost-effectiveness. In: Tyrer, P. and Creed, F. (eds), *Community Psychiatry in Action: Analysis and Prospects*. Cambridge: Cambridge University Press.

Maxwell, R.J. (1984) Quality assessment in health. *British Medical Journal*, 288, 1470–1472.

Mooney, G.H. (1986) *Economics, Medicine and Healthcare*. Brighton: Wheatsheaf Books.

Saarento, O., Oiesvold, T., Sytema, S., Gostas, G., Kastrup, M., Lonnerberg, O., Muus, S., Sandlund, M. and Hansson, L. (19998) The Nordic comparative study on sectorised psychiatry: continuity of care related to characteristics of the psychiatric services and the patients. *Social Psychiatry and Psychiatric Epidemiology*, 33, 521–527.

Sytema, S. and Burgess, P. (1999) Continuity of care and readmission in two service systems: a comparative Victorian and Groningen case-register study. *Acta Psychiatrica Scandanavica*, 100, 212–219.

Sytema, S., Micciolo, R. and Tansella, M. (1997) Continuity of care for patients with schizophrenia and related disorders: a comparative South-Verona and Groningen case register study. *Psychological Medicine*, 27, 1355–1362.

Tansella, M. and Thornicroft, G. (1998) A conceptual framework for mental health services. *Psychological Medicine*, 28, 503–508.

Thornicroft, G. and Tansella, M. (1999a) Can ethical principles become outcome measures for mental health service research? *Psychological Medicine* , 29, 761–767.

Thornicroft, G. and Tansella, M. (1999b) *The Mental Health Matrix. A Manual to Improve Services*. Cambridge: Cambridge University Press.

Westrin, C.-J., Nilstun, T., Smedby, B. and Haglund, B. (1992) Epidemiology and moral philosophy. *Journal of Medical Ethics*, 18, 193–196.

World Health Organisation/European Commission (1999). *Prevention of mental health problems: report of meeting in Brussels*. Geneva: WHO.

14 | *Balancing clinical values and finite resources*

Frank Holloway

Introduction

Mental health professionals frequently are placed in a dilemma: whose interests are they serving? This dilemma is readily apparent in debates surrounding coercion, confidentiality and the protection of others (Chapters 45 and 46). However, there is a largely unacknowledged major area of conflict of duty in the resource allocation role of mental health providers (Szmukler and Holloway, 1998). This chapter seeks to address the complex issues of how clinical activities within community mental health services can be prioritized and how these processes can be aided by application of evidence-based health and social care. It is written from a UK perspective although it is informed by developments in other countries, particularly the USA, which is showing significant signs of convergence with the UK despite apparently radically differing systems of health care (Newman, 1995). It should be read in conjunction with Chapter 44, which looks at the rationing of services from an ethical perspective.

The UK context

Health care in the UK is free at the point of delivery for the whole population, although an increasing minority opt to pay for health insurance that offers limited care in the private sector. Private insurance has a minimal impact on needs for treatment of psychotic illnesses, but in some affluent areas significantly decreases demand on services for non-psychotic disorders. At the time of writing, the 'health' and 'social' aspects of care are the responsibility of separate bodies, the National Health Service (NHS) and local authority Social Services Departments. A major thrust of recent mental health policy has been to bridge the health and social care divide (Department of Health, 1995), and there is increasing emphasis on joint working between health and social care agencies. Traditionally, access to all forms of health care is controlled by primary care doctors (Coulter, 1998), although people with a severe mental illness have always been able to by-pass this filtering mechanism (Goldberg and Huxley, 1980). Since the rise of the asylum in the 19th century, mental health care has been provided on a geographical basis, although the concept of localized 'District Psychiatry' only evolved during the 1950s (Freeman and Bennett, 1991).

Reforms to health and social care introduced in the 1990s brought in a divide between responsibility for the purchasing of care and its provision. Providers work to contracts negotiated with purchasers (Health and Social Services Authorities which are in turn responsible for disbursing monies almost entirely allocated by central government). The contracting process has similarities with managed care practices in the USA (Fairfield *et al.*, 1997a). Typically, in the UK, a single health care provider (an NHS Trust) will be responsible for the mainstream secondary mental health services to a geographical area, spanning the whole range of in-patient and community services. Specialist services may come from alternative providers. The geographical area is broken down further into local catchment areas or sectors provided for by community mental health teams in the models described throughout this book (see particularly Chapter 20). Generally, community teams work closely with in-patient services, often sharing key managerial and clinical personnel and a common budget for the locality or sector. The provision of social care is much more fragmented, operating as a deliberate policy within a 'mixed economy of care'.

Most health care providers are NHS employees, although purchasers may well contract for marginal activities (e.g. counselling, provision of welfare benefits advice, advocacy services) to voluntary sector agencies or private health care organizations. In a recent development, the purchasing responsibilities currently vested in Health Authorities (serving on average 500 000 people) may transfer to Primary Care Trusts, aggregations of local providers of primary care (serving on average 100 000 people) (Secretary of State for Health, 1997).

Three important features flow from the organization of mental health services in the UK. First, in contrast to insurance-based fee-for-service systems such as in France and Germany, there are no 'perverse incentives' for mental health providers or professionals to favour hospital over community care. Secondly, there currently are incentives to shift responsibility for patient care between 'health' and 'social' care sectors and between primary and secondary care, although all actors are supposed to co-operate and work within a National Service Framework set out by the Department of Health (Department of Health, 1999a). Thirdly, the autonomy of a provider is significantly limited by its contractual obligations to the purchaser. The UK system is therefore one of creative tension between stakeholders (which also increasingly include the non-statutory sector, service users and carers, and primary care doctors). The purchaser has the lead responsibility for change in the system (Gallagher, 1996). Central government, through the NHS Executive, can and will intervene to resolve conflicts, and closely monitors the performance of purchasers and providers.

Traditionally, funding streams have been relatively simple, flowing from central government according to centrally derived funding formulae to Health Authorities for health care and local authority Social Services Departments for social care. The latter are subject to the local political process and the former to the whole range of competing claims for health expenditure experienced by purchasers. There are sources of funding focused on areas of specific policy concern, such as the Mental Illness Specific Grant to Social Services Departments. Increasingly, additional funds are given to purchasers on the basis of competitive bids reflecting areas of innovation supported by government. Typically, these will require evidence of multi-agency engagement in the planning process. The bidding cycle for these funds, which represent a large proportion of the available growth monies, tends to be short.

Managed care

The structure of mental health services in the USA is highly complex, with multiple funding sources, competing providers and an array of purchasing responsibilities at national, state and local levels and within the private insurance sector (Santiago, 1992; Elpers and Levin, 1996). Government funds some 60% of US mental health and substance misuse services, with private insurance funding the balance. Managed care has developed "as a response to spiralling healthcare costs and dysfunctional fragmented services" (Fairfield, 1997a). It involves a variety of practices aimed at curbing costs by moving away from a demand-led fee-for-service system towards a system that constrains providers to offer a defined range of services within an overall budgetary allocation. Tight contracts are let with providers that specify entitlements. Strict treatment guidelines, management protocols and external review of entitlements and care plans are the norm. The penetration of the publicly funded mental health system by managed care has been rapid and dramatic (Hoge *et al.*, 1998). Gittleman (1998) provides a brief overview of the history and current practices of managed mental health care for the international reader.

The literature generated is vast, with numerous periodicals and books aimed at the mental health professional and administrator devoted to survival within a managed care environment (e.g. American Psychiatric Assiciation, 1996; Corcoran and Vandiver, 1996; Goodman *et al.*, 1996; Lazarus, 1996). One of the most startling aspects of managed mental health care from a European perspective is the practice of 'carve-outs', where the state mental health authorities subcontract the management of publicly funded mental health care (through Medicare, Medicaid and other programmes) to for-profit behavioural managed care companies. These large organizations then subcontract to provider organizations: overheads and profits must come from extracting increased 'efficiency' from providers.

Public sector-managed care in the US context, although in its infancy and rapidly evolving (Hoge *et al.*, 1999), arguably deserves a cautious welcome (Hoge *et al.*, 1998) in bringing some coherence to a fragmented and chaotic system. Preliminary evidence suggests that managed care has the capacity to reduce expenditure by trading-off increased access to care against reduced intensity of service provision, with little obvious impact on quality of care or service user satisfaction (Mechanic *et al.*, 1995). However, there are grounds for concern. Guze (1998) has asserted that psychotherapy is generally not integrated into overall managed care treatment plans and that the managed care model involves serious fragmentation of the overall care of patients. The National Alliance for the Mentally Ill concluded that treatment standards and practice protocols adopted by managed care organizations were out of date and unduly restrictive (Hall *et al.*, 1997). The implementation of for-profit managed care within the public sector has been highly controversial [see, for example, Fendell, 1998, who discusses very negatively the experience of a managed care 'carve-out' in Massachusetts which, in strict financial terms, has been reported as successful (Frank and McGuire, 1997)].

Working with limited resources

It is a truism that demand for health and social care outstrips the resources available to meet it. Health care expenditure within advanced economies has been steadily rising without ever quite matching the expectations of the population or of health care professionals. In the UK, mental health services have taken a progressively lower share of total health care spending since the inception of the National Health Service (from 15% of the total in the early 1950s to 11% in the late 1990s). A steady decline in hospital-based care has, however, allowed significant investment in community services. The technologies deployed within these services traditionally have been cheap. Community care has in general involved hard-pressed staff offering monitoring, medication and minimal support to patients and carers. New and more expensive treatment technologies that have been developed over recent years (e.g. atypical antipsychotic medication, family management strategies and psychological treatments for non-psychotic and psychotic disorder) are not widely available in the UK. This reflects both a lack of resources and lack of skills within the mental health workforce. (A similar bleak picture is painted in the USA by Lehman and Steinwachs, 1998a.)

UK policy has emphasized improving service structures, with expectations on providers to follow-up all people referred to secondary mental health services under the Care Programme Approach (Kingdon, 1994). This is officially defined as providing:

"a framework for care co-ordination of service users under specialist mental health services. The main elements are a care co-ordinator, a written care plan, and at higher levels, regular reviews by the multi-disciplinary health team and integration with the social services care management system" (Department of Health, 1999a, p. 129).

Policy has placed increasing emphasis on the assessment and management of risk (Holloway, 1996). The safety of the public is an explicit (if perhaps illusory) goal for the UK's 'safe, sound and supportive' mental health services (Secretary of State for Health, 1998), and decreasing the suicide rate is a key outcome indicator for the UK strategy on public health (Department of Health, 1999b). More recently, there has been pressure on providers to develop assertive outreach services [along the lines of assertive community treatment (Chapter 21)] for more vulnerable people with a severe mental illness, even in the absence of a local assessment of needs.

The provider of mental health services in the UK faces a range of demands in addition to the very evident needs of the clients or patients on the current caseload and those newly presenting for treatment and care. First, there are demands set out by government in statute, quasi-statute and policy guidance. The emphasis at this level is on targeting people with 'severe and enduring mental health problems' (the euphemism changes from time to time), ensuring follow-up, care planning and risk management services (Secretary of State for Health, 1998; Department of Health, 1999a). Diversion from in-patient beds, expensive and in the UK under increasing pressure, is seen as a major aim of service developments. Secondly, at a local level, there are the expectations of purchasers, GPs and the local community that the community mental health teams will respond to all requests for intervention when a 'mental health problem' has been identified. Reasons for referral from primary care are complex (see Chapter 36) but, in practice, the majority of referrals received by teams will not suffer from major mental illnesses. Thirdly, stakeholders are becoming more sophisticated and are beginning to expect mental health services to deploy modern treatments that are well publicized in the literature, on the Internet and by users' and carers' organizations such as the National Schizophrenia Fellowship (National Schizophrenia Fellowship, 1998). Fourthly, those providers who are not overwhelmed by the burden of day to day activity are frustrated at not being able to deploy their existing skills and develop new skills. Professionals want to improve their practice and in particular are unhappy at not being able to provide effective treatments to people in need because of arbitrarily imposed eligibility criteria (anecdotally, a particular concern in managed care). These potentially conflicting demands are compounded by another strand of UK government policy, the introduction of 'Clinical Governance' into the NHS (which in essence involves the introduction of a statutory duty on providers to pursue quality on an equal basis to the pre-existing

duty of financial probity) and an espousal of evidence-based practice (Secretary of State for Health, 1997). The National Service Framework (Department of Health, 1999a) refers throughout to the evidence base for the broad-brush national standards for mental health services it sets out, as well as containing numerous anecdotal descriptive accounts of services identified as examples of good practice.

In the face of a barrage of potentially conflicting demands, professionals can adopt a variety of well-worn pragmatic strategies (New, 1996). These are **deterrence** (service charges, gate-keeping by primary care, unfriendly staff, inconvenient appointment times, poor quality care environments); **deflection** (passing referrals to other agencies, shifting between 'health' and 'social' care); **dilution** (thinly spreading service provision, adopting minimal standards of care, reducing skill-mix in a nursing team); **delay** (waiting lists, which for psychological treatments can become infinitely long); and **denial**. The last involves not providing a treatment or service at all for more or less justifiable reasons. Most community mental health staff will recognize these strategies operating within their day to day work. The strategies are rarely acknowledged explicitly, with the exception of mechanisms of denial of care.

The ethics and economics of mental health care

There is an apparent tension between ethical and economic perspectives on mental health care. The ethical imperative for physicians to prescribe treatment to the best of their ability seems to be at odds with economic concepts such as cost containment, rationing and efficiency. Chisholm and Stewart (1998) challenge this assumption. Professionals generally see their role in terms of providing the best possible treatment for their individual patient or client (the traditional role of beneficence). However, this needs to be tempered by a consideration of the needs of other patients who potentially might benefit from care. Health and welfare services operate in conditions of resource scarcity. Any use of these resources carries with it an 'opportunity cost': what alternative use could be made of the resources allocated to a particular patient in a particular way? Principles of efficiency (making the best use of available resources) and welfare maximization (optimizing health and social welfare) can help structure debates at the level of national policy and large-scale purchasing. These will have to take account of the ethical principle of justice or fairness. More immediately, practitioners making the decision to admit a patient need to take account of the opportunity cost of that decision (not admitting someone with more urgent need). Taking a patient onto a caseload or into treatment is likely to mean that another patient is not taken on (or the quality of the overall service is diluted). Prescribing an atypical antipsychotic for a year to 10 patients has the opportunity cost of a community mental health worker in a hard-pressed team (at UK prices), unless there are efficiency benefits to the prescription (e.g. saving on bed utilization) which are recouped immediately by the services. In this analysis, engaging in ineffective practices, however much they reflect stakeholder demand and the predelictions of professionals, can be seen as unethical.

Professionals therefore have responsibilities not only to their individual patient but to the population as a whole. Operating in a system of scarcity they "find themselves in positions of deciding *who* receives *what* resources *when* and *how frequently*" (Christiansen, 1997a). Decisions are being made daily, albeit without conscious consideration, that balance beneficence and fairness. In the context of managed care, and indeed the practices of the purchaser–provider divide within a system funded through general taxation such as in the UK, professionals will also be mindful of organizational priorities. Within managed care services, there are clear incentives for not providing care (Chisholm and Stewart, 1998) and, unsurprisingly, the ethical practices of some managed care organizations have been questioned (Fairfield *et al.*, 1997b). Although there is scope for professionals to use their gate-keeping role creatively by ensuring that care for those who are "unnoticed, underserved, and unable to

negotiate passage into the health care system" (Christiansen, 1997b), the harsh reality is that a more strategic approach may be necessary. "To serve all her clients adequately, the provider needs to maintain a good reputation among those who allocate resources and who cannot meet all claims by all providers" (Backlar, 1996). Leaders within provider organizations have a complex task that includes both optimizing the efficiency and effectiveness of their staff and increasing the available local resources for care. Good relationships with purchasers, awareness of current policy trends, ability to react rapidly to funding opportunities and a willingness to accommodate the demands of stakeholders are all required if funding is to be maximized.

Rosenheck *et al.* (1998) have produced a number of key ethical principles in setting out mental health service priorities, emphasizing the obligation that exists to the least well-off and articulate members of society. These emphasize fairness of access to health care and fairness in decision making as priorities are set for different groups of people with a mental illness and between mental illness and other health problems.

Evidence-based mental health

Evidence-based medicine (EBM) is "the conscientious, explicit and judicious use of current best evidence in making decisions about the care of individual patients" (Sackett *et al.*, 1996), incorporating this evidence into the practical skills of the clinician. EBM is essentially about moving beyond received wisdom, custom and practice to take account of expanding knowledge. There is no analogous definition of 'evidence-based purchasing'. It must extend beyond the level of individual diagnosis and treatment into systems of care and difficult decisions about the relative value of differing forms of treatment and care within an area of activity (e.g. mental health services) and between areas of activity.

Key principles of EBM are set out in a pocketbook (Sackett *et al.*, 1997) which, given the alleged rate of advance in biomedical knowledge, consigns the textbook to the dustbin of history. A journal *Evidence Based Mental Health*, first published in 1998, outlines key papers in the field and offers structured commentaries. The clinician (and interested purchaser) can now have access to the overwhelming mass of data accumulated in the academic literature through databases such as Medline, Embase and PsychInfo, which are available on-line. A new technology, the systematic review, has been developed in an attempt to bring order to this potentially confusing mass of information. Systematic reviews seek to bring together all the available knowledge on a clearly formulated topic using explicit search criteria, sifting through it to identify methodologically sound studies and providing a balanced account of the findings in a statistically acceptable manner (Freemantle and Geddes, 1998; Geddes *et al.*, 1998). The Cochrane Collaboration [accessible through the Internet (www.update-software.com/ccweb/cochrane/cdsr.htm)] provides a library of systematic reviews of medical treatments, which includes many mental health topics. The UK is investing heavily in EBM. There is an NHS Centre for Reviews and Dissemination (www.york.ac.uk/inst/crd/srinfo.htm) based at the University of York. This collaborates with a Centre for Evidence Based Mental Health at the University of Oxford, which takes a lead in the mental health section of the UK National electronic Library for Health (NeLH) (www.psychiatry.ox.ac.uk/cebmh.htm).

Ready Internet access is also available to a wide range of clinical guidelines, which have been brought together in a variety of sites: a problem here is to winnow the evidence-based wheat from the opinionated chaff. There is an established good practice in the development of clinical guidelines relating to the process of guideline development and its format, the identification of evidence and its summary, and the formulation of recommendations. Published guidelines do not, in general, adhere to these standards (Shaneyfelt *et al.*, 1999) and should be treated with appropriate scepticism. Useful guidelines on treatment of schizophrenia utilizing EBM principles recently have been published (Lehman and Steinwachs, 1998b), as has a readable synthesis of the literature on the

management of deliberate self-harm (NHS Centre for Reviews and Dissemination, 1998).

Policy-relevant publications such as *New Directions for Mental Health Services* and *Effective Health Care* (not specifically devoted to mental health and available on-line via the Centre for Reviews and Dissemination) provide digests of the literature and review articles, as do more mainstream professional journals. Pressure groups and non-governmental organizations regularly produce reports on important issues that can inform policy makers at national and local level. These reports rarely if ever adhere to the tenets of EBM, providing commentaries on issues of concern from a particular perspective and quoting selectively from the research literature. They can, however, have influence on policy makers if they propose timely solutions to political dilemmas. Despite the contempt with which some EBM practitioners hold textbooks, these remain a useful source of information for purchasers and practitioners in synthesizing information, addressing complex and messy issues that tend not to achieve publication in academic journals and allowing fertilization between disciplines.

There are limitations to EBM as a tool for purchasing decisions (Conway *et al.*, 1996). In many areas of interest, the quality of the research evidence is poor, reflecting both failure to invest in research into service structures and psychological treatments compared with pharmacological treatments and the considerable methodological difficulties inherent in service research. Many mental health practices are almost unresearched. There is, for example, a dearth of well-designed studies on the value of the traditional out-patient clinic, on day care and sheltered work, on the decision to admit, on the role of in-patient care and on the outcome of compulsory treatment and coercion. Even when the *efficacy* of an intervention has been demonstrated in well-controlled research studies, this may not map onto *effectiveness* in clinical practice (Thornicroft *et al.*, 1998). Populations involved in research studies may differ markedly from the local population, and staff working in routine services may have very different motivations and capacities from those in short-term experimental programmes. Moreover, research into services will depend on the peculiarities of the cultural, legal and economic context of the study.

Further fundamental problems confront the EBM enthusiast. Service change may run ahead of the available evidence. As an example, there is good evidence that mental hospital closure can benefit existing hospital residents (Leff, 1997). However, hospital closure programmes throughout the western world have progressed without reference to these data on the basis of local concerns relating to cost, quality of care and the need to reinvest in community mental health services. Purchasers and practitioners may fundamentally disagree about the nature of the tasks being undertaken by mental health services. They may indeed view the 'evidence' being cited as irrelevant to their concerns and/or subsidiary to the other forms of 'evidence' with which they are faced. For purchasers, this will include demand as expressed by local 'stakeholders' and command from the centre to implement politically determined policies, procedures and service structures. One important issue is the development of an *agreed language* with which stakeholders can communicate (Conway *et al.*, 1996) and *a common understanding of need* (Holloway, 1994). Murphy (1992) gives an account of the practicalities of priority setting in an English context, showing how a range of information, both national and local, can be synthesized within a process that brings stakeholders together. This practical political approach supplements the rational planning approach advocated by Johnson *et al.* (1996), which draws heavily on epidemiological evidence.

Arguably the most important implication of EBM for practitioners and purchasers is in the identification of modalities of treatment that are not available or are highly rationed within a local community, and the consequent challenges this raises for the allocation of resources. For example, there is a sound evidence base for structured family and psychological treatments and vocational rehabilitation services for people with schizophrenia (see Lehman and Steinwachs, 1998b; Jones *et al.*, 1999; Pharoah *et al.*, 1999), but these are lacking within many services. Knowledge of EBM principles can also be used to crititicize demands on mental health services to manage risk, for example of self-harm or homicide, that are based on prejudice and woolly thinking rather than evidence (see Geddes, 1999). In reality, however, political considerations will always outweigh evidence in the formulation of public policy.

Prioritizing clinical activities within community mental health services

There are standard descriptions of the functions and components of a community mental health service (see, for example, Strathdee and Thornicroft, 1993, 1996; Chapters 20–27). These idealized descriptions rarely accommodate to the daily reality of response to chaotic and conflicting local demand by hard-pressed clinical staff. However, purchasers and providers have a common interest in addressing transparently the questions outlined by Christiansen (1997a): "*who receives what resources when and how frequently*". The first step in this process is to acknowledge the reality of scarcity of resources and the consequent need for hard choices. Next, there must be clarity over the nature of expressed and normative need for care, the activity of local services and the available resources. Without adequate information systems and access to relevant epidemiological data, the process becomes wholly subjective. One further vital step is assessing the competencies of local services: it is futile to demand access to cognitive behaviour therapy for the management of psychosis if these skills are not available locally. In a changing therapeutic world, prioritization of activity will include prioritization of training resources (see Chapter 18).

The traditional mechanisms of dealing with excessive demand (*deterrence, delay, deflection, dilution* and *denial*) will be operated by hard-pressed services irrespective of the explicit priorities of both purchasers and providers. It may be possible to negotiate eligibility criteria for a specific element of a local service, although this will result in shifting workload onto other services unless there is agreement that certain problems will not be addressed by mental health services.

Generic community mental health teams have perforce to work within a complex local system of demand that does not adhere to the tenets of rational planning.

Within community mental health teams that have a comprehensive remit, acknowledgement of the pressures and analysis of coping mechanisms that are employed may encourage a focus on the need explicitly to prioritize the work of the team. A hierarchy of activities can be determined fairly readily, which will relate to organizational and societal priorities. At the time of writing, people with 'severe and enduring mental health problems' are the UK priority (Gallagher, 1996) and, in parallel, the defensible management of clinical risk and offering rapid access to care for people in 'crisis'. Although meeting demand from primary care will be a significant priority, deploying effective treatments for non-psychotic disorders (e.g. behavioural treatment of anxiety and obsessive–compulsive disorder) within the local community will be of subsidiary importance. This raises ethical difficulties for practitioners, who are asked to spend time and effort in possibly futile but mandated activities relating to key organizational or medico-legal priorities, for example in carrying out procedures designed to assess and manage clinical risk, at the expense of providing evidence-based interventions for 'low risk' patients with treatable disorders. Strategically, community teams should give high priority to the recording of clinical activity and providers should be investing in measuring local demand for mental health services.

Managing the mental health budget

Financial management of mental health services requires both a strategic and an operational approach (Sorensen, 1996). Providers face constraints and opportunities that will reflect the vagaries of the local system of funding and the political process. In general terms, one needs to know where the money comes from, where new money can be found and where the threats to existing funding streams are located. Development or change requires either new external money or reallocation of resources from within existing budgets. In successful organizations, financial management will be an element of the overall strategic management of the organization and flow from its vision, values, goals and objectives. Only poor quality, failing services have as a primary goal balancing the books, although this will need to be a subsidiary objective if any provider is to survive.

Most practitioners will find the principles of financial accounting arcane, although it is of critical importance within a commercial environment in making decisions over whether a particular item of service should be embarked upon or dropped. Management accounts are, however, highly relevant to practitioners who have budgetary responsibility: these reflect the current expenditures under budget headings against planned budgets. Change in spending is only possible if new money flows in (creating new budget headings) or there is flexibility within the existing budgets. One obvious response to budgetary pressure is reviewing the skill-mix: are tasks being carried inappropriately out by staff of too high a grade (and consequently cost)?

Prioritization of spending is only possible if there is a degree of budgetary flexibility (possible only within a fairly large budget) that is combined with a detailed local knowledge of opportunities. Gallagher (1996) has argued that local community mental health services should have significant devolved budgets for discretionary spending on health and social care. However, devolution is only locally advantageous if it is not a 'devolution of debt' or there are mechanisms for risk sharing should expenditure exceed budgets. At an immediate practical level, services require at least minimal budgetary flexibility to foster small-scale innovation. One important, and often minimal, budget head is that devoted to training and continuing professional development. This will become increasingly significant as services struggle to recruit and retain staff and ensure that the workforce has skills relevant to contemporary demand.

Encouraging systems change

A major challenge is the reconfiguration of existing services in line with changing priorities. The extent of change that has already taken place should not be underestimated. The focus of mental health services has shifted from the mental hospital to the community, as a consequence of massive deinstitutionalization. Sectorization and local responsibility for a comprehensive mental health service has been generally adopted in economically advanced countries (see Chapter 20).

Hospital closure and developing community mental health teams are examples of clear and readily achievable service goals. Specific change issues, such as the development of a community mental health team base or the introduction of joint health/social services community teams, will require project management. The project manager (Reynolds and Thornicroft, 1999) will need to encourage a project group to define the problems to be addressed, generate alternative solutions, implement change and review progress. The review process depends crucially on identifying meaningful and measurable outcome indicators. Effective project management requires the structured use of problem-solving techniques leavened by an understanding of the need for a directive leadership role.

There is, however, a major difficulty in moving beyond introducing the obvious elements of community services towards the provision of sustained and high quality care. Significant improvement in care requires changing systems rather than change within systems (Berwick, 1996). Existing systems, Berwick argues, are perfectly designed to achieve the results they currently achieve. One important issue in systems change is clarity over goals, developing specific targets for improvement as opposed to vague aspirational statements. Aims should be measurable and ambitious, but achievable. Berwick stresses the importance of leadership in achieving systems change, although there are risks in over-reliance on a charismatic 'hero-innovator' figure encouraging unsustainable change that makes excessive demands on the workforce (Shepherd, 1984, pp. 101–117).

Purchasers can encourage systems change either by punishment for bad behaviour (likely to be ineffective) or by offering incentives for innovation and improvement. In the USA, highly assertive purchasing can be carried out through management of funding for those in receipt of public mental health care (largely the poor and indigent who are not privately insured) (Sabin and Daniels, 1999). Baron *et al.* (1998) provide a case study in the development of a comprehensive local mental health authority that sought to bring order to a fragmented and complex service system in Baltimore, USA. Within a more settled environment, such as the NHS, allocation of relatively small amounts of money can allow hard-pressed service systems to unfreeze (Gallagher, 1996). Providers that are aware of trends in fashions of treatment and care can attract funding by seeking to innovate: failure to innovate and invest in staff development will lead inevitably to relative decline in performance.

Conclusions

Clinicians have to move beyond their traditional concerns about treating the individual patient or client on the caseload, balancing the individual's needs with those of the whole community and the priorities of their organization. There is a need to be aware of developments at the level of policy and practice. Provider organizations need within them or to have access to a wide range of political, managerial, academic and technological skills. To be successful, it is vital that providers retain a firm commitment to training the workforce in the attitudes, practices and skills required in evolving mental health services.

References

American Psychiatric Association (1996) *The Psychiatrist's Managed Care Primer*. Washington, DC: American Psychiatric Press.

Backlar, P. (1996) Managed mental health care: conflicts of interest in the provider/client relationship. *Community Mental Health Journal*, 22, 101–106.

Baron, S.T., Agus, D.S., Osher, F. and Brown, D. (1998) The city of Baltimore, USA: the Baltimore experience. In: Goldberg, D. and Thornicroft, G. (eds), *Mental Health in Our Future Cities. Maudsley Monographs No 42.* Hove: Psychology Press.

Berwick, D.M. (1996) A primer on leading the improvement of systems. *British Medical Journal*, 312, 619–622.

Chisholm, D. and Stewart, A. (1998) Economics and ethics in mental health care: traditions and trade-offs. *Journal of Mental Health Policy and Economics*, 1, 5–62.

Christiansen, R.C. (1997a) Ethical issues in community mental health: cases and conflicts. *Community Mental Health Journal*, 23, 5–11.

Christiansen, R.C. (1997b) Psychiatrists as gatekeepers: a matter of perspective. *Psychiatric Services*, 48, 583.

Conway, M., Shepherd, G. and Melzer, D. (1996) Effectiveness of interventions for mental illness and implications for commissioning. In: Thornicroft, G. and Strathdee, G. (eds), *Commissioning Mental Health Services.* London: HMSO.

Corcoran, K. and Vandiver, V. (1996) *Manoeuvring the Maze of Managed Care: Skills for Mental Health Practitioners.* New York: The Free Press.

Coulter, A (1998) Managing demand at the interface between primary and secondary care. *British Medical Journal*, 316, 1974–1976.

Department of Health (1995) *Building Bridges.* London: HMSO.

Department of Health (1999a) *National Service Frameworks: Mental Health.* London: Department of Health.

Department of Health (1999b) *Saving Lives: Our Healthier Nation.* Cm 4386. London: HMSO.

Elpers, J.R. and Levin, B.L. (1996) Mental health services: epidemiology, prevention, and service delivery systems. In: Levin, B.L. and Petrila, J. (eds), *Mental Health Services. A Public Health Perspective.* New York: Oxford University Press, pp. 5–22.

Fairfield, G., Hunter, D.J., Mechanic, D. and Rosleff, F. (1997a) Managed care: origins, principles and evolution. *British Medical Journal*, 314, 1823–1826.

Fairfield, G., Hunter, D.J., Mechanic, D. and Rosleff, F. (1997b) Managed care: implications of managed care for health systems, clinicians and patients. *British Medical Journal*, 314, 1898–1901.

Fendell, S. (1998) Privately managed mental health care: shrinking services. *International Journal of Mental Health*, 27, 3–51.

Frank, R.G. and McGuire, T.G. (1997) Savings from a Medicaid carve-out for mental health and substance abuse services in Massachusetts. *Psychiatric Services*, 49, 1147–1152.

Freeman, H.L. and Bennett, D.H. (1991) Origins and development. In: Bennett, D.H. and Freeman, H.L. (eds), *Community Psychiatry. The Principles.* Edinburgh: Churchill Livingstone, pp. 40–70.

Freemantle, N. and Geddes, J. (1998) Understanding and interpreting systematic reviews and meta-analyses. Part 2: meta-analysis. *Evidence Based Mental Health*, 1, 102–104.

Gallagher, S. (1996) Implementing the core service components: commissioning and contracting. In: Thornicroft, G. and Strathdee, G. (eds), *Commissioning Mental Health Services.* London: HMSO, pp. 193–204.

Geddes, J. (1999) Suicide and homicide by people with mental illness. British Medical Journal, 318, 1225–1226.

Geddes, J., Fremantle, N., Reynolds, S. and Streiner, D. (1998) Understanding and interpreting systematic reviews and meta-anlayses. Part 1: rationale, search strategy and describing results. *Evidence Based Mental Health*, 1, 68–69.

Gittleman, M. (1998) Public and private managed care. *International Journal of Mental Health*, 27, 3–17.

Goldberg, D. and Huxley, P. (1980) *Mental Illness in the Community: The Pathway to Psychiatric Care.* London: Tavistock.

Goodman, M., Brown, J.A. and Deitz, P.M. (eds) (1996) *Managing Managed Care II: A Handbook for Mental Health Professionals.* Washington, DC: American Psychiatric Association Press.

Guze, S. (1998) Psychotherapy and managed care. *Archives of General Psychiatry*, 55, 490.

Hall, L.L., Edgar E.R., Micali P. and Palmer C. (1997) *Stand and deliver: Action call to a failing industry.* Arlington, VA: National Alliance for the Mentally Ill.

Hoge, M., Davidson, L., Griffith, E.E.H. and Jacobs, S. (1998) The crisis of managed care in the public sector. *International Journal of Mental Health*, 27, 52–71.

Hoge, M.A., Jacobs, S., Thakur, N.M. and Griffith, E.E.H. (1999) Ten dimensions of public-sector managed care. *Psychiatric Services*, 50, 51–55.

Holloway, F. (1994) The concept of need in community psychiatry: a consensus is required. *Psychiatric Bulletin*, 18, 321–323.

Holloway, F. (1996) Community psychiatric care: from libertarianism to coercion. 'Moral Panic' and mental health policy in Britain. *Health Care Analysis*, 4, 235–243.

Johnson, S., Thornicroft, G. and Strathdee, G. (1996) Population-based needs assessment. In: Thornicroft, G. and Strathdee G. (eds), *Commissioning Mental Health Services.* London: HMSO, pp. 37–52.

Jones, C., Cormac, I., Mota, J. and Campbell, C. (1999) Cognitive behaviour therapy for schizophrenia (Cochrane Review). In: *The Cochrane Library*, Issue 2, 1999. Oxford: Update Software.

Kingdon, D. (1994) Care programme approach. Recent Government policy and legislation. *Psychiatric Bulletin*, 18, 68–70.

Lazarus, A. (ed.) (1996) *Controversies in Managed Mental Health Care*. Washington, DC: American Psychiatric Press.

Leff, J. (ed) (1997) *Care in the Community – Illusion or Reality?* Chicester: Wiley.

Lehman and Steinwachs (1998a) Patterns of usual care for schizophrenia: initial results from the Schizophrenia Patient Outcomes Research Team (PORT) client survey. *Schizophrenia Bulletin*, 24, 11–20.

Lehman and Steinwachs (1998b) Translating research into practice: the schizophrenia patient outcomes research team (PORT) treatment recommendations. *Schizophrenia Bulletin*, 24, 1–10.

Mechanic, D., Schlesinger M. and McAlpine D.D. (1995) Management of mental health and substance abuse services: state of the art and early results. *Milbank Quarterly*, 73, 19–55.

Murphy, E. (1992) Setting priorities during the development of local psychiatric services. In: Thornicroft, G., Brewin, C.R. and Wing, J. (eds), *Measuring Mental Health Needs*. London: Gaskell, pp. 118–139.

National Schizophrenia Fellowship (1998) *Caring and Coping. A Resource Pack*. Kingston Upon Thames: National Schizophrenia Fellowship.

New, B. (1996) The rationing agenda in the NHS. *British Medical Journal*, 312, 1593–1601.

Newman, P. (1995) Interview with Alain Enthoven: is their convergence between Britain and the United States in the organisation of health services? *British Medical Journal*, 310, 1652–1655.

NHS Centre for Reviews and Dissemination (1998) Deliberate self-harm. *Effective Health Care*, 4, 6.

Pharoah, F.M., Mari, J.J. and Streiner, D. (1999) Family intervention for schizophrenia (Cochrane Review). In: *The Cochrane Library*, Issue 2, 1999. Oxford: Update Software.

Reynolds, A. and Thornicroft, G. (1999) *Managing Mental Health Services*. Buckingham: Open University Press.

Rosenheck, R, Armstrong, M., Callaghan, D. *et al.* (1998) Obligation to the least well off in setting mental health service priorities: a consensus statement. *Psychiatric Services*, 49, 1273–1274.

Sabin, J.E. and Daniels, N. (1999) Public-sector managed behavioural health care; II. Contracting for Medicaid services—the Massachusetts experience. *Psychiatric Services*, 50, 39–41.

Sackett, D.L., Rosenberg, W.M.C., Gray, J.A.M., Haynes, R.B. and Richardson, W.S. (1996) Evidence based medicine: what it is and what it isn't. *British Medical Journal*, 312, 71–72.

Sackett, D.L., Richardson, W.S., Rosenberg, W. and Haynes, R.B. (1997) *Evidence-based Medicine. How to Practice and Teach it*. New York: Churchill Livingstone.

Santiago, J. (1992) The fate of mental health services in health care reform: I a system in crisis. *Hospital and Community Psychiatry*, 43, 1091–1095.

Secretary of State for Health (1997) *The New NHS. Modern. Dependable*. Cm 3807. London: HMSO.

Secretary of State for Health (1998) *Modernising Mental Health Services. Safe, Sound and Supportive*. London: Department of Health.

Shaneyfelt, S., Mayo-Smith, M.F. and Rothangl, J. (1999) Are guidelines following guidelines? The methodological quality of clinical practice guidelines in the peer-reviewed literature. *Journal of the American Medical Association*, 281, 1900–1905.

Sorensen, J.E. (1996) Financial management in public mental health services: a strategic and operational approach. In: Levin, B.L. and Petrila, J. (eds), *Mental Health Services. A Public Health Perspective*. New York: Oxford University Press, pp. 138–160.

Strathdee, G. and Thornicroft, G. (1996) Core components of a comprehensive mental health service. In: Thornicroft, G. and Strathdee, G. (eds), *Commissioning Mental Health Services*. London: HMSO, pp. 71–84.

Szmukler, G. and Holloway, F. (1998) Ethics in community psychiatry. *Current Opinion in Psychiatry*, 11, 549–553.

Thornicroft, G., Strathdee, G., Phelan, M., Holloway, F. *et al.* (1998) Rationale and design: the PriSM Psychosis Study (1). *British Journal of Psychiatry*, 173, 363–370.

15 | *The planning process for mental health services*

Graham Thornicroft and Michele Tansella

Introduction

The aim of this chapter is to describe the process of planning mental health services for a defined community, taking into account temporal and geographical variables which may affect this process. *First*, we describe an overall conceptual model within which planning can be considered and organised, and we define the key relevant terms. *Secondly*, we describe in detail the sequential stages necessary for the planning of mental health services. This process of planning is considered as cyclical, rather than linear, beginning with establishing the service principles, moving to setting the boundary conditions, assessing population needs and the current service provision, formulating a strategic plan for a local system of services, implementing the service components at the local level, and ending with reviewing the service and monitoring the adequacy of provision. *Thirdly*, we discuss the ways in which planning at the local level differs from planning at the national and regional levels, illustrating this with examples from the epidemiological evidence referring to schizophrenia, one of the conditions making the most demands upon specialist mental health services. *Finally*, we deal with how faulty planning procedures, which fail to see service components within a wider systemic view, can lead to distorted and unbalanced services. In this respect, our approach will be to consider planning in relation to a whole community-orientated system of care, which includes both facilities and services at hospital and community sites.

A conceptual framework and key terms for planning mental health services

A conceptual model can be useful to establish a framework within which planning and implementation can be described and put into practice. We have created such a conceptual model which we recently have described in detail (Thornicroft and Tansella, 1999a). This 'matrix' model has two dimensions: the geographical and the temporal, as described in Chapter 16, and as illustrated in Table 16.6.

We define *planning* as 'a linked series of actions designed to achieve a particular goal, and which requires the completion of increasingly specific tasks within a given timescale'. In relation to the matrix model, 'planning is the process which intends to transform given inputs into optimum outputs'. On the other hand, the *Concise Oxford Dictionary* defines *process* as 'a course of action or proceeding, especially a series of stages in manufacture or some other operation' or as 'the progress or course of something'. Our conception of the entire system of mental health services is described in greater detail in Chapter 16. Briefly, we consider that *community-based mental health services* can be defined as those 'which provide a full range of effective mental health care to a defined population, and which are dedicated to treating and helping people with mental disorder, in proportion to their suffering or distress, in collaboration with other local agencies'.

Stages in planning mental health services

In the context of this conceptual framework and the definition of key terms that we have outlined, we now describe a seven-stage procedure to lead from planning to practice. This scheme is intended as a pragmatic guide to the key stages in the planning process. In real life, we expect that it will be rare for these stages to be followed sequentially, and in practice the order of events can change, or several stages may occur simultaneously (see Table 15.1).

Establishing the service principles

The *initial stage* refers to establishing the service principles, which can be seen as part of an ethical approach. We previously have described the combination of an evidence-based together with an ethical-based approach to planning (Thornicroft and Tansella, 1999a,b). Indeed, we would go further and place principles as the foundation stones for planning, and consider that the choice of using an evidence-based approach itself also demonstrates that evidence has been accorded high value, and accepted as a key principle.

Principles are more often implicit than explicit, and indeed their explicit identification is often excluded from the entire planning process. Even when principles are considered, most often at an early stage of planning, they remain without consequence for three reasons. (i) Those involved may assume that their colleagues share common ground and that such agreement goes without saying. (ii) They may tacitly acknowledge substantial differences in core values within the planning group, and reckon that better progress will be made by avoiding more than by addressing these differences. (iii) Planners may judge that discussion about underlying principles is not sufficiently important to take up scarce planning time. In our opinion, all three views, although common, are mistaken and will lead to the re-emergence of disagreements later in the planning process, when value differences become displaced onto operational matters. We can therefore identify four practical uses of principles in terms of planning (see Table 15.2), which are described in full in Chapter 13.

Table 15.1 *Seven stages in planning community services*

1 Establishing the service principles

2 Setting the boundary conditions

3 Assessing population needs

4 Assessing current provision

5 Formulating a strategic plan for a local system of mental health services

6 Implementing the service components at the local level

7 Monitoring and review cycle

Table 15.2 *Practical uses of principles in relation to mental health services*

Principles may be used in the *absence of evidence* (e.g. in establishing a service where no strong evidence exists) or *instead of evidence*, where evidence exists, but is discounted (e.g. on political or financial grounds)

Principles are often used *in conjunction with available evidence*. This may be: (i) to attach relative value to the results of research or (ii) to adjudicate where the research evidence is unclear or conflicting

Principles may be used to produce *new outcome measures*

Principles may orient decisions on *directions for research* funding and future scientific developments

Setting the boundary conditions

The *second stage* in planning is to *set the boundary conditions*. In terms of the general adult mental health services, two types of boundary are of particular concern: first, that between primary care and secondary care services; and secondly, within mental health services, the distinction in practice between the more and the less severely mentally ill. In terms of the former, since up to 25% of all adults suffer from some mental health problem in any year, and since the capacity of the specialist mental health services even in the most economically developed countries is to offer contact to 2–3% of the population in any year, it is clear that only about a tenth of all psychiatric morbidity can receive any clinical contact from specialist services (Office of Population and Census Surveys, 1995; Ustun and Sartorius, 1995). The central question then becomes: *which 10%?*

Regarding the second key boundary, the severity of mental health problems is in most areas poorly related to the intensity of care received (Goldberg and Gournay, 1997). As specialist services are relatively scarce and expensive, they should target their impact upon those with the most severe symptoms and the greatest degree of disability. To achieve this consistently, a service will need to set priorities for the groups of patients who should receive highest priority for contact. Figure 15.1 illustrates what we call a well targeted service in that the secondary (specialist) services concentrate their efforts entirely upon people with the most severe degrees of symptom/disability (area C). Primary care services then provide for all other patients with less severe conditions (area B). Even so, there is an oblique interface between C and B since some of the more severe cases will still be treated only by primary care services, towards the right side of the figure. The gradient of this interface will vary in different health systems, and for a well configured primary–secondary care interface is vertical. Area A represents true cases who are not receiving treatment, that is *untreated prevalence*. Such cases may not have presented to services, may have presented and not been recognized, or may have been identified and no treatment was given. The extent to which such morbidity, which is usually of relatively minor severity, is treated varies considerably between sites (Robins and Regier, 1991), as does

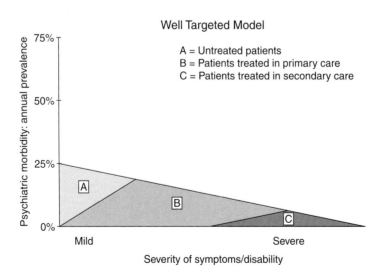

Figure 15.1 *Relationship between degree of disability and treatment setting (primary or secondary care) for a well targeted service.*

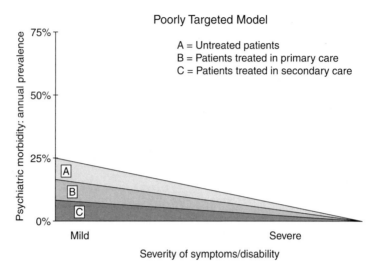

Figure 15.2 *Relationship between degree of disability and treatment setting (primary or secondary care) for poorly targeted services. (Taken from Thornicroft and Tansella, 1999a.)*

the gradient of the interface between A and B. In poorly targeted services, there may be horizontally parallel layers of A, B and C so that some very minor cases are treated by specialist services, and some severe cases go untreated, as shown in extreme form in Figure 15.2.

Targeting is necessary but not sufficient. A second key element is that the capacity of the secondary (specialist) service is large enough to absorb or accommodate all the cases who fulfil the entry criteria for the priority groups of patients (assuming that such entry criteria have been defined in advance). The third central characteristic of well functioning specialist services is that, once in contact with the target patient group, they deliver cost-effective (efficient) treatments, meaning that the cost implications should only be applied to treatments or services which are of already proven efficacy and effectiveness.

Assessing population needs

The *third stage* is to assess population needs. When assessing population-level needs for mental health services, it is useful first to define 'need'. There is at present no consensus on how needs

should be defined (Holloway, 1994; Slade, 1994; Slade *et al.*, 1998), and who should define them. The Oxford English Dictionary offers: 'necessity, requirement, essential'. Further, Stevens and Gabbay (1992) have introduced the idea of treatability by defining need as 'the *ability to benefit* in some way from health care'.

Assessing the needs for services for a defined population is closely related to targeting, since the degree of stringency necessary in defining the highest priority group in any service will depend upon three factors: (i) the *overall rates of psychiatric morbidity* in each local population; (ii) the *capacity of each local mental health service* in terms of the number of cases which can be treated at any one time; and (iii) the degree to which these services *effectively target* the severely mentally ill. A series of methods allows the measurement or the estimation of true (treated and untreated) prevalence, and the use of treated prevalence rates alone can produce a highly distorted picture of met and unmet need at the population level. At the same time, a population-based needs assessment only has value in terms of planning if it is more than an academic exercise, i.e. when it is an integral part of a programme of service

Table 15.3 *Proposed information pathway for planning mental health services*

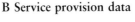

A Epidemiologically based data	B Service provision data
Population characteristics: in terms of the factors associated with psychiatric morbidity *Epidemiological data*: morbidity and disability for the particular area by age, sex and social status *Treated individuals*: appropriately/inappropriately *Place and type of treatment* *Untreated individuals*: those in need of treatment	*Define categories* of service components for primary, secondary and tertiary levels of care *Quantify the capacities* of the service components *Quality of care* of the service sites *Quantitative and qualitative* information on *Integration and co-ordination* of staff components into a service system

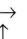 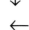

Planning process	C Service utilisation data
Constitution of a planning group representing a wide range of local interests group, including expert advisors *Selective assessment* of all data from A, B and C relevant for service planning *Setting* a *medium-term time scale* for service plans (3–5 years) *Identification of highest priority* service needs (both met and unmet) *Identification of highest priority unmet social needs* and information from relevant authorities *Planning of* (i) new service functions and necessary facilities (ii) extension of capacity of current services (iii) disinvestment from lower priority services *Collection* of new data necessary for the next planning cycle	*Event-based data* on clinical contacts by levels of care (in-patient, out-patient, etc.), numbers of events and rates per 10 000 population per year *Individual-based data* on both clinical contacts (as above) and on treatment episodes across different levels of care per year *Data on outcomes and costs* of different clinical contacts (disaggregated for subgroups of patients) with which to establish substitutability and complementarity of service components in terms of cost-effectiveness

From Thornicroft and Tansella (1999a)

development and reform. In practice, we propose a pragmatic strategy for the assessment of need which consists of using the best information available in each particular area. As correctly indicated by Wing (1989), this process is not linear but should be viewed as a circular pathway which can be followed more than once, as indicated in Table 15.3.

The feasibility of using epidemiological data may be limited because it will often be the case that no locally based epidemiological data are available, and the only practicable strategy is to make approximations using the results of national or international epidemiological studies, and applying these overall, or diagnosis-specific, rates to the local area

Simple estimates of the need for mental health services made from epidemiological data can be refined by weighting with socio-demographic variables to allow for factors such as social deprivation which are closely associated with variations in morbidity of the more disabling forms of mental illness. Table 15.4 shows census (predictor) variables which have been found to be significantly correlated with psychiatric service utilization, most often hospital in-patient admission rates (outcome variables), in five different studies.

Assessing current provision

Stage four is the assessment of current service provision. Having examined local population needs for mental health care, we now assess the nature and extent of existing services. Two separate exercises are necessary: first, the best possible description of the available services (structure) and secondly the description of the use of these resources (functioning).

For the description of local services in quantitative terms, we need to have an adequate method to describe their categories. Many standardised instruments have been established to measure individual psychiatric pathology, but in fact there is no accepted standard classification of mental health service components. An ambitious approach has been taken by de Jong (1990) who under the aegis of WHO developed the *International Classification of Mental Health Care* (WHO-ICMHC). A second possible approach is the *European Service Mapping Schedule* (Johnson *et al.*, 1997), which is being developed to allow international comparisons to be made. Although still at the pilot stage, and still to be fully standardised, it shows considerable promise for mental health service description in the future.

A third system is the *Basic Services Profile* (BSP), which shows the basic services we consider to be the essential elements in any system of care (Thornicroft and Tansella, 1999a). The BSP (see Table 15.5) is applicable to a wide range of service patterns at different stages of development.

Having established a system to categorise local services, the question of *service capacity* arises.

There is considerable debate about the numbers of psychiatric treatment and care places that are necessary (Wing, 1971, 1992). Targets for service provision based on likely prevalences of mental illness nationally have been proposed for England (Johnson *et al.*, 1996). These targets assume that community residential places and day care largely replace facilities for long-term patients in asylums. Wing (1992) provides figures for targets for day provision by mental health services, which again take account of the prevalence of severe mental illness in the community. The capacities given in Ramsay *et al.* (1997), for example, are intended to apply to a whole service where each of the other service components are present in the required capacities.

Recent experience suggests that figures of this sort may be of only limited use. They can be used for local comparisons between similar areas, but they become progressively less useful at the higher geographical levels. They are also open to misunderstanding or to misuse. For example, if used to calculate in-patient bed numbers alone in the absence of other related categories, then it will produce misleading results.

There is a strong relationship between service provision and service use, and it is somewhat similar to the economic relationship between supply and demand. It appears, *first*, that where psychiatric beds are available then they are filled, whatever the quantity of provision (see Chapter 28). *Secondly*, the categories of service used are usually governed entirely by the types of service available locally. If, for example, home treatment services are not provided in a given area, then the options available to staff when assessing a patient in crisis are normally restricted to in-patient or day-hospital admission. In this way, supply, in turn, also shapes demand in that the family of a patient in crisis may demand an admission, since in their experience this is the only option which can help. *Thirdly*, the use of the services provided depends to a large extent upon the system turnover, or, in the case of beds, for example, the average length of stay. In other words, both structural and dynamic aspects need to be considered simultaneously.

Table 15.4 *Recent examples of statistically significant socio-demographic predictors of mental health services use*

	Jarman, 1983	Thornicroft, 1991[a]	Jarman and Hirsch, 1992[b]	Thornicroft et al., 1993	Glover, 1996
Ethnic minorities	x	x			
Elderly living alone	x		x		
Children aged <5 years	x				
Single-parent families	x	x			
Unskilled workers	x				
Unemployed	x			x	x
Changed address	x	x			
Overcrowded	x			x	
Lack of internal amenities		x		x	
No car		x	x		x
Living in one room		x			
Population density		x		x	
Availability of general beds		x			
Household in single occupation			x	x	
Single, widowed or divorced			x	x	x
Illegitimacy index			x		
Private household with no car			x		
Dependency ratio[c]				x	
Registered as permanently disabled					x
Household not self-contained					x
Non-permanent accommodation[d]					x

[a]Correlation coefficient of >0.55 with standardized admission rate before principal components analysis.

[b]Six highest Pearson correlation coefficients of 169 variables entered into the model to predict standardized admission ratios based on district size and national overall rate.

[c]Percentage of persons aged <15 and aged 65 and over in relation to the population aged 15–64 years.

[d]Proportion of population resident in hostels, common lodging houses, miscellaneous establishments or sleeping rough.

Table 15.5 *The basic service profile*

Basic component	Variations
1. Out-patient and community services	mobile services for crisis assessment and treatment (including evening and weekend services) out-patient services for specific disorders or for specialized treatments consultations in general hospitals
2. Day services	sheltered workshops occupational and vocational rehabilitation supervised work placements co-operative work schemes self-help and user groups advocacy services training courses club houses/transitional employment programmes
3. Acute in-patient services	specialized units for specific disorders (e.g. intensive care and forensic) acute day hospitals crisis houses
4. Longer term residential services	unsupervised housing with administrative protection supervised housing (boarding out schemes) unstaffed group homes group homes with some residential or visiting staff hostels with day staff hostels with day and night staff hostels and homes with 24-hour nursing staff
5. Interfaces with other services	*Health services* forensic services old age services learning disability/mental handicap services/mental retardation specialized psychotherapies general physical and dental health consultation to primary care/GPs *Social services/Welfare benefits* income support domiciliary care (e.g. cleaning) holiday/respite care *Housing agencies* unsupervised housing/apartments *Other government agencies* police prison probation *Non-governmental agencies* religious organization voluntary groups for-profit private organizations

From Thornicroft and Tansella (1999a).

Formulating a strategic plan for a local system of mental health services

After collecting this background information, *stage five* is the formulation of a strategic plan for the local system of mental health services. Such a written plan will usually involve the setting of short- and long-term objectives, and widespread consultation and involvement in the plan. The strategic plan: (i) estimate deficiencies in the capacity of services; (ii) will include a specific costing; (iii) and will set out a detailed project management timetable which indicates the time points at which each service change will take place. A basic decision to be made at this stage is to choose between a systemic and a component planning approach. This will be elaborated upon below.

Working at the local community level makes building links with key local figures and agencies desirable (see Chapter 36). They will most often include family doctors, general hospital and other health service clinicians, social service and housing department staff, patients and their representatives, family members and carer groups, local politicians, local newspapers and radio stations. However, a wider array of stakeholders may also wish to have their interests represented and respected. This wider set of constituencies can include: neighbourhood or residents' associations; local school staff; governors and parents; shopkeepers; local politicians; church ministers; and police officers. The importance of these stakeholders emerges particularly at times when plans are being developed to open new mental health facilities. Our experience leads us to the view that treating neighbours openly, as potential partners, and seeking their early informed consent for proposals at the planning stage is pragmatic, principled and a proper base for mental health services that are fully integrated within their local communities.

Implementing the service components at the local level

The *sixth stage* in planning is the implementation of the essential service components. The decisions relevant here will follow on from the previous stages, especially the identification of unmet needs at the population level. Pragmatically, planners often consider that several service components are absent, weak or inappropriately provided, and so the question arises of how to set priorities between competing components in the sequence of implementation. We suggest that there should be some provision in each category of the basic service components (see Table 15.5). If any single category is totally absent in a local area, then the planning team will need to consider whether the provision of some capacity in this missing category should be one of the highest priorities. Again it will be important to use a systems perspective so that priorities are conceptualised as lying not *only* within the same categories as those in which the problem is identified, but also within the wider system as a whole. For example, the provision of high staffed residential care should usually be considered for individual patients only if lesser degrees of support have proven insufficient.

Monitoring and review cycle

Finally, the *seventh stage* is that of monitoring and conducting a review cycle. This stage is often forgotten so that there is a discrepancy between the resources invested in changing and maintaining health services, and the budget dedicated to evaluate the effect of these interventions. This is shortsighted because a proper review needs to address the following questions: have the services provided benefits to patients and, if so, how efficiently? We refer the reader to Chapters 6 and 7 which consider the evaluation of services in detail.

Planning at the national/regional level

So far, our discussion of planning has addressed issues mainly in relation to what we refer to as the local level. In this section, we will refer to those factors which are of more relevance to the national/regional level.

At the local level, the primary concerns are to use data specific to that area where possible and to tailor services to the specific needs of the local populations, according to the locally agreed service development priorities, which may be quite different even from those of adjoining areas. One evidence-based approach to assessing local needs is to refer to epidemiological knowledge, and Table 15.6 gives examples of which epidemiological findings about one particular example, schizophrenia, may be relevant for service planning purposes.

In comparison, planning at the national level will usually need to attain a lesser level of specificity. National strategic plans, for example, may indicate the need for local services to comply with agreed guidelines or protocols, but attempts to overspecify the exact components and models which should be provided in every local area within a country are likely to prove to be somewhat irrelevant to those areas in which current services are very different from the model proposed, or where the assumptions upon which the proposals are based (e.g. from urban settings) do not hold (e.g. rural areas). Once again, epidemiological

data may be useful, and Table 15.7 gives examples of which data, when aggregated to a higher level of analysis, may still be able to inform planning.

Planning tools relevant to the national/regional level tend to be less specific than those useful at the local level. One recent example of this is the National Service Framework for Mental Health in England, published in 1999. This is a national blueprint for mental health services for adults of working age and sets seven standards to apply at the national level (see Table 15.8).

Systemic versus segmental approaches to planning

We have dealt above with some of the operational stages of planning in detail, but at the same time we wish to emphasize the need for a wider strategic approach to service planning, one that considers the components as part of a *whole system* of treatment and care (Breakey, 1996). As we

Table 15.6 *Epidemiological findings with implications at the local level*

Epidemiological findings/risk factors	Service planning implications
Onset in early adulthood, males earlier than females	Organize services to identify prodromes in teenagers and young adults, and related to life cycle problems
Delay of treatment associated with poorer course	Provide easy access to services
High risk groups: ethnic minorities, prisoners and dual diagnosis	Targeted services, acceptable to specific high risk groups
Geographical mobility: immigrants and internal migration	Target services acceptable to immigrants, and organize services to minimize loss to treatment
Urban excess and changes in age/social class structure	Monitor changing population structure and target more resources and staff in urban, poor areas
Increased mortality and physical morbidity rates physical health assessment and treatment	Provide services for health promotion and for regular

From Thornicroft and Tansella (2000).

Table 15.7 *Epidemiological findings with implications at the national/regional level*

Epidemiological findings/risk factors	Service planning implications
Urban excess of schizophrenia	Funding formula adjusted for urbanicity and social deprivation
High unemployment rates	Specific programme for vocational rehabilitation
Fluctuating course of relapses and remissions	Change pension and disability social security payment systems to allow more flexible movement into and out of the 'disabled' category

From Thornicroft and Tansella (2000).

indicated earlier, there are two types of planning approach: (i) the *service component* (segmental) view and (ii) the *system* view. The former considers each treatment facility or programme as essentially a separate functioning entity, with specific aims, operational policies, funding sources and selection criteria. The latter sees each individual facility or programme as a part of the wider system of care, and explicitly takes account of the inter-relationships between the constituent parts.

The strength of the segmental approach is that it allows more specific and detailed planning for the separate service components. Its weakness is that it does not provide a framework to understand interactions between these components. It cannot explain, for example, how the lack of provision of long-term residential care can mean that acute beds are used inappropriately for new long-term patients, leaving no capacity for acute crisis care.

We therefore propose that the totality of mental health service components be considered as a series of inter-related elements, in which the behaviour of each affects (directly or indirectly) all the others within, in a sense, a *hydraulic system* (see Table 15.9). Such a view allows us to speak of the volume and the capacity of components and of the whole system (for both under- and overcapacity), to calculate rates of flow between components, to build in control taps and safety valves for periods of expected and unexpected excess pressure, and to make allowance for overflow

capacity in times of excess volume, for the 'leakage' of some patients out the system (when patients may be lost inappropriately to contact with services). Such a metaphor also allows us to consider the need for routine and emergency maintenance in order to avoid system breakdowns, and to build in sentinel events or alarm systems to warn of incipient system failures. While not wishing to overstretch this parallel, we do find that such a view helps to understand the links between service components.

Conclusion

In this chapter, we have discussed the contribution of evidence to planning. We need, in conclusion, to put this in the wider context of the other key stakeholders in the planning process. These stakeholders are: (i) researchers; (ii) politicians; (iii) service users (Beeforth *et al.*, 1990; Andrews *et al.*, 1994; Chapter 39); (iv) carers (Hogman and Pearson, 1995); (v) public opinion; (vi) clinicians and practitioners; and (vii) administrative and financial managers. The relative influence of each of these stakeholders, and their practical impact, will vary according to local circumstances. While we propose that evidence be included in the planning process, it is still often true that evidence of the type we have described in this chapter is seen to be neither necessary nor sufficient for planning We are therefore describing a paradigmatic shift—

Table 15.8 *National Service Framework for Mental Health (Department of Health, 1999)*

Standard 1: Mental health promotion
Health and social services should:
    promote mental health for all, working with individuals and communities
    combat discrimination against individuals and groups with mental health problems, and promote
    their social inclusion

Standard 2: Primary care and access to services
Any service user who contacts their primary health care team with a common mental health
problem should:
    have their mental health needs identified and assessed
    be offered effective treatments, including referral to specialist services for further assessment,
    treatment and care if they require it

Standard 3: Primary care and access to services
Any individual with a common mental health problem should:
    be able to make contact round the clock with the local services necessary to meet their needs and
    receive adequate care
    be able to use NHS Direct, as it develops, for first-level advice and referral on to specialist
    helplines or to local services

Standard 4: Severe mental illness
All mental health service users on the Care Programme Approach (CPA) should:
    receive care which optimizes engagement, anticipates or prevents a crisis, and reduces risk
    have a copy of a written care plan which:
        includes action to be taken in a crisis by service user, their carer and care co-ordinator
        advises their GP how they should respond if the service user needs additional help
        is regularly reviewed by their care co-ordinator
    be able to access services 24 hours a day, 365 days a week

Standard 5: Severe mental illness
Each service user who is assessed as requiring a period of care away from their home should have:
    timely access to an appropriate hospital bed or alternative bed or place, which is:
        in the least restrictive environment consistent with the need to protect them and the public
        as close to home as possible
    a copy of a written aftercare plan agreed on discharge which sets out the care and rehabilitation
    to be provided, identifies the care co-ordinator and specifies the action to be taken in a crisis

Standard 6: Caring about carers
All individuals who provide regular and substantial care for a person on CPA should:
    have an assessment of their caring, physical and mental health needs, repeated on at least an
    annual basis
    have their own written care plan which is given to them and implemented in discussion with them

Standard 7: Preventing suicide
Local health and social care communities should prevent suicides by:
    promoting mental health for all, working with individuals and communities (Standard 1)
    delivering high quality primary mental health care (Standard 2)
    ensuring that anyone with a mental health problem can contact local services via the primary care
    team, a helpline or an A & E department (Standard 3)
    ensuring that individuals with severe and mental illness have a care plan which meets their specific
    needs, including access to services round the clock (Standard 4)
    providing safe hospital accommodation for individuals who need it (Standard 5)
    enabling individuals caring for someone with severe mental illness to receive the support which
    they need to continue to care (Standard 6)

Table 15.9 *The metaphor of the 'hydraulic model' for a mental health system*

volume and capacity of different components, as well as of the whole system of care

rates of flow between components

control taps and safety valves for periods of expected or unexpected pressure

overflow capacity in times of excess volume

'leakage' of some patients out of the system (patients inappropriately lost to contact with services)

need for routine and maintenance to avoid system breakdowns

From Thornicroft and Tansella (1999a).

from planning as a solely political process to one which is, in a sense, a multiple simultaneous equation.

References

Andrews, G., Peters, L. and Teesson, M. (1994) *Measurement of Consumer Outcome in Mental Health: A Report to the National Mental Health Information Strategy Committee*. Report to the Australian Government, posted on the Worldwide Web at the University of New South Wales site.

Beeforth, M., Conlan, E., Field, V., Hoser, B. and Sayce, L. (1990) *Whose Service is it Anyway? Users' Views on Co-ordinating Community Care*. London: Research and Development for Psychiatry.

Breakey, W. (1996) *Integrated Mental Health Services*. Oxford: Oxford University Press.

de Jong, P. (1990) *International Classification of Mental Health Settings*. Geneva: WHO.

Department of Health (1999) *The National Service Framework for Mental Health. Modern Standards and Service Models*. London: Department of Health.

Glover, G. (1996) Health service indictors for mental health. In: Thornicroft, G. and Strathdee, G. (eds), *Commissioning Mental Health Services*. London: HMSO, pp. 311–318.

Goldberg, D. and Gournay, K. (1997) *The General Practitioner, the Psychiatrist and the Burden to Mental Health Care*. Maudsley Discussion Paper No 1. London: Institute of Psychiatry.

Hogman, G. and Pearson, G. (1995) *The Silent Partners. The Needs and Experiences of People who Provide Informal Care to People with a Severe Mental Illness*. London: National Schizophrenia Fellowship.

Holloway, F. (1994). Need in community psychiatry: a consensus is required. *Psychiatric Bulletin*, 18, 321–323.

Jarman, B. (1983) Identification of underprivileged areas. *British Medical Journal*, 286, 1705–1709.

Jarman, B. and Hirsch, S. (1992) Statistical models to predict district psychiatric morbidity. In: Thornicroft, G., Brewin, C. and Wing, J.K. (eds), *Measuring Mental Health Needs*. London: Royal College of Psychiatrists, Gaskell Press, pp. 62–80.

Johnson, S., Thornicroft, S. and Strathdee, G. (1996) Population-based assessment of needs for services. In Thornicroft, G. and Strathdee, G., (eds) *Commissioning Mental Health Services*. HMSO London, pp. 37–51.

Johnson, S., Kuhlmann, R. and the EPCAT group (1997) *The European Service Mapping Schedule*. Version 3. London: Section of Community Psychiatry, Institute of Psychiatry.

Office of Population and Census Surveys (1995) *National Psychiatric Morbidity Survey*. London: HMSO.

Ramsay, R., Thornicroft, G., Johnson, S., Brooks, L. and Glover, G. (1997) Levels of in-patient and residential provision throughout London. In: Johnson, S. et al. (eds), *London's Mental Health*. London: King's Fund, pp.193–219.

Robins, L.N. and Regier, D.A. (1991) *Psychiatric Disorders in America*. New York: The Free Press.

Slade, M. (1994) Needs assessment: who needs to assess? *British Journal of Psychiatry*, 165, 287–292.

Slade, M., Phelan, M. and Thornicroft, G. (1998) A comparison of needs assessed by staff and by an epidemiologically representative sample of patients with psychosis. *Psychological Medicine*, 28, 543–550.

Stevens, A. and Gabbay, J. (1992) The purchasers' information requirements on mental health needs and contracting for mental health services. In: Thornicroft, G., Brewin, C. and Wing, J.K. (eds), *Measuring Mental Health Needs*. London: Royal College of Psychiatrists, Gaskell Press, pp. 42–61.

Thornicroft, G. (1991). Social deprivation and rates of treated mental disorder: developing statistical models to predict psychiatric service utilisation. *British Journal of Psychiatry*, 158, 475–484.

Thornicroft, G. and Tansella, M. (1999a) *The Mental Health Matrix. A Manual to Improve Services*. Cambridge: Cambridge University Press.

Thornicroft, G. and Tansella, M. (1999b) Translating ethical principles into outcome measures for mental health service research *Psychological Medicine*, 29, 761–767.

Thornicroft, G. and Tansella, M (2000) The implications of epidemiology for service planning in schizophrenia. In: Murray, R. Jones,P. Susser, E., van Os, J. and Cannon, M. (eds), *Epidemiology of Schizophrenia*.Cambridge: Cambridge University Press, in press.

Thornicroft, G., De Salvia, G. and Tansella, M. (1993) Urban–rural differences in the associations between social deprivation and psychiatric service utilisation in schizophrenia and all diagnoses: a case-register study in Northern Italy. *Psychological Medicine*, 23, 487–469.

Ustun, B. and Sartorius. N. (1995) *Mental Illness in General Health Care. An International Study.* Chichester: Wiley.

Wing, J. (1971) How many psychiatric beds? *Psychological Medicine*, 1, 189–190.

Wing, J.(ed.) (1989) *Health Services Planning and Research. Contributions from Psychiatric Case Registers.* London: Gaskell.

Wing, J. (1992) *Epidemiologically Based Needs Assessment. Report 6. Mental Illness.* Leeds: NHS Management Executive.

16 | *Service responses to cultural diversity*

Harry Minas

"Matters of practical conduct have nothing invariable about them, any more than matters of health. This is true of ethics in general, and it is true even more of moral issues arising in particular cases. These are not a scientific or technical matter: rather as in medicine or navigation, they require human beings to consider what is appropriate to specific circumstances and to specific occasions."

Aristotle, *Nicomachean Ethics* (II.2.1104a).
(Cited in: Jonsen, 1990).

The question facing mental health services in multi-cultural societies is how to deal effectively with cultural complexity. While it is now widely acknowledged that culture is important in understanding mental health and illness, and in the development of mental health services, it is necessary to transform such awareness into action at the levels of policy, service design and evaluation, and the clinical encounter. In this chapter, I will outline an ethical basis for, and a practical approach to, the development of mental health services in a multi-cultural society.

Cultural pluralism and justice

The term culture, as used here, includes the shared language, beliefs, values and rules that characterize a distinctive community and that enable individuals within that community to live, work, communicate, and to anticipate and interpret each other's intent and behaviour. Until confronted by a different and unfamiliar culture, our own is largely hidden from view, unobtrusive. While cultures are dynamic and constantly changing, core elements are preserved and provide for continuity of identity of the culture. Culture is learned in one's family and through contact with the culture's core institutions, for example the systems of education, law, religion and medicine, and through sustained participation in customary events and practices. Every culture is, to a greater or lesser extent, heterogeneous. While membership of a particular ethnic group is important in shaping culture, a person's beliefs, values, behaviour and identity are also profoundly influenced by gender, class, education and religion. We will focus here on the cultural diversity that is associated with the ethnic pluralism that is such a prominent feature of most contemporary societies, particularly those that have accepted large numbers of immigrants and refugees.

Most contemporary societies are culturally diverse. The world's 190-odd independent states contain approximately 600 living language groups and 5000 ethnic groups (Huntington, 1996). Such diversity confronts societies with a series of important challenges and potentially divisive questions. These questions include issues of national and regional identity; distribution of resources; the legitimate role of government; and the purposes, structure and operations of social institutions. Health services are not exempt from these debates, although it has to be said that the fact of linguistic and cultural diversity has had surprisingly little impact on our conceptions of health and illness, the structure and operations of health institutions and health care systems, professional education and clinical practice.

The key political and ethical question that is raised by cultural pluralism is this: "How is it possible that there may exist over time a stable and just society of free and equal citizens profoundly divided by reasonable though incompatible religious, philosophical and moral doctrines? This is a problem of political justice ... Among our most basic problems are those of race, ethnicity and gender." (Rawls, 1993, pp. xxii–xxx). The task of finding morally defensible and politically viable answers to this question is among the greatest challenges currently facing liberal democracies (Kymlicka, 1995). In seeking an answer to this question, Rawls (1993, p. 5) suggests two principles of justice:

"a. Each person has an equal claim to a fully adequate scheme of basic rights and liberties, which scheme is compatible with the same scheme for all ...

b. Social and economic inequalities are to satisfy two conditions: first, they are to be attached to positions and offices open to all under conditions of fair equality of opportunity; and second, they are to be *to the greatest benefit of the least advantaged members of society*." (my emphasis)

This aspect of Rawls' theory of justice (Rawls, 1971, 1993) requires that groups that are among the most disadvantaged (e.g. indigenous groups, immigrants, asylum seekers and refugees) are accorded priority in the framing of political and social arrangements that are intended to ensure justice.

The paradox of multi-cultural states is that a wide variety of (sometimes incompatible) normative or ethical cultures exist within a unitary legal/state framework. The ethical basis for a liberal, democratic society is belief in the primacy of individual autonomy and freedom, and in the equality of its citizens. On this basis, it frequently is asserted that common citizenship and the protection of individual rights is all that needs to be done to ensure justice. However, a majoritarian democracy can systematically ignore the voices of minorities. Decision making by the majority within a state, which often means universalizing the cultural beliefs, values and commitments of the majority (Murphy, 1995), renders cultural minorities vulnerable to significant injustice at the hands of the majority, resulting in systematic disadvantage. In the context of this discussion, this

means to provide to all a health service that has been designed by and for the majority, and then to be satisfied with the assertion that every individual, regardless of cultural background, English proficiency and so on, has equal access to this system. Kymlicka (1995) suggests that it is legitimate, and indeed unavoidable, to supplement traditional individual human rights with minority rights.

A comprehensive theory of justice in a multicultural state will include both universal rights, assigned to individuals regardless of group membership, and certain group-differentiated rights for minority cultural groups. Group-differentiated rights can be made to compensate for unequal circumstances which put members of minority cultures at a systematic disadvantage regardless of their personal choices. The freedom and autonomy of individual members of minority groups require not identical treatment but rather differential treatment in order to accommodate differential needs (Barry, 1990). Such differential treatment can support the common rights of citizenship through promoting equal access to mainstream culture and its benefits (Kymlicka, 1995).

In a society of free and equal citizens, health is a primary good as it is a fundamental condition for the full exercise of rights and liberties. Basic institutions and social arrangements are inherently unjust if those institutions and arrangements themselves result in systematic disadvantage accruing to some social groups. If such systematic disadvantages exist, it is the duty of a just society to eliminate such group disadvantage. This may require that priority is accorded to disadvantaged groups on the principle of equity that "equals should be treated equally, and unequals unequally" (Barry, 1990).

If it is the case that cultural minority groups are subject to systematic disadvantage as a result of social arrangements, including the organization and delivery of mental health services, then these ethical considerations have direct implications for the distribution of resources, and the establishment and support of services that meet the needs of particular groups.

Cultural minorities and systematic disadvantage

There is now a substantial (and often confusing) literature on the mental health of indigenous and immigrant populations, and on the variation, across different cultural groups, of prevalence of mental illness among adults, children and adolescents and the elderly; rates of suicide among different ethnic groups; conceptions of health and illness and of illness causation, and the experience and expression of illness; patterns of primary care and specialist mental health service utilization; rates of compulsory admission; and the specific problems of refugees and asylum seekers. There has, as yet, been relatively little work done on the effectiveness or otherwise of various forms of psychiatric treatment of people from cultural minorities.

Prevalence of mental disorders

The results of prevalence studies vary widely according to the disorder being studied, particular ethnic or country of birth groups and the location of the study. It is possible to find reports of higher and lower prevalence of various disorders in various groups, and numerous studies where no difference has been found between (for example) immigrant groups and host populations. (Kemp et al., 1987; Krupinski and Burrows, 1987; Eisenbruch, 1988; Gupta, 1991; Mutchler and Burr, 1991; King et al., 1994; Klimidis et al., 1994; Yamamoto et al., 1994; Cheung, 1995; Cheung and Spears, 1995; Dassori et al., 1995; Trauer, 1995; Mui, 1996; McDonald and Steel, 1997; Nesdale et al., 1997; Stuart et al., 1998). Reports of higher prevalence of schizophrenia among black Caribbeans in the UK than among the white population (McGovern and Cope, 1987; Fernando, 1988), particularly among people of Caribbean origin born in Britain (Harrison et al., 1988; McGovern and Cope, 1991), have aroused substantial controversy. Numerous hypotheses advanced to explain these findings have not withstood scrutiny (Jablensky, 1999). Psychiatrists do not appear to display a greater propensity to diagnose schizophrenia in Afro-Caribbean patients; there is not a greater proportion of acute transient psychoses or drug-induced psychoses in Afro-Caribbean patients, or a greater incidence of schizophrenia in the Caribbean countries from which the immigrants have come; there do not appear to be increased perinatal problems among Afro-Caribbeans; and possible underestimations of the denominator size of the Afro-Caribbean population in the UK have been corrected. Jablensky (1999) concludes that the "causes of the Afro-Caribbean phenomenon remain obscure". As yet unidentified environmental factors are likely to be particularly important.

Among the groups most vulnerable to the development of mental health problems are refugees and asylum seekers. The rates of depression, anxiety and post-traumatic stress disorder were between three and four times higher among Tamil asylum seekers in Australia than the rates of these problems among immigrants (Silove and Steel, 1998; Silove et al., 1998). Despite these very high rates of psychiatric disorder, asylum seekers experienced considerable difficulties in gaining access to mental health and social services (Silove and Steel, 1998).

Service utilization

A pattern of underutilization or overutilization of mental health services by particular groups may point to systematic inadequacies of a service system and raise important questions concerning needs for service, community attitudes towards and beliefs about mental illness and psychiatric treatment, barriers to service access, difficulties in diagnosis, and racism.

Numerous studies have demonstrated differential service utilization by immigrant groups (Sue et al., 1991; Bruxner et al., 1997; McDonald and Steele, 1997; Klimidis et al., 1999a,b). There are three broad factors that will influence the patterns of service use by different sections of the community. They are differences in prevalence of mental illness, different rates of entry into the service system and different rates of exit from the service system.

It is now clear that immigrant status, in itself, is not associated with either a higher or lower prevalence of mental disorder (Klimidis *et al.*, 1994). There are, however, many factors that are a part of the experience of some immigrants (such as pre-migration trauma or torture, disrupted families, maltreatment of various kinds in the host society, unemployment and poverty) that may be associated with increased vulnerability (Silove and Steel, 1998; Silove *et al.*, 1998).

Reduced rates of voluntary entry (Harvey *et al.*, 1990; McGovern and Cope, 1991) into the service system may occur as a result of many factors, including greater stigmatization of mental illness and psychiatric treatment (Ng, 1997; Tabora and Flaskerud, 1997); lack of knowledge of the availability of mental health services and of how to gain access to them; a preference for other forms of assistance (e.g. herbalist, priest); and failure of recognition of the presence of mental disorder at a primary care level. Increased rates of entry may occur as a result of misdiagnosis, lack of other more appropriate service options, greater rates of compulsory admission (Littlewood, 1986;

McGovern and Cope, 1987; Owens *et al.*, 1991; McKenzie *et al.*, 1995; Davies *et al.*, 1996 and admission to secure units (Davies *et al.*, 1996).

Increased rates of exit from the service system (Sue *et al.*, 1991) may occur as a result of dissatisfaction with important elements of the service (Parkman *et al.*, 1997), services being seen as culturally insensitive (Lefley, 1986; Flaskerud and Hu, 1994) and increased stigma being associated with psychiatric treatment.

The most consistent pattern reported is one of underutilization of mental health services by many ethnic communities in many different mental health service systems. Figures 16.1 and 16.2 show a summary of the pattern of mental health service by country of birth and by English proficiency in Victoria, Australia. It can be seen that there is a general pattern of underutilization of services although there is considerable variation by country of birth and, more particularly, by level of English fluency.

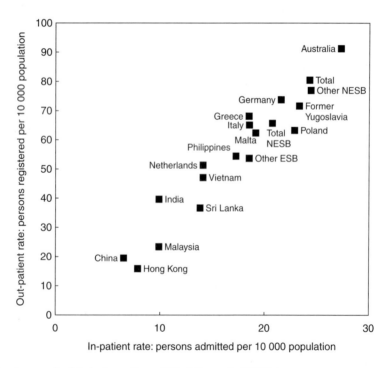

Figure 16.1 *Service use by birthplace. From Klimidis et al. (1999a).*

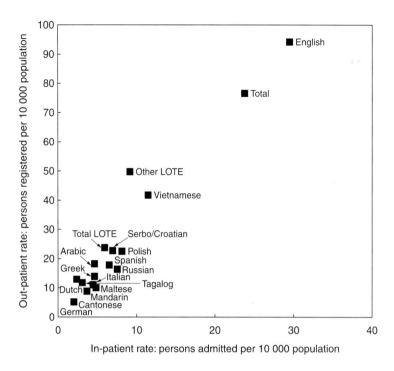

Figure 16.2 *Service use by language. From Klimidis et al. (1999a).*

Treatment outcomes

There is relatively little information available on the quality of treatment outcome among cultural minority groups, although there are suggestions that outcome is generally poorer for immigrants (Minas *et al.*, 1994).

Variation in findings

A striking characteristic of this body of research is the great variation in findings. There are several possible reasons for this lack of consistency. The first is the wide variation in the demographic, cultural and migration profiles of the groups being studied and the wide variation in national and regional mental health service systems. The second is the many methodological difficulties that exist in cross-cultural mental health research (Minas, 1996). These difficulties include lack of common definitions of the populations being studied, including problems with the concept of

ethnicity (McKenzie and Snowcroft; 1994; Senior and Bhopal, 1994); problems in sampling ethnic communities; lack of cross-culturally reliable and valid research instruments (Abiodun, 1994; Gregory, 1994; Janca *et al.*, 1994; Chan, 1995; El-Rufaie and Absood, 1995; Lewis and Araya, 1995); problems associated with cross-cultural diagnosis (Westermeyer, 1985, 1987; Zheng *et al.*, 1994; Alarcon, 1995; Manson, 1995; Mezzich, 1995); the lack of generally acceptable methods for studying culturally derived concepts of mental illness (Pfeiffer, 1994; Patel, 1995; Patel *et al.*, 1995; Weiss *et al.*, 1995); and wide variations in clinical presentation across cultural groups and health systems (Sue and Sue, 1987; Goodman and Richards, 1995).

Despite this variation, it is reasonable to conclude that many (although certainly not all) cultural minority groups in many different service systems experience difficulty in gaining access to culturally appropriate and effective mental health services (Canadian Task Force on Mental Health

Issues Affecting Immigrants and Refugees, 1988; Human Rights and Equal Opportunity Commission, 1993; Minas *et al.*, 1993; Klimidis *et al.*, 1999a). The social arrangements (including the structure and operations of mental health service systems) of many multi-cultural societies systematically disadvantage ethnic and other cultural minorities. In these circumstances, the principles of justice outlined above (Barry, 1990; Rawls, 1993; Kymlicka, 1995) demand that particular efforts are made to redress this disadvantage. It is necessary, in this regard, to shift from an almost exclusive focus on the characteristics of ethnic communities to include consideration of the structure and operations of health systems (Minas, 1991; Sue *et al.*, 1991; Minas *et al.*, 1995) and the relatively neglected issue of translating policies into actual practice (Minas *et al.*, 1996; Ziguras, 1997; Ziguras *et al.*, 1999).

Developing appropriate and effective services

Several authors (Minas, 1991; Sue *et al.*, 1991; Dana *et al.*, 1992; Bhui *et al.*, 1995; Minas *et al.*, 1996) have set out their views concerning the key features of equitable and effective mental health services for culturally diverse societies (Table 16.1). Considerations such as these recently have been incorporated into Australian national

Table 16.1 *Some defining characteristics of an effective and equitable mental health service*

The mental health service needs of the community are defined jointly by the community (including service recipients) and service providers.

The types of services offered, their location and the skills of professionals working in the service are all issues which are determined by the needs of the community to be served. Where there is a disjunction between any of the above characteristics of the service and community needs, the service recognizes that it is its responsibility to develop the capacity to meet diverse needs effectively.

As well as effectively responding to clinical needs, the service will take into account the various religious, cultural and communication needs of service recipients.

Those who may require the service:
    know of its existence;
    regard it as being appropriate to their needs;
    can gain easy and timely access to the service;
    can communicate adequately with service providers;
    can gain access to the full range of services which are appropriate to their needs; and
    are treated with respect and without prejudice.

External outcome indicators demonstrate that the service is achieving the clinical and other goals of service providers and recipients, e.g. the resolution of acute illness, the diminution of disability, the achievement of maximal functioning, the prevention of chronicity, etc.

The quality of outcome is not determined or influenced substantially by factors such as English language fluency or membership of any particular ethnic or social group;

Community, and consumer and carer, representatives are involved in the continuing evaluation, and redesign where necessary, of the service.

Source: Minas *et al.* (1996).

standards for mental health services (Mental Health Branch, Department of Health and Family Services, 1996).

The process of developing services such as these requires action at multiple levels—national, state/regional and local—and must involve all who have a legitimate interest, including consumers and carers, community organizations, mental health professionals, service managers and policy makers. This process will be either facilitated or constrained by the broad political, economic and socio-cultural environment.

Thornicroft and Tansella (1999) have set out a framework that is intended to guide attempts to improve mental health services. The framework is organized around a 3×3 matrix of two dimensions—geographical (1 country/regional, 2 local and 3 patient) and temporal (A inputs, B processes and C outcomes). The use of the 3×3 matrix that is generated can assist in identifying existing problems with services and with the reform of mental health services. Using this framework, I will outline the major requirements that should be met if we are to develop effective, appropriate and equitable mental health services for a culturally diverse society.

National level

Input phase

The first requirement at a national level is a political, socio-cultural and ethical framework for constructive social (including health service) responses to the reality of cultural diversity. A political and ethical framework that reflects the Rawlsian notion of justice as fairness (Rawls, 1971, 1993) will incorporate considerations of diversity into all relevant legislative, policy and programme activities at national, regional and local levels. Particularly important in this regard are national and state/regional mental health policies, and mental health legislation that protects the rights of citizens and of groups that are disadvantaged systematically (Kymlicka, 1995).

Centrally important at this level is the availability of research data on needs of ethnic communities, effective responses to needs, and on approaches to service development and the means for such knowledge to influence policy.

Resources should be allocated in a manner that will give effect to policy intentions, including the allocation of additional resources where necessary to initiate and firmly embed service reforms, and to provide services of equal effectiveness to different sections of the population. A common example is the need to fund professional interpreting services. Among the most important resources are the knowledge, skills and commitment of mental health professionals. The development of an awareness of cultural diversity (and the equity implications of such diversity) and the development of appropriate professional skills through education and training programmes is essential. An input that is no less crucial than professional skills and commitment is a knowledgeable community, one that can participate in mental health promotion programmes, that can recognize mental health problems early and that knows how to gain access to effective and appropriate services. The development of national and regional mental health awareness programmes that are tailored to the needs of diverse ethnic communities requires appropriate resourcing. The involvement of communities in the design and delivery of such programmes is crucial to their success.

National or regional policy intent, a commitment to equity, and current professional and community knowledge may be distilled in a set of national standards for mental health services. Such standards are only useful if there is regular audit of whether the standards are being achieved. An example of such standards is Standard 7 (Cultural Awareness) of the Australian National Standards for Mental Health Services (Mental Health Branch, Department of Health and Family Services, 1998).

Process phase

An important component of the process phase at a national or regional level is the collection of comprehensive data to monitor equity in service provision and to identify whether effective practice is being implemented. The promulgation of standards of care, the process of ensuring that service agencies and clinicians are familiar with and are working towards meeting these standards, and the monitoring of the extent to which agreed standards are being met is also important in this phase. A common experience in mental health service reform is the development of good policies followed by a failure of implementation (Ziguras, 1997). Clear implementation strategies for diversity policies, and provision of the resources necessary for implementation, are essential. This may require the establishment of a policy implementation and research group or unit that will consult with stakeholders, inform policy development and resolve implementation problems and bottlenecks.

Outcome phase

The outcomes should include more equitable and effective mental health services for cultural and linguistic minorities as indicated by the relevant national and regional data collections, including epidemiological, service use and treatment outcome data.

Local level

Input phase

The inputs at a local (e.g. agency) level include agency policies and procedures that give effect to national or regional policies and that reflect local realities, such as the composition of the population served, the profile of available professional, cultural and linguistic skills among staff, and other available resources. Such resources include professional interpreters for the language groups represented in the population, translated information materials, etc. A vital resource or input is the quality of the relationships and patterns of collaboration between local mental health service agencies and the communities being served. Such collaborative relationships will enable service agencies to acquire the necessary knowledge about community structure, needs and resources, and to support communities in their full involvement in service design and evaluation.

Process phase

Processes at a local level include frequent discussions between service agencies and community representatives so as to foster mutual trust and collaboration. These should include both formal (e.g. membership of management committees, participation in service audits, etc.) and informal processes. The quality of linkages between various sections of the service system is also crucial. The key issue in these processes is the extent of the agencies' willingness to share power in decision making with consumers, carers and communities. Token relationships and endless consultations without real power sharing will not do.

Outcome phase

Positive outcomes will include more appropriate patterns of service use by the various communities the agency serves, ready and timely access to services and the developing capacity of the agency to meet a wider range of community needs. A robust collaborative network with communities, community organizations and other service agencies enables a broader and deeper response to varying service needs.

Patient level

Input phase

The key inputs at the patient level are staff attitudes and skills. Attitudes of respect for cultural difference, genuine curiosity and a willingness to learn, and a reflective and critical stance in relation to one's own beliefs and commitments (moral and professional) are indispensable for effective cross-cultural clinical work. Such attitudes will promote a focus on the needs of the patient and flexibility in response to those needs. Such attitudes, in combination with a broad range of clinical and communication skills (see Minas *et al.*, 1996, Table 5.1), will enable the establishment of effective cross-cultural therapeutic relationships.

Process phase

The central process at this level is negotiation between clinician and patient of their respective conceptions of the nature and probable origins of the clinical problem and beliefs concerning the most appropriate and effective intervention. Such negotiations must be genuine, that is with the possibility that both participants in the process will shift from their initial positions. This is a process of mutual education that will influence each person's understanding of the problem, both constrain and extend (in different ways) what is therapeutically possible, serve as the basis for setting priorities and deciding on methods of treatment, and will establish the criteria for evaluating the success of treatment interventions. It will often be necessary to include other key people in this process, usually family members. Clinicians frequently will need to re-examine the place of their own taken-for-granted beliefs about a number of issues (e.g. confidentiality, autonomy and interdependence of patients in relation to their families, and the possible role of traditional–alternative practitioners and non-standard methods of treatment) as well as questioning and, where necessary, challenging patients' and families' beliefs concerning the illness and treatments.

Outcome phase

The outcome of such a process is a robust therapeutic relationship based on mutual respect in which the needs of the patient take precedence and the patient's beliefs and values shape the nature of the therapeutic intervention in a manner that is acceptable to both patient and clinician. The application of the clinician's knowledge and skill within the framework of this kind of therapeutic relationship is likely to lead to better clinical and social outcomes while supporting and enhancing the patient's agency in relation to his illness.

Programme elements

It is not likely that models of transcultural mental health service developed in one place can be implemented successfully elsewhere since so much is dependent on local circumstances. It may be useful, however, to outline some of the more important programme elements or modules that

may be combined in very many different ways to produce a comprehensive response to the needs of culturally diverse societies. I will describe here what I regard as essential elements of such a comprehensive response.

Community development

Informed, confident communities, capable of advocating on their own behalf and of participating fully in policy development, service design and evaluation, will ensure that they are heard at all levels from national policy development to the details of the operations of local service agencies. In order to achieve this, programmes of community development and community support are essential. The goal of such programmes is to build capacity for full participation by minority communities. Such programmes are often best developed and carried out by a wide variety of non-government and ethno-specific organizations. In addition to the activities of non-government organizations (NGOs), there is a clear place for community information and education programmes that are best carried out in partnership between government agencies, specialist transcultural organizations, NGOs and the ethnic media (print and radio).

Patient and carer support

Specific patient and carer support programmes, run in the preferred language of patients and carers and in settings that are culturally familiar, are very important. NGOs are best at developing and sustaining such programmes if they can get access to sufficient financial resources and crucial support from mental health agencies in the design and operation of such programmes.

Support of clinicians in mainstream mental health services

The great majority of people with mental illness from cultural minority groups are assessed and treated by mainstream psychiatric service agencies. This will continue to be the case regardless of the existence of specialist transcultural mental health services. It is neither possible nor desirable to set up a parallel system of mental health services for minority communities. Specialist transcultural mental health services can support mainstream agency clinicians by providing supervision of transcultural clinical work and information about cultural issues that are relevant to particular ethnic communities, assisting with information about bilingual and bicultural clinicians to whom patients can be referred, and providing secondary consultation clinical services. A variety of other approaches have been taken to supporting clinicians in mainstream services, including the appointment of bilingual case managers to work together with clinicians and patients, and the training of professional interpreters as co-therapists. Provision of such support enhances the capacity of mainstream agencies to provide appropriate and effective mental health services to minority communities.

Ethno-specific clinical service

It will sometimes be appropriate to establish mental health services for specific ethnic and linguistic groups. This is only possible where there are large concentrations of particular ethnic groups and the bilingual professionals required to staff such services are available. It is very important that such services, and the professionals working in them, do not become isolated from mainstream services.

Specialist services for particularly vulnerable groups

An example of such services is the various programmes that have been developed around the world to deal with the particular problems of survivors of torture and trauma. Such services are required because of the highly specialized nature of the work. Again it is essential that there are strong linkages between such specialist services and mainstream agencies.

Service innovation and evaluation

There is a continuing need for service innovation and evaluation. This usually occurs through the establishment and evaluation of pilot programmes. A particular problem is that such pilot programmes are often funded only on a short-term basis and it is often difficult for even successful pilot programmes to be incorporated as continuing components of mainstream services. Specialist transcultural mental health input is important for such innovation and for evaluation.

Policy analysis, development and implementation

Analysis of existing policy and its impact on the availability and quality of services for cultural minorities is a crucially important task. An often neglected component of such work is economic analysis of various policy and service options. It is very common for excellent policy documents to have been prepared in the area of transcultural mental health. It is very unusual to have a clear implementation strategy and a commitment of resources to implementation.

Transcultural mental health research

There are numerous methodological and practical difficulties in carrying out transcultural mental health research. There are also great difficulties in securing adequate funding for such work from the standard research funding bodies. There is a great need for well-designed studies, with clear theoretical questions and adequate sample sizes. Replication studies are extremely uncommon. With the increasing (and justified) insistence on evidence, this is a crucial problem for this area of work. There is a great need for cross-regional and cross-national collaborative studies that will answer important questions.

Professional education and training

Education of mainstream mental health professionals in transcultural mental health practice in undergraduate, postgraduate and continuing education programmes will improve the capacity of the general mental health system (where most people from cultural minority communities will be assessed and treated) to provide responsive and effective services. Although there are examples of such education programmes (e.g. the University of Melbourne Graduate Diploma in Transcultural Mental Health [http://www.cimh.unimelb.edu.au/graddip/]), they are not easily accessible by all who require them. The development and widespread delivery of such educational programmes are a high priority.

Specialist transcultural mental health units

The creation of specialist units (as part of state mental health service organizations or within university departments) can bring together the critical mass of researchers, educators and policy analysts in order to carry out the sustained work that is necessary to influence service systems and governments. Such units have the capacity to work collaboratively with ethnic communities, policy makers and service managers in a way that will bring about systemic change. The work of such units may include basic theoretical and services research, policy analysis and policy development, development of educational curricula and delivery of educational programmes, design and piloting of service innovations, and evaluation of service models and treatment approaches. The size and scope of each such unit will depend on local circumstances; however, such units generally should have cross-regional (or perhaps even national) responsibilities if they are to have the capacity to transform accumulated clinical experience, research results and minority community inputs into policies and programmes which can be implemented and evaluated by mainstream service agencies.

Co-ordination of programmes

It is important that there is co-ordination of the various programme elements so that each contributes to a broader process of service reform. Such co-ordination must occur across a number of levels, including the national level. An example of such national co-ordination and transcultural mental health development is the Australian Transcultural Mental Health Network [http://www.atmhn.unimelb.edu.au/].

Conclusion

The development of mental health services that are responsive, accessible, culturally appropriate and effective should not be an add-on or an afterthought. It is not a distraction from the 'core business' of mental health services. It is one expression of the extent to which a society values justice and equity. Even though knowledge about culture, migration and mental health is partial and sometimes inconsistent, there is enough known about how to provide equitable culturally acceptable services. Still often missing is the political will and the commitment of service agencies and mental health professionals to develop such services. Working through the process of reforming services so that they are capable of meeting the diverse needs of a culturally diverse society will have the added benefit of making those services more flexible and responsive to the needs of all members of the community.

References

Abiodun, A. (1994) A validity study of the Hospital Anxiety and Depression Scale in general hospital units and a community sample in Nigeria. *British Journal of Psychiatry*, 165, 669–672.

Alarcon, R.D. (1995) Culture and psychiatric diagnosis: impact on DSM-IV and ICD-10. *Psychiatric Clinics of North America*, 18, 449–465.

Barry, B. (1990) *Political Argument*. Berkley: University of California Press.

Bhui, K., Christie, Y. and Bhugra, D. (1995) The essential elements of culturally sensitive psychiatric services. *International Journal of Social Psychiatry*, 41, 242–256.

Bruxner, G., Burvill, P., Fazio, S. and Febbo, S. (1997) Aspects of psychiatric admission of migrants to hospitals in Perth, Western Australia. *Australian and New Zealand Journal of Psychiatry*, 31, 532–542.

Canadian Task Force on Mental Health Issues Affecting Immigrants and Refugees (1988) *Review of the Literature on Migrant Mental Health*. Ottawa: Health and Welfare Canada, Minister of Supply and Services Canada, Cat. No. Ci96-37/1988E.

Chan, D.W. (1995) The two scaled versions of the Chinese General Health Questionnaire: a comparative analysis. *Social Psychiatry and Psychiatric Epidemiology*, 30, 85–91.

Cheung, P. (1995) Acculturation and psychiatric morbidity among Cambodian refugees in New Zealand. *International Journal of Social Psychiatry*, 41, 108–119.

Cheung, P. and Spears, G. (1995) Illness constructs, health status and use of health services among Cambodians in New Zealand. *Australian and New Zealand Journal of Psychiatry*, 29, 257–265.

Dana, R.H., Behn, J.D. and Gonwa, T. (1992) A checklist for the examination of cultural competence in social service agencies. *Research on Social Work Practice*, 2, 220–233.

Dassori, A.M., Miller, A.L. and Saldana, D. (1995) Schizophrenia among Hispanics: epidemiology, phenomenology, course, and outcome. *Schizophrenia Bulletin*, 21, 303–312.

Davies, S., Thornicroft, G., Leese, M. *et al.* (1996) Ethnic differences in risk of compulsory psychiatric admissions among representative cases in London. *British Medical Journal*, 312, 533–537.

Eisenbruch, M. (1988) The mental health of refugee children and their cultural development. *International Migration Review*, 22, 282–297.

El-Rufaie, O.E.F. and Absood, G.H. (1995) Retesting the validity of the Arabic version of the Hospital Anxiety and Depression (HAD) scale in primary health care. *Social Psychiatry and Psychiatric Epidemiology*, 30, 26–31.

Fernado, S. (1988) *Race and Culture in Psychiatry.* London: Routledge.

Flaskerund, J.H. and Hu, L. (1992) Racial/ethnic identity and amount and type of psychiatric treatment. *American Journal of Psychiatry*, 149, 379–384.

Flaskerud, J.H. and Hu, L.T. (1994) Participation in and outcome of treatment for major depression among low income Asian-Americans. *Psychiatry Reports*, 53, 289–300.

Goodman, R. and Richards, H. (1995) Child and adolescent psychiatric presentations of second-generation Afro-Caribbeans in Britain. *British Journal of Psychiatry*, 167, 362–369.

Gregory, R.J. (1994) The Zung Self-Rating Depression Scale as a potential screening tool for use with Eskimos. *Hospital and Community Psychiatry*, 45, 573–575.

Gupta, S. (1991) Psychosis in migrants from the Indian Subcontinent and English-born controls. *British Journal of Psychiatry*, 159, 222–225.

Harrison, G., Owens, D., Holton, A. *et al.* (1988) A prospective study of severe mental disorder in Afro-Caribbean patients. *Psychological Medicine*, 18, 643–657.

Harvey, J., Williams, M., McGuffin, P. *et al.* (1990) The functional psychoses in Afro-Caribbeans. *British Journal of Psychiatry*, 157, 515–522.

Humans Rights and Equal Opportunity Commission (1993) *Human Rights and Mental Illness: Report of the National Inquiry into the Human Rights of People with Mental Illness.* Canberra: Australian Government Publishing Service.

Huntington, S.P. (1996) *The Clash of Civilisations and the Remaking of World Order.* New York: Simon and Schuster.

Jablensky, A. (1999) Schizophrenia: epidemiology. *Current Opinion in Psychiatry*, 12, 19–28.

Janca, A., Ustun, T.B. and Sartorius, N. (1994) New versions of World Health Organization instruments for the assessment of mental disorders. *Acta Psychiatrica Scandinavica*, 90, 73–83.

Jonsen, A.R. (1990). *The New Medicine and the Old Ethics.* Cambridge, MA: Harvard University Press.

Kemp, B.J., Staples, F. and Lopez-Aqueres, W. (1987) Epidemiology of depression and dysphoria in an elderly Hispanic population. *Journal of the American Geriatrics Society*, 35, 920–926.

King, M., Coker, E., Leavey, G. *et al.* (1994) Incidence of psychotic illness in London: comparison of ethnic groups. *British Medical Journal*, 309, 1115–1119.

Klimidis, S., Stuart, G., Minas, I.H. and Ata, A.W. (1994) Immigrant status and gender effects on psychopathology and self-concept in adolescents: a test of the migration-morbidity hypothesis. *Comprehensive Psychiatry*, 35, 393–404.

Klimidis, S., Lewis, J., Miletic, T., McKenzie, S., Stolk, Y. and Minas, I.H. (1999a) *Mental Health Service Use by Ethnic Communities in Victoria: Part I, Descriptive Report.* Melbourne: Victorian Transcultural Psychiatry Unit. [http://www.ccsh.unimelb.edu.au/vtpu/mhsu/leader.pdf]

Klimidis, S., Lewis, J., Miletic, T., McKenzie, S., Stolk, Y. and Minas, I.H. (1999b) *Mental Health Service Use by Ethnic Communities in Victoria: Part II, Statistical Tables.* Melbourne:Victorian Transcultural Psychiatry Unit. [http://www.ccsh.unimelb.edu.au/vtpu/mhsu/leader.pdf]

Krupinski, J. and Burrows, G. (eds) (1987) *The Price of Freedom.* Sydney: Pergamon Press.

Kymlicka, W. (1995) *Multicultural Citizenship: A Liberal Theory of Minority Rights.* Oxford: Clarendon Press.

Lefley, H.P. (1986) Why cross-cultural training? Applied issues in culture and mental health service delivery. In: Lefley, H.P. and Pederson, P.B. (eds), *Cross Cultural Training for Mental Health Professionals.* Springfield, IL: Charles C. Thomas. pp. 11–46.

Lewis, G. and Araya, R.I. (1995) Is the General Health Questionnaire (12 item) a culturally biased measure of psychiatric disorder? *Social Psychiatry and Psychiatric Epidemiology*, 30, 20–25.

Littlewood, R. (1986) Ethnic minorities and the Mental Health Act. Patterns of explanation. *Bulletin of the Royal College of Psychiatrists* 10, 306–308.

Manson, S.M. (1995) Culture and major depression: current challenges in the diagnosis of mood disorders. *Psychiatric Clinics of North America*, 18, 487–501.

McDonald, B. and Steel, Z. (1997) *Immigrants and Mental Health: An Epidemiological Analysis.* Sydney: Transcultural Mental Health Centre.

McGovern, D. and Cope, R. (1987) The compulsory detention of males of different ethnic groups, with special reference to offender patients. *British Journal of Psychiatry*, 150, 505–512.

McGovern, D. and Cope, R. (1991) Second generation of Afro-Caribbeans and Whites with first admission diagnosis of schizophrenia. *Social Psychiatry and Psychiatric Epidemiology*, 26, 95–99.

McKenzie, K.J. and Snowcroft, N.S. (1994) Race, ethnicity, culture, and science. *British Medical Journal*, 309, 286–287.

McKenzie, K., van Os, J., Fahy, T. *et al.* (1995) Psychosis with good prognosis in Afro-Caribbean people now living in the United Kingdom. *British Medical Journal*, 311, 1325–1328.

Mental Health Branch, Department of Health and Family Services (1996) National Standards for Mental Health Services. http://www.atmhn.unimelb.edu.au/research/guidelines/ns_mhs.html

Mezzich, J.E. (1995) Cultural formulation and comprehensive diagnosis: clinical and research perspectives. *Psychiatric Clinics of North America*, 18, 649–657.

Minas, I.H. (1991) Inequalities in mental health care based on language and culture. Submission to the Human Rights and Equal Opportunity Commission National Inquiry Concerning the Human Rights of People with Mental Illness.

Minas, I.H. (1996) Transcultural psychiatry. *Current Opinion in Psychiatry*, 9, 144–148.

Minas, I.H., Silove, D. and Kunst, J.-P. (1993) *Mental Health for Multicultural Australia: A National Strategy.* Report of a consultancy to the Commonwealth Department of Human Services and Health. Melbourne: Victorian Transcultural Psychiatry Unit.

Minas, I.H., Stuart, G.W. and Klimidis, S. (1994) Language, culture and psychiatric services: a survey of Victorian clinical staff. *Australian and New Zealand Journal of Psychiatry*, 28, 250–258.

Minas, I.H., Ziguras, S., Klimidis, S, Stuart, G.W. and Freidin, S.P. (1995) *Extending the Framework: A Proposal for a State-wide Bilingual Clinical Support and Development Program.* Melbourne: Victorian Transcultural Psychiatry Unit.

Minas, I.H., Lambert, T.J.R., Kostov, S. and Boranga, G. (1996) *Mental Health Service for NESB Immigrants: Transforming Policy Into Practice.* Canberra: Australian Government Publishing Service.

Mui, A.C. (1996) Depression among elderly Chinese immigrants: an exploratory study. *Social Work*, 41, 633–644.

Murphy, P. (1995) The body politic. In Komesaroff, P.A. (ed.), *Troubled Bodies: Critical Perspectives on Postmodernism, Medical Ethics, and the Body.* Melbourne: Melbourne University Press, pp. 103–124.

Mutchler, J.E. and Burr, J.A. (1991) Racial differences in health and health care utilisation in later life: the effect of socioeconomic status. *Journal of Health and Social Behaviour*, 32, 342–356.

Nesdale, D., Rooney, R. and Smith, L. (1997) Migrant ethnic identity and psychological distress. *Journal of Cross-cultural Psychology*, 28, 569–588.

Ng, C.H. (1997) The stigma of mental illness in Asian cultures. *Australian and New Zealand Journal of Psychiatry*, 31, 382–390.

Owens, D., Harrison, G. and Boot, D. (1991) Ethnic factors in voluntary and compulsory admissions. *Psychological Medicine*, 21, 185–196.

Parkman, S., Davies, S., Leese, M., Phelan, M. and Thornicroft, G. (1997) Ethnic differences in satisfaction with mental health services among representative people with psychosis in South London: Prism Study 4. *British Journal of Psychiatry*, 171, 260–264.

Patel, V. (1995) Explanatory models of mental illness in sub-Saharan Africa. *Social Science and Medicine*, 40, 1291–1298.

Patel, V., Musara, T, Butau, T., Maramba, P. and Futane, S. (1995) Concepts of mental illness and medical pluralism in Harare. *Psychological Medicine*, 25, 485–493.

Pfeiffer S. (1994) Belief in demons and exorcism in psychiatric patients in Switzerland. *British Journal of Medical Psychology*, 67, 247–258.

Rawls, J. (1971) *A Theory of Justice.* Cambridge, MA: Harvard University Press.

Rawls, J. (1993) *Political Liberalism.* New York: Columbia University Press.

Senior, P.A. and Bhopal, R. (1994) Ethnicity as a variable in epidemiological research. *British Medical Journal*, 309, 327–330.

Silove, D. and Steel, Z. (1998) *The Mental Health and Well-being of On-shore Asylum Seekers in Australia.* Sydney: Psychiatry Research and Teaching Unit, University of New South Wales.

Silove, D., Steel, Z., McGorry, P. and Mohan, P. (1998) Psychiatric symptoms and living difficulties in Tamil asylum seekers: comparisons with refugees and immigrants. *Acta Psychiatrica Scandinavica*, 97, 175–181.

Stuart, G.W., Klimidis, S. and Minas, I.H. (1998) The treated prevalence of mental disorder amongst immigrants and Australian-born: community and primary care rates. *International Journal of Social Psychiatry*, 44, 22–34.

Sue, D. and Sue, S. (1987) Cultural factors in the clinical assessment of Asian Americans. *Journal of Consulting and Clinical Psychology*, 55, 479–487.

Sue, S., Fujino, D.C., Hu, L., Takeuchi, D.T. and Zane, N.W.S. (1991) Community mental health services for ethnic minority groups: a test of the cultural responsiveness hypothesis. *Journal of Consulting and Clinical Psychology*, 59, 533–540.

Tabora, B. and Flaskerud, J.H. (1997) Mental health beliefs, practices and knowledge of Chinese American immigrant women. *Issues in Mental Health Nursing*, 18, 178–189.

Thornicroft, G. and Tansella, M. (1999) *The Mental Health Matrix: A Manual to Improve Services*. Cambridge: Cambridge University Press.

Trauer, T. (1995) Ethnic differences in the utilisation of public psychiatric services in an area of suburban Melbourne. *Australian and New Zealand Journal of Psychiatry*, 29, 615–623.

Weiss, M.G., Raguram, R. and Channabasavanna, S.M. (1995) Cultural dimensions of psychiatric diagnosis: comparison of DSM-III-R and illness explanatory models in South India. *British Journal of Psychiatry*, 166, 353–359.

Westermeyer, J. (1985) Psychiatric diagnosis across cultural boundaries. *American Journal of Psychiatry*, 142, 798–805.

Westermeyer, J. (1987) Clinical considerations in cross-cultural diagnosis. *Hospital and Community Psychiatry*, 38, 160–165.

Yamamoto, J., Rhee, S. and Chang, D.S. (1994) Psychiatric disorders among elderly Koreans in the United States. *Community Mental Health*, 30, 17–27.

Zheng, Y.-P., Lin, K.-M., Zhao, J.-P., Zhang, M.-Y. and Yong, D. (1994) Comparative study of diagnostic systems: Chinese Classification of Mental Disorders—Second Edition versus DSM-III-R. *Comprehensive Psychiatry*, 35, 441–449.

Ziguras, S. (1997) Implementation of ethnic health policy in community mental health centres in Melbourne. *Australian and New Zealand Journal of Public Health*, 21, 323–328.

Ziguras, S.J., Stankovska, M. and Minas, I.H. (1999) Initiatives for improving mental health services to ethnic minorities in Australia. *Psychiatric Services*, 50, 1229–1231.

17 | *The multi-disciplinary team*

John Øvretveit

Introduction

Teams are ways in which people can work with others to do things which they cannot do alone. Most of this chapter is about clinical community mental health teams for organizing and providing services to people with mental health problems. However, there are other types of teams, such as project teams, and other ways of co-ordinating care, such as case management. The chapter considers why we need teams as an organizational arrangement for providing services and gives some concepts for understanding the structure and dynamics of a community mental health team.

There are many different types of clinical teams for different purposes. One type of team is a grouping of personnel who are all employed by different agencies or are self-employed. Anther type is where all in the team are employed by one agency and the team leader is the manager of all the personnel in the team. This is one dimension for distinguishing teams which we will consider later—the dimension of team member's management. Table 17.1 shows some of the main types of teams and co-ordination in mental health services.

Do *we really need teams?*

It is fashionable to undertake many tasks by setting-up or using a team, but we need to remember that a team is just one of many ways of getting work done. A team is a method for organizing the contributions of different people to carry out a task. The first consideration should be 'what are the needs' either a patient's needs or the needs of a task. The second is 'what resources—mainly expertise and skills—are required to meet these needs or to carry out this task?'

Once these questions are clear, we can consider what might be the best or most feasible way to organize the different contributions of people or services which are required. A team is one of the methods of organization. Other methods are for one person to seek out and co-ordinate the contributions of others (e.g. a case manager, or a project officer without a defined team), or to create a 'working forum' or 'loose network' if flexibility and autonomy are important or as a possible stepping stone to a more permanent and formal team.

Teams, in the sense of a relatively permanent grouping of different disciplines, can be an efficient and a satisfying form of work organization. However, they can also be a disaster, hiding disrespect with the pretence of co-operation, or can be rent with conflict. Both patients and health workers can benefit and grow from teamwork, and they can also suffer from poor teamwork. This chapter takes the view that much depends on clear structure and good leadership. Later, we consider some of the factors which are essential to team success.

Teams are for matching and co-ordination

Two of the most important functions of teams are 'matching' and 'co-ordination'. 'Matching' is where we can get the quickest and best match between the client's needs and the skills available. If specialist mental health professionals are organized, financed and managed separately, then it takes time to get the client to the person with the best expertise to help them. The client may be referred a number of times and never get to the best person, especially if there are financial incentives to treat. This experience can not only delay treatment but can itself exacerbate many client's condition. A much quicker and effective way is to

Table 17.1 *The main types of teams in mental health services*

Type of team	Purpose	Example
Case manager's team or client's team	Organize and co-ordinate different services to one person	The different people providing help to a schizophrenic patient who are co-ordinated by one case manager.
Network team	Easy exchange of information and referral, sometimes through 'network meetings'	Some primary health care teams. Some loose-knit large community mental health teams with little formal structure
Formal service delivery team	Provide a range of services to a defined population and manage the resources within the team	A community mental health team with a collective responsibility for providing a specialist mental health service to a population of 60 000 people, and with an accountable team leader and budget
Project team	Carry out a task within a set time period	A working group set up to make proposals for improving liaison between primary health care and specialist mental health services
Management team	Collectively accountable for providing a specified service within a defined budget, or for advising a general manager who is accountable for this service	The management team of a sector mental health service or division, or the top management team of a mental health service

bring all the specialists into the same team, and channel all referrals to this team. It is easier within a team to agree which specialist is most suited to the clients needs, or to do a quick specialist assessment to decide who will work with the client. It is also easier to adjust for workload differences amongst the specialists to ensure that the client gets a service.

Effective matching requires good organization (discussed below) and an acceptance amongst specialists to give up a degree of autonomy in favour of some of the benefits from working in a team. Matching is in fact one type of co-ordination, but there are other co-ordination functions which

teams perform. One is where two or more people in the team are working with the same client. If the practitioners are in the team, it is easier for them to know who else is or has been working with the client and to liaise, and to agree joint treatment plans. It is also often easier to co-ordinate others outside of a team or to ensure good transfer if a team member presents themselves as being the teams' client co-ordinator.

Both good matching and good co-ordination depend on organizational arrangements being set up in the team—they need to be agreed, explicit, understood and managed if these arrangements are to work.

Making sense of a community mental health team

In the last 20 years, many different types of community mental health teams have been formed or have evolved. There are four main ways in which these teams differ, which are described presently. These concepts are part of the language for discussing and understanding teams. Using this way of describing a team can help us to see the underlying structure, gives tools to explain and solve problems, and also gives a language to communicate with others in the team about how to make improvements.

Accountability

The first of these ways of describing a team is to clarify whether it is clear and agreed that the team is a collectively accountable service provision team (CAT) or a co-ordinated profession team (CPT). A collective accountability team is one where team members are assigned to a group which is collectively accountable for using the groups resources to provide a defined service to a defined population. Each person in the team has an employment contract or an agreement that they serve as part of this group to provide a specialist service to this population.

Teams with 'collective population responsibility' are teams in which members are accountable as a group for pooling and using their collective resources in the best way to meet the most pressing special needs of the population which they serve. This does not mean that members are responsible as a group for a clinical decision, just that they are responsible for how they allocate their collective resources in a management sense. In any team, each individual member is always professionally and legally accountable for their own casework and clinical omissions.

One of the consequences of this is that the group has to decide how best to use its resources to meet the most pressing specialist needs of this population. The group is forced to agree and implement collective priorities—to manage its resources as a collective—and individuals cannot opt out. If fact, there are few teams where this is clear and agreed, but all teams have an element of collective responsibility which translates into resource management issues, and these issues need to be confronted and debated if the team is not to suffer from some individuals opting out.

Membership

The second set of concepts for describing a team define different types of team membership. Distinguishing different types of membership is important when teams are large or involve members from different organizations. Membership defines a group's boundaries. The moment we talk of network 'membership', we imply less fluidity and more permanence and stability. We begin to think of a group with regular attenders and the concepts of attender's obligations to the group and their rights and commitments.

The question of team membership often arises when a group is evolving from a network into a formal team. Agreeing membership is a way of drawing boundaries around the group. Typically, in the early stages, everyone is a member and no distinctions are made. Making distinctions threatens the weak bonds holding the group together. Later, when important decisions have to be made, for example about priorities or whether to have self-referral or crisis intervention, the meaning of membership becomes more important. People ask if it is right that people who are not affected by the decision, or who often do not come to meetings, should have an equal vote to those whose working week will be profoundly affected by the decision. Are those not affected in fact real members of the group?

Clarifying membership often marks a transition from an informal loose-knit group to a more formal and organized team. It often happens as a result of, or as part of a process of clarifying the purpose of the group. This transition is helped by being able to assign different categories of membership, so as to recognize differences in the group and keep valued contributors. The most common membership distinction is between 'core' and 'associate' (or 'extended team'), usually meaning full-time in the team or part-time.

One membership issue is which mix of different professions and other staff should be in the team and how many of each. Often team membership is the result of historic staffing decisions and arbitrary fate. Managers work with what they have and, if they are able, change professions and staff grades when people leave in order to get a better match between the demands on the team and the range of skills available (Patmore and Weaver, 1991).

Another aspect of membership is the more personal characteristics of members: their skills apart from profession-specific skills, and their experience, status and seniority. In the same way as there is a tendency to avoid defining membership in developing teams, there is also a tendency to avoid recognizing real and important seniority and status differences between team members. Perhaps recognizing these differences within a team may undermine a tentative consensus about purpose which is essential to holding the group together. Another hypothesis is that team member's fear that recognizing payment and status differences may release destructive feelings of jealously and envy which cannot be contained by the fragile mechanisms which exist within the team. A third is that teams which wish to establish participatory and more equal relationships with clients also stress equality and democracy within the team. It is curious that some teams find it easy to recognize sex and race differences in a team and try to appoint new members to ensure the 'right balance', yet deny differences in experience, status and seniority.

Pathway and decision-making process

The third dimension for clarifying how a team works and how it could be improved is the pathway and decision-making process in the team (Øvretveit, 1993). We noted earlier that co-ordination of resources and skills is a key function in teams and that co-ordination had to be created, managed and improved. The concepts of patient pathway and decision-making methods help us to describe how the team works now and how co-ordination could be improved. In some teams, all referrals are made to the team and practitioners take most or all of their work from the team allocation meeting. These 'single entry teams' then vary in terms of whether the practitioner reports back to the team at later stages of the client's pathway, or whether the client is managed within a professional service pathway.

We can consider the patient's pathway in terms of the following stages: source of referral; reception or short-term team response; allocation; assessment; intervention; review; closure; and, sometimes, follow-up. Some teams have one general pathway for all clients: all clients receive an assessment, have a care plan, get a review and are closed to the team according to the same general procedure and decision-making process. Some teams have different pathways for different clients, such as for long-term or acute clients in mental health teams—they have different 'care programme pathways' (Patmore and Weaver, 1991; Sayce *et al.*, 1991).

Type 1: parallel pathway

Most network teams have this type of multiple pathway. Each profession has their own pathway, and team meetings are for cross-referrals.

Type 2: allocation or 'postbox' pathway

A second type of pathway is followed in the 'postbox team'—the team meeting serves as a point where professionals can pick up referrals which they then take back to the separate professional pathways. In this type of team, there are usually two pathways for clients to get to the team. In one, the client is referred to a team secretary or a team leader, who then brings the referral to a team meeting. In the other, the team member takes the referral and brings it to the team meeting, if they do not decide to 'take the case' themselves.

Type 3: reception and allocation pathway

The third type of pathway is different from the second in that the team has a team short-term response at the 'reception' stage. Team members take turns on a duty rota to staff the reception stage.

Type 4: reception–assessment–allocation pathway

In this process, there are two allocation stages, one for assessment and one for longer term work. Clients are allocated first for an assessment which is more detailed than the one done at 'reception'. This assessment is used to decide whether to allocate for longer term work, and who should do this work. The team does not assume that the person doing the assessment will do longer term work, if any is called for, although for continuity it is better that it is the same person.

Type 5: reception–assessment–allocation–review pathway

In this type of pathway, the team has a review stage, in addition to the stages of the Type 4 pathway team. At the review, the team member working on the case presents a report to the team: they report their progress in carrying out the care plan and the client's current needs, and make recommendations to the team about any further work. Teams which are careful about managing their resources assume that team members have to justify 'keeping a case open' to the team—the team may be struggling to allocate other clients with greater needs. Some Type 5 teams also influence the decision by the practitioner to finish casework ('closure').

Justifying keeping the case open and review reports are ways of ensuring practitioner accountability to the team after intervention. They help the team to monitor client care, and to increase control over team resources. It also calls for closer team integration, which requires a more bureaucratic structure, and reduces team member's autonomy. In practice, many team are of the sixth type, i.e. a mixture.

Type 6: hybrid parallel pathway

This process is quite common, and is a mixture of separate profession pathways for some professions (e.g. psychology and psychiatry), and a team pathway such as Type 5 or Type 4. Professionals who work in professional services separate from the team refer patients to the team and take patients from the team at different stages in the pathway.

Management

The fourth way to understand a team is by clarifying who manages and employs each member. It is common to down-play the structural features of teams such as management and employment, but these features can assert themselves at critical times and are an underlying reality which can constrain the degree of teamwork which is possible, separate from the personalities involved.

Traditionally, health and social services have managed practitioners within professional structures, at least up to a certain level, above which general management took over. In these structures, profession heads have been responsible for assessing the needs for the profession's services and allocating practitioners to areas of work to meet the most pressing needs. Lower down the profession-managed structure, operational profession managers have directed staff, and, in professions with less practitioner autonomy, have decided how many hours staff would spend on different activities or on particular clients (Øvretveit, 1992). This type of structure is simple, clear and well understood, but can limit interprofessional working in some types of teams. It is one of five subcategories of management structure for teams described below (Øvretveit, 1993).

To clarify a team management structure, we need to consider the management work which needs to be done to manage practitioners in a team. Although the details vary between professions and according to the level of seniority of the practitioner, in principle someone has to be responsible for carrying out each of the following eight key management tasks: (i) drafting job description; (ii) interviewing and appointing; (iii) introducing the person to the job; (iv) assigning work; (v) reviewing work (holding accountable); (vi) annual performance appraisal and objectives setting; (vii) ensuring practice quality, training and professional development; and (viii) disciplinary action. Traditionally, profession managers have been responsible for each of these tasks, and profession management is still an option for some types of team—this is the Type 1 structure.

Type 1: profession-managed structure

Practitioners are managed by their profession managers, each of whom undertakes the eight personnel management tasks listed above, but each in a slightly different way because of differences between professions in practitioner's autonomy. This structure is most common in network teams.

Type 2: single manager structure

At the other extreme from the profession-managed structure is the team where all practitioners are managed by one manger, who undertakes all the eight personnel management tasks in relation to each practitioner. This model is common in the USA, Australia and in some European countries, but less common in the UK, apart from in some community health locality teams. In some variations of this model, the team manager and practitioners may have access to a senior profession advisor to help the manager with certain personnel tasks such as performance appraisal.

Type 3: joint management structure

This structure was popular in joint health and social service teams in the 1980s. A team co-ordinator and a professional superior, who is sometimes also a team member, agree who will carry out which of the eight management tasks, or which tasks will be shared.

Type 4: team manager-contracted structure

There has been a trend towards having a team manager with a budget, who contracts-in some or all team members. Team members are often part of profession-managed services (e.g. a physiotherapy service) which may be organized within the same service as the team manager, as for example in an NHS Community Health Trust. This model

gives team managers control over team members through contracts, although the bureaucracy of contracts can approach that of the joint management agreements. It also allows team mangers the flexibility to contract-in the skills that they need, especially when professions cannot recruit staff, and the opportunity to use private practitioners and others under short-term contracts. Profession managers retain the management of their staff, which can make it easier to recruit staff who prefer to work in a profession-managed service.

Type 5: hybrid management structure

An increasing number of teams have a mixed management structure, with the team manger managing core staff, co-ordinating some staff under a joint management agreement and contracting-in others.

One challenge in creating a management structure for a multi-disciplinary team is establishing management which allows appropriate autonomy for practitioners from different professions and with different levels of seniority. A second is establishing responsibility for managing the total resources of the team: for assessing needs and ensuring that practitioners time is allocated to where the needs are most pressing. Each profession and each practitioner has their own views on these issues, often leading to disagreements about the role of team leader, or people avoiding clarifying the role. Team management is a controversial subject, raising issues of practitioner autonomy and control over their time, and of professions self-image and status.

Other issues in teamwork

Structure is one aspect of teams, and to conclude this chapter we note some other aspects and issues which need to be considered in setting up or improving a team. Getting the right balance of roles and behaviours in a team is important to success. Above we considered the disciplinary background and expertise of team members, but we also need to consider people's 'team style'.

Psychologists have given a number of characterizations of the different roles which people may play in any group, and in working groups in particular (e.g. Belbin, 1981). Some teams have an imbalance of critical behaviours over positive and constructive problem solving. Others have an imbalance of too many proposals without discussion of priorities and what is feasible. In part, these imbalances are due to missing behaviours and roles in the team such as 'critical assessor'. Sometimes it is possible to analyse the missing behaviours and persistently intervene in ways which lead in time to permanent changes in culture. Are some of the following roles/behaviours under-represented in the team: ideas generation, support of different contributions, concern for feelings, task orientation, co-ordination, evaluation of past actions, completer–finisher (concerned with ensuring that the action is carried through), time-keeper, responsibility assigned for tasks?

Some of the other subjects which need to be considered in setting up and running a team are how the team assesses the needs of the population it serves and makes changes in response (Øvretveit, 1993), team member's motivation, how team members get feedback about their individual professional performance and their team performance (Iles, 1997), how to develop facilitation skills for managing teams as a team leader (Hunter *et al.*, 1992; Fisher and Sharp, 1998), conflict management (Fisher *et al.*, 1991), how power works inside and outside of teams (Iles, 1997), and how to evaluate team performance and services (Øvretveit, 1998).

Conclusions

The chapter concentrated on concepts for understanding the underlying structure of a team. The reason that many team problems arise is because structural issues are ignored, and also because agreeing structure is how we ensure that the potential benefits of teams are in fact realized. We noted earlier that matching and co-ordination are two of these benefits, but good matching and co-ordination have to be created, organized and continually managed in a team—they do not just happen when a group of specialists are put in the same room, even if they agree a chairperson. To be successful, teams have to agree and continually review their organization, and concepts to describe the organization are essential tools for this process.

References

Belbin, M. (1981) *Management Teams: Why they Succeed or Fail*. Oxford: Heinemann.

Fisher, R. and Sharp, A. (1998) *Getting it Done*. New York: Harper Collins.

Fisher, R., Ury, W. and Patton, B. (1991) *Getting to Yes*. London: Century Business Books.

Hunter, D., Bailey, A. and Taylor, B. (1992) *The Art of Facilitation*. Auckland: Tandem Press.

Iles, V. (1997) *Really Managing Health Care*. Milton Keynes, UK: Open University Press.

Øvretveit, J. (1992) *Therapy Services: Organisation, Management, and Autonomy*. London: Harwood Academic Press.

Øvretveit, J. (1993) *Coordinating Community Care: Multidisciplinary Teams and Care Management*. Milton Keynes, UK: Open University Press.

Øvretveit, J. (1998) *Evaluating Health Interventions*. Milton Keynes, UK: Open University Press.

Patmore, C. and Weaver, T. (1991) *Community Mental Health Teams: Lessons for Planners and Managers*. London: Good Practices in Mental Health.

Sayce, L., Craig, T. and Boardman, A. (1991) The development of community health centres in the UK. *Social Psychiatry and Psychiatric Epidemiology*, 26, 14–20.

18 | Sectorization

Lars Hansson

What is a sectorized service?

The replacement of care in psychiatric hospitals with care in community-based psychiatric services during the last decades has been a major trend in the development of mental health care systems. The general aims of deinstitutionalization were to prevent inappropriate mental hospital admissions through the provision of community-based alternatives for treatment; to discharge to the community all institutionalized patients who had been given adequate preparation for such a change; and to establish and maintain community support systems for people receiving mental health services in the community (Bachrach, 1977). This movement was founded in, and reinforced by, a number of social, political and economical trends, of which an emphasis on civil rights and the pressure to reduce spending on mental health care may have been the most important (Breakey, 1996). A number of principles have evolved, guiding the building up of psychiatric service systems for care in the community. Some of these principles have been related to the organization of care, while others have expressed public policy, ideology or a philosophy of care, relying on evolving social values consistent with the development of these new services. The principles identified in this process have been that psychiatric services should be comprehensive, co-ordinated, accessible, acceptable, accountable, efficient and effective (Huxley, 1990). These principles have been related to the organization and content of services, but have also been seen as a means to increase effectiveness and outcome of treatment of individuals.

The concept of sectorization, or sectorized services, has been used to denote an organizational framework that can underpin the development and maintenance of a community-based service system, consistent with aims of the deinstitution-

alization movement. However, the concept has since become somewhat ambiguous. It is therefore preferable to conceive of sectorization as a way of organizing a local service system, which has the potential to support community-based service models. A sectorized service might be characterized by the adherence to the following principles:

(i) *The catchment area principle:* the organization of psychiatric services is related to a specific geographic area.

(ii) *The population responsibility principle:* the psychiatric services are responsible for care of the total population within the catchment area.

(iii) *The comprehensiveness principle:* the psychiatric care organization is specified in a range of differentiated services covering all levels of mental health services for the population under responsibility.

A sectorized psychiatric service can therefore be seen as an important and necessary (but not sufficient) premise for the implementation of a community-based service system.

Objectives of sectorized psychiatric services

The objectives of sectorized psychiatric services have been intertwined with the objectives of the deinstitutionalization process. The general objective of a sectorized service, as for any other rational model of organization of psychiatric services, is to improve the mental health in the target population, focusing on prevention and the reduction of prevalence and incidence of mental illness. The reduction of needs of care in the population and that services should be delivered in a cost-effective way may be seen as objectives related to this.

However, such health-related objectives seldom are stated clearly or operationalized by the services (Falloon *et al.*, 1987). Rather, there has been a reliance on intermediate (process) objectives, which at their best have only a potential relationship with the mental health in the target population. Common process aims used have been to reduce rates of in-patient treatment, length of in-patient stay or rates of readmission. A related objective has been to keep the patient in the community and to avoid in-patient treatment as much as possible (Häfner and an der Heiden, 1991).

Proposed advantages and drawbacks of sectorization

The advantage of sectorized services is that it is a population-based system with a defined responsibility of a comprehensive care organization. This may have relevance for the effectiveness of care, because it can increase accessibility, availability and co-operation with other mental health-related agents within the local community. A sectorized service system may also counteract the risk of fragmentation of community-based services. From a system level point of view, a sectorized service enables a population-based monitoring of the effectiveness of the service system. The evaluation and monitoring of the mental health of the population within a defined psychiatric sectorized service is improved by using local data on process outcome. A number of other advantages for sectorized services have been proposed (Tansella, 1991; Strathdee and Thornicroft, 1992; Johnson and Thornicroft, 1993). Planning of services may be improved by high identification rates of patients, it may assist the development and integration of local service components, the knowledge and use of community resources may be better, and it may also result in a greater budgetary clarity. Service delivery advantages may be that fewer patients are lost to follow-up, integration of inter-agency patient programmes, and clarity of functions of the different parts of the service

system. Regarding quality of care, it may result in a better-defined responsibility of the individual patient, an improvement in patient education and intervention, and a greater support for relatives. It may also give opportunities for an improved communication between staff and users and a better communication between primary care and secondary care services. Some disadvantages with services organized according to the principles of sectorization have also been put forth (Lindholm, 1983; Johnson and Thornicroft, 1993). A sectorized service limits the patient's choice of services and care-giver, and it may also promote generalist services rather than specialist services. Staff may not be so specialized or experienced in particular areas of work as the staff in specialist services, and they also have to set priorities among competing client groups in a way which may not be necessary in specialist services.

Models of catchment area-based services

Sectorization provides an organizational and structural framework for the establishment of community-based services. However, it does not imply *per se* any specific arrangements of the catchment area-based services. Some general principles may, however, be linked as intermediate objectives to the sectorization of services. The promotion of continuity of care, co-ordination of care and integration of care have been put forward as such general principles (Walsh, 1987). Continuity of care is important to ensure that persons have access to care at all stages and levels of illness, and ideally is dealt with by the same team or service. Co-ordination of care is seen as important since mental illness often has a complex and broad impact on the life situation and needs of the afflicted individuals with disabilities and impairments in several functional areas. A multi-disciplinary approach is therefore essential.

The integration of care refers both to integration between specialist psychiatric services and other community services in contact with the mentally ill, and to the integration of care within specific parts of the psychiatric services. From this, it is clear that the basic tasks in a sectorized service are fulfilled by multi-disciplinary teams which might be looked upon as a cornerstone for the implementation of a sectorized service. However, as vividly shown by the WHO multi-centre study (Giel *et al.*, 1987), sectorized services are organized very differently and the allocation of resources to specific types of services shows a great variation due to differences in priorities with regard to target population, client group and functions of the services. Sectorized services might be categorized *ad hoc* into four models (Strathdee and Thornicroft, 1992).

- The hospital core model, which advocates that the hospital base should be the core of the system with a close co-ordination with services such as community clinics, mental health centres and day care units located in strategic parts of the catchment area.

- The community mental health centre model, which is using a community base for both acute and continuing care services of the catchment area, providing both a location for services and a base for outreach services, and linking to other local services outside the psychiatric services.

- The integrated primary care model, which is based on the fact that first contact sites, such as the primary care service or social service, is the base and location for assessment and treatment. The staff of the psychiatric services have a specific liaison with these services both concerning acute and crisis interventions and continuing care. A range of in-patient facilities for both acute and chronic patients may remain on hospital-based services run by the psychiatric service.

- The assertive outreach or home-based treatment model. This model may not be suitable as a general model for a sectorized service, but may be used rather for a core client group with severe needs and who are unable or unwilling to attend the regular services. As an approach, it emphasizes care in the community and avoiding hospital treatment.

Effects of sectorization

Research on the effects of sectorization may be divided into two kinds of studies, one is concerned with outcome in relation to changes of the service system into a sectorized service, and the second evaluates the outcome of a service in operation. In studies related to the changes into a sectorized service, it is also of great importance to differentiate methodologically between research on effects of organizational change and research on the outcome to individuals.

Studies on the implementation of a sectorized service have been concerned mainly with intermediate process objectives of reducing in-patient care in favour of the use of alternative services, and consequently have been discussing 'outcome' in terms of changes in utilization rates on different service levels. Utilization rates, which strictly speaking are measures of care processes, have been used as proxies for outcome, and these studies have reported changes in bed day utilization, changes in rates of admissions, length of in-patient treatment, readmission rates, changes in day- and out-patient contact patterns, and in survival measures such as time in the community. There has been a clear tendency to view these measures as if they are outcome measures, sometimes clearly stated and sometimes implicit. However, utilization is not cure, nor is it necessarily related to needs, and these measures have been strongly criticized as measures of process rather than outcome (Rosenblatt and Mayer, 1974; Turner, 1979; Bachrach, 1982; Falloon, 1984).

As far as in-patient treatment indices are concerned, the best predictor of being admitted to hospital has been shown to be a history of earlier admissions, rather than level of symptoms or psychopathology. These measures are also highly influenced by a number of other variables such as bed capacity, availability of alternative services, social characteristics of the patients, level of tolerance in the community, and administrative and discharge policies (Zohar *et al.*, 1987; Häfner and an der Heiden, 1991). Furthermore, since reduction in the numbers of hospital beds has been a major feature of the deinstitutionalization process, irrespective of sectorization, it often is hard to distinguish the effects of this process on use of beds from effects stemming from the sectorization of the services.

A number of studies on the transition to a sectorized service have shown changes in utilization rates. Results have been divergent, but generally there has been an increase in total rates of utilization as well as in rates of use of out-patient services (Tischler *et al.*, 1972; Babigian, 1977; NIMH, 1977; Häfner and Klug, 1982; British Psychiatric Register Group, 1984). Concerning bed use, there generally have been reports of a decrease in admissions (Babigian, 1977; Stefansson, 1985; Tyrer *et al.*, 1985; Hansson, 1989), although an increase has also been reported (Holsten and d'Elia, 1984). An initial increase in admissions has been demonstrated (Babigian, 1977; Hansson, 1989). In these instances, it was related to an increased geographical accessibility of out-patient services, and discussed in terms of previously unmet needs for care. Readmissions have been shown to both increase and decrease. The findings are also divergent concerning changes in patterns of clinical characteristics of admitted patients. In some reports, there has been an increase in patients with non-psychotic disorders and in some an increase in patients with psychotic disorders. The point of departure in changing the service system and the specific accessibility and availability of care facilities in the new services seem crucial for the outcome in this respect.

Outcome studies of sectorized services in operation are also scarce. The studies performed have been process studies analysing care utilization data. The increased treated prevalence or incidence of patients in sectorized services has raised the question of utilization of resources when the patient has entered the service system. This has to be studied in individual patient-linked studies of utilization of services or of individual patterns of care. Patterns of care reflect the interaction of features of the psychiatric care organization and the needs and help-seeking behaviour of the patient. The concept of pattern of care has several dimensions such as type of care, setting, intensity and duration of care (Sytema and ten Horn, 1989). The utilization of care may then be weighted, classified and/or categorized, resulting in individual patterns of care or consumption scores.

A review of eight system level studies of psychiatric services investigating utilization of services revealed that none of these studies included outcome measures pertaining to mental health (Hansson and Sandlund, 1992). The results from these studies show that a small proportion of patients use a large proportion of the resources of the services. In some of the studies, social characteristics such as living alone or having no occupation predicted a higher utilization. Only one study reported sex differences, male patients being more common among heavy users. In most of the studies, psychosis predicted higher utilization. A multi-centre study performed by WHO of mental health in pilot study areas (Giel *et al.*, 1987) did not derive generally interpretable and meaningful analyses of the utilization data gathered. Another multi-centre study comparing sectorized services in the Nordic countries showed no uniform patterns of service use in the included comprehensive sectorized services. There was great variation in contact rates as well as in use of services, which were only moderately associated with service characteristics such as rates of bed provision, rates of staff and geographical or procedural accessibility (Saarento, 1996; Sandlund, 1998).

In a review article, Bachrach (1982) stated six major methodological problems concerning studies of community support programmes:

(i)   The goals of the community support programmes were not clearly stated.

(ii) The major outcome measure used was recidivism.

(iii) If other outcome measures were used, they were largely unstandardized and of questionable adequacy (which could be seen in connection with the goal problem).

(iv) Interactive and combined effects of multiple interventions were not studied, which excludes conclusions concerning impact of interventions on a system level.

(v)   Study groups were standardized inadequately with regard to diagnosis, psychopathology, symptomatology, institutional history and other patient characteristics.

(vi) The time frame of the studies was not adequate.

Many of these problems are also valid for research done on the system level.

Research on sectors which also investigates health-related outcomes is still lacking. This is true concerning both studies of the effects of an organizational change and studies of sectorized services in operation. An analysis of the effectiveness of utilization and of specific patterns of care requires measurement of the benefits or outcome of care. Conclusions concerning the optimality of resource allocation and use of services require an analysis of the relationship of costs to the effectiveness and benefits of care. Since no comprehensive studies of utilization have related care patterns to costs or outcome/benefits of care, conclusions concerning efficiency or effectiveness of specific patterns of care for specific groups of patients cannot be made at present. After several decades of this international transitional process, we still lack the basic scientific evidence of the sectorized services efficacy and effectiveness in terms of impact on the mental health status of the target population (Johnson and Thornicroft, 1993).

One study which did investigate the effects of introducing community mental health teams to a whole sector catchment area was the PRiSM Psychosis Study. The aims were to answer three questions: could the gains of experimental studies which have demonstrated benefits arising from treatment by community mental health teams be translated to routine settings? If so, were the benefits diluted in ordinary clinical practice? What were the costs? The study design was a prospective non-randomized controlled trial of two types of community mental health service. The study had two phases: case identification and patient interviews. For the case identification, the research team conducted the complete ascertainment of all prevalent cases of psychosis in the two study catchment areas in the index year in South London.

From all 514 patients with psychotic disorders known from the case identification stage, 302 patients were allocated randomly for interview, along with a key informant clinician and a carer. Interviews were undertaken at two time points. At time 1 (1992–1993 for Nunhead and 1993–1994 for Norwood), in-patient and out-patient services were largely provided to patients at the Maudsley Hospital site. At time 2, which was 2 years after time 1 for each patient included for interview, provision had changed to include a wide range of community-orientated services (Thornicroft *et al.*, 1998a).

The main findings were that: (i) the types of patient gain reported in experimental studies of community mental health services were replicable in ordinary clinical settings, in other words, these forms of community care are somewhat more effective than the hospital-orientated services which they had replaced; (ii) dilution did occur, in other words, these gains were less pronounced than in experimental (efficacy) studies; (iii) both models of clinical service studied produced a pattern of improvements; (iv) there were some limited extra advantages in terms of met needs, improved quality of life and social networks for the more expensive service in the intensive sector; (v) careful scrutiny of possible adverse outcomes did not find any clear evidence that community-orientated services (which included a complement of in-patient beds) failed their patients, their families or the wider public; and (vi) taking into account the more disabled patient population in the intensive sector, on balance, the results weighed very slightly in favour of the two-team model (for acute and continuing care) in terms of clinical effectiveness, but the generic model was almost as effective and was clearly less expensive (Thornicroft *et al.*, 1998b).

Boundaries between primary and secondary care

Considering that primary care services are in contact with the majority of individuals with a mental illness, and the psychiatric services only a minority, issues of integration, co-operation, co-ordination and boundaries between the two become essential. According to the Goldberg–Huxley model (Goldberg and Huxley, 1980), there is a pathway from the community through the GP level in order to access the psychiatric services. The GP is seen as a filter and a gate-keeper to the psychiatric services. Since one of the general aims of sectorization has been to increase the accessibility of psychiatric services, an open referral system with the opportunity of direct access to services has been used in many instances, in contrast to a closed referral system where a medical referral from the GP is required. There have been reports that one result of an increased accessibility has been the inflow of patients with more minor mental illness, while the situation has become more cumbersome for patients with a severe illness, resulting in a greater burden on these patients and their relatives (Braun *et al.*, 1981; Lehman *et al.*, 1982). It has been proposed that a closed referral system to the specialist psychiatric services, to a larger extent, would divert patients with a minor illness to the generalist or primary care level, and that patients with a severe illness would be prioritized within the specialist services (Stefansson *et al.*, 1990). This was not confirmed in a Nordic multi-centre study (Hansson *et al.*, 1995) or in a study by Marriott *et al.* (1993). The latter study concluded that milder cases of mental illness were referred more often from doctors than from other agencies, and that those with more severe mental health problems were largely by-passing the GP. There is no single best solution to this issue. It has rather to be resolved within the framework of the overall model of sectorized services applied in a specific catchment area.

Catchment area size and resource allocation

Establishing the optimal population size of a service catchment area, given a certain allocation of resources, is a complicated issue since the catchment area size is dependent on the specific service functions, factors in the population and factors in the organization of services. The prevalence of mental illness is not distributed uniformly in the population. It has been shown that social and demographic characteristics of the population are related to psychiatric morbidity and to psychiatric admission rates (Thornicroft, 1991; Jarman and Hirsch, 1992). As an example, Jarman developed an index where estimates of social deprivation

have been shown to be correlated to use of psychiatric services. The index includes variables such as elderly alone, people living in one-parent families, unemployed, unskilled workers, housing mobility, immigrants and living in overcrowded households. The age and sex structure of the population is also of importance. Factors of importance with regard to the organization of services are the boundaries and organization of local social services and primary care services together with factors such as the presence of mental hospitals and district general hospitals within the catchment area. Furthermore, services directed towards clients with needs with a low prevalence require a greater population base in order to be feasible and cost-effective.

Looking at it the other way around, the question is what the service demands are for a given population. Of course this is related to what has been said above, but some indications might be given from Table 18.1, adopted from Strathdee and Thornicroft (1992). The table gives ranges of places of different service components, considering the variation of required places due to differences in morbidity, in a catchment area population of 250 000.

Table 18.1 *Provision of inpatient and residential facilities in a catchment area with a population of 250 000*

Type of provision	Range of places needed
24-hour staffed residences	40–150
Day staffed residences	30–120
Acute psychiatric care	50–150
Unstaffed group homes	48–80
Adult placement schemes	0–15
Local secure places	5–10
Respite facilities	0–5
Regional secure unit	1–10

Summary

It is evident from this chapter that sectorization is not an unambiguous and clear-cut concept. It has been blurred with deinstitutionalization and the establishment of community-based care models. Partly due to this, the early optimism concerning the effects of the reorganization of psychiatric services into a sectorized model has not been fulfilled. It has been overlooked that sectorization is an important means and a prerequisite for the development of community-based care, but does not imply anything more specific concerning the structure and content of the service model or content of services. A sectorized service is consistent both with service models using the mental hospital as the main base for services and interventions and with service models depending almost solely on community-based care facilities.

Research on sectorization has targeted mainly intermediate objectives and process characteristics, such as changes in flows of patients at different service levels. Outcome studies on the system level of sectorized services, using health-related or cost-related measures of outcome, are still lacking, and have a high priority. The widespread and long-lasting clinical development and implementation of sectorized services throughout the western world is therefore in great contrast to the lack of scientific evidence for the effectiveness and efficiency of sectorized services. If future decisions and policies are to be based on rational evidence of the effectiveness of sectorization, such studies must be the principal guide for the further development of these services.

References

Babigian, H.M. (1977) The impact of community mental health centers on the utilization of services. *Archives of General Psychiatry*, 34, 385–394.

Bachrach, L. (1977) *Deinstitutionalization: An Analytical Review and Sociological Perspective.* Rockville, MD: National Institute of Mental Health, Division of Biometry and Epidemiology.

Bachrach, L. (1982) Assessment of outcomes in community support programs: results, problems and limitations. *Schizophrenia Bulletin*, 8, 39–60.

Braun, P., Kochansky, G. and Shapiro, R. (1981) Overview: deinstitutionalization of psychiatric patients, a critical review of outcome studies. *American Journal of Psychiatry*, 138, 736–749.

Breakey, W.R. (1996) The rise and fall of the state hospital. In: Breakey, W.R. (ed.), *Integrated Mental Health Services*. New York: Oxford University Press, pp. 15–28.

British Psychiatric Register Group (1984) *Psychiatric Care in 8 Register Areas: Statistics From 8 Psychiatric Case Registers in Great Britain, 1976–1981.* Southampton: British Psychiatric Register Group, Knowle Hospital.

Falloon, I. (1984) Relapse: a reappraisal of assessment of outcome in schizophrenia. *Schizophrenia Bulletin*, 10, 293–299.

Falloon, I. (1987) Evaluation in psychiatry: planning, developing and evaluating community based services for adults. In: Milne, J. (ed.), *Evaluating Mental Health Practice. Methods and Applications.* Beckenham: Croom Helm, pp. 196–238.

Giel, R., Hannibal, J.U., Henderson, H H. and ten Horn, G.H.M.M. (eds) (1987) *Mental Health Services in Pilot Study Areas.* Copenhagen: WHO.

Goldberg, D. and Huxley, P. (1980) *Mental Illness in the Community: The Pathways to Psychiatric Care.* London: Tavistock.

Häfner, H. and an der Heiden, W. (1991) Methodology of evaluative studies in the mental health field. In: Freeeman, H. and Henderson, J. (eds), *Evaluation of Comprehensive Care of the Mentally Ill.* London: Gaskell, pp. 1–23.

Häfner, H. and Klug, J. (1982) First evaluation of the Mannheim community mental health service. *Acta Psychiatrica Scandinavica*, 62 (Suppl. 285), 67–78.

Hansson, L. (1989) Utilization of psychiatric inpatient care. A study of changes related to the introduction of a sectorized care organization. *Acta Psychiatrica Scandinavica*, 79, 571–578.

Hansson, L. and Sandlund, M. (1992) Utilization and patterns of care in comprehensive psychiatric care organizations. A review of studies and some methodological considerations. *Acta Psychiatrica Scandinavica*, 86, 255–261.

Hansson, L., Öiesvold, T., Göstas, G., Kastrup, M., Lönnerberg, O., Saarento, O. and Sandlund, M. (1995) The Nordic Comparative Study on Sectorized Psychiatry. Part I: treated point-prevalence and characteristics of the psychiatric services. *Acta Psychiatrica Scandinavica*, 91, 41–47.

Holsten, F. and d'Elia, G. (1984) Sectorized psychiatry. Some characteristics of patient population after reorganization. *Nordic Journal of Psychiatry*, 38, 603–611.

Huxley, P. (1990). *Effective Community Mental Health Services*. Avebury/Gower, Aldershot.

Jarman, B. and Hirsch, S. (1992) Statistical models to predict district psychiatric morbidity. In: Thornicroft, G., Brewin, C.R. and Wing, J. (eds), *Measuring Mental Health Needs*. London: Gaskell, pp. 62–80.

Johnson, S. and Thornicroft, G. (1993) The sectorisation of psychiatric services in England and Wales. *Social Psychiatry and Psychiatric Epidemiology*, 28, 45–47.

Lehman, A.F., Ward, N.C. and Linn, L.S. (1982) Chronic mental patients: the quality of life issue. *American Journal of Psychiatry*, 139, 1271–1276.

Lindholm, H. (1983) Sectorized psychiatry. A methodological study of the effects of reorganization on patients treated at a mental hospital. *Acta Psychiatrica Scandinavica*, 67 (Suppl. 304).

Marriott, S., Malone, S., Onyett, S. and Tyrer, P. (1993) The consequences of an open referral system to a community mental health service. *Acta Psychiatrica Scandinavica*, 88, 93–97.

National Institute of Mental Health (1977) *Psychiatric Services and the Changing Institutional Scene, 1950–1975*. DHEW Publication no. 77-433. Washington, DC; US Government Printing Office.

Rosenblatt, A. and Mayer, J.E. (1974) The recidivism of mental patients. A review of past studies. *American Journal of Ortopsychiatry*, 44, 697–706.

Saarento, O. (1996) Factors related to treated incidence in psychiatric services and utilization of psychiatric inpatient care. A Nordic comparative study on sectorised psychiatry. Doctoral thesis. Finland: Department of Psychiatry, University of Oulu, Oulu.

Sandlund, M. (1998) A Nordic multicenter study on sectorized psychiatry. Contact rates, accessibility and quality of care. Doctoral thesis. Sweden: Department of Psychiatry, Umeå University, Umeå.

Stefansson, C.G. (1985) A case register as a tool for studies in sectorised psychiatry. Doctoral thesis. Sweden: Department of Social Medicine, Karolinska Institute.

Stefansson, C.G., Cullberg, J. and Steinholtz-Ekecrantz, L. (1990) From community mental health services to specialized psychiatry: the effects of a change in policy on patient acessibility and care utilization. *Acta Psychiatrica Scandinavica*, 82, 157–164.

Strathdee, G. and Thornicroft G. (1992) Community sectors for needs-led mental health services. In: Thornicroft, G., Brewin, C.R. and Wing, J. (eds), *Measuring Mental Health Needs*. London: Gaskell, pp. 140–162.

Sytema, S., Giel, R. and ten Horn, G.H.M.M. (1989) Patterns of care in the field of mental health. Conceptual definitions and research methods. *Acta Psychiatrica Scandinavica*, 79, 1–10.

Tansella, M. (1991) Community-based psychiatry: long-term pattern of care in South Verona. *Psychological Medicine*, Supplement 19.

Thornicroft, G. (1991) Social deprivation and rates of treated mental disorders. *British Journal of Psychiatry*, 158, 475–484.

Thornicroft, G., Strathdee, G., Phelan, M., Holloway, F. *et al.* (1998a) Rationale and design: the PriSM Psychosis Study (1). *British Journal of Psychiatry*, 173, 363–370.

Thornicroft, G., Wykes, T., Holloway, F., Johnson, S. and Szmukler, G. (1998b) From efficacy to effectiveness in community mental health services. PRiSM Psychosis Study 10. *British Journal of Psychiatry*, 173, 423–427.

Tischler, G.L., Henisz, J., Myers, J.K. and Garrsion, V. (1972) Catchmenting and the use of mental health services. *Archives of General Psychiatry*, 27, 389–392.

Turner, A.J. (1979) Readmisson rates to community mental health centers as a measure of programme effectiveness. *Evaluation and the Health Professions*, 1, 20–31.

Tyrer, P., Turner, R. and Johnsson, A. (1989) Integrated hospital and community psychiatric services and use of inpatient beds. *British Medical Journal*, 299, 298–300.

Walsh, D. (1987) Mental health service models in Europe. In: Giel, R., Hannibal, J.U., Henderson, H.H. and ten Horn, G.H.M.M. (eds), *Mental Health Services in Pilot Study Areas*. Copenhagen: WHO, pp. 53–76.

Zohar, M., Hadaz, Z. and Modan, B. (1987) Factors affecting the decision to admit mental patients in a community hospital. *Journal of Nervous and Mental Disease*, 175, 301–305.

Balancing the service elements

Tom Burns

Introduction

This would have been an easy chapter to write 40 years ago. The elements of a mental health service would be readily identified as doctors, nurses, in-patient beds with associated clinical psychologists and occupational therapists. The range of treatments essentially would be restricted to the hospital, and the only controversies would focus on the respective merits of art therapy or industrial placements for the patients. Now the whole remit of mental health services is open for debate and along with it the content and configuration of those services to meet modern demands. Indeed, how much of that remit should be met from statutory mental health services and how much from social services, the voluntary sector, and increasingly from user and carer self-help groups is far from clear.

The recently published *National Service Framework for Mental Health* (Department of Health, 1999) exemplifies this broad approach. It envisages the future configuration of mental health services as encompassing health promotion, housing provision, primary care, etc. Along with the increasing complexity of modern mental health services and the broader remit ascribed to them, there has also developed a wider range of perspectives from which their 'fitness for purpose' can be assessed. While ensuring that effective, evidence-based treatments are offered remains the core measure, a whole range of other parameters have acquired prominence. These include accessibility, cultural sensitivity, flexibility with an increased measure of choice (Department of Health, 1999). There is unlikely to be a simple definitive answer to balancing the service elements or a universally applicable template for an optimal mental health service.

The fundamental aims of a balanced portfolio of services, however, have not moved that much in practice despite this increasing complexity. The priorities of mental health staff are surprisingly similar the world over, and often shine through the rhetoric of service description. They are ethical values, values of the whole society but also incorporated into professions with a century or more of evolving consensus on their roles and purpose. The six standards in the National Service Framework are examples of such values but are probably too non-specific to define or measure the configuration of mental health services. Three more fundamental values stand out as determining priorities:

- A commitment to prioritize those conditions where there is most to gain from treatment and most to be lost if treatment is not forthcoming. Thus, brief, but potentially catastrophic, disorders such as post-partum psychosis or severe depression are accorded an importance that is related to neither their obvious disturbance nor their resource implications.

- A commitment to minimize long-term disability resulting from mental illness and to protect the personal dignity (both within the treatment process and in the wider context) of patients.

- A recognition of the need to protect the public from danger and severe nuisance from those whose mental illness may pose such risks. This is essential both to avoid excessive stigmatization and abuse of the mentally ill and also to secure society's continuing support of mental health services.

A reading of current government pronouncements would include these values but (certainly in the UK) would appear to reverse their order of importance. There is a necessary tension between this narrow, professionally determined, approach to priority setting and the need to encompass a wider societal view. The application of a more structured approach, such as the mental health matrix model (Tansella and Thornicroft, 1998; Thornicroft and Tansella, 1999) has much to recommend it. Identifying and setting out the parameters with which to test a system for its completeness, strengths and weaknesses at national, regional and local levels ensures both a consistency of approach and a comprehensive assessment. It may also alert the planner to potential knock-on effects of service changes. It is not, however, an alternative to making judgements about priorities.

Such judgements often need to be made with imperfect or absent scientific evidence. The evidence base for comparing mental health services is very small indeed. The subject of service evaluation is in its infancy and dogged by overinterpretation of meagre results (Burns *et al.*, 1999a). All too often, conclusions are drawn from head to head comparisons of services where the control service is unknown (Burns and Priebe, 1996) and the stimulus to introduce the experimental service has been a recognition of the inadequacy of local provision. To date, there have been very few studies where only individual elements of the service have been tested so that genuinely causal conclusions can be drawn (Burns *et al.*, 1999a). A further limitation to a consistent, scientific approach to service development is the need to take account of local traditions and expertise. Where a day hospital or rehabilitation service are local jewels in the crown, it is illogical to dismiss the expertise they bring, even at the cost of distorting the balance of service provision.

Judgements around balancing the service elements inevitably are going to be complex and conditional. Issues around the multi-disciplinary team, the balance of generic and specialized provision and the interface with tertiary services are dealt with elsewhere in this volume. What follows is an examination of the dominant themes in such a process of which the most pressing is inevitably that of in-patient care. Although the focus of mental health services has shifted fundamentally from hospital beds to community provision over

the last 40 years, the proportion of spend absorbed by in-patient services has remained stubbornly high at around 80% (Knapp *et al.*, 1990). The difficulty of shifting this spend from beds to community services is cited repeatedly as a major impediment to the development of adequate comprehensive services. The fixed costs of continuing to fund enormous institutions with a shrinking patient population is one driver in this equation. Another is the improvement in staffing on the wards in these hospitals. An examination of the staffing and skill levels in mental hospitals in the 1950s and 1960s makes sobering reading, and it is no surprise that the reduction in patients was not paralleled by a reduction in staff.

The scale of in-patient provision

The argument for reduction in long-stay beds has been essentially won, and few would insist that there should be hospital-based provision for patients with long-term disabilities from mental illness. The studies from the TAPs project in North London (Geddes *et al.*, 1994; Leff *et al.*, 1996a,b) have confirmed the feasibility of cost-effective and high quality reprovision in a range of sheltered living situations for previously long-stay patients. An adequate range of supported and affordable independent accommodation is clearly an essential component of comprehensive mental health services. The nature and extent of such provision will depend on the area served. In many settings, housing associations or the local council can provide accommodation for patients with a range of supports from social services and some input from the mental health services. In inner city areas, health services may staff such accommodation themselves, reflecting the greater degree of disturbance and clinical need of the residents. Hospital hostels are particularly valuable in allowing patients to receive treatment under sections of the Mental Health Act without having to come into the ward. While such health-driven arrangements undoubtedly are effective in managing difficult patients, the benefits of a health and voluntary sector–social services partnership extend beyond the purely financial. Direct responsibility from such services for social care in this group increases their confidence and reduces stigmatization and social marginalization of individuals with enduring mental illnesses. Not all long-term patients can survive in the community, however, and neither the financial nor social cost of striving to keep the most disabled and disruptive out of hospital can be justified (Knapp *et al.*, 1990). The impact of this 'new long-stay' group on service provision is out of proportion to their number, and they are often overlooked. Hirsch (1988) has drawn attention to how short-term studies of 'community-based' services underestimate their impact because of their slow build up, and how only a few such patients can profoundly unbalance careful planning.

Despite these caveats, the move to community care is nearly always associated with a reduction in in-patient bed provision and use. As mental health technologies improve, fewer and fewer treatments require in-patient care. A reduction in beds is therefore to be desired both because it allows resources to be transferred from 'hotel' costs to treatment costs and also because we know that patients do not like being in hospital. They consistently prefer treatment in the community when it is available (Grad and Sainsbury, 1968; Hoult, 1986; Knapp, 1998). A reduction in the number of beds in a service must, however, follow a shift in practice, not vice versa. The Italian approach (Mangen, 1985; Fioritti *et al.*, 1997) exemplified this. A change in provision to reduce the need for admission was introduced 3 years before any reduction in the number of beds was undertaken.

There have been numerous examples in the UK of beds being closed in an attempt to force a change of practice. These usually have been unsuccessful, leading to overoccupancy and inefficient and expensive use of private resources to meet need (Tyrer *et al.*, 1989; Lelliott *et al.*, 1995; Tyrer, 1998). The National Service Framework emphasizes the need to run in-patient services below full occupancy if they are to be efficient. Calculating bed requirements needs some slack incorporated both for safety to cover inevitable fluctuations and to avoid staff burn-out.

Much of the planning directed towards calculating minimum bed requirements draws heavily upon 'alternatives to hospitalization studies'. While there is a wide range of possible service models which have been used (Hoult, 1986; Merson *et al.*, 1992; Burns *et al.*, 1993; Dean *et al.*, 1993; Tyrer *et al.*, 1998), attention has focused increasingly on intensive case management and forms of assertive outreach (Holloway *et al.*, 1995; Marshall *et al.*, 1997; Marshall and Lockwood, 1998; Mueser *et al.*, 1998). Although these studies have produced equivocal findings (in particular the discrepancy between US and European studies), their earlier US results have been regularly interpreted to predict a substantially reduced need for acute in-patient beds.

Where European studies fail to replicate the bed savings of the early US studies, there is often a call for an examination of treatment fidelity (Teague *et al.*, 1995, 1998; Burns *et al.*, 1999b). What seems to be overlooked is the much greater potential variation in the control services—especially since many of the original experimental services were responses to significant failures in local practice. If a reduction in bed numbers is to be planned for in the light of service changes, then detailed local benchmarking may be of much greater value than extrapolation from published studies conducted in very different settings. Such benchmarking requires a careful inventory of local needs and of local resources, both those that support the mental health services (housing, social services day centres, etc.) and those within the mental health services (including the skill-mix of the staff). A particularly revealing study in this context is the comparison between Australian and New Zealand mental health services in the late 1980s where the higher bed usage in New Zealand was associated with having fewer psychiatrists, not having more (Sims, 1991).

A paradox in UK services is the commonly observed lower bed usage when the community team is responsible for in-patient care as well as the outreach (Marks *et al.*, 1994). It could be anticipated that having a team whose full attention was directed at providing home-based or community care should reduce bed need. However, separating in-patient and out-patient responsibility often results in a drift in focus, with energies being directed to less needy patients. This was certainly the experience in US Community Mental Health Centers (Talbott *et al.*, 1987). It also makes effective discharge planning more difficult, introducing delays and carrying significant risks (Appleby *et al.*, 1999). The importance of provision for the 'new long-stay' patients is often overlooked in calculations of in-patient provision.

Out-of-hours services

The importance of out-of-hours services has become increasingly central to much of the debate about resource allocation. User and carer groups have emphasized their relevance to quality of care, and this, allied with research findings from crisis services (Hoult, 1986), has been used to support the value of out-of-hours crisis services to reduce the need for hospital admissions. There can be little doubt that an emergency response is a necessary component of any comprehensive service. The availability of an adequately trained psychiatrist to make an emergency assessment [and an Approved Social Worker (ASW) in the UK] is clearly a minimal standard of care, a safety net. However, is there really any indication for a more extensive 24-hour service? Despite the clearly and eloquently expressed opinions of carers, there is very little such evidence. Where services are fragmented and inadequate, a crisis service does, undoubtedly, meet a need and probably reduces admissions.

The call for 24-hour services, especially where the implication is for an equal service around the clock, could be viewed as evidence of an extreme 'medical model' approach to mental health care. The idea that there is a mental health equivalent of a myocardial infarction or perforated ulcer simply does not withstand scrutiny. Psychiatric crises evolve over days (and indeed weeks) not minutes or hours. Whenever crisis services have been set up, they often soon find themselves redundant (Cooper, 1979). The availability of a mental health assessment within a day or two soon obviates the need for one within an hour or so. There are now several anecdotal reports of crisis services (including my own) establishing good working relationships with primary care such that the need for GPs to 'dress up' referrals as crises soon evaporated. In large metropolitan areas, immediate access to psychiatric assessment is still of paramount importance for the itinerant and the homeless, but this is probably best met through Accident and Emergency departments and the capacity for mental health act assessments.

Local audits of 24-hour telephone lines and assessment within well-functioning services regularly demonstrate low usage. Where day staff are involved in these services, they regularly report dissatisfaction with their work and a sense that they are being used inefficiently. Given that so much of modern mental health practice involves multi-agency work, out-of-hours practice is perforce narrow and limited. Cooper's review (Cooper, 1979) of crisis services (most of which were committed to a 24-hour approach) found that few were still in existence 5 years after their initiation, although it is unclear whether they disbanded because they had reduced the need or whether they were unsustainable. Cullberg (personal communication) has reported that the commitment to a full 24-hour service was one of the principle causes of the unsustainability of the Nacka project.

Clearly a 24-hour service of some form is an essential component of modern mental health care but exemplifies the difficulties of comprehensive plans to balance service components. In many of those services which have reported building their configuration around this provision, its value has shrunk as better integration has been achieved. Indeed, there may be a case for using it to spearhead such integration. A rigid commitment to its provision may lead ultimately to an unbalanced, inefficient service model.

Interface with Accident and Emergency (A&E) departments and social work

Service planners are often overoptimistic when they design mental health provisions. A common feature of this overoptimism is to overlook the importance of A&E. No matter how accessible a mental health service is, a significant number of very needy and complex patients will arrive at A&E. Provision of psychiatric support to A&E is generally less academically interesting to Liaison psychiatrists than that to other hospital departments, and the rapid staff turnover makes adequate support difficult. An identified input to A&E which is provided ungrudgingly is an essential component of service. Its extent will depend on local circumstances—greater in Metropolitan areas where there is poorer primary care and more homelessness and individual mobility.

Similar provision needs to be made for involvement with social services, beyond the issues of care management and social work involvement in community mental health teams (CMHTs). Housing departments and homelessness units often have to deal with some of the most intractable mental health problems, often with patients and families who adamantly refuse referral to mental health services. Only in exceptional circumstances would there be a need for a dedicated independent service, but most need a mechanism for regular communication and support. Such consistent support can be very cost-effective but probably needs to be conducted by a relatively senior or experienced team member. Ethical problems are often severe in this area, especially those around issues of confidentiality, and require careful thought.

Specific homelessness teams, operated jointly with social services, may be a real option in some large city centres. Overall, the benefits of specific 'liaison' teams need to be carefully weighed against the investment of staff time and the risks of fragmentation and information transfer costs.

Day care

An expansion in day care (both day hospitals and day centres) was seen as the alternative to in-patient care in the 1960s and 1970s. The provision of day places lagged significantly behind the closure of beds and has been criticized as one of the failings of community care. It is not clear, however, that current thinking places the same priority on day hospitals. Research into day hospitals is not representative of their practice. Most of the recent published studies relating to day hospitals have focused on their role as alternatives to admission (Hirsch *et al.*, 1979; Creed *et al.*, 1989a,b, 1990), yet the 'acute' day hospital is a rare specimen (Creed *et al.*, 1991). Most day hospitals provide rehabilitation for patients as they are discharged from in-patient wards or provide care and treatment for patients who would otherwise not have been admitted (Burns *et al.*, 1993). They are competing, therefore, with CMHTs and day centres, not beds, for resource allocation. Even where they are attempting to replace in-patient care, simple per diem cost comparisons can be misleading. Day hospitals tend to keep people much longer than in-patient units (Hirsch *et al.*, 1979; Burns *et al.*, 1993), and while the referral process is usually under the control of the CMHT (and occasionally the ward), discharge tends to rest with day hospital staff. Ease of access is crucial for the successful functioning of both day hospitals and day centres. Few patients will change buses to attend for any length of time, so either transport has to be provided or units need to be small and well dispersed.

When balancing the service elements, it is the needs that they meet, not the resource that they replace, that should be considered. Indeed, a recent unpublished study of the closure of a day hospital demonstrated little need that could not be met within a well established service, only half of the patients transferring to the other day hospital in the district.

For day centres, the evidence base is even less available. While there have been some studies of patient characteristics in individual day centres (Brewin *et al.*, 1988; Brugha *et al.*, 1988; Holloway, 1988), a recent Cochrane collaboration survey (Catty *et al.*, 1999) found not a single controlled study of day centres in the care of severe mental illness. Beecham (Beecham *et al.*, 1999) has shown a range of provision of day care by local authorities. The current emphasis on contracting day care out to voluntary bodies may make identification of their service profile even more difficult. Generally, day centres offer structured daily activity over very extended periods to people with long-term disabilities, a high proportion of whom have a psychotic illness. The flexibility of this care is valued by patients, but as yet there is little published work from which estimate the overlap between social services-provided day care and that which should be provided by health care. Anecdotally, it does seem that where there is generous provision of day centres then day hospitals can more easily profile their services and consequently have greater scope for varying their call on local resources.

The importance of day hospitals as 'places to go to', to structure the day and give it meaning may be less pressing when there is adequate day centre provision. The current consideration of differing forms of day hospital (partial hospitalization, clubhouses, etc.) needs to be in the context of the range of treatments offered, and rehabilitative opportunities provided, rather than of containment and support.

Conclusions

The considerations for balancing the elements for planning a community mental health service are potentially endless. This review has emphasized the central significance of in-patient beds and the CMHT. These are the twin pillars without which no system will work effectively. They need to be resourced adequately and well integrated with each other. Overoptimistic expectations that their functions will soon be replaced by highly tailored interventions should be resisted—at least until such interventions have demonstrated sustained reductions in the calls made on routine services. In dispersed rural settings, the availability of specialized interventions may never be a reality. A well resourced, flexible CMHT which manages its own beds with some facility for partial hospitalization or day care from the ward may, then, be the best solution.

Decisions around the extent of day care, rehabilitation and crisis care will depend very much on local circumstances. Some provision for all three is clearly needed, but whether as a function within a generic team (the CMHT social worker acting as duty ASW) or a dedicated and self-contained

service (a rehabilitation or an assertive outreach team) will have to be decided locally by those who know the setting. With current expectations, it would be difficult to consider any local service complete without dedicated resources for long-term sheltered accommodation and some forms of structured day care.

The arrival of a series of external bodies to advise will not remove the need for local decision making about balancing service elements. On the contrary, the range of advice offered both locally and nationally will require an on-going capacity to weigh and apply it. Local leadership will be needed to balance the understandable belief that what works in one place will work in another if carefully transferred. The very need to achieve consistency requires careful attention to implementation.

Difficult decisions have to be made if services are not to be flabby and unfocused. Even worse, if difficult decisions about conflicting priorities are not addressed openly and resolved honestly, then discord and inefficiency can persist. This can take the form of the competing elements of the service striving to 'overperform' in terms of engaging patients to demonstrate the overwhelming need. This is rarely good for patients or staff. Our local experience of having to make savings that resulted in the closure of a day hospital demonstrated that, once the issues were acknowledged honestly, staff could work through their disappointment and then collaborate to find safe and acceptable solutions for the patients. An initial option appraisal (using techniques similar to, but more modest than, those outlined by Thornicroft and Tansella, 1999) established the basis on which the decision could be made. Having established the basis for making the decision, this did not, however, produce a simple, quantifiable 'right answer' acknowledged by all involved. There was still a need for judgement in the final decision. What it did achieve was to remove a sense of arbitrariness or vindictiveness than can otherwise sour working relationships for long periods.

These decisions may be informed by an increasingly sophisticated technology of mental health services evaluation, but they will remain essentially ethical decisions. Balancing the value of day care against rapid response in the night cannot draw on a single, undisputed outcome measure. Expertise, honesty and openness to a wide range of perspectives are still required. Nowhere will these be tested more than in the decisions that have to be made around the care provided for the very small number of patients whose severity of illness and persisting behavioural problems are resistant to current treatments and make them unacceptable to their neighbourhoods.

References

Appleby, L., Shaw, J., Amos, T., McDonnell,R., Harris, C., McCann, K., Kiernan, K., Davis, S., Bickley, H. and Parsons, R. (1999) Suicide within 12 months of contact with mental health services: national clinical survey. *British Medical Journal*, 318, 1235–1239.

Beecham, J., Schneider, J. and Knapp, M. (1999) Survey of day activity settings for people with mental health problems. *Mental Health Research Review*, 6, 18–22.

Brewin, C.R., Wing, J.K., Mangen, S.P., Brugha, T.S., MacCarthy, B. and Lesage, A. (1988) Needs for care among the long-term mentally ill: a report from the Camberwell High Contact Survey. *Psychological Medicine*, 18, 457–468.

Brugha, T.S., Wing, J.K., Brewin, C.R., MacCarthy, B., Mangen, S., Lesage, A. and Mumford, J. (1988) The problems of people in long-term psychiatric day care. An introduction to the Camberwell High Contact Survey. *Psychological Medicine*, 18, 443–456.

Burns, T. and Priebe, S. (1996) Mental health care systems and their characteristics: a proposal. *Acta Psychiatrica Scandinavica*, 94, 381–385.

Burns, T., Raftery, J., Beadsmoore, A., McGuigan, S. and Dickson, M. (1993) A controlled trial of home-based acute psychiatric services. II: treatment patterns and costs. *British Journal of Psychiatry*, 163, 55–61.

Burns, T., Creed, F., Fahy, T., Thompson, S., Tyrer, P. and White, I. (1999a) Intensive versus standard case management for severe psychotic illness: a randomised trial. *Lancet*, 353, 2185–2189.

Burns, T., Fahy, T., Thompson, S., Tyrer, P. and White, I. (1999b) Intensive case management for severe psychotic illness (Authors' reply to letter from McGovern D., Owen A.). *Lancet*, 354, 1384–1386.

Catty, J., Burns, T. and Comas, A. (1999) Day centres for severe mental illness (Protocol for a Cochrane Review). *The Cochrane Library*. Oxford: Update Software

Cooper, J.E. (1979) Crisis admission units and emergency psychiatric services. In: Anonymous, *Public Health in Europe*, No. 2. Copenhagen: WHO.

Creed, F., Anthony, P., Godbert, K. and Huxley, P. (1989a) Treatment of severe psychiatric illness in a day hospital. *British Journal of Psychiatry*, 154, 341–347.

Creed, F., Black, D. and Anthony, P. (1989b) Day-hospital and community treatment for acute psychiatric illness. A critical appraisal. *British Journal of Psychiatry*, 154, 300–310.

Creed, F., Black, D., Anthony, P., Osborn, M., Thomas, P. and Tomenson, B. (1990) Randomised controlled trial of day patient versus inpatient psychiatric treatment. *British Medical Journal*, 300, 1033–1037.

Creed, F., Black, D., Anthony, P., Osborn, M., Thomas, P., Franks, Polley, R., Lancashire, S., Saleem, P. and Tomenson, B. (1991) Randomised controlled trial of day and in-patient psychiatric treatment. 2: comparison of two hospitals. *British Journal of Psychiatry*, 158, 183–189.

Dean, C., Phillips, J., Gadd, E.M., Joseph, M. and England, S. (1993) Comparison of community based service with hospital based service for people with acute, severe psychiatric illness. *British Medical Journal*, 307, 473–476.

Department of Health (1999) *Modern Standards and Service Models: National Service Framework for Mental Health*. London: Department of Health.

Fioritti, A., Lo, R.L. and Melega, V. (1997) Reform said or done? The case of Emilia-Romagna within the Italian psychiatric context. *American Journal of Psychiatry*, 154, 94–98.

Geddes, J., Mercer, G., Frith, C.D., MacMillan, F., Owens, D.G.C. and Johnstone, E.C. (1994) Prediction of outcome following a first episode of schizophrenia: a follow-up study of Northwick Park first episode study subjects. *British Journal of Psychiatry*, 165, 664–668.

Grad, J. and Sainsbury, P. (1968) The effects that patients have on their families in a community care and a control psychiatric service—a two year follow-up. *British Journal of Psychiatry*, 114, 265–278.

Hirsch, S. (1988) Psychiatric *Beds and Resources: Factors Influencing Bed Use and Service Planning*. London: Gaskell (Royal College of Psychiatrists).

Hirsch, S.R., Platt, S., Knights, A. and Weyman, A. (1979) Shortening hospital stay for psychiatric care: effect on patients and their families. *British Medical Journal*, 1, 442–446.

Holloway, F. (1988) Prescribing for the long-term mentally ill. A study of treatment practices. *British Journal of Psychiatry*, 152, 511–515.

Holloway, F., Oliver, N., Collins, E. and Carson, J. (1995) Case management: a critical review of the outcome literature. *European Psychiatry*, 113–128.

Hoult, J. (1986) Community care of the acutely mentally ill. *British Journal of Psychiatry*, 149, 137–144.

Knapp, M. (1998) Making music out of noise—the cost function approach to evaluation. *British Journal of Psychiatry*, 173, 7–11.

Knapp, M., Beecham, J., Anderson, J., Dayson, D., Leff, J., Margolius, O., O'Driscoll, C. and Wills, W. (1990) The TAPS project. 3: predicting the community costs of closing psychiatric hospitals. *British Journal of Psychiatry*, 157, 661–670.

Leff, J., Trieman, N. and Gooch, C. (1996a) Team for the Assessment of Psychiatric Services (TAPS) Project 33: prospective follow-up study of long-stay patients discharged from two psychiatric hospitals. *American Journal of Psychiatry*, 153, 1318–1324.

Leff, J., Dayson, D., Gooch, C., Thornicroft, G. and Wills, W. (1996b) Quality of life of long-stay patients discharged from two psychiatric institutions. *Psychiatric Services*, 47, 62–67.

Lelliott, P., Audini, B. and Darroch, N. (1995) Monitoring inner London mental illness services. *Psychiatric Bulletin*, 19, 276–280.

Mangen, S.P. (1985) Psychiatric policies: development and constraints. In: Mangen, S.P. (ed.), *Mental Health Care in the European Community*. London: Croom Helm.

Marks, I.M., Connolly, J., Muijen, M., Audini, B., McNamee, G. and Lawrence, R.E. (1994) Home-based versus hospital-based care for people with serious mental illness. *British Journal of Psychiatry*, 165, 179–194.

Marshall, M. and Lockwood, A. (1998) Assertive community treatment for people with severe mental disorders (Cochrane Review). *The Cochrane Library* (3): Oxford: Update Software.

Marshall, M., Gray, A., Lockwood, A. and Green, R. (1997) Case management for severe mental disorders. *The Cochrane Collaboration* (2): Oxford: Update Software.

Merson, S., Tyrer, P., Onyett, S., Lack, S., Birkett, P., Lynch, S. and Johnson, T. (1992) Early intervention in psychiatric emergencies: a controlled clinical trial. *Lancet*, 339, 1311–1314.

Mueser, K.T., Bond, G.R., Drake, R.E. and Resnick, S.G. (1998) Models of community care for severe mental illness: a review of research on case management. *Schizophrenia Bulletin*, 24, 37–74.

Sims, A. (1991) Even better services: a psychiatric perspective. *British Medical Journal*, 302, 1061–1063.

Talbott, J.A., Clark, G.H.J., Sharfstein, S.S. and Klein, J. (1987) Issues in developing standards governing psychiatric practice in community mental health centers. *Hospital and Community Psychiatry*, 38, 1198–1202.

Tansella, M. and Thornicroft, G. (1998) A conceptual framework for mental health services: the matrix model. *Psychological Medicine*, 28, 503–508.

Teague, G.B., Drake, R.E. and Ackerson, T.H. (1995) Evaluating use of continuous treatment teams for persons with mental illness and substance abuse. *Psychiatric Services*, 46, 689–695.

Teague, G.B., Bond, G.R. and Drake, R.E. (1998) Program fidelity in assertive community treatment: development and use of a measure. *American Journal of Orthopsychiatry*, 68, 216–232.

Thornicroft, G. and Tansella, M. (1999) *The Mental Health Matrix: A Manual to Improve Services*. Cambridge: Cambridge University Press.

Tyrer, P. (1998) Cost-effective or profligate community psychiatry? *British Journal of Psychiatry*, 172, 1–3.

Tyrer, P., Turner, R. and Johnson, A.L. (1989) Integrated hospital and community psychiatric services and use of inpatient beds. *British Medical Journal*, 299, 298–300.

Tyrer, P., Coid, J., Simmonds, S., Joseph, P. and Marriott, S. (1998) Community mental health team management for those with severe mental illnesses and disordered personality (Cochrane Review). Oxford: The Cochrane Library.

20 | *Generic versus specialist mental health teams*

Tom Burns

Introduction

The last 100 years has witnessed a steady development from generalist to specialist throughout medicine, reflecting an exponential growth of knowledge plus vested professional interests. This pressure is most in chronic diseases, which dominate the clinical challenge in the developed world where the 'epidemiological transition' has occurred (Davis *et al.*, 1999). It is argued that generalists do not provide high quality care for chronic or complex disorders and, in the USA, disease management companies provide separate programmes of care for specific disorders, threatening the continuity of the doctor–patient relationship (Bodenheimer, 1999). Psychiatry, a long established medical specialty (Lewis, 1963), is currently experiencing similar pressures.

The rise of evidence-based medicine (EBM) is a powerful force shaping mental health services. The research advantages of a defined target patient population, with similar problems and relevant outcome measures, favour specialized services. One example is the rapidly expanding literature on Assertive Community Treatment (ACT) teams for psychotic patients (Solomon, 1992; Burns and Santos, 1995; Holloway *et al.*, 1995; Mueser *et al.*, 1998). These replication studies reflect the clarity of definition of the approach and target group. Studies of generic teams (with their broad range of patients) are understandably rarer (Tyrer *et al.*, 1998; Burns *et al.*, 1993a,b), implying less EBM support.

Despite EBM, mental health services organization is highly susceptible to local culture. European psychiatry has strong roots in mental hospitals, and its intellectual base in phenomenology and the treatment of psychoses. The emphasis on severe mental illness in northern Europe has been promoted by extensive development in primary care where most self-limiting and minor disorders are managed. In France and the UK, generic mental health services have been consolidated by the sector movements of the 1960s. An emphasis on providing a comprehensive service for a geographically defined area characterized developments in both countries during this period. Both sought to bring care closer to patients and their families, reflecting strong influences from social psychology and sociology, and both sought to ensure transparency of responsibility and accountability for care. In France, the 'secteur' approach spread slowly from Paris (Kovess *et al.*, 1995) and has been focused almost exclusively upon severe psychotic illnesses. The availability of private psychotherapy by psychiatrists and separate private in-patient facilities (both funded by social security reimbursement), have lifted most minor and short-term disorders out of the 'secteur' provision.

In the UK, sectorized services have become the norm (Johnson and Thornicroft, 1993), serving over 80% of the population. Their establishment can be traced to the 1959 Mental Health Act. This Act required that all hospitals must provide an out-patient clinic. This ensured that an assessment could be obtained without admission, and some rudimentary follow-up provided for discharged patients. It also reduced the isolation and narrow professional perspective common in remote mental hospitals and established a professional expectation that psychiatrists would work in both hospital and community settings. It also required health and local authority social services to work together, authorizing social service spending on mental health. At its simplest, this is manifest in the central role of social workers in initiating compulsory psychiatric care. At a policy level, there are efforts to integrate social services' 'care management' with health services' 'care programme approach' (Department of Health, 1990; Burns, 1997). In day to day practice, many social workers have been integrated into community mental health teams (CMHTs) for several decades, although the degree of integration has varied considerably.

The development of generic mental health teams on both sides of the Atlantic received powerful endorsement from the Therapeutic Community movement of the 1960s and 1970s. This emphasized the social determinants of mental illness stressing the role of relationships in treatment. This focus on the working alliance (Priebe and Gruyters, 1993, 1994), plus the centrality of 'role blurring' in therapeutic community thinking (Rapoport, 1960) together with the need to ensure co-ordinated health and social care for the severely mentally ill, has established the multi-disciplinary team as a central feature of virtually all forms of modern mental health care.

The 'role blurring' and 'democratization' that were so characteristic of therapeutic communities live on in generic multi-disciplinary teams although their original purposes often are obscured. The persistence of role blurring in mental health teams may reflect realistically the state of current therapeutic specificity and sophistication. Democratization (or at least the remarkable level of egalitarianism in teams) deprives hierarchy of its potentially destructive interpersonal impact and recognizes the corrosive influence of stigma and low self-esteem on patients with mental illness.

Whether or not the generic CMHT remains an appropriate form to deliver mental health care will rest on its strengths and weaknesses for the task in hand. Specialized services are also organized as multi-disciplinary teams, though generally with less role blurring. As patient problems can be predicted more accurately (or indeed prescribed), the roles of team members can be defined ahead. The roles of the doctor, nurse and therapist can be highly specified in advance of meeting the individual patient. There is little dispute over the need for such tertiary teams for highly specialized services (e.g. anorexia nervosa) and access is via, not instead of, the generic team.

Current controversy centres on whether 'specialized' teams, defined either by patient characteristics (e.g. 'first break' schizophrenia) or by team activity (e.g. crisis intervention), should replace generic CMHTs, totally or in good measure. This implies the replacement of a patchwork of small teams, each serving a limited and defined population, with a system of two, three or even four teams each with a specific task, all covering one larger area. The commonest format is to separate acute, crisis work from continuing care (Hoult, 1986). This approach, with one team for crisis and short-term interventions and one for community support and rehabilitation, has been recently evaluated extensively and described (Thornicroft *et al.*, 1998).

The research literature is rich in descriptions of the functioning and merits of specialized or experimental teams but is remarkably deficient in descriptions of the standard, generic team so often designated the 'control' service (Burns and Priebe, 1996). Despite considerable consensus on generic team functioning, this has evolved over several decades from clinical experience rather than controlled evaluations. To balance a discussion of the relative merits of the two approaches, the features of a standard, generic CMHT are first summarized.

A typical generic CMHT

Composition

A multi-disciplinary team needs at least three disciplines (Teague *et al.*, 1995a). Psychiatrists and nurses make up the backbone. Without psychiatrists, a team cannot offer a comprehensive mental health assessment or prescribe medicines. Without nurses, it cannot deliver and monitor such care. The administration of maintenance antipsychotics by nurses was a driving force for the development of their community role (Pasamanick *et al.*, 1964).

Clinical Psychology and Occupational Therapy are increasingly regarded as essential. Local practice confirms psychiatrists and nurses as 'core' to CMHT practice, with cross-cover within the same discipline invariably needed. For psychologists and occupational therapists, internal cross-cover by other disciplines is common.

Social workers are not employed by health services, so their integration is variable. Well functioning CMHTs are usually jointly managed with fully integrated social workers. They are located in the CMHT base, but receive professional supervision and management from social work. Their routine work, however, is dictated by the demands of the team, as for other members. This involves both generic activity (assessment and monitoring of clients who they keywork) and discipline-specific tasks, such as care management and statutory mental health legislation tasks. The different responsibilities within social work, the need for note keeping to be integrated with a separate management structure, and the purchaser–provider tension inherent in care management complicates effective integration. The ideological battles of the past are, however, replaced by differing priorities and accountabilities to separate employing organizations.

Boundaries

Probably the most stressful aspect of modern mental health care is establishing thresholds for care and maintaining boundaries for the team's responsibilities. The universal experience of CMHTs, starting with those established by President Kennedy's mental health centres (Talbott *et al.*, 1987), has been of most pressure on their resources from individuals with mild, self-limiting, disorders. Such patients are eloquent in their requests for help and powerfully supported from primary care. They are also rewarding to treat as they recover quickly. The severely mentally ill, on the other hand, are often reluctant to ask for help, require protracted care and are easily ignored. Mental health services can easily drift 'up market' and become overloaded, generating long waiting lists. CMHTs must establish and maintain clinically responsive boundaries,

balancing new patients with discharges. This threshold is not easily prescribed and requires constant negotiations if it is to be consistent.

Assessments

Despite several attempts to define entry criteria to secondary mental health services, none are entirely successful, and a comprehensive clinical assessment remains the only reliable way to ensure that serious illnesses are not missed. CMHTs take their referrals predominantly from GPs. A vogue in the 1980s for self-referrals swamped teams with inappropriate work. Most now require GP referral except for patients well known to the team. Referrals from police, social services or homelessness units are common for patients who are not registered with GPs. The number of referrals varies markedly but in our South-west London service these have averaged around 10 per week (Burns *et al.*, 1993 a,b). Originally all patients were assessed by a psychiatrist, but there is now considerable variation. In some CMHTs, the GP can determine who sees the patient and most include assessments by non-medical staff. Assessments may be conducted jointly and these are often in the patients' homes or GP surgeries (Tyrer *et al.*, 1990; Burns *et al.*, 1993a,b; Strathdee, 1994).

GP liaison

Not all referred patients suffer from a diagnosable mental illness. A significant proportion are referred back to the GP with advice on management. For those accepted for care, a letter is sent to the GP outlining the proposed treatment and delineating the extent of shared care. CMHTs can exploit their restricted population bases to establish regular liaison meetings (Strathdee and Williams, 1984; Burns and Bale, 1997), further facilitated by aligning CMHTs with GP lists (Burns, 1998).

Review process

CMHT patients require periodic review and most teams meet weekly to do this (Burns, 1990). These periodic reviews [regulated through the Care Programme Approach (Department of Health, 1990) in the UK] foster skill sharing and tailor treatment for each patient. They also develop and define the threshold for discharge to primary care and manage and supervise caseloads. A single point of entry for patients to the team consolidates this clinical management process.

Team leadership

Generic CMHTs are often ambivalent about leadership. Most evolve a hierarchy so impasses can be arbitrated, but the form of this hierarchy is often obscure. There is no consensus on the management structure for such teams, with their parallel lines of accountability to health or social services. A tension between team accountability and professional accountability is normal in such teams and rarely leads to dysfunction. Regular team-building days and repeated redrafting of the operational policy is a feature.

The UK has different generic CMHTs for different age groups. Child and adolescent teams care for individuals up to either 16 or 18 years of age, and old age psychiatry from the age of 65 years. In their assessment, review and organizational features, they echo CMHTs for working age adults. They relate to GPs, offer continuity of care and experience substantially the same levels of role blurring and role conflict.

Specialist mental health teams

Specialist mental health teams differ from generic CMHTs in a number of important respects:

- They have clear definitions of their target patient group (based, for example, on diagnosis, age or gender).
- They usually have an explicit range of treatments that they offer (e.g. family therapy, medication regimes) and may exclude patients unable to engage with these interventions.
- Their treatments often are based on research evidence.

- Patients who fail to respond to the offered treatments will usually be discharged to another secondary care system.
- They have a fixed capacity and may only accept patients when there is a vacancy.
- Roles and responsibilities are generally well clarified with minimum role blurring or conflict.
- Training and skill levels within these defined roles are very high.

Most UK specialized teams operate as tertiary services, accepting all, or the bulk of their referrals from CMHTs. They can, therefore, reserve their skills and resources for those patients which CMHTs cannot manage effectively. If a patient does not respond to the specialized treatments offered, there is an agreed exit plan which provides a safety net. It is not always possible (or sensible) to hold rigorously to this division. For example, mother and baby units usually take referrals of post-partum psychoses direct from GPs because of the urgency of the situation but then establish the normal secondary–tertiary relationship with the CMHT for ongoing care. Forensic services receive most of their patients from CMHTs but also a significant proportion from the courts, and then negotiate a secondary–tertiary relationship with the relevant CMHT.

Drug and alcohol teams and some psychotherapy services may operate as either secondary or tertiary services. Depending on local arrangements, different approaches have advantages and disadvantages. Access is improved by direct referrals, but there can be problems of capacity and potential overtreatment if the highly developed skills and time-consuming procedures of such teams are provided for patients whose problems would have responded quickly to brief, economical interventions.

Which specialized teams are *essential* for a district service rather than simply *desirable*, is a vexed question. A Royal College of Psychiatrists (UK) working party on community care identifies three specialized services which are considered *essential* for comprehensive mental health care:

- Rehabilitation services, providing both sheltered accommodation and assertive community treatment
- Forensic services, including medium and minimum secure provision
- Drug and alcohol services, including capacity for dually diagnosed patients with severe mental illness.

In highly dispersed rural services, these specialized functions may have to be provided via specialized staff in CMHTs. They, along with the three generic CMHTs (child and adolescent, adults of working age, old age), are unchallenged as essential components of a comprehensive district service. Depending on need and resources, the following special services are usually available:

- mothers and babies
- eating disorders
- liaison
- psychotherapy.

There are also highly specialized services which are not possible on a district basis but require a regional or national catchment area and often reflect the initiative of specific individuals. These include specialized services for personality disorders, for ethnic minorities, highly specialized in-patient psychotherapy units, challenging behaviour units, services for the pre-lingually deaf and those for young brain-damaged individuals.

Generic versus specialist teams

Specialized team functioning varies according to their target groups and remits, but there are some relatively consistent differences between them and generic teams. These differences should not be exaggerated but provide a framework to examine the balance between specialist and generic teams as *alternative provision*.

- The target population served by a specialist team is determined almost exclusively by that team. Based on its remit and skills, the team will define the patients it will accept. This is in contrast to generic teams where referrers have the major say in the team's practice.
- Therapeutic interventions and component skills are pre-determined to a greater extent. The team will reflect a perceived need for a form of intervention (e.g. cognitive behavioural therapy) or a target group known to require specific skills (e.g. vocational counselling for rehabilitation patients).
- Operational policies are more detailed and prescriptive. There may be a degree of 'manual-led' practice rare in generic CMHTs.
- Skill levels in these interventions are highly developed, often explicitly at the cost of a wider competence.
- Individual skills are identified with specific training. Role definition is greater than with generic CMHTs, with less role conflict and greater clarity over hierarchy and responsibilities.
- The review process is often more predictable, determined by anticipated transitions in treatment (e.g. when an anorexic patient reaches target weight) rather than crises.

These differences suggest that specialized teams are more comfortable to work in, more able to reflect changes in the current evidence base, deliver more consistent treatments and are more easily audited. This contributes to interest in replacing the generic team with a range of such specialized teams. The teams most often proposed are:

- A continuing community support team for patients with long-standing psychotic disorders, usually a modified form of ACT. These teams are multi-disciplinary; have small caseloads (1:10); high contact frequency; manage patients assertively in their own homes; focus on medication compliance, community stabilization and remain involved during hospitalization (Teague *et al.*, 1995a; Stein and Test, 1980; Burns and Guest, 1999).
- Crisis intervention teams are 24-hour mobile teams who deal with the full range of mental health emergencies. They provide immediate,

flexible support including intensive pharma-cotherapy and counselling but for a limited time (Ratna, 1981; Auerbach and Stolberg, 1986; Hoult, 1986; Parad and Parad, 1990; Dean *et al.*, 1993; Joy *et al.*, 1998). Involvement varies from a few days up to about 3–6 weeks. For most psychotic relapses, the crisis intervention team would hand the patient on to the 'standard' team either when the immediate crisis has settled or after at 3 weeks if still unresolved.

- Home nursing teams are much less researched than ACT or crisis intervention, but are valued by users and strongly advocated in recent years (Dean, 1991). They avoid in-patient care by providing round the clock supervision and treatment in the patient's home. They reduce hospitalization but can only treat few patients at a time, are costly and there is no firm evidence of their sustainability. They also hand on to standard services after the immediate high dependency period.

Apart from the ACT or community support team, these teams must refer on to 'standard' service to provide continuity of care. The issue is not, therefore, specialist versus generic teams but to what extent generic teams can be replaced more effectively by these specialist teams. This question cannot be answered in a vacuum—context is crucial. What is appropriate for an inner city area with a high rate of psychosis, homelessness and rootlessness may appear clumsy and unnecessary in a more stable area. It may also be simply impractical in highly dispersed rural areas. North Birmingham currently is evaluating a model which brings together a range of specialist teams to provide a comprehensive service. The service comprises a home treatment team, a continuing care (ACT-like) team, a crisis team and a 'primary care liaison' team (a modified CMHT), all covering the same patch.

Strengths and weaknesses

The strengths of specialized teams in terms of high skilling, predicable treatments, responsiveness to accruing evidence and relative ease of audit and

evaluation have been rehearsed above. Are there any drawbacks, and how can their relative contribution, compared with generic teams, be assessed? Six dimensions of this decision-making process are outlined below.

Cost and efficiency

A publicly funded health service must invest in maximal health gain for its population. Generic teams have evolved within highly accountable, public sector services and, not surprisingly, they appear less expensive than specialist services. This does not necessarily mean that they are better value for money. There is often compelling evidence for increased longer term costs associated with poor or partial treatment. Costing mental health services, however, is not straightforward and does not substitute for value judgements (Knapp and Beecham, 1990). Benefits from one service must be weighed against the opportunity costs of not investing in others (e.g. how is an improvement in the quality of life of a schizophrenia patient to be compared with delay in treating someone with depression?). Cost-effectiveness analysis needs to encompass broader impacts on the system as well as outcomes for a specific service on its target patient group. The era of simple overall, cost savings demonstrated by earlier American ACT services (Weisbrod *et al.*, 1980) is long past (Knapp *et al.*, 1998; Mueser *et al.*, 1998) and cost–benefit decisions are rarely easy or clear cut.

The efficiency of a mental health team is influenced by its liaison with the other essential services (social services, voluntary agencies, housing, primary care, etc.). Good care depends on this liaison being more than just a list of telephone numbers. Personal relationships are needed to assess other agencies. One GP's competence with mental health problems is very different from another's; a voluntary day centre needs to be visited before a patient is referred if disasters are to be avoided. These agencies also need to assess the mental health staff before they will rely on advice. There are only so many relationships one can maintain, and sector teams have the enormous advantage of local knowledge.

Accessibility and accountability

For the patient, family and referrer, a great advantage of the CMHT is its simplicity and accessibility. It is the mental health equivalent of 'one stop shopping'. The GP referral should activate a thorough assessment and an appropriate (if sometimes limited) response to the patient's needs. GP, patient and family know who to approach and the accessibility can be written into service specifications. There can be some confusion (because of role blurring) about responsibility within the team at any given time, but the care programme approach is reducing this. Within the specialist system, accessibility is equally good, but getting there can be long-winded and confusing. There is a real risk of ending up in the wrong service if the CMHT does not 'gate-keep' specialist teams to avoid attendant clinical risks (e.g. a depressed patient waiting several months for a chronic fatigue clinic). There is also a significant risk of loss to care at each referral process (explored further below in '*skills*').

Accountability to the referrer is less in specialist teams, but internal accountability to explicit standards of care is higher. The introduction of clinical governance, by which local clinical practice will be assessed regularly against nationally set standards, should improve the CMHT's accountability for the quality of its care. The accountability of CMHTs to their referrers (especially where the service is sectorized) has helped anchor their practice in the mental health priorities of the local population. This anchoring reduces the tendency to select more attractive, less needy and more easily treated patients, which threatens virtually all mental health services (Talbott *et al.*, 1987). CMHT staff complain that specialist teams exclude the difficult and unrewarding patients who then become their responsibility. There is some substance to this, with little evidence that parallel mental health services (whether in secondary or in primary care) significantly reduce CMHT workload. Resourcing of specialist teams from within a total mental health budget requires careful monitoring of workloads if CMHT staff are not to feel exploited and risk burn-out.

Flexibility

Specialist teams are only slowly responsive to fluctuations in demand—it is not easy to expand or contract the team. The commitment to service provider-determined standards makes it only rarely possible to 'cut corners' to deal with temporary increases in referrals. CMHTs, on the other hand, are extraordinarily flexible. Basic standards for waiting times are agreed with purchasers, so CMHTs must vary the rate of assessments to reflect demand. It is not unusual for this demand and that for beds to vary by up to 100%, and CMHTs must alter work schedules and thresholds accordingly. From the purchaser's and referrer's perspective, this must be one of the major strengths of the generic team. For the patient needing urgent attention, it is equally an advantage, but for the patient currently in treatment this flexibility can only be achieved by compromise around the clinical quality of their care. Variations in the extent and quality of care offered over time, and between areas of differing morbidity, are major problems with generic teams. Many inner city teams can offer little more than a basic psychosis service, whereas most teams are able to offer a broad range of interventions for a variety of mental illnesses.

This flexibility imposes demands that can, at times, seem impossible and are stressful. On the other hand, the sheer variety and unpredictability of the work is often cited as a major attraction of the job. The need to address widely differing problems can be refreshing and rewarding—both by feeling fully stretched and from the life-long learning that comes from such work. Reports of 'burn-out' in CMHTs are rare.

Skills

The acquisition and maintenance of highly developed therapeutic skills and practices are the major reasons for specialist teams. An earlier excessive insistence on generic working, however, has given way in CMHTs to a judicious mix of generic and specific work. Clinical psychologists will keywork a small number of patients but undertake specific psychological treatments for a greater number; a community psychiatric nurse may develop a specific expertise in behavioural family management or vocational placement. Despite this, there is still a significant gap between the levels of expertise generally offered in the two types of teams.

There may be some advantages to the less sophisticated generic approach. Patients prefer relating to fewer staff—even if interventions could be better delivered by other team members. In a study of home-based assessment (Burns *et al.*, 1993a,b), both staff and patients attributed the uni-disciplinary working in the standard care service to a resistance in the individual assessing them to refer patients on for treatment by another member of the team. The assessment process was acknowledged as an emotionally powerful experience, establishing a rapport which they did not want broken. As the average number of contacts per patient in that study was six, the disruption of a repeat assessment could be considerable.

A generic caseload also offers some protection against an overtechnical or impersonal approach and helps staff members maintain a sense of perspective. A narrowly focused, intense involvement with one type of problem can lead to a lack of proportion. Regular exposure to minor and short-lived problems reinforces the human dimension of mental health care (e.g. a referral of a suddenly bereaved woman can sensitize a staff member to losses currently being experienced by one of their patients suffering from chronic schizophrenia).

A research-based service

The fundamental question is whether the advantages of a generic caseload can balance the potential health gain from a specific highly skilled intervention. This question requires a careful evaluation of the evidence for each intervention and not a structural or ideological response. We need health services research which goes beyond evaluation of efficacy to that of effectiveness (Thornicroft *et al.*, 1998). The heterogeneity of generic CMHT practice makes it notoriously difficult to research. The implications of research evidence from specialized services require careful appraisal if the baby is not to be thrown out with the bathwater—demonstrated gains must be

weighed carefully against the disruption to existing services. This interpretation also requires careful attention to the contribution of charismatic leaders and to the exclusion of difficult patients (Coid, 1994). Translation from one setting to another calls for recognition of the differing contexts (Burns and Priebe, 1996).

Roles and structures

The high priority for flexibility in generic teams has fostered a skill-sharing model where most members have to be able to do most things, often at short notice. The result is a rather flattened management structure with few internal boundaries and often an unclear hierarchy. This can be unnecessarily stressful, and extensive role blurring is unlikely to survive. Advances in evidence-based practice means that nobody can adequately acquire the full range of expertise to manage all routine conditions optimally. Role blurring is also threatened by the increasing accountability of mental health services. Generic teams are likely to organize roles and responsibilities in a more transparent and less stressful manner than previously. They have much to learn from specialist services in this regard, but will need to adapt the structures to the more uncertain demands of their work.

Conclusions

Improvements in mental health treatments have become measured in more sophisticated and precise ways. Increasingly precise measurements of health gain as a result of specific treatments will shift the balance between those gains and the benefits of accessibility and flexibility. There are no universal or permanent formulae for such decisions. A proposal to restrict surgery for breast cancer to surgeons who perform a stated minimum of such operations a year will depend not simply on an audit of survival rates. It also needs to be sensitive to the availability of such surgeons, the likely waiting times for care and the impact on surgical capacity of district general hospitals. So it is with the relative contribution of specialist and generic mental health teams.

The comparison in mental health care is complex. 'Patient-based' outcome measures, while vastly superior to what they were 30 years ago, are nowhere near as robust as the survival rates and complication rates used in medical and surgical evaluations. Indeed, there remains as much debate about what to measure as about how best to measure it. Is symptom resolution more important than residual disability? Is quality of life independent of symptom resolution and, if so, which should take precedence, and so on?

Evaluations needed to advance this question are also generally not of treatments, but of systems of care. These currently are poorly described and defined (Burns and Priebe, 1996), and even where they are, there is rarely effective programme fidelity monitoring (Teague *et al.*, 1995b). To compound matters further, there is almost never an equally detailed description, definition or monitoring of content in the control service. Systematic reviews such as those carried out by the Cochrane Collaboration are of limited value in resolving such questions. As most health care service developments and reforms are politically and socially driven rather than evidence led, researchers cannot embargo change until they have defined systems. Control services are likely to change as rapidly as experimental services. Accumulating evidence from sequential studies will still require judgement and interpretation.

Professions may also be increasingly out of step with what patients want. Doctors and researchers focus on the outcomes of treatments, often at the expense of the experience of these treatments. The public portrayal of medicine and the current interests in alternative medicines confirm the value placed on a relationship between a patient and a doctor which is less technical and more holistic. Patients increasingly assert their preference for being treated as unique individuals when they consult a professional, rather than increasing life expectancy by 2% within a remote and complex health care 'industry'.

This is probably most important in mental health care. The severely mentally ill often come to treatment with damaged self-esteem and a history of social marginalization. Core experiences of their illnesses are located in self-understanding and relationships, and most current treatments are dependent on establishing a trusting and respectful relationship (either as the therapeutic tool itself or as the medium for ensuring collaboration with the treatment).

Genericism in mental health care has a double advantage in this respect. Firstly, it protects the patient from feeling they are simply an object, passed from expert to expert. They engage with a skilled individual, explore their problems with that person and negotiate a treatment plan. The very process of mutually defining the problem emphasizes the uniqueness of the patient and their importance and competence in the exchange. Secondly, the range of issues that the staff have to deal with ensures that they are kept in touch with the common human problems that lie at the centre of the experience of most mental illnesses. They are more likely to conceptualize the experience of the illness within the framework of a broadly normal psychology rather than purely of psychopathology and abnormal psychology. In short, they may empathize more readily with patient's problems than a staff member with a highly developed intervention scheme which anticipates the consultation.

It is not possible to rank the importance of these dimensions of evaluation to satisfy all involved parties. Even if it were possible at present, priorities would soon change as treatments and skills evolve. Policy for service delivery must set research evidence in a realistic context. Decisions should follow explicit criteria which may include values and knowledge not obtained through randomized control trials.

Quality mental health care is based on a relationship between at least two individuals (patient and mental health worker) which respects the experiences and knowledge of both. Successful mental health service planning must incorporate the experience of care as much as measures of outcome. There may be life left in generic teams after all.

References

Auerbach, S. and Stolberg, A. (1986) *Crisis Intervention with Children and Families.*, Washington, DC: Hemisphere Publishing.

Bodenheimer, T. (1999) Disease management: promises and pitfalls. *New England Journal of Medicine*, 340, 1202–1205.

Burns, T. (1990) Community ward rounds. *Health Trends*, 22, 62–63.

Burns, T. (1997) Case management, care management and care programming. *British Journal of Psychiatry*, 170, 393–395.

Burns, T. (1998) Inner-city general practice population with schizophrenia. *Psychiatric Bulletin*, 22, 639–642.

Burns, T. and Bale, R. (1997) Establishing a mental health liaison attachment with primary care. *Advances in Psychiatric Treatment*, 3, 219–224.

Burns, T. and Guest, L. (1999) Running an assertive community treatment team. *Advances in Psychiatric Treatment*, in press.

Burns, T. and Priebe, S. (1996) Mental health care systems and their characteristics: a proposal. *Acta Psychiatrica Scandinavica*, 94, 381–385.

Burns, B.J. and Santos, A.B. (1995) Assertive community treatment: an update of randomized trials. *Psychiatric Services*, 46, 669–675.

Burns, T., Beadsmoore, A., Bhat, A.V., Oliver, A. and Mathers, C. (1993a) A controlled trial of home-based acute psychiatric services. I: clinical and social outcome. *British Journal of Psychiatry*, 163, 49–54.

Burns, T., Raftery, J., Beadsmoore, A., McGuigan, S. and Dickson, M. (1993b) A controlled trial of home-based acute psychiatric services. II: treatment patterns and costs. *British Journal of Psychiatry*, 163, 55–61.

Coid, J. (1994) Failure in community care: psychiatry's dilemma. *British Medical Journal*, 308, 805–806.

Davis, R.M., Wagner, E.H. and Groves, T. (1999) Managing chronic disease. *British Medical Journal*, 318, 1090–1091.

Dean, C. (1991) Home treatment for acute psychiatric illness. *Nursing Times*, 87, 47–48.

Dean, C., Phillips, J., Gadd, E.M., Joseph, M. and England, S. (1993) Comparison of community based service with hospital based service for people with acute, severe psychiatric illness. *British Medical Journal*, 307, 473–476.

Department of Health (1990) *The Care Programme Approach for People with a Mental Illness Referred to the Special Psychiatric Services.* London: Department of Health.

Holloway, F., Oliver, N., Collins, E. and Carson, J. (1995) Case management: a critical review of the outcome literature. *European Psychiatry*, 113–128.

Hoult, J. (1986) Community care of the acutely mentally ill. *British Journal of Psychiatry* 149, 137–144.

Johnson, S. and Thornicroft, G. (1993) The sectorisation of psychiatric services in England and Wales. *Social Psychiatry and Psychiatric Epidemiology*, 28, 45–47.

Joy, C.B., Adams, C.E. and Rice, K. (1998) Crisis intervention for severe mental illness. *The Cochrane Library*, in press.

Knapp, M. and Beecham, J. (1990) Costing mental health services. *Psychological Medicine*, 20, 893–908.

Knapp, M., Marks, I., Wolstenholme, J., Beecham, J., Astin, J., Audini, B., Connolly, J. and Watts, V. (1998) Home-based versus hospital-based care for serious mental illness: controlled cost-effectiveness study over four years. *British Journal of Psychiatry*, 172, 506–512.

Kovess, V., Boisguerin, B., Antoine, D. and Reynauld, M. (1995) Has the sectorization of psychiatric services in France really been effective? *Social Psychiatry and Psychiatric Epidemiology*, 30, 132–138.

Lewis, A. (1963) *Medicine and the Affections of the Mind.* London: British Medical Association.

Mueser, K.T., Bond, G.R., Drake, R.E. and Resnick, S.G. (1998) Models of community care for severe mental illness: a review of research on case management. *Schizophrenia Bulletin*, 24, 37–74.

Parad, H.J. and Parad, L.G. (1990) Crisis intervention Book 2. In: Anonymous, *The Practitioner's Source Book for Brief Therapy.* Milwaukee, USA: Family Service America.

Pasamanick, B., Scarpitti, F.R. and Leyton, M. (1964) Home versus hospital care for schizophrenics. *Journal of the American Medical Association*, 187, 177–181.

Priebe, S. and Gruyters, T. (1993) The role of the helping alliance in psychiatric community care. A prospective study. *Journal of Nervous and Mental Disease*, 181, 552–557.

Priebe, S. and Gruyters, T. (1994) Patients' and caregivers' initial assessments of day-hospital treatment and course of symptoms. *Comprehensive Psychiatry*, 35, 234–238.

Rapoport, R.N. (1960) *Community as Doctor.* London: Tavistock.

Ratna, L. (1981) *The Practice of Psychiatric Crisis Intervention.* London: Nabsbury Hospital League of Friends.

Solomon, P. (1992) The efficacy of case management services for severely mentally disabled clients. *Community Mental Health Journal*, 28, 163–180.

Stein, L.I. and Test, M.A. (1980) Alternative to mental hospital treatment. I. Conceptual model, treatment program, and clinical evaluation. *Archives of General Psychiatry*, 37, 392–397.

Strathdee, G. (1994) The GP, the community and shared psychiatric care. *Practitioner*, 238, 751–754.

Strathdee, G. and Williams, P. (1984) A survey of psychiatrists in primary care: the silent growth of a new service. *Journal of the Royal College of General Practitioners*, 34, 615–618.

Talbott, J.A., Clark, G.H.J., Sharfstein, S.S. and Klein, J. (1987) Issues in developing standards governing psychiatric practice in community mental health centers. *Hospital and Community Psychiatry*, 38, 1198–1202.

Teague, G.B., Drake, R.E. and Ackerson, T.H. (1995a) Evaluating implementation of a modified PACT model for people with co-occurring severe mental disorder and substance use disorder. *Hospital and Community Psychiatry*, 46, 689–695.

Teague, G.B., Drake, R.E. and Ackerson, T.H. (1995b) Evaluating use of continuous treatment teams for persons with mental illness and substance abuse. *Psychiatric Services*, 46, 689–695.

Thornicroft, G., Wykes, T., Holloway, F., Johnson, S. and Szmukler, G. (1998) From efficacy to effectiveness in community mental health services. PRiSM Psychosis Study 10. *British Journal of Psychiatry*, 173, 423–427.

Tyrer, P., Ferguson, B. and Wadsworth, J. (1990) Liaison psychiatry in general practice: the comprehensive collaborative model. *Acta Psychiatrica Scandinavica*, 81, 359–363.

Tyrer, P., Coid, J., Simmonds, S., Joseph, P., and Marriott, S. (1998) Community mental health team management for those with severe mental illnesses and disordered personality (Cochrane Review). Oxford: The Cochrane Library.

Weisbrod, B.A., Test, M.A. and Stein, L.I. (1980) Alternative to mental hospital treatment. II. Economic benefit–cost analysis. *Archives of General Psychiatry*, 37, 400–405.

21 | *Training for competence*

Kevin Gournay

Introduction

Mental health services face two fundamental challenges. First, as many have noted (Lewis et al 1997), the evidence base for interventions in mental health care is sparse, to say the least. Secondly, we know very little about how these interventions can be delivered in services. A report by the Clinical Standards Advisory Group (CSAG) Schizophrenia Committee (Department of Health, 1995), for example, demonstrated that this leap from evidence to implementation had not been made by British mental health services. CSAG carried out detailed visits to 11 services across the four countries of the UK and found that effective treatments, such as family interventions and cognitive behaviour therapy, were virtually absent from all of the services studied.

More recently, an even more alarming picture has been painted of our in-patient services by two reports, the first by the Sainsbury Centre (1998) and the second by the Standing Nursing Midwifery Advisory Committee (Department of Health, 1999) (the source of advice on nursing for English Health Ministers). Both of these reports painted a very depressing picture of custodial, rather than therapeutic care and, as in the work by CSAG, the authors noted an absence of evidence-based interventions. This chapter sets out to identify a number of areas in community psychiatry where training should be a priority. In turn, it will examine some of the issues noted above regarding the gap between research evidence and implementation in day to day practice.

Prior to examining these areas in detail, it may be worth reflecting on the specific issues of the workforce and describing some of the professional difficulties, to put the issue of the specific interventions in context.

The workforce

There is no doubt that the nature of all of the professions in mental health care has changed considerably over the past three decades, although the changes in some have been more radical than in others. We have entered an age where multidisciplinary education and training is seen as the optimum approach. However, a comprehensive review of the training for the workforce commissioned by the Sainsbury Centre for Mental Health, *Pulling Together* (Sainsbury Centre, 1997), pointed out that the rhetoric of multi-disciplinarity in education and training has yet to be translated into widespread practice. It is true that there exist one or two exemplary programmes of training at post-registration level which operate a common gate of entry for doctors, nurses, psychologists and for people with no professional background, who are committed to working in mental health care. One of the best examples of this approach is to be seen at Birmingham University. There are similar initiatives at Universities in Sheffield, Middlesex and Manchester. However, these programmes are exceptional, and initial evidence from those involved in the design and delivery of such courses reports implementation difficulties, such as different funding streams for different professions, and a variation in the quality of partnerships between the university provider and the NHS trusts, which send their students.

It is notable that the gap between universities and NHS trusts is often wide in both a geographical and a philosophical sense. As we shall note below, training for competence requires educational programmes to be inextricably linked with service settings, so that relevant skills can be taught, transferred to practice and supervised in an appropriate manner.

Of all of the professions, perhaps the most significant changes in education have occurred in nursing. Project 2000 in England, which set out to transfer all nursing education into universities, has now completed this task, with the final transfers occurring in Northern Ireland in 1998. This move to Higher Education has brought with it a wide range of changes to the education and training of the mental health nursing workforce.

Overall, there has been a great shift of emphasis towards a more theoretical education, and a shift away from an apprenticeship model. The restructuring of courses has led to students being required to undertake an 18-month Common Foundation Programme which, in some universities, will have virtually no mental health content. After this generic nursing preparation, those students who wish to qualify in mental health will then receive 18 months further education, of which only a modest amount will actually be spent in clinical environments. Thus, students qualifying from these programmes will have had much less clinical experience than students who attended the traditional RMN programmes, which trained all psychiatric nurses across the British Isles until the beginning the 1990s.

While Project 2000 programmes will produce academically able graduates with arguably a much wider and deeper knowledge base, there are also major drawbacks. It is true to say that many University departments of nursing are still staffed by mental health lecturers who maintain an anti-psychiatry stance and who themselves have little, if any, current or recent contact with clinical services. A major review of nursing education is being conducted by the United Kingdom Council for Nursing, Midwifery and Health Visiting (UKCC), which is examining these issues both for mental health nursing and for nursing in general. The overwhelming consensus is that we should retrieve those elements of apprenticeship which are so valuable to the training of nurses and balance this practical experience with an appropriate theoretical background.

The problems in the psychiatric training of medical staff were noted in *Pulling Together*. One of the biggest criticisms in the report was of the relatively poor Community Psychiatry content in both basic and higher psychiatric training for doctors. Thus, it was argued in the report, it is still possible to appoint someone to a consultant post whose knowledge and skills of community psychiatry are rudimentary because they may have received the majority of their training in specialities and hospital-based work. One other shortcoming of psychiatric training is the limited access of psychiatrists in training to educational programmes which teach skills in evidence-based interventions. It is certainly true that until very recently there were few psychiatrists who possessed higher level skills in cognitive behaviour therapy or evidence-based family interventions.

However, the picture is changing gradually. The recent experience on courses which have opened their doors to medically qualified staff (e.g. at the Institute of Psychiatry, Sheffield and Manchester) is that psychiatrists seem to greatly value courses which offer them skills training. However, at present, funding arrangements within the NHS are such that there is a separation between medical and non-medical staff, and paying for doctors to attend multi-disciplinary courses is fraught with difficulty.

Clinical psychology is a central component of mental health services. However, it has long been acknowledged that there are great shortages of clinical psychologists in Britain. Recent estimates suggest that the 3000 psychologists on the register of the British Psychological Society who hold a clinical qualification, have a broad array of skills and spread themselves over a wide spectrum of clinical areas (Goldberg and Gournay, 1997). Unfortunately, there is no information regarding the distribution of psychologists within mental health services, but there is very widespread anecdotal evidence that clinical psychology input with the seriously mentally ill is minimal. With regard to social work, outside of their statutory work in relation to the Mental Health Act, there is little evidence that social workers are employed in the use of psychosocial interventions or in other 'therapeutic' roles.

Occupational therapists are a small workforce, but they have a significant impact on people with mental illness. A recent survey (Filson and Kendrick, 1997) showed that community occupational therapists often occupy roles in community mental health teams which overlap considerably with community psychiatric nurses (CPNs). However, as Goldberg and Gournay (1997) note, we do not know how many occupational therapists are employed in mental health services.

Training initiatives in nursing

Any discussion of the contemporary picture of training must take account of the evolution of such programmes. At the end of the 1980s, a census of the then 5000 CPNs in the UK (White, 1990) showed that approximately 40% of CPN's work was located in primary care, and their focus was on populations with anxiety, depression and adjustment disorders. In turn, the survey showed that client-centred counselling was the central therapeutic approach used by CPNs with these populations. Later estimates, derived from this survey, revealed that 80% of patients in the community with schizophrenia received no services whatsoever from a CPN (Department of Health 1994). Without clear direction from central government, CPNs had developed their own methods of working. The net effect of this shift of emphasis by CPNs was that the seriously mentally ill were very often neglected. The results of research conducted between 1988 and 1992 (Gournay and Brooking, 1994, 1995) showed that CPNs' work in primary care was largely ineffective and very expensive. The beginning of the 1990s saw the development of the Thorn Initiative. This was funded by the Sir Jules Thorn Charitable Trust, who wished to facilitate the development of training courses for nurses in research-based interventions in schizophrenia. In turn, the foundation for this training came from courses in family work in schizophrenia (Barrowclough and Tarrier, 1992; Brooker *et al.*, 1994). The Thorn funding enabled the Institute of Psychiatry and the University of Manchester to run three 1-year part-time courses between 1992 and 1995. The programme comprised three core modules of training based on research evidence. These were:

- clinical case management (assertive community treatment)
- psychological interventions
- family interventions for schizophrenia.

Since 1995, the programme has become self-funding and the two original centres at the Institute of Psychiatry and University of Manchester have now spawned a number of similar programmes, set up at other universities in England and Northern Ireland. While there is some variation in the content and form of these programmes, they share a number of common elements. These are:

- a focus on severe and enduring mental illness;
- the use of a biopsychosocial model of mental illness;
- a focus on the evidence base;
- an emphasis on skill acquisition
- the use of structured clinical supervision;
- the use of valid and reliable measures of change;
- the use of a cognitive behavioural model as a broad base for intervention, including the notion of working collaboratively with the patient and their carers;
- multi-disciplinarity, in terms of student intake and teaching.

The first 3 years of the programme were evaluated by two independent research assistants who followed-up the progress of four patients identified by each student at the beginning of their programmes. The evaluation comprised the repeated use of a range of measures of symptoms and social functioning. In the first 3 years, approximately 100 trainees completed the course and their knowledge and skill acquisition were also measured by the evaluation team. Initial findings show positive outcomes for trainees and patients, and the overall results of the study are very likely to mirror earlier reports of the analyses of smaller data sets (Lancashire *et al.*, 1997).

Seven years after Thorn training commenced, the evidence base continues to expand. The three core modules serve as a reasonable basis for training in community interventions and are worth describing in more detail.

Clinical case management (assertive community treatment)

This module focuses on assertive community treatment skills, as broadly defined by the Marshall and Lockwood (1998) Cochrane Review. Thus, students are trained in the use of various assessment protocols so that they can reliably rate symptoms and social function and are also to use standardized measures of need, e.g. the Camberwell Assessment of Need (Phelan *et al.*, 1995). Skills training involves time spent on practical exercises, such as using video tapes of patient interviews to assist students to become more proficient at using valid and reliable measures. In turn, students practise their newly acquired skills in their clinical setting. Students are also taught theory and skills regarding other aspects of clinical case management, including brokering, networking and engagement with other agencies. Considerable attention is also given to team-working and clinical supervision. Obviously the course contains a number of important core case management skills relating to medication. Recent research (e.g. Kemp *et al.*, 1996) has demonstrated the need to use a range of interventions to improve adherence to medication programmes. The core components of medication management training include:

- Education of the student regarding the nature and action of various medications;

- The use of educational methods for patients and carers;

- The use of valid and reliable measures of medication side-effects;

- The use of cognitive behavioural techniques, such as motivational interviewing, to deal with non-compliance.

Psychological interventions

Although it is only recently that cognitive behavioural interventions for schizophrenia have received widespread attention, effective psychological interventions are not at all new in the treatment of schizophrenia. For example, Ayllon and Azrin (1968) used operant conditioning techniques as the basis for the token economies which were so much part of psychiatric rehabilitation in the 1960s and 1970s. Indeed social skills training has been used for many years as a method of tackling the deficits seen in schizophrenia, which either are caused by the illness itself or are consequences of long periods of institutionalization (Brady, 1984). Smith *et al.* (1996) pointed to the fact that there have been a number of randomized controlled trials testifying to the efficacy of this technique. Latterly, there have been a number of specific cognitive behavioural strategies which principally target the distress caused by hallucinations and delusions. Although the cognitive theories regarding schizophrenic thinking are complex, it has to be said that many of the psychological strategies currently used in the management of hallucinations and delusions are simple, and many involve common-sense techniques such as distraction and alternative activities.

Thorn students receive a basic training in the fundamentals of psychological interventions, so that by the end of the course they can use some of the procedures under supervision. The aim of the Thorn Programme is not to develop high level cognitive behavioural practitioners, but to familiarize students with a range of techniques available based on the research literature and to deliver the common procedures with competence. The central elements of training in psychological interventions received by Thorn students are:

- The principles of functional analysis;

- The use of simple behavioural strategies;

- The use of social skills training methods;

- The application of cognitive methods;

- The use of valid and reliable measures of cognitive and behavioural change.

Family interventions for schizophrenia

Initially, as noted above, the Thorn Programme was greatly influenced by the work on training in family interventions (Brooker *et al.*, 1994) and this, in turn, was prompted by the work on expressed emotion (Leff *et al.*, 1982) and more behaviourally based family approaches (Tarrier *et al.*, 1988). Students on the Thorn Programme acquire skills in a number of key areas in family interventions, and these include:

- Assessment methods
- Providing families with education
- Family problem solving
- Family stress management
- Providing families with practical support.

Students attending the Thorn Programme today are expected to carry out a significant amount of work with families during their training, and the important role of the family in caring for people with schizophrenia in the community is emphasized continually throughout the course. In accord with the principle of collaborative working with patients and their families, the Thorn Programme encourages students not only to develop strong relationships with their families, but also to work with the voluntary agencies which support carers, notably the National Schizophrenia Fellowship.

Dual diagnosis

There is a great deal of research which shows that up to 40% of people with schizophrenia in the community may have a drug and alcohol problem (e.g. Menezes *et al.*, 1996). We also know that such populations have higher rates of non-compliance (Bebbington, 1995), stay in hospital for longer periods and have high levels of violent behaviour (Gournay *et al.*, 1997). At the same time, services find increasing difficulty coping with this population, and that there is very little relevant training available We have some evidence from the USA that properly trained and prepared teams may have an impact on this population (Drake *et al.*, 1993; Bartels *et al.*, 1995).

The training that has been developed (e.g. at the University of Wollongong in New South Wales, and at the Institute of Psychiatry in London) focuses on a number of areas including detection, the use of valid and reliable methods of assessment, and interventions based on the motivational interviewing paradigm (Rollnick and Miller, 1995), and emphasizing a non-confrontational approach. Training programmes emphasize the need to target both the serious mental illness and the substance abuse within the *same* service, and also emphasize the need to use engagement strategies, and maintain people within the service network. It is likely that there will be a need to ensure that such training becomes widely available in future.

Training users

One possibility for expanding the workforce may lay in the training of user case manager aides. In the USA, there have been training initiatives for many years with case manager aides, who themselves have had a mental health problem. The first programme began in Denver, Colorado, and an evaluation of this programme was first reported by Sherman and Porter (1991). The Denver training consists of a comprehensive programme, which includes an initial analysis of the prospective students' learning needs, and then a year long part-time course which includes both theory and skills, but with a great emphasis on working within community mental health teams. Students are provided with a range of knowledge ranging from models of mental illness, to drug treatments and legal aspects. The experience from Denver has shown that one of the major difficulties in setting up user case management aide programmes is resistance from other mental health workers. The Denver Programme deals with this by preparation of the team, and careful thought to the allocation of the user case manager aide to a suitable worker who then acts as a mentor. The Sherman and Porter evaluation shows that user case management aides enhance the benefits of the service given to clients, and at the same time their own health status is improved. There seems to be little evidence that the work causes unacceptable levels of stress or burn-out, and, provided that the initiative is planned properly and sustained with supervision, it has many advantages. These projects are now beginning to develop outside of the USA, and in the UK.

Nurse behaviour therapy

CPNs have, in the last decade, refocused their efforts on those with serious mental illnesses in Britain. However, it seems likely that the growing influence of primary care on mental health services will again emphasize more common mental health disorders. Nevertheless, as Goldberg and Gournay (1997) have pointed out, these conditions are so common in the community that only a proportion of those who need treatment will receive it. Indeed, the problem is complicated by other factors. For example, some severe neurotic conditions will remit without professional treatment, and many of the conditions which do persist and cause considerable handicap will respond in a very variable way to both drug treatment and psychological interventions.

Goldberg and Gournay (1997) have proposed a matrix for deciding where the interventions of the workforce should be targeted. This decision matrix takes into account diagnosis, handicap caused, evidence for efficacy of various drug and non-drug treatments, and likelihood of spontaneous remission. For such a matrix to be of use, we are in need of a workforce with skills in the use of effective interventions. However, the recognition of this need occurred long ago. At the beginning of the 1970s, Professor Isaac Marks at the Institute of Psychiatry recognized that the evolving effective behavioural therapies for neurosis could not be delivered by the existing workforce of clinical psychologists and psychiatrists, who were interested in psychological interventions, and concluded that a more numerous workforce was necessary. He piloted a 3-year full-time training for nurses in behavioural psychotherapy, targeting a number of core conditions (e.g. agoraphobia, obsessive–compulsive disorder, specific phobias, habit disorders) which were known to be responsive to behavioural methods. These conditions were also notoriously treatment-resistant to other methods, and had very low rates of spontaneous remission. Marks showed conclusively (Marks *et al.*, 1977; Marks, 1985) that nurses could be trained to deliver such treatment. Since 1975, the Nurse Therapy Programme has run as an 18-month full-time training and, for the whole

of that 25-year period, courses have been run at the Maudsley Hospital, training approximately 12 nurses in every 18-month, full-time course.

There have been several other nurse behavioural therapist training centres set up across the UK, and by 1998 a survey conducted by Gournay *et al.* (2000) showed that there are approximately 200 nurse therapists working in the NHS. This survey, and previous work (Newell and Gournay, 1994) showed that psychologists complete treatment on approximately 50 000 patients a year. Therefore, between nurses and psychologists with cognitive behavioural training, something approaching 65 000 patients a year receive evidence-based cognitive behavioural treatment for neurotic disorders. One needs to put this figure of 65 000 into the context of the very high prevalence rates of neurotic disorders. For example, based on epidemiological evidence (e.g. Marks, 1987), the point prevalence of panic disorder with agoraphobia is approximately 300 000 in the UK. In turn, there will be similar numbers of people with obsessive–compulsive disorder, and literally many times that number with depressive illnesses, post-traumatic stress disorder, social phobias, and so on. This, therefore, leaves the NHS with a considerable problem. The training provided to small numbers of nurses and only slightly larger numbers of clinical psychologists needs to be extended dramatically.

The growing efficacy of computer-assisted methods of treatment (Marks *et al.*, 1998) may provide some additional treatment resource. However, there is also a need to consider whether more brief training in cognitive behavioural methods for more numerous groups, such as CPNs, practice nurses and lay counsellors, is necessary. To put the problem into context, there currently are 57 000 nurses in the UK with a mental health qualification, but probably only 8000 of these work as CPNs (Brooker and White, 1998). In turn, there are approximately 25 000 nurses employed as practice nurses, who, *de facto*, carry out many mental health tasks without adequate training (Gray *et al.*, 1999). It is clear that, while the rhetoric of evidence-based interventions is to be welcomed, there are clearly many problems with increasing the capacity to deliver these interventions equitably across the country.

Fidelity to training

Given the huge amount of money spent on training, there is only a minute amount of work which has actually followed-up mental health professionals who have received training, and examined their work later. Kavannagh and colleagues (1993) followed up a group of mental health professionals who had received family intervention training in New South Wales. They found that in the period after training, graduates of the programme either carried out very little of the interventions in which they were trained, or were using the interventions in an altered way. Such research obviously needs to be replicated in training programmes such as that of Thorn. However, various Thorn training sites have provided a great deal of anecdotal evidence that some graduates of the programme return to their services, and fail to apply the model with which they were trained. The reasons for this include difficulties with continuing supervision, workload problems or quite simply that the service to which these workers return has a model of service delivery which is incompatible with the graduate using their newly acquired skills.

Future research on new interventions needs to include follow-up of trainees after completion of training. The only other area where such work has been carried out in any detail is within nurse behaviour therapy, and there are now three studies (Brooker and Brown, 1986; Newell and Gournay, 1994; Gournay *et al.*, 2000) which have followed up all nurse therapy course completers from the beginning of the training in 1972. Although there is a need to approach the findings of these surveys with caution, as they consist entirely of self-report, the results are encouraging, Overall, the surveys show that, even many years after training, a majority of course graduates continue working with the populations targeted during their training, and continue using a range of evidence-based interventions. In turn, course graduates report continuing to use outcome measures routinely as part of clinical practice.

Staff morale

Are community mental health teams sustainable? Is their viability susceptible to diminishing morale and increasing 'burn-out' among mental health staff (Dedman *et al.*, 1994; Connolly *et al.*, 1996)? Such teams entail new staff roles and responsibilities in multi-disciplinary teams. Relatively new professions such as community psychiatric nursing have developed.

Carson *et al.* (1995) have found high levels of 'emotional exhaustion' in CPNs, and also moderate levels of 'depersonalization' alongside high levels of personal accomplishment. Compared with in-patient nurses, community mental health nurses had worse psychological health (GHQ; Goldberg and Williams, 1988), but better job satisfaction and less 'depersonalization'. Onyett *et al.* (1997) also reported high levels of emotional exhaustion in members of CMHTs, once more accompanied by high levels of job satisfaction and personal accomplishment .

A study in South London suggested that reported stress due to work overload was particularly common in the community, and was associated with emotional exhaustion and worse mental health (Prosser *et al.*, 1997, 1999). Qualitative methods were used with a purposive sample of 30 mental health staff selected to include junior and senior members of each profession in both hospital and community settings. For most, contact with colleagues was a major reward of the job. There was little evidence of conflict or difficulties defining roles between disciplines, except for the social workers, for whom difficulty in defining roles in relation to other professions was a major issue. Stresses differed between community and hospital. Community staff tended to find their contacts with patients rewarding, but they also felt burdened by a sense of responsibility for their clients' well-being and behaviour. Ward staff, on the other hand, identified as major drawbacks a lack of autonomy, responsibility and scope for developing an independent therapeutic role. They felt demoralized by 'revolving door' patients and by violence and the need to restrain patients (Reid *et al.*, 1999a).

Informal contacts with colleagues were the most common means of coping with the demanding aspects of work in both hospital and community settings, closely followed by time management techniques. The main formal sources of support described by staff were individual supervision and staff support groups. Accounts of the former were generally positive, but opinions varied about the value of staff support groups. Most believed that further training would improve their jobs. For community mental health staff, the main training gaps identified were skills in specific clinical interventions, whilst ward staff identified the need for further skills in diffusing potentially violent situations (Reid *et al.*, 1999b). There is as yet insufficient evidence available about how far training mediates or reduces levels of stress and burn-out experienced by staff.

Future directions

In the UK, there are two major government initiatives which indicate the way forward. The first is the National Service Framework for Mental Health, which aims to secure equity of access to effective interventions for people with mental health problems. The second initiative, the National Institute for Clinical Excellence, emphasizes the need to improve standards in health care delivery, by defining both effective treatments and models of delivery. Many reports, such as that of the Clinical Standards Advisory Group in Schizophrenia (Department of Health 1995), emphasize the patchy distribution of mental health services and the poor availability of evidence-based approaches. Training is one of the keys to the solutions to these problems. There has already been some work to identify core competencies for the training of mental health professionals (Sainsbury Centre, 1997). The conclusions of this review include increased multi-disciplinarity of approach, training in teams and training methods which are relevant to service location. This means that we have to shift from the position where training is delivered in University Departments (which are often many miles from

the service setting), by lecturers who are largely out of touch with day to day clinical practice. There is also a need for governments to invest relatively heavily to ensure that there is an adequate infrastructure not only to prepare the workforce but also to ensure that skills are updated and refreshed continually.

Finally, until now, good quality research on training which examines patient outcomes and skill and knowledge acquisition in trainees has not existed. Given that, worldwide, we spend many hundreds of millions of pounds training mental health workforces, this is an omission which must be rectified.

References

Ayllon, T. and Azrin, N. (1968) *The Token Economy: A Motivational System for Therapy and Rehabilitation*. New York: Appleton-Century-Crofts.

Barrowclough, C. and Tarrier, N (1992) *Families of Schizophrenic Patients: Cognitive Behavioural Interventions*. London: Chapman and Hall.

Bartels, S., Drake, R. and Wallach, M. (1995) Long term course of substance use disorder among patients with severe mental illness. *Psychiatric Services*, 46, 248–251.

Bebbington, P. (1995) The content and context of compliance. *International Clinical Psychopharmacology*, 9, 41–50.

Brady, J. (1984) Social skills training for psychiatric patients. I: concepts, methods and clinical results. *American Journal of Psychiatry*, 141, 333–340.

Brooker, C. and Brown, M. (1986) Survey of nurse therapists. In Brooking, J. (ed.), *Readings in Psychiatric Nursing Research*. London: John Wiley, pp. 177–194.

Brooker, C. and White, E. (1998) *Fourth Quinquennial Survey of CPN's in England and Wales*. Manchester: University of Manchester: Department of Nursing Monograph.

Brooker, C., Faloon, I., Butterworth, A. *et al.* (1994) The outcome of training community psychiatric nurses to deliver psychosocial interventions. *British Journal of Psychiatry*, 165, 222–230.

Carson, J., Fagin, L. and Ritter, S. (1995) *Stress and Coping in Mental Health Nursing*. London: Chapman Hall.

Dedman, P. (1993) Home treatment for acute psychiatric disorder. *British Medical Journal*, 306, 1359–1360

Department of Health (1994) *Working in Partnership: A Review of Mental Health Nursing.* London: HMSO.

Department of Health (1995) *Clinical Standards Advisory Group: Schizophrenia.* London: HMSO.

Department of Health (1999) *Addressing Acute Concerns.* Report of the Standing Nursing Midwifery Advisory Committee. London: Department of Health.

Drake, R. and Noordsy, D. (1994) Case management for people with co-existing severe mental disorder and substance abuse disorder. *Psychiatric Annals*, 24, 427–431.

Filson, P. and Kendrick, T. (1997) Survey of roles of community psychiatric nurses and occupational therapists. *Psychiatric Bulletin*, 1, 70–73.

Goldberg, D. and Gournay, K. (1997) *The GP, the Psychiatrist and the Burden of Mental Health Care. Maudsley Discussion Paper.* London: Institute of Psychiatry/Maudsley Hospital Publications.

Gournay, K. and Brooking, J. (1994) Community psychiatric nurses in primary health care. *British Journal of Psychiatry*, 165, 231–238.

Gournay, K. and Brooking, J. (1995) The community psychiatric nurse in primary care: an economic analysis. *Journal of Advanced Nursing*, 22, 769–778.

Gournay, K., Sandford, T., Johnson, S. and Thornicroft, G. (1997) Dual diagnosis of severe mental health problems. *Journal of Psychiatric and Mental Health Nursing*, 4, 89–95.

Gournay, K., Denford, L., Parr, A.M. and Newell, R. (2000) Nursing in behavioural psychotherapy: a 25 year follow up. *Journal of Advanced Nursing*, 32(2), 343–351.

Gray, R., Parr, A.M., Plummer S. *et al.* (1999) A national survey of practice nurses' involvement in mental health. *Journal of Advanced Nursing*, 30, 901–906.

Kavannagh, D., Clark, D. Piatkowska, O. *et al.* (1993) Application of cognitive behavioural family interventions for schizophrenia: what can the matter be? *Australian Psychologist*, 28, 1–8.

Kemp, R., Hayward, P., Applewhaite, G. *et al.* (1996) Compliance therapy and psychotic patients: a randomised controlled trial. *British Medical Journal*, 312, 345–349.

Lancashire, S., Haddock, J. and Tarrier, N. (1997) Effects of training in psychological interventions for community psychiatric nurses in England. *Psychiatric Services*, 48, 39–41.

Leff, J., Kuipers, L., Berkowitz, R. *et al.* (1982) A controlled trial of intervention in the families of schizophrenic patients. *British Journal of Psychiatry*, 141, 121–134.

Lewis, G., Churchill, R. and Hotopf, M. (1997) Editorial: systematic reviews and meta-analysis. *Psychological Medicine*, 27, 3–7.

Marks, I. (1985) *Nurse Therapists in Primary Care.* London: RCN Publications.

Marks, I. (1987) *Fears, Phobias and Rituals.* Oxford: Oxford Medical.

Marks, I., Connolly, J., Hallam, R. and Phillpott, R. (1977) *Nursing in Behavioural Psychotherapy.* London: RCN Publications.

Marks I., Baer L., Greist J. *et al.* (1998) Home self-assessment of obsessive compulsive disorder—use of a manual and a computer conducted telephone interview: two UK–US studies. *British Journal of Psychiatry*, 172, 406–412.

Marshall, M. and Lockwood, A. (1998) *Assertive Community Treatment for People with Severe Mental Disorders.* London: The Cochrane Library, British Medical Journal Publications.

Menezes, P.R, Johnson, S., Thornicroft, G. *et al.* (1996) Drug and alcohol problems among people with severe mental illnesses in south London. *British Journal of Psychiatry*, 168, 612–619.

Newell, R. and Gournay, K. (1994) British nurses in behavioural psychotherapy: a twenty year follow up. *Journal of Advanced Nursing*, 20, 53–60.

Onyett, S., Pillenger, T. and Muijen, M. (1997) Job satisfaction and burnout among community mental health teams. *Journal of Mental Health*, 6, 55–66.

Phelan, M., Slade, M., Thornicroft, G. *et al.* (1995) The Camberwell assessment of need. *British Journal of Psychiatry*, 167, 589–595.

Prosser, D., Johnson, S., Kuipers, E., Szmukler, G., Bebbington, P. and Thornicroft, G. (1997) Perceived sources of work stress and satisfaction amongst hospital and community mental health staff, and their relation to mental health, burnout and job satisfaction. *Journal of Psychosomatic Research*, 43, 51–59.

Prosser, D., Johnson, S., Kuipers, E., Dunn, G., Szmukler, G., Reid, Y., Bebbington, P. and Thornicroft, G. (1999) Mental health, 'burnout' and job satisfaction in a longitudinal study of mental health staff. *Social Psychiatry and Psychiatric Epidemiology*, 34, 295–300.

Reid, Y., Johnson, S., Morant, N., Kuipers, E., Szmukler, G., Thornicroft G., Bebbington, P. and Prosser, D. (1999a) Explanations for stress and satisfaction in mental health professionals: a qualitative study. *Social Psychiatry and Psychiatric Epidemiology*, 34, 301–308.

Reid, Y., Johnson, S., Morant, N., Kuipers, E., Szmukler, G., Bebbington, P., Thornicroft, G. and Prosser, D. (1999b) Improving support for mental health staff; a qualitative study. *Social Psychiatry and Psychiatric Epidemiology*, 34, 309–315.

Rollnick, S. and Miller, N. (1995) What is motivational interviewing? *Behavioural and Cognitive Psychotherapy*, 23, 325–334.

Sainsbury Centre for Mental Health (1997) *Pulling Together*. London: Sainsbury Centre Publications.

Sainsbury Centre for Mental Health (1998) *Acute Problems*. London: Sainsbury Centre Publications.

Sherman, P. and Porter, R. (1991) Mental health consumers as case manager aides. *Hospital and Community Psychiatry*, 42, 494–498.

Smith, T., Bellack, A. and Liberman, R. (1996) Social skills training for schizophrenia: review and future directions. *Clinical Psychology Review*, 16, 599–617.

Tarrier, N., Barrowclough, C., Vaughn, C. *et al.* (1988) The community management of schizophrenia: a controlled trial of a behavioural intervention with families to reduce relapse. *British Journal of Psychiatry*, 153, 532–542.

White, E. (1990) *Third Quinquennial Survey of Community Psychiatric Nurses in the United Kingdom*. Manchester: University of Manchester, Department of Nursing, Monograph.

22 | *Case management and assertive community treatment*

Jack E. Scott and Anthony F. Lehman

Introduction

With the advent of deinstitutionalization during the 1950s, care for persons with severe mental illnesses (SMI) has shifted increasingly to community settings. While this change has conferred some important benefits, it has also revealed some critical problems in the organization and delivery of community services. Adequate resources to fund and support needed levels of care have not followed this shift to the extent necessary to meet demand. At the same time, individuals with SMI require a variety of treatment, rehabilitation and support services to function in the community. Typically these services are provided by different agencies operating from several service delivery systems (e.g. medical, mental health, substance abuse, social services, housing and vocational rehabilitation), each with its own set of contact persons, eligibility requirements, and rules and procedures. A mechanism is needed to integrate and co-ordinate this care. In the absence of natural mechanisms for navigating across these systems, persons with SMI typically did not obtain or maintain the services they needed. This reflected both the complexity of these service delivery systems and the inability of many persons with SMI to assume responsibility for initiating and co-ordinating their own care within these systems. As a result, they tended to use services only during emergencies, leading to patterns of service use that were crisis-oriented, highly costly and lacking in follow-up and transition to regular, ongoing community-based care. Often these individuals cycled rapidly between an absence of care within the community, different psychiatric emergency services, in-patient psychiatric hospital units and a return to the community without provision for aftercare.

During the 1970s, two organizational mechanisms evolved to address these problems. *Case management* emerged as one means for helping clients to access and co-ordinate services across different service delivery systems. Orwin *et al.* (1994, p. 154) noted that a common theme underlying various models of case management is the "... provision for some greater continuity of care through periodic contact between the case manager(s) and the client that produce greater (or longer) coordination and brokerage of services than the client could be expected to obtain without case management." Several different models have been developed, and we describe some of these later in this chapter.

A second mechanism emerging during the 1970s was *assertive community treatment* (ACT). First developed at the Mendota State Hospital in Madison, Wisconsin as the *Training in Community Living* (TCL) model by Leonard Stein, Mary Ann Test and their colleagues, the model later came to be known as the *Program of Assertive Community Treatment* (PACT) or, more generally, ACT (the latter designation will be used in this chapter). ACT was developed originally to provide the service integration of a 'hospital without walls' for newly discharged individuals with SMI who were at high risk for repeated rehospitalization. ACT achieves integration of services through the direct provision of various treatment, rehabilitation and support services by a multi-disciplinary team of providers that is available 24 hours per day for an indefinite period of time. Olfson (1990) defines ACT as a set of interventions based upon direct assistance to persons with SMI, instruction in basic living skills and social support.

Both interventions have become mainstays in the community-based care of persons with SMI. Moreover, both interventions are now being applied more broadly to other special populations, such as persons who are homeless (Burns and Santos, 1995; Meisler *et al.*, 1998), individuals with co-occurring mental illnesses and substance use disorders (Drake *et al.*, 1998), and those involved with the criminal justice system (Scarpitti *et al.*, 1994; Solomon and Draine, 1995). In this chapter, we discuss various models of case management and ACT, and present a brief summary of research on the impact of case management and ACT on several kinds of outcome domains.

Defining case management and assertive community treatment

Case management

Bachrach (1993) has noted the absence of a consensus about the definition of case management in the care of long-term mentally ill patients. This confusion partially reflects different usages of the phrase in the public and private mental health sectors. In the public mental health sector, case management traditionally has been concerned with promoting access to and continuity of community-based care to persons with SMI and other underserved populations (Sledge *et al.*, 1995). On the other hand, in the private sector, case management has often been viewed as a mechanism for utilization review and for limiting access to scarce and more costly resources. With the advent of managed care, case managers must now find ways to integrate both of these functions (Dixon and Scott, 1997). Definitional confusion can also arise when treatment and rehabilitation services are provided directly by the case manager, as in some of the models to be discussed below.

Case management models traditionally have included at least five core functions (assessment, planning, advocacy, linkage and monitoring) (Scott and Dixon, 1995). Different models combine these functions in different ways; two examples are brokered models and intensive case management models.

Brokered (or generalist) models

One of the first models to emerge in the mental health field, the *brokered* (sometimes called *generalist*) model is very similar to social casework. A non-clinician case manager (often someone with a bachelor's degree in the human services) does not provide direct treatment or rehabilitation services herself. Rather, the case manager works with clients to identify unmet clinical and social service needs, develops a treatment plan, refers clients to appropriate community agencies, advocates on a client's behalf and monitors receipt of services to ensure that linkage has occurred (Intagliata, 1982). Typically, caseloads in this model tend to be larger than other models (e.g. 1:40 clients or more). The generalist model has four basic service objectives: continuity of care, accessibility of services, accountability and efficiency. Dixon and Scott (1997) observe that the generalist model can only be as effective as the surrounding service delivery system; if needed services are not available, case managers operating from this model cannot access services that do not exist. This problem has emerged in some of the evaluations of this approach, in which the service-richness (or poorness) of the community services is confounded with the effectiveness of the case management.

Intensive case management models

As the needs of individuals with SMI in the community became better understood, some case management programmes began to include the direct provision of clinical services, assertive outreach and *in vivo* provision of services to clients in their homes and other settings within the community. As these additional activities were added to the traditional generalist model, caseloads were reduced in size to provide more time for the provision of these services (e.g. 1:10–1:20 clients), and the types of providers delivering these services shifted to those with greater clinical training, now working as part of a team of clinical professionals. These intensive case management programmes often include components common to ACT (see below), and it can be difficult at times to discern clear differences between them. One difference which applies to many intensive case management programmes is that they tend to utilize individual caseloads in contrast to the shared caseloads found in ACT multi-disciplinary teams (Mueser *et al.*, 1998).

Within the overall category of intensive case management are several subtypes that differ somewhat in terms of theoretical rationales and values. *Social network case management* (Bebout, 1993), for example, attempts to improve and expand the client's social network as a major resource for providing the client with social, material and emotional support. By strengthening the willingness and capacity of others to cope with and support the client, the social network model seeks to adapt the social environment to compensate for the client's disability while helping the client gain mastery and independence. The *rehabilitation model* (Anthony *et al.*, 1993) emphasizes the learning of skills and development of appropriate environmental supports to compensate for the illness. The *personal strengths* model (Rapp, 1993) focuses on the client's personal strengths and preferences to help the client achieve the goals and objectives he or she views as important. Like other intensive case management models, the personal strengths model includes assertive outreach and frequent contact but, unlike many intensive case management programmes, the personal strengths model is meant to be independent of (and in addition to) the provision of mental health services.

While these descriptions represent 'pure' models of case management, in practice case management programmes may look more alike than these models suggest. In a national survey of 323 programmes in 1991, Ellison *et al.* (1995) at the Center for Psychiatric Rehabilitation reported that the primary mission of most programmes was stated as 'preventing hospitalization', followed by 'improving quality of/satisfaction with life'. Ellison and her colleagues note that in practice, case management programmes tend toward an 'ideal type' in terms of functions (keeping clients in the community, minimizing hospital costs, promoting cost efficiency) and programme focus (assessing client needs, planning, linking and monitoring client services; focusing on practical problems of daily living and using a multi-disciplinary

team approach). Most programmes did not identify with a specific theoretical model. While these data reflect a period just before the greatest impact of managed mental health care, it nonetheless is worth noting that case management programmes appeared to be converging toward some level of 'more or less' intensive case management.

Assertive community treatment (ACT)

As noted earlier, ACT represents a change in how mental health, substance abuse and supportive services are organized. In contrast to case management, which seeks to access most or all of the needed services from other community agencies, ACT brings together a multi-disciplinary treatment team which together can provide most or all of these services directly. As a service (and systems) integration strategy, ACT is intended to be a more intensive intervention.

The early history of this intervention was outlined previously; Thompson *et al.* (1990) and Drake (1998) provide historical summaries of the development of the ACT model. Following a pilot evaluation of the original TCL model (Marx *et al.*, 1973), Stein and Test reported results from a successful formal randomized controlled trial in the late 1970s (Stein and Test, 1980; Test and Stein, 1980) and a cost–benefit study (Weisbrod *et al.*, 1980; Weisbrod, 1983). Subsequent independent experimental replications using the TCL model were conducted in Michigan (Mulder, 1982, 1985) and Sydney, Australia (Hoult *et al.*, 1983; Hoult and Reynolds, 1984).

There have been a number of modifications and adaptations of this model as clinicians have applied it to different populations (e.g. Scarpitti *et al.*, 1994; Dixon *et al.*, 1995) and within different agencies and settings. An important example of the latter is the *assertive outreach* or *assertive case management model* first developed within the Thresholds Bridge psychosocial rehabilitation programme in Chicago (Witheridge *et al.*, 1982). This model differs from the original TCL model in several respects, including a focus on persons with SMI who are homeless, a stronger 'survival' orientation that emphasizes helping people obtain entitlements, housing and direct assistance with basic needs in daily life; staffing and team size; and 24-hour availability (Bond *et al.*, 1995). These modifications and others related to adaptation of the ACT model to special populations prompt the question of how much can a particular programme vary from the original ACT framework and still be considered ACT.

McGrew and Bond (1995) asked 20 experts on ACT to rate the importance of 73 programme elements characterizing ACT. The experts were able to achieve a high level of agreement on specific organizational and staffing characteristics that reflect ACT. Among the more important characteristics ratified by these experts were: assistance in obtaining basic needs and entitlements; a focus on increasing client functioning; medication and symptom management; assertive and persistent engagement and follow-through; a 'no-close' policy with respect to length of treatment; a multidisciplinary team which includes a psychiatrist, a registered nurse and a social worker; shared caseloads; small client:staff caseloads of limited size; and an *in vivo* treatment focus. McGrew *et al.* (1994) reported results from the creation and application of a fidelity measure derived from these elements that showed that ACT programmes that obtained higher fidelity scores on this measure were associated with greater reductions in psychiatric hospitalization for their clients. Teague *et al.* (1995, 1998) developed and validated a second fidelity measure for a modified ACT programme that serves individuals with SMI and co-occurring mental disorders. This work is important because it reflects a general level of agreement about the ACT model and the emergence of standards that can be used to guide the development and monitoring of ACT programmes for quality assurance and research purposes.

The ACT programme model has had an important effect on treatment for persons with SMI. Case management models are gradually incorporating elements of the ACT intervention, thus slowly narrowing the range of differences between the two. ACT programmes are also spreading throughout the USA. Deci *et al.* (1995) reported that more than 30 states now have at least one ACT team, and 14 states are implementing ACT on a statewide basis (Meisler, 1997). Federal, con-

sumer and family, and research groups have advocated for wider adoption of ACT programmes (Gilbert, 1997; Flynn *et al.*, 1997; Lehman *et al.*, 1998), and the recent publication of two clinical manuals will help provide technical assistance in programme development and implementation (Allness and Knoedler, 1998; Stein and Santos, 1998). There are, however, important problems to be resolved if ACT is to receive wider implementation, particularly how these programmes will be financed (Clark, 1997).

Efficacy and effectiveness of ACT and case management

During the past 25 years, an extensive research literature on these interventions has accumulated. We reviewed this literature as it related to the treatment of schizophrenia through 1995 as part of the work of the Schizophrenia Patient Outcomes Research Team (PORT) Project (see Scott and Dixon, 1995; Lehman *et al.*, 1998). The most recent comprehensive literature review on this topic (Mueser *et al.*, 1998) included 75 studies through 1997, with 44 of these studies addressing the efficacy or effectiveness of ACT. Studies of case management models for individuals with SMI have been far less numerous (except as comparisons for ACT). This literature is becoming increasingly international (with studies published from the USA, UK, Australia and Canada), which introduces interesting interpretative issues arising from differences in national systems of mental health care. There has also been an increasing focus on special populations, such as persons who are homeless, those with co-occurring mental and substance use disorders, and those involved within the criminal justice system. Interested readers are referred to the following recent reviews (Bond *et al.*, 1995; Burns and Santos, 1995; Holloway *et al.*, 1995; Rapp, 1995; Scott and Dixon, 1995; Meisler and Santos, 1996; Dixon and Scott, 1997; McHugo *et al.*, 1998; Mueser *et al.*, 1998).

Here we provide a selective overview of the findings for ACT, focusing on rehospitalization, housing and residential stability, costs and other outcomes. These outcomes have received the most attention and, in the case of the first two, have yielded the most consistent results.

ACT findings on rehospitalization

Past research on ACT has yielded consistent findings regarding its positive effect in reducing psychiatric rehospitalizations. Both ACT and intensive case management models resembling ACT appear to reduce the rate and duration of rehospitalizations among individuals with SMI who are at substantial risk for rehospitalization relative to control groups. Mueser *et al.* (1998) noted that 14 of 23 (or 61%) controlled studies of ACT or intensive case management that used rehospitalization as an outcome found a significant decrease in the number of readmissions compared with the control group. In a meta-analysis of nine studies involving the assertive case management model, Bond *et al.* (1995; p. 12) concluded that "as a rule of thumb, providing assertive outreach programs for frequent users of hospitals can be expected to reduce inpatient days by about 50%." Burns and Santos (1995) concluded that the impact of ACT on use of in-patient psychiatric services is stronger for the number of days of hospital use than for the number of admissions.

There are several points that should be considered in interpreting the effect of ACT on rehospitalization, however.

(i) Rehospitalization is not always an adverse outcome. Most studies in which it is used as an outcome fail to distinguish between in-patient episodes that reflect a negative outcome and those that may represent a more positive event.

(ii) This outcome is most likely to be observed when persons participating in the study are at major risk for rehospitalization, an important point to consider as ACT programmes are extended to newer populations.

(iii) The reduction in use of in-patient services is observed most often when the treatment team can control the hospital admissions and discharge process. For example, in a British study of the Daily Living Programme (DLP), Marks *et al.* (1994) reported that the DLP team initially could control the length of in-patient stays for team patients. During this period, hospitalizations for DLP patients occurred at about the same rate as observed for controls, but the DLP team was able to reduce the length of these rehospitalizations by about 80%. When control over admissions and discharge decisions was assumed subsequently by a non-DLP group, the average lengths of stay increased markedly.

(iv) One way by which rehospitalization can be prevented (or delayed) is through the use of community-based alternatives such as 24-hour crisis intervention services, or residential programmes. If these resources are not available within a community, reductions in rehospitalization rates may be harder to achieve.

(v) There is evidence that the effects of ACT on rehospitalization may be mediated by the extent of fidelity to the ACT model. McGrew *et al.* (1994) examined the effect of programme fidelity with the ACT model in a study of 18 programmes and reported a statistically significant association between several measures of programme fidelity and reductions in hospital days.

(vi) Several studies have shown that rehospitalization rates tend to return to pre-ACT levels after ACT treatment is discontinued (Scott and Dixon, 1995). In contrast, evidence for the effects of case management programmes on the use of in-patient psychiatric services is more limited and mixed, reflecting an absence of replication studies of clearly defined case management models.

A question that is receiving recent attention is whether there are specific client-level or organizational characteristics that might predict which individuals are most likely to experience a reduction in risk for rehospitalization through ACT. For example, we have already seen that clients who have been rehospitalized more frequently in the past are more likely to experience fewer and/or shorter rehospitalizations through ACT programmes. Work by McGrew *et al.* (1994) showed that programmes with increased fidelity to the 'critical ingredients' of ACT achieved greater reductions in rehospitalizations for their clients. Salkever *et al.* (1999) found that the reduction in risk of rehospitalization (but not the length of hospitalization) was greatest among older clients and those with diagnoses of schizophrenia or schizoaffective disorders. They also found that higher programme staffing levels were associated with lower rates of rehospitalization. In a multi-site evaluation of intensive case management programmes in VA neuro-psychiatric and general medical/surgical facilities, Rosenheck *et al.* (1995) also found that ACT programmes in VA neuro-psychiatric facilities attained greater reductions in rehospitalization than those in general medical/surgical facilities, and that patients over the age of 45 years and those with higher than median pre-treatment days of in-patient care exhibited the most pronounced reductions. The increasing use of newer antipsychotic medications such as clozapine and olanzapine is likely to be an important variable in future studies. As Salkever *et al.* (1999) note, the capacity to examine these predictive relationships in a particular study requires a larger sample size that can support the necessary multi-variate analyses given the number of potential predictive characteristics. They suggest the desirability of looking for ways to pool data across study samples, programmes and sites.

ACT and housing status and residential stability

Previous research also consistently documents that ACT programmes produce improvements in housing status, residential stability and independent living. Mueser *et al.* (1998) report that nine of 12 controlled studies of ACT and intensive case management found significant improvements in this area. At least one study (Test *et al.*, 1985) found that recipients of ACT significantly reduced the number of nights participants reported being homeless or utilizing homeless shelters.

Cost and cost-effectiveness studies of ACT

The impact of ACT on the costs of treatment has been examined through a number of studies of costs, cost–benefits and cost-effectiveness. In the original cost–benefit evaluation of the TCL model, Weisbrod (1980, 1983) reported that the average direct treatment cost per client per day during the first year of treatment was higher among the TCL patients than among the control subjects, but these higher costs were offset by a higher level of benefits (including a doubling of work productivity) among the experimental TCL group. This resulted in a small but significant and positive cost–benefit ratio favouring TCL. In the Australian TCL replication study, Hoult and Reynolds (1984) found that the average annual direct and indirect treatment costs were significantly lower for TCL subjects than controls, a result attributable to reductions in the use of in-patient psychiatric care by the former group. Subsequent studies generally have shown that TCL programmes tend to be no more costly than (or even less costly than) their comparison conditions, typically due to fewer rehospitalizations. The findings for the assertive case management model are somewhat less consistent (Scott and Dixon, 1995), but this may reflect differences in the type of patient targeted and variations in the programme model. Bond *et al.* (1988) have argued that model fidelity may be an important factor in the realization of any prospective savings.

Recent economic research on ACT has elaborated these findings within the traditional ACT target population or extended these findings to different treatment populations. Salkever *et al.* (1999) examined two ACT programmes in Charleston (South Carolina) that worked with inner-city persons with SMI and a history of or high risk for high service use patterns (long-term or multiple hospitalizations). Patients who received ACT were 40% less likely to be rehospitalized during an 18-month follow-up than a standard care group, although the groups did not differ on the number of days hospitalized for patients who were admitted to a hospital. The age of the patients and higher staff:patient ratios significantly affected the probability of readmission. In a study of ACT at three sites in Connecticut, Essock *et al.* (1998) reported that ACT significantly decreased days of hospital use and increased days of residential stability at no additional cost to the public mental health system, the state or society when compared with a mobile, assertive individual case management programme. An important finding was that the ACT intervention was cost-effective for patients who had been hospitalized at the time of their entry into the study; for those who had not, the intervention was cost-neutral. Essock *et al.* emphasize the importance of reserving scarce ACT slots for individuals who have been recent and heavy users of hospital services.

Clark *et al.* (1998) examined the extension of the ACT model to persons with SMI and co-occurring substance use disorders. This experimental study compared an ACT programme model implemented in seven community mental health centres in New Hampshire with a standard case management model that incorporated some aspects of ACT but did not share the team focus and provided a lower intensity of treatment. Clark and his colleagues found that both programmes significantly improved quality of life and achieved significant reductions in substance use from pre-treatment levels over a 3-year period, but did not differ from each other on these measures. The two conditions were not significantly different in costs of treatment, although ACT became significantly more cost-efficient during the third year of treatment as a result of decreases in costs among ACT patients during the final year of treatment. These cost decreases were particularly evident for housing support, day treatment and arrest-related costs. This study supports the widely held belief that intensive treatment may be more expensive than standard treatment in the short run, but equally or less costly in the long run.

Lehman *et al.* (1999) (also Lehman *et al.*, 1997) compared an ACT programme adapted to the needs of homeless persons with SMI with usual community services for this population. Costs for mental health in-patient days and mental health emergency room care were significantly lower among the ACT patients compared with usual care. Conversely, costs for out-patient services were higher among the ACT patients. ACT patients spent 31% more days in stable community housing and experienced significantly greater improvements in symptoms, life satisfaction and perceived health status. The cost-efficiency of the programmes in assisting these homeless patients in achieving stable housing favoured ACT, with ACT spending 42% less to achieve each day of stable housing.

ACT and other outcome domains

Evidence for the effectiveness of ACT and other outcome areas is much less consistent. Results for outcomes such as decreased psychiatric symptomatology, reductions in substance use and improvements in social functioning and quality of life have been mixed (Scott and Dixon, 1995; Mueser *et al.*, 1998). There may be several reasons for these inconsistent findings. Certain domains are hard to measure reliably (e.g. medication compliance). Some domains (e.g. vocational functioning, social functioning) may represent categories of services that are absent and should be incorporated into the ACT model (e.g. vocational rehabilitation, social learning or social skills training). Domains such as reductions in psychiatric symptomatology (e.g. negative symptoms) may require longer intervals to produce than are often assessed in follow-up studies.

Discussion

Case management and ACT represent attempts to integrate the wide range of treatment and support services that individuals with SMI require in order to live successfully in the community. Case management models evolved from initial social casework approaches designed to help clients identify and plan for service needs, access and link with agencies that provide these services, and monitor receipt of services. Over time, this initial model evolved to include direct provision of clinical treatment services, the development of a clinical team, assertive engagement, *in vivo* service provision and other features. Today, as Ellison *et al.*

(1995) have noted, what we know as 'standard case management' has moved considerably beyond the original generalist model.

The in-patient psychiatric hospital represented an important, but costly and restrictive, model of service integration. In an effort to achieve the integrative effects of a 'hospital without walls' in community settings, the first ACT programmes were developed during the 1970s and 1980s. These programmes emphasized the use of a multidisciplinary team that provided and co-ordinated the care of individuals with SMI who were at substantial risk for subsequent rehospitalization in the community. Research over the past 25 years has provided considerable support for the ACT model, and Lehman *et al.* (1998) conclude that ACT is one of only two psychosocial interventions for persons with SMI with strong empirical support.

Research on these interventions has focused on ACT (although case management in various forms is used as a comparison in many studies). One result of this is that there has been relatively little investigation of less intensive alternatives to ACT for individuals who may not require the intensity of services afforded by ACT. Not all patients require ACT; in fact, some estimates suggest that the target population may only comprise 15–20% of individuals with SMI (Drake, 1998). An important issue for future research concerns the types of case management models that might be appropriate for this larger group of patients.

Research on ACT has established that it consistently can reduce the use of in-patient psychiatric care and promote residential stability and independent living among selected patients. Its effect on other outcomes is not as clear and consistent. One reason may be a lack of adequate programme theory that links the activities of the intervention to the effects they are supposed to produce (McHugo *et al.*, 1998). Psychiatric symptomatology affords a good example of an outcome for which better explication of the programme theory underlying the expected effects of ACT would improve our research. What are the mechanisms within ACT by which we would expect it to reduce psychiatric symptoms? Does symptom reduction have something to do with

staffing levels, or frequency or location of contact, or other components of the ACT intervention? Which types of symptoms (e.g. positive or negative) do we expect to improve, and why? Is there an inter-relationship among various intervention outcomes such that some outcomes have to be achieved *before* positive or negative symptoms improve (e.g. stable housing, enrolment in entitlements, adequate medication compliance)? Over what time frame should we anticipate improvement in negative symptoms? Are clinically adequate and appropriate levels of medication being prescribed? How will the use of newer antipsychotic medications such as clozapine or olanzapine affect these issues? Similar questions can be asked for each type of outcome. Attempting to provide an answer to these questions in the form of a set of testable assumptions about ACT would provide a more rigorous conceptualization of this intervention and its effects.

Research on ACT is likely to become more challenging to conduct in the future. Changing practice patterns (and managed mental health care) are reducing the length of psychiatric hospitalization for all patients. As 'standard case management' incorporates more of the features of ACT, it could become harder to show pronounced differences between those receiving ACT and those receiving standard care. However, research on these interventions appears likely to become even more exciting in the future, as practitioners seek to open the 'black boxes' of case management and ACT to find out which aspects of these interventions produce which effects for which types of patients.

References

Allness, D.J. and Knoedler, W.H. (1998) *The PACT Model of Community-based Treatment for Persons with Severe and Persistent Mental Illnesses: A Manual for PACT Start-up.* Arlington VA: NAMI Anti-Stigma Foundation.

Anthony, W.A., Forbess, R. and Cohen, M.R. (1993) Rehabilitation-oriented case management. In: Harris, M. and Bergman, H.C. (eds), *Case Management for Mentally Ill Patients: Theory and Practice.* Langhorne, PA: Academic Publishers.

Bachrach, L.L. (1993) Continuity of care and approaches to case management for long-term mentally ill patients. *Hospital and Community Psychiatry*, 44, 465–468.

Bebout, R. (1993) Contextual case management: restructuring the social support networks of seriously mentally ill adults. In: Harris, M. and Bergman, H.C. (eds), *Case Management for Mentally Ill Patients: Theory and Practice*. Langhorne, PA: Academic Publishers.

Bond, G.R., Miller, L.D., Krumweid, R.D. and Ward, R.S. (1988) Assertive case management in three CMHCs: a controlled study. *Hospital and Community Psychiatry*, 39, 411–418.

Bond, G.R., McGrew, J.H. and Fekete, D.M. (1995) Assertive outreach for frequent users of psychiatric hospitals: a meta-analysis. *Journal of Mental Health Administration*, 22, 4–16.

Burns, B.J. and Santos, A.B. (1995) Assertive community treatment: an update of randomized trials. *Psychiatric Services*, 46, 669–675.

Clark, R.E. (1997) Financing assertive community treatment. *Administration and Policy in Mental Health*, 25, 209–220.

Clark, R.E., Teague, G.B., Ricketts, S.K., Bush, P.W., Xie, H., McGuire, T.G., Drake, R.E., McHugo, G.J., Keller, A.M. and Zubkoff, M. (1998) Cost-effectiveness of assertive community treatment versus standard case management for persons with co-occurring severe mental illness and substance use disorders. *Health Services Research*, 33, 1285–1308.

Deci, P.A., Santos, A.B., Hiott, D.W., Schoenwald, S. and Dias, J.K. (1995) Dissemination of assertive community treatment programs. *Psychiatric Services*, 46, 676–678.

Dixon, L. and Scott, J. (1997) Case management. In: Sederer, L.I. and Rothschild, A.J. (eds), *Acute Care Psychiatry: Diagnosis and Treatment*. Baltimore, MD: Williams and Wilkins.

Dixon, L.B., Krauss, N., Kernan, E., Lehman, A.F. and DeForge, B.R. (1995) Modifying the PACT model to serve homeless persons with severe mental illness. *Psychiatric Services*, 46, 684–688.

Drake, R.E. (1998) Brief history, current status, and future place of assertive community treatment. *American Journal of Orthopsychiatry*, 68, 172–175.

Drake, R.E., McHugo, G.J., Clark, R.E., Teague, G.B., Xie, H., Miles, K. and Ackerson, T.H. (1998) Assertive community treatment for patients with co-occurring severe mental illness and substance use disorder: a clinical trial. *American Journal of Orthopsychiatry*, 68, 201–215.

Ellison, M.L., Rogers, E.S., Sciarappa, K., Cohen, M. and Forbess, R. (1995) Characteristics of mental health case management: results of a national survey. *Journal of Mental Health Administration*, 22, 101–112.

Essock, S.M., Frisman, L.K. and Kontos, N.J. (1998) Cost-effectiveness of assertive community treatment teams. *American Journal of Orthopsychiatry*, 68, 179–190.

Flynn, L., Bevilaqua, J., Meisler, N., Knoedler, W., Allness, D. and Steinwachs, D. (1997) NAMI Anti-Stigma Foundation, NAMI/PACT initiative for national dissemination of the PACT model. *Community Support Network News*, 11, 10–11.

Gilbert, D. (1997) States helping states: PACT and managed care. *Community Support Network News*, 11, 1, 16.

Holloway, F., Oliver, N., Collins, E. and Carson, J. (1995) Case management: a critical review of the outcome literature. *European Psychiatry*, 10, 113–128.

Hoult, J. and Reynolds, I. (1984) Schizophrenia: a comparative trial of community-oriented and hospital-oriented psychiatric care. *Acta Psychiatrica Scandinavia*, 69, 359–372.

Intagliata, J. (1982) Improving the quality of community care for the chronically mentally disabled: the role of case management. *Schizophrenia Bulletin*, 8, 655–674.

Hoult, J., Reynolds, I., Charboneau-Powis, M., Weekes, P. and Briggs, J. (1983) Psychiatric hospital versus community treatment: the results of a randomized trial. *Australian and New Zealand Journal of Psychiatry*, 17, 160–1673.

Lehman, A.F., Dixon, L.B., Kernan, E., DeForge, B.R. and Postrado, L.T. (1997) A randomized trial of assertive community treatment from homeless persons with severe mental illness. *Archives of General Psychiatry*, 54, 1038–1043.

Lehman, A.F., Steinwachs, D.M. and the Co-Investigators of the PORT Project (1998) Translating research into practice: the Schizophrenia Patient Outcomes Research Team (PORT) treatment recommendations. *Schizophrenia Bulletin*, 24, 1–10.

Lehman, A.F., Dixon, L.B., Hoch, J.S., DeForge, B., Kernan, E. and Frank, R. (1999) Cost-effectiveness of assertive community treatment for homeless persons with severe mental illness. *British Journal of Psychiatry*, 174, 346–352.

Marks, I.M., Connolly, J., Muijen, M., McNamee, G. and Lawrence, R.E. (1994) Home-based versus hospital-based care for people with serious mental illness. *British Journal of Psychiatry*, 165, 179–194.

Marx, A.J., Test, M.A. and Stein, L.I. (1973) Extrahospital management of severe mental illness: feasibility and effects on social functioning. *Archives of General Psychiatry*, 29, 505.

McGrew, J.H. and Bond, G.R. (1995) Critical ingredients of assertive community treatment: judgements of the experts. *Journal of Mental Health Administration*, 22, 113–125.

McGrew, J.H., Bond, G.R., Dietzen, L. and Salyers, M. (1994) Measuring the fidelity and implementation of a mental health program model. *Journal of Consulting and Clinical Psychology*, 62, 670–678.

McHugo, G.J., Hargreaves, W., Drake, R.E., Clark, R.E., Xie, H., Bond, G.R. and Burns, B.J. (1998) Methodological issues in assertive community treatment studies. *American Journal of Orthopsychiatry*, 68, 246–264.

Meisler, N. (1997) Assertive community treatment initiatives: results from a survey of state mental health authorities. *Community Support Network News*, 11, 3–5.

Meisler, N. and Santos, A.B. (1996) Case management of persons with schizophrenia and other severe mental illnesses in the USA. In: Moscarelli, M., Rupp, A. and Sartorius, N. (eds), *Handbook of Mental Health Economics and Health Policy, Volume I, Schizophrenia*. Chichester, UK: Johns Wiley and Sons.

Meisler, N., Blankertz, L., Santos, A.B. and McKay, C. (1998) Impact of assertive community treatment on homeless persons with co-occurring severe psychiatric and substance use disorders. *Community Mental Health Journal*, 33, 113–122.

Mueser, K.T., Bond, G.R., Drake, R.E. and Resnick, S.G. (1998) Models of community care for severe mental illness: a review of research on case management. *Schizophrenia Bulletin*, 24, 37–74.

Mulder, R. (1982) *Final Evaluation of the Harbinger Program as a Demonstration Project*. Lansing, MI: Kent County Community Mental Health Center.

Mulder, R. (1985) *Evaluation of the Harbinger Program, 1982–1985*. Lansing, MI: Kent County Community Mental Health Center.

Olfson, M. (1990) Assertive community treatment: an evaluation of the experimental evidence. *Hospital and Community Psychiatry*, 41, 634–641.

Orwin, R., Sonnefeld, L.J., Garrison-Mogren, R. and Smith, N.G. (1994) Pitfalls in evaluating the effectiveness of case management programs for homeless persons: lessons from the NIAAA Community Demonstration Program. *Evaluation Review*, 18, 153–185.

Rapp, C.A. (1993) Theory, principles, and methods of the strengths model of case management. In: Harris, M. and Bergman, H.C. (eds), *Case Management for Mentally Ill Patients: Theory and Practice*. Langhorne, PA: Academic Publishers.

Rapp, C.A. (1995) The active ingredients of effective case management: a research synthesis. In: Rapp, C.A., Manderscheid, R.W., Henderon, M.J., Hodge, M., Knisely, M.B., Penny, D.J., Stoneking, B.B., Hyde, P. and Geisler, L.J. (eds), *Case Management for Behavioral Managed Care*. Rockville, MD: Center

for Mental Health Services (SAMHSA) and the National Association of Case Management.

Rosenheck, R., Neale, M., Leaf, P., Milstein, R. and Frisman. L, (1995) Multi-site experimental cost study of intensive psychiatric community care. *Schizophrenia Bulletin*, 21, 129–140.

Salkever, D., Domino, M.E., Burns, B.J., Santos, A.B., Deci, P.A., Dias, J., Wagner, H.R., Faldowski, R.A. and Paolone, J. (1999) Assertive community treatment for people with severe mental illness: the effect on hospital use and costs. *Health Services Research*, 34, 577–601.

Scarpitti, F.R., Inciardi, J.A. and Martin, S.S. (1994) Assertive community treatment: obstacles to implementation. In: Fletcher, B.W., Inciardi, J.A. and Horton, A.M. (eds), *Drug Abuse Treatment: The implementation of Innovative Approaches*. Westport, CT: Greenwood Press.

Scott, J.E. and Dixon, L.B. (1995) Assertive community treatment and case management for schizophrenia. *Schizophrenia Bulletin*, 21, 657–668.

Sledge, W.H., Astrachan, B., Thompson, K., Rakfeldt, J. and Leaf, P.J. (1995) Case management in psychiatry: an analysis of tasks. *American Journal of Psychiatry*, 152, 1259–1265.

Solomon, P. and Draine, J. (1995) One year outcomes of a randomized trial of case management with seriously mentally ill clients leaving jail. *Evaluation Review*, 19, 256–273.

Stein, L.I. and Santos, A.B. (1998) *Assertive Community Treatment of Persons with Severe Mental Illness*. New York: Norton.

Stein, L.I. and Test, M.A. (1980) Alternative to mental hospital treatment: I. Conceptual model, treatment program, and clinical evaluation. *Archives of General Psychiatry*, 37, 392–397.

Teague, G.B., Drake, R.E. and Ackerson, T.H. (1995) Evaluating use of continuous treatment teams for persons with mental illness and substance abuse. *Psychiatric Services*, 46, 689–695.

Teague, G.B., Bond, G.R. and Drake, R.E. (1998) Program fidelity in assertive community treatment: development and use of a measure. *American Journal of Orthopsychiatry*, 68, 216–232.

Test, M.A., Knoedler, W.H. and Allness, D.J. (1985) The long-term treatment of young schizophrenics in a community support program. *New Directions for Mental Health Services*, 26, 17–27.

Test, M.A. and Stein, L.I. (1980) Alternatives to mental hospital treatment: III. Social costs. *Archives of General Psychiatry*, 37, 409–412.

Thompson, K.H., Griffith, E.E.H. and Leaf, P.J. (1990) A historical review of the Madison model of community care. *Psychiatric Services*, 41, 625–634.

Weisbrod, B.A. (1983)A guide to benefit–cost analysis, as seen through a controlled experiment in treating the mentally ill. *Journal of Health, Policy and Law*, 7, 808–846.

Weisbrod, B.A., Test, M.A. and Stein, L.I. (1980) Alternative to mental hospital treatment: II. Economic benefit–cost analysis. *Archives of General Psychiatry*, 37, 400–405.

Witheridge, T.F., Dincin, J. and Appleby, L. (1982) Working with the most frequent recidivists: a total team approach to assertive resource management. *Psychosocial Rehabilitation Journal*, 5, 9–11.

23 | *Emergency psychiatric services*
Richard E. Breslow

Introduction

Emergency psychiatric services are the part of the system of psychiatric services responsible for responding to psychiatric emergencies (Gerson and Bassuk, 1980). The psychiatric emergency is a serious, acute situation which has arisen that requires immediate assessment and treatment. The common emergencies are suicide, acute psychosis, other mental status change, substance abuse and behavioural disturbance. Any marked change in a person's mental status that activates a response in the support system to seek help may come under the purview of the emergency psychiatric system (Munizza *et al.*, 1993).

It may be helpful to think in terms of an initial change, usually on the part of an individual, along the lines listed above (Thienhaus *et al.*, 1995). Sometimes the change involves a couple or a group. Next comes the detection of the change by the person, the support system or the community at large. There are definite signal detection characteristics in this phase. The same behavioural disturbance may activate a response in one community and get very little reaction in another. Even within a family at different stages, there may be emergency responses or not (Slaby, 1981). Once the disturbance has been detected, there is a response by the person, support system, therapist, clinic, family doctor, police, mobile team, emergency room, insurance company or managed care organization. The response generally is referral for emergency psychiatric evaluation where the change can be assessed. This may be done by a psychiatric consultant in an emergency room, a private psychiatrist, a community-based psychiatric agency or a comprehensive psychiatric emergency service. In the final stage, this evaluation is used to produce a referral to one of many possible settings including out-patient treatment, substance abuse treatment, social service organizations or in-patient psychiatric hospitalization (Way *et al.*, 1992). One variant on this is the capacity for extended evaluation, where in a more comprehensive service, time can be provided to observe the patient and note changes in clinical status (Ianzito *et al.*, 1978). Further history and contacts with family and other informants can be obtained to clarify the clinical situation and then referral can be accomplished.

Importance of emergency room/casualty facilities

Hospital emergency departments have become the focus of health care in medical emergencies and for more general medical problems when there are access problems to other components of the health system (Bell *et al.*, 1991). Problems of lack of health insurance, poverty, limited education, membership of a vulnerable population or limited hours of operation of health care facilities (Johnson and Thornicroft, 1995) throw the burden of enormous amounts of general medical care on the emergency department. Since emergency departments generally have been mandated to provide a medical screening examination and treatment for all patients who present themselves for care, the emergency service may have become the only guaranteed access point to the health care system (Linn, 1971). Many of these trends are intensified even more when it comes to psychiatric emergencies. Firstly, many psychiatric emergencies start off as medical emergencies such as serious overdoses or the psychological reaction to physical or emotional trauma. Next, these emergencies sometimes can involve management of out of control behaviour. Also, psychiatric patients are particularly prone to access problems such as those delineated above. Finally, other components of the psychiatric health care system often tend to be ill suited to the handling of emergencies (Wellin *et al.*, 1987).

The general model for rendering of psychiatric services in a medical emergency room is the consultant relationship. After the patient is medically stabilized, the psychiatrist, who has general coverage duties elsewhere, comes to the emergency department to see the patient, make an assessment, propose treatment recommendations and help plan a disposition (Stebbins and Hardman, 1993). This remains the most common model for delivery of care in psychiatric emergencies. It has the advantage of flexibility of use of physician time. Physicians can cover many different services and may be based on the in-patient unit or the out-patient clinic. In the after-hours situation, the physician can cover from home or private office. Nursing staff needs are minimized since the emergency department staff are responsible for all care. A general medical evaluation is guaranteed on all patients. This is quite important since mental status changes so frequently can be from organic aetiologies. There should be good communication between medicine and psychiatry, since all parties to the consultation are physically located in the emergency department (McClelland, 1983).

The deficits in this model are also compelling to the point where major modifications have been needed (Oldham *et al.*, 1990; Surles *et al.*, 1994). There is a fundamental clash in attitude between the medical emergency room with its emphasis on rapid treatment and disposition to make space for the next emergency and the needs of psychiatric evaluation (Baxter *et al.*, 1968; Goss *et al.*, 1971). The organization of space in the emergency room does not allow for the privacy and ability to separate out conflicting parties that may be so crucial to a proper assessment. Psychiatric patients tend to be regarded as a nuisance or, even worse, a hindrance to the work of the emergency service since they frequently have accompanying behavioural disturbance (Comstock, 1983). There is a negative mind-set towards those with psychiatric emergencies with the assumption that these emergencies are more volitional and less 'genuine' than a true medical emergency. The negative set extends to family members as well who cannot be handled adequately in the available space and can be viewed as obstacles to rapid disposition. This may even include a negative attitude towards the psychiatric consultant; there is an implicit or at times more overt demand to 'get your patient out of my emergency room'. The time course of evaluations presents perhaps the most fundamental conflict between the medical and the psychiatric emergency (Breslow *et al.*, 1997). In the medical emergency, the high acuity patient is generally in a life-threatening situation and must be seen and treated as rapidly as possible (Saunders, 1987; Hu, 1993). The high acuity psychiatric emergency may need rapid attention to prevent self-harm or harm to others. Once this is accomplished, longer time periods can be very helpful in allowing the immediate crisis to pass, letting acute intoxication resolve, noting and tracking changes in mental status, getting additional history and records, making contact with family members and re-approaching the patient after some calming down to better establish a therapeutic alliance.

Development of psychiatric emergency services

There was a tremendous impetus for the development of more comprehensive psychiatric emergency services in response to the problems described (Hughes, 1993; Breslow *et al.*, 1996a). These comprehensive services usually are hospital based and have sufficient space to allow for privacy, confidentiality and enough calm and quiet to conduct an evaluation. The separation in space has many beneficial aspects, but perhaps the most important is the provision of adequate time to observe the patient and to remove the urgency of the medical emergency atmosphere. The chance to separate the behaviourally disturbed patient helps the operation of the medical emergency room and benefits the patient as well by providing a quieter area in which to calm down (Hankoff *et al.*, 1974). This ensures less 'scapegoating' of psychiatric patients and staff as well. It also provides a better opportunity to pay attention to the needs of patient's families. Their questions can be answered and their participation utilized to improve the treatment plan (Barton, 1974). A separate emergency facility also involves separate staffing. This enables recruitment of nurses and social workers with an interest in psychiatric emergencies who will be able to see these patients not as 'nuisances', but as having illnesses requiring treatment (Blais and Georges, 1969). This also allows staff over time to develop the specialized skills necessary to treat these patients.

A key advantage of this specialization of services is the opportunity to have full-time attending psychiatric coverage. This elevates the prestige of the discipline and has changed the whole mind-set with respect to delivering emergency psychiatric care. In the prior model, the psychiatrist was always pulled from other clinical services to see an emergency and would have an urgency to get back to the original service. The whole process would be viewed as at best a nuisance and at worst a critical disruption, rather than as an end in itself. This also has enabled the emergency service to develop into an important training setting (Hillard *et al.*, 1993). In the older model, emergency work was regarded as undesirable and relegated to the most junior staff. Frequently, staff in training such as residents would be handling emergencies largely on their own with limited or no back-up and little chance to use it as a learning experience.

The organization of a separate service with specialized attending psychiatrists providing the supervision has made it possible to uncover the strengths of the emergency service as a psychiatry teaching setting. The trainee has a chance to see all stages of psychiatric illness, particularly the acute initial phase, and not just already stabilized patients. The resident or student can gain experience in dealing with first episodes of illness, interpersonal crises, families and acute substance abuse issues. There are more opportunities to observe the supervisor doing interviews and practising psychiatry in the emergency service than in other settings. In addition, the supervisor gets many opportunities to observe the work of the trainee directly. The emergency service is an excellent

introduction to the mental health system, since it interfaces with so many elements of it. The flexibility of this setting also enables training of many different specialties and disciplines in addition to the primary goal of training of psychiatric residents. At various times, medical students, nursing students, social work students, psychology interns, family practice residents, emergency medicine residents and internists have benefited from exposure to the emergency service.

There is a negative side to the development of separate psychiatric emergency services. Setting up such services involves increased expense in this era of competition amongst various community psychiatric service needs with decreasing financial resources available to meet these needs. Services separated from medical emergency room/casualty facilities require hiring specialized nursing and social work staff. It always requires more staffing to cover a separate service than a combined service. Full-time psychiatric coverage can also add a major operating expense. There is also the possibility of less thorough medical evaluations as medical staff hurry to get behaviourally disturbed patients out to the psychiatric emergency facility as soon as possible (Breslow *et al.*, 1999). Patients who present first to the psychiatric emergency service might not get the medical evaluation needed at all unless psychiatric staff are particularly attuned to the issue of possible underlying organic dysfunction. Communication might not be as good between medical and psychiatric staff when the services are separated, and the possibility of misunderstandings is increased. Patients and families may feel stigmatized by being sent to a psychiatric emergency service, rather than just being treated in the medical emergency room. Sometimes they state that they do not want to be in that place with 'crazy people'. If they observe some disturbed behaviour or locked doors, they may find the experience frightening.

Crisis hospitalization and crisis residential services

The most important aspect of the development of a separate psychiatric emergency service is the flexibility it provides in meeting the needs of the community (Oldham and DeMasi, 1995). Sometimes increased time is needed to deal with a crisis beyond the usual emergency room time frame. Additional time allows staff to gather information from family and treating clinicians to compare with the patient's own statements. It permits the programme to provide targeted interventions for patients where symptoms can be ameliorated quickly. Some psychiatric emergencies involve rapid changes of mental status over a relatively brief period of time such as happens when substance abuse is an issue. In this case, additional time can change the entire psychiatric evaluation. Finally, the possibility of a more extended time period for evaluation can give respite to both caregivers and patients in the community and allow resources to be reordered or restored to allow maintenance of the patient in the community (Breslow *et al.*, 1993).

The emergency service can provide the increased time in a number of ways. One is through an extended evaluation capacity. In many services, this includes the ability to hold the patient overnight, if necessary, to make community contacts in the morning. More flexibility is provided if patients can actually be admitted for a few days to the psychiatric emergency service. The same utilization review criteria as used for standard in-patient admissions apply. Patients must have significant functional impairment or mental illness with threats to self or others sufficient to warrant in-patient treatment. A number of psychiatric beds, usually 2–12 and sometimes called 'holding beds', are designated for the purpose of these 'very short hospitalization' units. It is usually best for these beds to have their own identity by being physically located on or near the emergency service (Weisman *et al.*, 1969; Rhine and Mayerson, 1971; Walker *et al.*, 1973).

Crisis hospitalization can be effective in managing psychiatric emergencies, and it provides a useful intermediate alternative to out-patient referral or to longer term hospitalization. The majority of patients are dischargeable in the short time frame, so many avoid longer term hospitalization (Gillig *et al.*, 1989). The patients who cannot be discharged require transfer to standard units for further care and treatment.

It must be stressed that the patients who could benefit would be those who require hospitalization for a condition that might be expected to improve in 2 or 3 days. For example, personality disorder patients, who by definition have limited personality coping resources, frequently will develop suicidal ideation or gestures under stress. These patients respond dramatically to the short, focused nature of crisis hospitalization. The chronically mentally ill, if they are well connected with community treatment programmes and are reacting to acute but transient stressors, may also respond favourably to crisis hospitalization. The patient who is abusing alcohol or other drugs but is no longer acutely intoxicated may still have substantial changes in mental status in the 2 or 3 days following an acute episode. Crisis hospitalization makes possible a longer period in which to allow evaluation and resolution of these changes.

The availability of crisis hospitalization provides benefits to the mental health system as well. It permits increased census flexibility. When all in-patient units are full, a patient can be admitted to await the next available bed. Community service providers such as supervised apartment programmes, halfway houses, out-patient clinics and continuing treatment programmes also view the possibility of crisis hospitalization as beneficial. The programme maintains the morale of both the patient and his or her community supports. Community service providers and patients often see rehospitalization as a failure. Crisis hospitalization allows both parties respite and time to mobilize defences or to adjust treatment strategies to allow the patient to return to the community rapidly. We have found that patients already well connected with treatment in the community can be discharged much more readily (Breslow *et al.*, 1995).

Another alternative available to the psychiatric emergency service as part of a comprehensive system of treatment is crisis respite care (Stroul, 1988). The variety of programmes is enormous, but the intention is to provide diversion from the emergency service to an acute care residential service, rather than utilizing psychiatric hospitalization. Patients are referred to a specially prepared residential setting which may consist of a foster home setting for up to two individuals or a larger group home model of 6–15 clients. In the family-based crisis home, carefully selected and trained families provide short-term housing and support to persons in acute psychiatric crisis. Professional staff support the family sponsors with case management services, nursing and psychiatric back-up to adjust medication, maintain compliance and provide emergency hospitalization if needed. The advantage is in providing a less restrictive, less stigmatizing, less traumatic, more normative environment for the patient to resolve the psychiatric crisis. The economic benefit of avoiding hospitalization and perhaps shortening the duration of treatment may be considerable. The group home model (Fields and Weisman, 1995) adds the elements of therapeutic milieu, group support and feedback and indigenous paraprofessional staffing to help in resolution of the psychiatric emergency. The emphasis is on a problem-solving approach and the need to work on a task in co-operation with others to get the patient to focus more quickly, avoiding the regression that institutionalization fosters. Programmes may exclude the most severe emergencies such as the acutely suicidal or violent patient or the patient with significant medical problems. The usual time frame for resolution of the emergency is up to 2 weeks when the expectation is for discharge to another level of care.

Mobile teams

Mobile emergency treatment teams have become a prominent part of the mental health system. Usually these teams have been developed on a local basis in response to the individual needs of each community. The original systems developed over 25 years ago based on an 'activist' approach to the problems of mental illness and their relationship to social problems. One of the early units described reliance on a family system perspective as the model for care (Bengelsdorf and Alden, 1987). The idea was to see the patient in the midst of the support system to intervene at an early stage and prevent further deterioration. Assessment and treatment could be directed towards the system

itself to help resolve a family crisis, to connect patients with clinics or social service resources or to advocate for the patient. The widespread belief was that such systems prevent in-patient psychiatric admission. It was thought that they could even be able to eliminate the need for more traditional sources of emergency care, such as emergency rooms and comprehensive psychiatric emergency services (Ruiz *et al.*, 1973; Granovetter, 1975; West *et al.*, 1980).

A survey of mobile crisis services found that they are prevalent throughout the emergency care system and felt to be helpful in a general sense, but there are few actual data demonstrating their effectiveness (Geller *et al.*, 1995). A controlled study of localities with and without mobile teams failed to demonstrate an impact on admission rates to psychiatric hospitals (Fisher *et al.*, 1990). Most of the other data collected are uncontrolled, where counts are provided of the number of mobile contacts and each is considered a prevention of hospitalization without consideration of base rates of hospitalization or what happens to the patient on longitudinal follow-up. One well designed randomized study of community outreach versus hospital-based care did demonstrate greater symptom improvement, more patient satisfaction and dramatically less use of in-patient psychiatric services with those assigned to the outreach care (Merson *et al.*, 1992). Patients were randomized to a multi-disciplinary community-based early intervention team or a conventional hospital-based psychiatric service with clinic facilities. The authors felt that the better outcome in the community group was from a greater ability to ensure follow-up with the outreach team compared with the clinic where many did not keep or receive continuing appointments.

Systems of care have become more sophisticated and it is now possible to differentiate types of mobile crisis services having different rationales underlying the service (Gillig, 1995). The most common demands for service are usually acute emergencies in the community involving the suicidal, acutely psychotic behaviourally disturbed or threatening patient. Frequently this involves either a police emergency or a 'mobile team' intervention to prevent a police emergency. The general public demand for such a service often stems from an incident in the community that became high profile and helped to create the demand. This type of service does not function to prevent admission, but rather works in the opposite sense of a 'case finder' for the emergency service since most of these patients are referred to the emergency service. Subsequently, they are held for stabilization and in many cases admitted to the psychiatric in-patient unit.

The team consists of one or two mobile workers, usually with training in community work through a social work degree, who can intervene in emergencies in the community by negotiating with the people involved or, if needed, work with police agencies to set limits on situations which are getting out of control. The emergency nature of the work makes it necessary to have 24-hour, 7 days per week availability of services, so the workers work in shifts that parallel the nursing shifts in the emergency service. They receive calls for help from the community at the psychiatric emergency service and go out by car for on-site visits with communication back to the service via cell phone. In some cases, such as overdoses, the patient is brought to the medical emergency room and later transferred for psychiatric evaluation. Otherwise the patient is transported directly to the psychiatric emergency service for further management if the issue cannot be settled in the community.

An approach has been developed to deliver 'at-home' treatment for psychiatric patients by a mobile crisis unit (Soreff, 1983; Tufnell *et al.*, 1985; Chiu and Primeau, 1991). This was designed as a formal 'mobile unit' to compensate for the fact that a tradition of psychiatric 'house calls' has never been popular in some settings. Home treatment is beneficial in engaging reluctant patients, strengthening the support network, working with the entire environment, collaborating with the family in therapy, dealing with the social service system and providing medication for non-responders to hospitalization. This mobile approach has even been adapted by the use of vans and good communication equipment to provide the benefits of the home visit approach to the homeless (Cohen *et al.*, 1984). The multi-disciplinary team approach has been the prevailing

model, with a psychiatrist, a psychiatric nurse and a social worker comprising the mobile unit. Units are only available when the mobile team members are working. Referrals come from phone calls to the mobile unit made by family members, neighbours, clergymen and assorted others. Hospitalization is usually regarded as a last resort, and treatment can be time limited or indefinite. One group has raised the question of whether a controlled study would be helpful to determine guidelines for how long such treatment should last and how effective it is (Chiu and Primeau, 1991).

A different level of care is involved in an 'outreach team'. In this case, the team sees a lower acuity patient than described above, but renders care to those who do not keep traditional clinic appointments or even use emergency room services. The team can help maintain the patient in the community and is well suited to providing care for less well served populations such as the homeless, the elderly and mentally ill substance abusers (Gillig *et al.*, 1990). This type of outreach lends itself as well to aftercare services for patients who are readmitted repeatedly because they discontinue their medication and relapse (Rubinstein, 1972). Another variant on this approach is the 'admission diversion team', which strives to provide psychotherapy, interim medication and support to connect the patient to social service and housing options. The team intervention is designed to be time limited, with treatment continuing in more standard out-patient settings. When housing is an issue, some teams assist in shelter placement and follow-up with regular shelter rounds to track the patients and provide supportive services. Emergency case management and provision for transportation to and from services can be part of the overall team responsibility. The variety of different types of mobile teams undoubtedly allows a wider and more diverse population to be served by the emergency mental health system.

Impact of managed care

Managed care has had a dramatic effect on delivery of psychiatric services. Most managed care is delivered through private insurance providers—health maintenance organizations, preferred provider organizations and health insurance companies contracting with outside managed care companies. The public entitlement health coverage is also increasingly adopting this model, sometimes contracting with private companies to manage the care or developing their own parallel systems (Stroup and Dorwart, 1995). The management of psychiatric care often is 'carved out' from general health care (Marshall, 1992). Managed care relies on gate-keeping, prior authorization of services, concurrent utilization review and constraints on choice of providers to attain its goal of cost-effective, high quality care. More sophisticated plans provide active case management services. Basic plans restrict admission to contracting hospitals and control utilization by requiring telephone authorization for services. The overall effect has been huge reductions in the use of in-patient psychiatric services and much closer monitoring of the treatment goals and time limits of out-patient treatment.

The relationship of managed care to emergency psychiatric services is complex. On the one hand, managed care borrows heavily from the emergency psychiatry model in devising its data collecting and triage services, while on the other hand the two systems can come into substantial conflict, since both exercise gate-keeping functions, but from different perspectives (Schuster, 1995). Managing care of the medically ill can result in 'dumping' of medically ill patients by redefining them as psychiatric emergencies (Lazarus, 1994). Deficits in managed care systems for the mentally ill can lead to overutilization of psychiatric hospitalization in emergencies (Fink and Dubin, 1991). One plan had no provision for out-patient psychiatric consultation, hiring only psychologists, social workers and bachelor's-level therapists to provide out-patient care to save money. The affiliated hospital was overwhelmed with admissions because all more difficult mentally ill patients and psychiatric emergencies were referred for immediate in-patient care. The existence of the managed care system can lead to discordance between where emergency care is sought and the resources of the managed care network (Lazarus,

1993). A suicidal patient may seek assistance at the nearest psychiatric emergency service, but the network may have an affiliation with an entirely different hospital, leading to what can be difficult negotiations concerning where the psychiatric care should be provided.

It is unclear whether managed care programmes lead to an increase or a decrease in the use of psychiatric emergency services. One expert maintains that the psychiatric emergency service has the potential to take on the major role in rationing treatment through managed care programmes (Hillard, 1994). These programmes may encourage expansion of emergency services to minimize use of more expensive systems of care such as in-patient hospitalization. However, many systems establish procedures such as 24-hour emergency hotlines to obtain referrals and approval of services to help their patients avoid use of psychiatric emergency care. The use of these services may short-cut the emergency service by providing rapid access to out-patient care or pre-approving an in-patient stay. The patient may be able to go directly to the in-patient unit or may come to the emergency service just for the admission paperwork.

The two systems can work in synergy. Thus, the existence of managed care has been a strong stimulus for the development of extended evaluation beds and mobile outreach to deal with acute situations while avoiding the use of more expensive systems of care such as in-patient hospitalization. Innovative emergency services such as definitive emergency treatment (Forster and King, 1994a,b) and use of the emergency service for an aftercare role in the recently discharged patient can facilitate the transition to out-patient services and shorten the length of treatment for many diagnoses. In the definitive treatment model, medications and psychotherapy are begun in the emergency service to shorten the total time needed to ameliorate the presenting problem. The existence of a managed care system can also make the referral work of an emergency room easier. It helps in obtaining more rapid appointments with private practitioners in the plan. Many plans utilize a case manager approach. The manager can become a potent ally of the emergency psychiatrist in finding services to maintain the patient in the community.

One study demonstrated that managed care patients do need to use psychiatric emergency services (Breslow *et al.*, 1996b). The impression was that the enrolled patients who do visit an emergency service may be less able to understand the network procedures of the managed care company or may be in too much of a crisis to use them. Many of the plan patients who used the emergency service were referred from medical emergency rooms after overdoses, and a substantial number were brought in by the mobile team or the police. The managed care patients who presented did constitute a more functional group than the non-managed care patients because they were the privately insured who were more likely to have current employment and intact families. Many received crisis services and subsequently were discharged. The contact time for managed care patients may be lengthened by the need to negotiate with the managed care system to obtain approval for hospitalization or out-patient services. Frequently this involves making many phone calls. A major concern is the instance when the two systems come to differing clinical conclusions and the emergency service feels that in-patient hospitalization is warranted, while the managed care reviewer denies approval for services. This may make the work of the emergency service especially difficult because the clinical and legal responsibility for the patient's care remains with the emergency service (Bitterman, 1994; Marder, 1997).

Substance abuse issues

Substance abuse appears to add the problems of disruptive, disinhibited, non-compliant behaviours to chronic mental illness, which then leads to frequent use of the psychiatric emergency service by chronically and persistently mentally ill patients (Barbee *et al.*, 1989). Additionally, individuals who are primary substance abusers often present to the psychiatric emergency service with psychotic or mood disturbances of either a transitory

or persistent nature (Helzer and Pryzbeck, 1988). A number of studies have demonstrated the potentiating effect of substance abuse and mental disorder, with two studies showing an incidence of about one-third of patients presenting to the emergency service (Atkinson, 1973; Szuster *et al.*, 1990a). Many are using alcohol and/or illegal drugs such as cocaine, cannabis, heroin, amphetamines and hallucinogens (Miller *et al.*, 1994).

The high prevalence of alcohol and substance abuse in those showing behavioural disturbance sufficient to mobilize community attention means that substance abuse should always be part of the differential diagnosis for a patient who presents to the emergency service. The underdiagnosis of psychoactive substance-induced organic mental disorders in emergency psychiatry has been documented (Szuster *et al.*, 1990b; Elangovan *et al.*, 1993). There are those who maintain that the purely substance-abusing population should not be treated in the psychiatric emergency setting, but this does not take into account that these patients are brought to the emergency service for the behavioural disturbances they display in the community. In addition, many of the mentally ill require use of emergency services because of problems with substance abuse.

The effects of intoxication, withdrawal and neuro-cognitive abnormalities secondary to substance use may be difficult to differentiate from primary psychiatric disorder when examining the patient in the acute state. The time course of symptomatology is crucial in making a proper diagnosis since the substance-related symptoms pass more quickly. Past history is an important guide as well. Since the substance-abusing patient may be a poor historian during a phase of acute intoxication or withdrawal, records of previous visits to the emergency service may be especially useful. Behavioural manifestations and physical signs of intoxication or withdrawal must be noted carefully because, with the limited information available, they may be the most reliable guides to the diagnosis (Currier *et al.*, 1995). Laboratory and breathalyser determinations supplement the clinical findings. Studies have shown that there are 'false-negative' patients where the interview and clinical assessment have failed to pick up current substance abuse, while the laboratory does reveal it (Wilkins *et al.*, 1991; Sanguineti and Samuel, 1993).

One of the most important uses of extended evaluation capacity and crisis hospitalization is to enable the emergency service to have sufficient time to observe the patient until the acute effects of substances of abuse have worn off. During this time, the emergency service will need to manage the effects of the acute intoxication or the withdrawal. Clear rules and communication by staff are important for the patient who may have some associated mental clouding or confusion. Provision of clean, quiet areas may also be helpful in aiding recovery. Behaviour management in the form of sedating medication or physical restraint is sometimes necessary to prevent the patient from harming himself or others. Mental status, physical condition and vital signs are monitored at frequent intervals by nursing staff. This is particularly important in the case of the alcohol-dependent patient who might slip into acute withdrawal, a potentially life-threatening medical emergency. This requires intensive support and may indicate rapid transfer to an acute care medical facility. Careful monitoring of vital signs and physical signs or withdrawal can prevent this since chlordiazepoxide or lorazepam can be administered to maintain the patient in a pre-withdrawal state until the risk of withdrawal has subsided. Caution must be used in the use of antipsychotics, particularly low potency agents, because of their seizure threshold-lowering effects, which may exacerbate withdrawal.

One study demonstrated that the acutely intoxicated and substance-abusing patients presenting to the psychiatric emergency service require more behaviour management and take more time to be evaluated in the emergency service. However, they have much reduced need for psychiatric hospitalization (Breslow *et al.*, 1996c). A method of approach is to wait until effects of intoxication are over (e.g. breathalyser alcohol determinations read zero) before conducting the psychiatric evaluation and deciding on disposition. What is found in many instances is that the acutely suicidal intoxicated patient may give up the suicidality on sobering up, enabling referral to more appropriate

alcohol and drug treatment facilities. This may help to avoid unnecessary hospitalization. It also indicates that a very important role of the psychiatric emergency service is to act as a 'filter' for the mental health system. The service can prevent waste of scarce in-patient and out-patient resources designated specifically for the mentally ill and it can enable triage of patients to the treatment system most specific to their needs.

Future directions

The psychiatric emergency service seems on first view to be a wonderful resource for psychiatric research, including clinical trials of the effectiveness of treatment alternatives, services research and outcomes studies (Thienhaus, 1995). The advantages are the size of the databases, how quickly data accumulate and how well collection of data fits in with normal emergency room data gathering. However, the nature of the emergency service with its emphasis on rapid diagnostic assessment, stabilization and disposition makes it difficult to control enough variables to carry out detailed studies in this setting. There are further problems of patient acuity, sampling problems, time constraints and resource constraints. The issue of patient consent is a particularly thorny one since the patient in crisis may by definition be unable to give informed consent. Many studies have appeared, but it has been difficult to be systematic. Services research, descriptive studies and studies of decision making have been well represented. More work must be done in the study of evaluation, treatments, substance abuse and special populations. There is a great need for creative approaches to using the strengths of the emergency service as a research setting, while compensating for the obvious weaknesses. This may enable us to move the field forward in finding what works and what does not work in emergency psychiatric intervention.

Emergency psychiatric services will continue to develop in the next decade or so along the lines already outlined. There will be an emphasis on separate and more comprehensive services with extended evaluation capacity and the ability to initiate more treatment options. There will be more demand for mobile outreach into the community as the benefits become more apparent. Managed care will have substantial impact on service delivery. The psychiatric emergency service will play an ever-growing role as the 'filter' for the mental health system with respect to the substance-abusing patient. Underserved populations such as children, the mentally retarded and the elderly will present in increasing numbers.

The emergency service has strong potential as a locus of education and research. Technology may begin to transform the emergency service with advances in communication, safety, computerized records and databases. Cell phones and fax machines have already enabled better communication with the mobile team, increased ability to obtain old records and better co-ordination of services. Cameras and computerized alarm systems have permitted better safety on the unit. The computerized record can serve as a prompt to the staff of all areas where information should be collected and, in a more sophisticated system, may even allow 'calling up' just the crucial information from the past records relating to past suicide episodes or violence towards others. The emergency service database can be a vital tool for tracking what transpires on the service to make improvements and research important questions about service delivery. In the future, it may be possible to integrate this database with other databases such as the pharmacy database to help make emergency medication decisions. Other databases could contribute by giving information on substance abuse history, criminal history and past history of high-risk behaviour. This ability to search and perhaps even combine databases collected in many diverse areas undoubtedly will raise some complex issues of consent and potential invasion of privacy which will necessitate development of regulatory mechanisms. These developments raise the possibility that the emergency psychiatrist of the future will have some wonderful new tools to perform the psychiatric evaluation, initiate treatment and manage risk for the community.

References

Atkinson, R.M. (1973) Importance of alcohol and drug abuse in psychiatric emergencies. *California Medicine*, 118, 1–4.

Barbee, J.G., Clark, P.D.and Crapanzano M.S. (1989) Alcohol and substance abuse among schizophrenic patients presenting to an emergency psychiatric service. *Journal of Nervous and Mental Disease*, 177, 400–407.

Barton, G.M. (1974) A hospital's political environment and its effect on the patient's admission. *Hospital and Community Psychiatry*, 25, 156–169.

Baxter, S., Chodorkoff, B. and Underhill, R. (1968) Psychiatric emergencies: dispositional determinants and the validity of the decision to admit. *American Journal of Psychiatry*, 124, 1542–1546.

Bell, G., Reinstein, D.Z., Rajiyah, G. and Rosser, R. (1991) Psychiatric screening of admissions to an accident and emergency ward. *British Journal of Psychiatry*, 158, 554–557.

Bengelsdorf, H. and Alden, D.C. (1987) A mobile crisis unit in the psychiatric emergency room. *Hospital and Community Psychiatry*, 38, 662–665.

Bitterman, R.A. (1994) Dealing with managed care under COBRA parts I and II. *Emergency Physician Legal Bulletin*, 7, numbers 4 and 5.

Blais, A. and Georges, J. (1969) Psychiatric emergencies in a general hospital outpatient department. *Canadian Psychiatric Association Journal*, 14, 123–133.

Breslow, R.E., Klinger, B.I. and Erickson, B.J. (1993) Crisis hospitalization on a psychiatric emergency service. *General Hospital Psychiatry*, 15, 307–315.

Breslow, R.E., Klinger, B.I. and Erickson, B.J. (1995) Crisis hospitalization in a psychiatric emergency service. *New Directions for Mental Health Services*, 67, 5–12.

Breslow, R.E., Klinger, B.I. and Erickson, B.J. (1996a) Trends in the psychiatric emergency service in the 1990's. *Emergency Psychiatry*, 2, 4.

Breslow, R.E., Klinger, B.I. and Erickson, B.J. (1996b) Characteristics of managed care patients in a psychiatric emergency service. *Psychiatric Services*, 47, 1259–1261.

Breslow, R.E., Klinger, B.I. and Erickson, B.J. (1996c) Acute intoxication and substance abuse among patients presenting to a psychiatric emergency service. *General Hospital Psychiatry*, 18, 183–191.

Breslow, R.E., Klinger, B.I. and Erickson, B.J. (1997) Time study of psychiatric emergency service evaluations. *General Hospital Psychiatry*, 19, 1–4.

Breslow, R.E., Klinger, B.I. and Erickson, B.J. (1999) The disruptive behavior disorders in the psychiatric emergency service. *General Hospital Psychiatry*, 21, 214–219.

Chiu, T.L. and Primeau, C. (1991) A psychiatric mobile crisis unit in New York City: description and assessment. *International Journal of Social Psychiatry*, 37, 251–258.

Cohen, N., Putnam, J. and Sullivan, A. (1984) The mentally ill homeless: isolation and adaptation. *Hospital and Community Psychiatry*, 35, 922–924.

Comstock, B. (1983) Psychiatric emergency intensive care. *Psychiatric Clinics of North America*, 6, 305–316.

Currier, G.W., Serper, M.R. and Allen, M.H. (1995) Diagnosing substance abuse in psychiatric emergency service patients. *New Directions for Mental Health Services*, 67, 57–63.

Elangovan, N., Berman, S. and Meinzer, A. (1993) Substance abuse among patients presenting at an inner-city psychiatric emergency room. *Hospital and Community Psychiatry*, 44, 782–784.

Fields, S. and Weisman, G.K. (1995) Crisis residential treatment: an alternative to hospitalization. *New Directions for Mental Health Services*, 67, 23–31.

Fink, P.J. and Dubin, W.R. (1991) No free lunch: limitations on psychiatric care in HMO's. *Hospital and Community Psychiatry*, 42, 363–365.

Fisher, W.H., Geller, J.L. and Wirth-Cauchon, J. (1990) Empirically assessing the impact of mobile crisis capacity on state hospital admissions. *Community Mental Health Journal*, 26, 245–253.

Forster, P. and King, J. (1994a) Definitive treatment of patients with severe mental disorder in an emergency service, part I. *Hospital and Community Psychiatry*, 45, 867–869.

Forster, P. and King, J. (1994b) Definitive treatment of patients with severe mental disorder in an emergency service, part II. *Hospital and Community Psychiatry*, 45, 1177–1178.

Geller, J.L., Fisher, W.H. and McDermeit, M. (1995) A national survey of mobile crisis services and their evaluation. *Psychiatric Services*, 46, 893–897.

Gerson, S. and Bassuk, E. (1980) Psychiatric emergencies: an overview. *American Journal of Psychiatry*, 137, 1–11.

Gillig, P.M. (1995) The spectrum of mobile outreach and its role in the emergency service. *New Directions for Mental Health Services*, 67, 13–21.

Gillig, P.M., Hillard, J.R., Bell, J., Combs, H.E., Martin, C. and Deddens, J.A. (1989) The psychiatric emergency service holding area: effect on utilization of inpatient resources. *American Journal of Psychiatry*, 146, 369–372.

Gillig, P.M., Dumaine, M. and Hillard, J.R. (1990) Whom do mobile crisis services serve? *Hospital and Community Psychiatry*, 41, 804–805.

Goss, M.E., Reed, J.I. and Reader, G.G. (1971) Time spent by patients in emergency room: survey at the New York Hospital. *New York State Journal of Medicine*, 71, 1243–1246.

Granovetter, B. (1975) The use of home visits to avoid hospitalization in a psychiatric case. *Hospital and Community Psychiatry*, 26, 645–646.

Hankoff, L.D., Mischorr, M.T. and Tomlinson, K.E. (1974) A program of crisis intervention in the emergency medical setting. *American Journal of Psychiatry*, 131, 47–50.

Helzer, J.D. and Pryzbeck, T.R. (1988) The co-occurrence of alcoholism with other psychiatric disorders in the general population and its impact on treatment. *Journal of Studies in Alcoholism*, 49, 219–224.

Hillard, J.R. (1994) The past and future of psychiatric emergency services in the U.S. *Hospital and Community Psychiatry*, 45, 541–543.

Hillard, J.R., Zitek, B. and Thienhaus, O.J. (1993) Residency training in emergency psychiatry. *Academic Psychiatry*, 17, 125–129.

Hu, S.C. (1993) Computerized monitoring of emergency department patient flow. *American Journal of Emergency Medicine*, 11, 8–11.

Hughes, D.H. (1993) Trends and treatment models in emergency psychiatry. *Hospital and Community Psychiatry*, 44, 927–928.

Ianzito, B.M., Fine, J., Sprague, B. and Pestana, J. (1978) Overnight admission for psychiatric emergencies. *Hospital and Community Psychiatry*, 29, 728–730.

Johnson, S. and Thornicroft, G. (1995) Emergency psychiatric services in England and Wales. *British Medical Journal*, 311, 287–288.

Lazarus, A. (1993) Managed competition and access to emergency psychiatric care. *Hospital and Community Psychiatry*, 44, 1134–1136.

Lazarus, A. (1994) Dumping psychiatric patients in the managed care sector. *Hospital and Community Psychiatry*, 45, 529–530.

Linn, L. (1971) Emergency room psychiatry: a gateway to community medicine. *Mount Sinai Journal of Medicine*, 38, 110–120.

Marder, D. (1997) Hospital policy: responding to COBRA. *Emergency Psychiatry*, 3, 31–33.

Marshall, P.E. (1992) The mental health HMO: capitation funding for the chronically mentally ill. *Community Mental Health Journal*, 28, 111–120.

McClelland, P.A. (1983) The emergency psychiatric system. *Psychiatric Clinics of North America*, 6, 225–232.

Merson, S., Tyrer, P., Onyett, S., Lack, S., Birkett, P., Lynch, S. and Johnson, T. (1992) Early intervention in psychiatric emergencies: a controlled clinical trial. *Lancet*, 339, 1311–1314.

Miller, N.S., Owley, T. and Eriksenn, A. (1994) Working with drug/alcohol addicted patients in crisis. *Psychiatric Annals*, 24, 592–597.

Munizza, C., Furlan, P., d'Elia, A. and D'Onofrio, M. (1993) Emergency psychiatry: a review of the literature. *Acta Psychiatrica Scandinavica*, 885, 1–51.

Oldham, J.M. and DeMasi, M.E. (1995) An integrated approach to emergency psychiatric care. *New Directions for Mental Health Services*, 67, 33–42.

Oldham, J.M., Lin, A. and Breslin, L. (1990) Comprehensive psychiatric emergency services. *Psychiatric Quarterly*, 61, 57–66.

Rhine, M.W. and Mayerson, P. (1971) Crisis hospitalization within a psychiatric emergency service. *American Journal of Psychiatry*, 127, 1386–1391.

Rubinstein, D. (1972) Re-hospitalization versus family crisis intervention. *American Journal of Psychiatry*, 129, 715–720.

Ruiz, P., Vazquez, W. and Vazquez, K. (1973) The mobile unit: a new approach in mental health. *Community Mental Health Journal*, 9, 18–24.

Sanguineti, V.R. and Samuel, S.E. (1993) Reported prevalence of drug abuse comorbidity in a city-wide emergency room system. *American Journal of Drug and Alcohol Abuse*, 19, 443–450.

Saunders, C.E. (1987) Time study of patient movement through the emergency department: sources of delay in relation to patient acuity. *Annals of Emergency Medicine*, 16, 1244–1248.

Schuster, J.M. (1995) Frustration or opportunity? The impact of managed care on emergency psychiatry. *New Directions for Mental Health Services*, 67, 101–108.

Slaby, A.E. (1981) Emergency psychiatry: an update. *Hospital and Community Psychiatry*, 32, 687–688.

Soreff, S. (1983) New directions and added dimensions in home psychiatric treatment. *American Journal of Psychiatry*, 140, 1213–1216.

Stebbins, L.A. and Hardman, G.L. (1993) A survey of psychiatric consultants at a suburban emergency room. *General Hospital Psychiatry*, 15, 234–242.

Stroul, B.A. (1988) Residential crisis services: a review. *Hospital and Community Psychiatry*, 39, 1095–1099.

Stroup, T.S. and Dorwart, R.A. (1995) The impact of a managed mental health program on medicaid recipients with severe mental illness. *Psychiatric Services*, 46, 885–889.

Surles, R.C., Petrila, J. and Evans, M.E. (1994) Redesigning emergency room psychiatry in New York. *Administration and Policy in Mental Health*, 22, 97–104.

Szuster, R.R., Schanbacher, B.L. and McCann, S.C. (1990a) Characteristics of psychiatric emergency room patients with alcohol or drug-induced disorders. *Hospital and Community Psychiatry*, 41, 1342–1345.

Szuster, R.R., Schanbacher, B.L. and McCann, S.C. (1990b) Underdiagnosis of psychoactive substance induced organic mental disorders in emergency psychiatry. *American Journal of Drug and Alcohol Abuse*, 16, 319–327.

Thienhaus, O.J. (1995) Academic issues in emergency psychiatry. *New Directions for Mental Health Services*, 67, 109–114.

Thienhaus, O.J., Ford, J. and Hillard, J.R. (1995) Factors related to patients' decisions to visit the psychiatric emergency service. *Psychiatric Services*, 46, 1227–1228.

Tufnell, G., Bouras, N., Watson, J. and Brough, D. (1985) Home assessment and treatment in a community psychiatric service. *Acta Psychiatrica Scandinavica*, 72, 20–28.

Walker, W.R., Parsons, L.B. and Skelton, W.D. (1973) Brief hospitalization on a crisis service: a study of patient and treatment variables. *American Journal of Psychiatry*, 130, 896–900.

Way, B.B., Evans, M.E. and Banks, S.M. (1992) Factors predicting referral to inpatient or outpatient treatment from psychiatric emergency services. *Hospital and Community Psychiatry*, 43, 703–708.

Weisman, G., Feirstein, A. and Thomas, C. (1969) Three-day hospitalization: a model for intervention. *Archives of General Psychiatry*, 21, 620–629.

Wellin, E., Slesinger, D.P. and Hollister, C.D. (1987) Psychiatric emergency services: evolution, adaptation and proliferation. *Social Science and Medicine*, 24, 475–482.

West, D.A., Litwok, E. and Oberlander, K. (1980) Emergency psychiatric home visiting: report of four years' experience. *Journal of Clinical Psychiatry*, 41, 113–118.

Wilkins, J.N., Shaner, A.L., Patterson, C.M., Seruda, D. and Gorelick, D. (1991) Discrepancies between patient report, clinical assessment and urine analysis in psychiatric patients presenting during inpatient admission. *Psychopharmacology Bulletin*, 27, 149–154.

24 | *Out-patient psychiatric services*
Thomas Becker

Introduction

Specialist psychiatric out-patient services are not discussed in many current comprehensive accounts of community mental health care (e.g. Shepherd, 1998), and there are no previous reviews of studies evaluating psychiatric out-patient clinics. In spite of this low profile in the literature, they constitute a standard component of most community mental health care systems, and have long been considered an important element in professional training and psychiatric practice. In some mental health care systems which are not part of a national, taxation-funded health service, out-patient care is provided by office-based psychiatrists. Thus, most of out-patient psychiatric care in Germany, for example, is provided by office-based psychiatrists (who are often both psychiatrists and neurologists; 'niedergelassene Nervenärzte') . This chapter reviews the relevant research on the nature and outcomes of out-patient psychiatric care.

Historical development

In the UK, out-patient mental health care was offered by some asylum psychiatrists in the 19th century. They described the importance of continuity of care for those with long-term mental illness. Initiating out-patient psychiatric clinics was an important step in 20th century mental health care reform, which started in the 1930s and continued to be a key element in the process of reform of mental hospitals in England during the 1930s through to the 1960s (Freeman and Bennett, 1991).

Functions of out-patient services

Psychiatric out-patient clinics have been a standard service provided for a long time, but there is little evidence regarding their efficacy or effectiveness. In a comparative cross-national study in Scandinavian countries, an eightfold variation in out-patient service use was found (Hansson *et al.*, 1998). In a study in Ireland, attendances at psychiatric out-patient services over a 3-year period were analysed retrospectively, and a new episode attendance rate of 3.7/1000 population per year was shown. The area adult attendance rate was 3.1/1000 population per year, and 90% of patients were referred by GPs. The predominant diagnosis was affective psychosis followed by neuroses. Group practices tended to make fewer referrals to psychiatric out-patient services, and there was a significant tendency for GPs with vocational or psychiatric training to make more referrals (which suggests difficulties in identifying mental disorders). Other studies have shown that referrals to psychiatric clinics in primary care settings are higher than to hospital-based clinics (Cooper *et al.*, 1992).

International variations

The German mental health care system has office-based psychiatrists throughout the country who provide out-patient clinics. This is part of an insurance-based health care system with much weaker secondary, hospital-based out-patient services. Office-based psychiatrists used to be single-handed, but now increasingly tend to be in joint practices of at least two (neurologists and) psychiatrists (Rössler and Salize, 1996). With virtually every citizen having health insurance in

Germany, office-based psychiatrists provide free services with unrestricted physician choice by patients. However, both psychiatric and neurological out-patient clinics are held in these practices. Psychiatrists working exclusively in private practice are very rare. From 1980 to 1993, the number of office-based (neuro-) psychiatrists increased from about 1480 to 4145, and there is now a ratio of about one psychiatrist per 17 500 population (Rössler and Salize, 1996).

Dittmann *et al.* (1997) assessed antidepressant drug use by GPs/internists and psychiatrists/neurologists in Germany, and patients of the latter presented with more severe depression and more suicidality, required more medication and showed with poorer outcomes. This supports the view that there is some selection, with the more severely ill usually treated by specialists. In Germany, there are also community mental health-type services (Institutsambulanzen, Sozialpsychiatrische Dienste) which aim to meet the needs of those with severe mental illness who have difficulty in attending out-patient clinics at office-based practices. In the East part of the country, psychiatric polyclinics (Polikliniken, Dispensaires) have (with a very few exceptions such as Leipzig) not survived reunification, but have been closed and superseded by a network of office-based psychiatrists. The loss of this service component has been felt by some to have negative effects on care for the severely mentally ill, but new community-type services have attempted to take over their role (Bundesminister für Gesundheit, 1991).

What is the service context for out-patient services?

Specialist psychiatric out-patient services are a key service component for those less severely ill, with fewer needs in domains other than symptoms/medication, or for those without symptoms who are socially disruptive. However, this focus in service delivery may conflict with the aim of community services targeting those patients who are most severely and chronically ill. Siddique and Aubry (1997), in a study of 7220 admissions to three community mental health centres in semi-rural Canada, found patients presenting with problems related to marital relationships, family circumstances, interpersonal relationships, or stressful life events not attributable to a mental disorder (DSM-III-R V-code conditions) to represent one-third of psychiatric out-patient admissions. These patients consumed treatment resources comparable with those needed by patients with mental disorders, and they were evaluated by their therapists as experiencing similar levels of improvement in the course of treatment (Siddique and Aubry, 1997).

There is some evidence of both intensive out-patient services and intensive case management (ICM) increasing service utilization as patients formerly not seen by specialist mental health services are seen in such out-patient service settings (Ford *et al*, 1997); this effect may offset any cost saving due to a reduction of bed days (an der Heiden, 1996). In the ICM study, clients receiving this type of case management received more psychiatric out-patient, primary health, residential and social services care, in addition to high levels of input from case managers (Ford *et al.*, 1997).

Does out-patient care need to be linked to other elements?

A cross-national Scandinavian study which investigated the likelihood of aftercare following hospitalization found such follow-up to be more probable if the out-patient services were located geographically close to the patients, if hospitalization lasted between 2 and 4 weeks, if there was a community care contact shortly before hospital admission and if the patient was not retired or not divorced (Saarento *et al.*, 1998b). Out-patient services appear to be important for the overall performance of the mental health care system. Thus, a lack of 24-hour emergency settings, in the Nordic Comparative Study on Sectorized Psychiatry, was found to correlate positively with the use of in-patient care alone (Saarento *et al.*, 1998a). This indicates that having extended availability of out-patient services in the community for people in crisis may facilitate comprehensive utilization of mental health services.

How difficult is it to establish out-patient services?

Out-patient services are to be found in most current mental health care systems in economically developed countries. The trend in contemporary community mental health care may be to reduce traditional out-patient clinics as some studies have indicated that out-patient service provision by community mental health teams is more successful (Goldberg *et al.*, 1996; Lehman *et al.*, 1997). However, out-patient clinics are considered a key component of care by many community mental health teams. Out-patient clinics can be held in community mental health centres, and so community teams can provide single-handed out-patient care for patients who do not need multi-disciplinary team input, and multi-disciplinary care during crises and for people with multiple needs.

Evaluation of out-patient services

There are randomized controlled trials (RCTs) relevant to the topic. In a controlled intervention study of the management of non-compliance with referral to out-patient aftercare among attempted suicide patients in Gent, Belgium, patients in the experimental group were visited in their homes by a community nurse in order to assess reasons for non-compliance and to motivate patients to comply with referral (van Heeringen *et al.*, 1995). At 1-year follow-up, a significant beneficial effect of the intervention on compliance with referral was found, and there was a near-significant effect on the rate of repetition of suicidal behaviour (11% in the intervention group versus 17% in the control group). The authors argued that future research of this kind should best be conducted with a more carefully focused intervention with step-by-step guidelines for the intervening nurses (van Heeringen *et al.*, 1995).

In a further RCT (Spooren *et al.*, 1998), the same group assessed the effect of a combination of several strategies (fixed appointment, family involvement, presence of aftercare person and motivational counselling) on referral compliance and continuity of aftercare in patients referred to three general hospital psychiatric emergency clinics. They found a beneficial effect on referral compliance in two and a near-significant effect in the third centre. The effect on adherence to treatment persisted for 3 months in two out of three services.

There is some evidence that drug refusal (non-compliance) in the community is managed mostly by community keyworkers, and without recourse to the Mental Health Act in the UK (Macpherson *et al.*, 1998). This might help in understanding both the success of interventions such as the above and the difficulties of traditional out-patient clinics in addressing the issue. Tyrer *et al.* (1998), in an RCT in London, compared the clinical outcome and costs of care of psychiatric patients allocated to community multi-disciplinary teams or to hospital-based out-patient care programmes after discharge from in-patient care. The clinical outcomes were similar, but admission to hospital during follow-up was more likely in the hospital-based care group.

Is there any other evidence supporting its effectiveness?

Psychiatric out-patient clinics in general practice (Strathdee and Williams, 1984) have been termed the 'shifted out-patient clinic' by Tyrer (1984). Visiting psychiatrists operate clinics within health centres and see both new and follow-up patients. Treatment is independent of the GP, and the shifted out-patient clinic has much in common with a hospital-based out-patient service (Gask *et al.*, 1997). Psychiatric out-patient clinics in general practice were found to lead to a 20% reduction in admission rate (Tyrer *et al.*, 1984).

Goldberg *et al.* (1996) compared a community team based in primary care with a traditional hospital-based service in the care offered to people with common mental disorders (anxiety and depression). Non-urgent cases were seen more quickly in the community although the response time of each service was prompt with cases rated as urgent. Only 45% of the patients seen by the community team saw a psychiatrist for out-patient appointments, with a further 29.5% seeing a psychologist, whereas all the controls saw one or the other. The community service offered fewer changes of staff without therapeutic advantage to the patient (e.g. seeing another junior doctor because of the training rotation). Patients in the community were more likely to have been visited at home, and they were significantly more satisfied with the service on nine separate aspects of satisfaction. Patients of the hospital-based service more frequently had failed to attend for an out-patient appointment because of problems with the journey. Overall performance favoured the primary care-based community team (with no overall cost advantage due to more patients seen), and satisfaction was higher. However, data analysis did not focus on comparing types of out-patient contact specifically.

Lehman *et al.* (1997), in a randomized trial of assertive community treatment (ACT) for homeless persons with severe mental illness, reported subjects in the ACT programme using more psychiatric out-patient visits than the comparison subjects in usual community services. Thus, intensive community treatment is likely to foster out-patient service attendance.

Summarizing the research literature

Psychiatric out-patient services provide a key element of community mental health care although they consume only a small proportion of the cost of care for people with serious mental illness. Ford *et al.* (1997) found the proportion to be about 1%. There is some evidence that out-patient service contacts help to establish and maintain continuity of care. Community-based teams may be better equipped to ensure attendance at out-patient appointments. There are innovative interventions to ensure out-patient attendance following suicide attempts and emergency clinic contacts. Current evidence and practice favour the integration of out-patient clinics as a service provided by comprehensive community mental health teams.

It is important, in this context, to see that service users/patients focus on social issues, and give positive ratings of help provided by non-professional community support workers when they assess community care (Shepherd *et al.*, 1995; Murray and Shepherd, 1996). At the other end of the spectrum of interventions for people with severe mental illness, traditional out-patient clinics provide a professional service focused on a one-to-one therapeutic relationship, psychotherapy and/or pharmacotherapy. The difficulties that community care is facing may be related, among other factors, to the quality of therapeutic face-to-face contact. Therapeutic relationships of the kind offered in traditional out-patient clinics may, therefore, contribute substantially to the success of community intervention programmes.

Conclusions

What is the place of the out-patient component in psychiatric services?

Psychiatric out-patient clinics are a standard service component, but they are not very well researched. There is now a focus on the fidelity to treatment interventions and on what makes an intervention work (Becker and Thornicroft, 1998). In this perspective, we can expect renewed interest in out-patient clinics, the type of face-to-face contact they offer, the interventions which are being discussed with patients and what makes them work.

The effectiveness of out-patient services is related both to the treatment package offered and to the working alliance between the individual user/patient and professional. Research methodology, in this field, is deficient in some studies. Dowdney *et al.* (1993), in analysing influences upon attendance at child guidance clinics, have pointed out that inadequate statistical procedures may hamper the detection of influences upon attendance at out-patient facilities. Siddique and Aubry (1997), in a study of patients with conditions other than a diagnosable DSM-III R mental disorder on the caseloads of Canadian community mental health centres (CMHCs), argue that in order to target interventions adequately, professional time could be allocated according to some criterion of the severity of presenting problems. CMHCs would thus provide limited out-patient treatment or refer patients with non-specific 'problems in living' or life crises to appropriate outside services upon initial assessment. This strategy would enable CMHCs to devote most of their treatment resources to patients with serious mental disorders. The allocation of service interventions according to the severity of presenting problems would serve as the guiding principle, and alternative services which people might be referred to would include self-help groups, psychoeducational programmes and self-help books, using out-patient care for those with serious, but not the most serious, forms of mental illness.

References

an der Heiden, W. (1996) Do outpatient measures reduce inpatient treatment? *Gesundheitswesen*, 58, 38–43.

Becker, T. and Thornicroft, G. (1998) Community care and management of schizophrenia. *Current Opinion in Psychiatry*, 11, 49–54.

Bundesminister für Gesundheit (1991) Zur Lage der Psychiatrie in der ehemagaligen DDR – Bestandsaufnahme und Empfehlungen. Gutachten. Bonn: Bundesministerium für Gesundheit.

Cooper, S.J., Gilliland, A. *et al.* (1992) Primary care based psychiatric clinics: observations on a one year cohort of referrals. *Irish Journal of Psychological Medicine*, 9, 13–16.

Dittmann, R.W., Linden, M., Osterheider, M., Schaaf, B., Ohnmacht, U. and Weber, H.J. (1997) Antidepressant drug use: differences between psychiatrists and general practitioners. Results from a drug utilization observation study with fluoxetine. *Pharmacopsychiatry*, 30 (Suppl. 1), 28–34.

Dowdney, L, Rogers, C. and Dunn, G. (1993) Influences upon attendances at out-patient facilities—the contribution of linear-logistic modelling. *Psychological Medicine*, 23, 195–201.

Ford, R., Raftery, J., Ryan, P., Beadsmoore, A., Craig, T. and Muijen, M. (1997) Intensive case management for people with serious mental illness—site 2: cost-effectiveness. *Journal of Mental Health*, 6, 191–199.

Freeman, H. and Bennett, D.H. (1991) Origins and development. In: Bennett, D.H. and Freeman, H.L. (eds),*Community Psychiatry*. Edinburgh: Churchill Livingstone, pp. 40–70.

Gask, L., Sibbald, B. and Creed, F. (1997) Evaluating models of working at the interface between mental health services and primary care. *British Journal of Psychiatry*, 170, 6–11.

Goldberg, D., Jackson, G., Gater, R., Campbell, M. and Jennett, N. (1996) The treatment of common mental disorders by a community team based in primary care: a cost-effectiveness study. *Psychological Medicine*, 26, 487–492.

Hansson, L., Muus, S., Vinding, H.R., Göstas, G., Saarento, O., Sandlund, M. *et al.* (1998) The Nordic Comparative Study on Sectorized Psychiatry: contact rates and use of services for patients with a functional psychosis. *Acta Psychiatrica Scandinavica*, 97, 315–320.

Lehman, A.F., Dixon, L.B., Kernan, E., DeForge, B.R. and Postrado, L.T. (1997) A randomized trial of assertive community treatment for homeless persons with severe mental illness. *Archives of General Psychiatry*, 54, 1038–1043.

Macpherson, R., Alexander, M. and Jerrom, W. (1998) Medication refusal among patients treated in a community mental health rehabilitation service. *Psychiatric Bulletin*, 22, 744–748.

Murray, A. and Shepherd, G. (1996) Support workers. Suspicious minds. *Health Services Journal*, 106, 27.

Rössler, W. and Salize, H.J. (1996) *Die psychiatrische Versorgung chronisch psychisch Kranker—Daten, Fakten, Analysen*. Schriftenreihe des Bundesministeriums für Gesundheit, Band 77. Baden-Baden: Nomos.

Saarento, O., Kastrup, M., Lönnerberg, O., Göstas, G., Muus, S., Sandlund, M. *et al.* (1998a) The Nordic Comparative Study on Sectorized Psychiatry: patients who use only psychiatric in-patient care in comprehensive community-based services—a 1-year follow-up study. *Acta Psychiatrica Scandinavica*, 98, 98–104.

Saarento, O., Öiesvold, T., Sytema, S., Göstas, G., Kastrup, M., Lönnerberg, O. *et al.* (1998b). The Nordic Comparative Study on Sectorized Psychiatry: continuity of care related to characeristics of the psychiatric services and the patients. *Social Psychiatry and Psychiatric Epidemiology*, 33, 521–527.

Shepherd, G. (1998) Models of community care. *Journal of Mental Health*, 7, 165–177.

Shepherd, G., Murray, A. and Muijen, M. (1995) Perspectives on schizophrenia: a survey of user, family carer and professional views regarding effective care. *Journal of Mental Health*, 4, 403–422.

Siddique, C.M. and Aubry, T. (1997) Use of mental health resources in the treatment of adult out-patients with no diagnosable mental disorders. *Acta Psychiatrica Scandinavica*, 95, 19–25.

Spooren, D., van Heeringen, C. and Jannes, C. (1998) Strategies to increase compliance with out-patient aftercare among patients referred to a psychiatric emergency department: a multi-centre controlled intervention study. *Psychological Medicine*, 28, 949–956.

Strathdee, G. and Williams, P. (1984) A survey of psychiatrists in primary care: the silent growth of a new service. *Journal of the Royal College of General Practitioners*, 34, 615–618.

Tyrer, P. (1984) Psychiatric clinic in general practice: an extension of community care. *British Journal of Psychiatry*, 145, 9–14.

Tyrer, P., Sievewright, N. and Wollerton, S. (1984) General practice psychiatric clinics, impact on psychiatric services. *British Journal of Psychiatry*, 145, 15–19.

Tyrer, P., Evans, K., Gandhi, N., Lamont, A., Harrison-Read, P. and Johnson, T. (1998) Randomised controlled trial of two models of care for discharged psychiatric patients. *British Medical Journal*, 316, 106–109.

Van Heeringen, C., Jannes, S., Buylaert, W., Henderick, H., De Bacquer, D. and van Remoortel, J. (1995) The management of non-compliance with referral to out-patient after-care among attempted suicide patients: a controlled intervention study. *Psychological Medicine*, 25, 963–970.

25 | *Partial hospitalization*

Aart H. Schene

Introduction

Partial hospitalization (PH) as a treatment modality for psychiatric disorders has evolved over more than 50 years. In terms of treatment intensity, PH aims to fill the wide gap between in-patient or full-time hospitalization (FTH) on the one hand and out-patient or community mental health care on the other. As a part of the comprehensive psychiatric services, PH has the potential for patients, carers and professional staff to offer more than low frequency out-patient visits while at the same time it prevents the disadvantages of a hospital admission.

Although PH has come of age during the last decades, there are still many questions with regard to its current status and future development. In this chapter, I discuss some main issues: history, development, conceptual issues and definition, different types of PH programmes, effectiveness of PH in comparison with FTH and out-patient treatment, cost-effectiveness, selection criteria, treatment models and therapeutic factors. In the last paragraph, I discuss the place of this component in the total of psychiatric services.

History

The history of PH goes back to the 1930s. Shortage of money urged Dzhagarov (1937) in 1932 in Moscow to open a hospital without beds. Next, Adams House started in Boston in 1935 and, in the UK, Lady Chichester Hospital in Hove was first in 1938. After the Second World War, PH at first saw a slow development: Marlborough Day Hospital in London (1946), Allan Memorial Institute in Montreal (1946), Yale University Clinic (1948), Menninger Clinic (1949), Bristol Day Hospital (1951), Massachusetts Mental Health Center (1952) and the Maudsley Day Hospital (1953).

The two pioneers of PH, Bierer and Cameron, deserve mention. Bierer (1951) initiated a Social Psychotherapy Centre (later the Marlborough Day Hospital) in London in 1946. In his view, the day hospital was the predecessor of the era of social psychiatry. Later, he described the day hospital as an independent treatment centre with preventive, out-patient and temporary in-patient services (Bierer, 1961). In his view, the day hospital was based on the principles of the therapeutic community and was to function independently of the hospital. The main focus was to keep patients in contact with their normal living environment.

Cameron (1947) introduced the term day hospital in 1946 when he opened such a service as part of the Allan Memorial Institute of Psychiatry, being part of a large general hospital. Cameron described it as an extension of and addition to FTH. In comparison with Bierer, whose ideas very much resemble the later philosophy of the US Community Mental Health Centers, Cameron had a more medical view of psychiatry. Without knowing it, these two pioneers represented two distinct visions of the later development of PH, namely that of the day hospital and day treatment.

Further development of PH differed greatly between different countries. For the UK, Farndale (1961) described the rapid increase of day hospital settings in the late 1950s as a 'day hospital movement'. Between 1959 and 1979, the number of day hospitals increased from 58 to 303 (Brocklehurst, 1979). 'Better Services for the Mentally Ill' (1975) had mentioned a ratio of day hospital places of 30 per 100 000 and of day centre places of 60 per 100 000. Between 1974 and 1982, day hospital places rose from 9400 to 15 300, a short-fall of 1200 in comparison with the 1975 targets. For day care centres, the rise in that period was from 3600 to 5000, a shortfall of 28 000.

The USA saw the growth of PH in the 1960s mainly as a result of the 1963 Community Mental Health Center Construction Act, while countries such as The Netherlands and Germany started to develop PH as late as the 1970s and 1980s (Bosch and Veltin, 1983; Schene, 1985; Schene *et al.*, 1986). Dutch figures, for instance, show a rise of day hospital places from 100 in 1965, to 1400 in 1980, and to 3700 in 1996. In 1996, about 16 500 patients were treated. Day care services rose from 12 in 1987 to 170 in 1996. About 13 000 long-term patients were using these services in 1996.

Development and further growth

During its first decades, the development of PH was initiated and stimulated by different motives. First, the post-war period saw a growing optimism about the possibilities of treating mental disorders, not only by biological methods but also by individual and group psychotherapeutic techniques as well as occupational, family and social psychiatric methods. Secondly, PH pioneers saw the hospital setting with its strong boundaries against the outside world as a less adequate structure in which to use these new type of treatments. Thirdly, during the 1960s, it became clear that PH could have an important and specific role in the run-down of large mental hospitals and in the further development of community-oriented psychiatry. Finally, effectiveness studies such as those of Kris (1960), Zwerling and Wilder (1962), Meltzhoff and Blumenthal (1966) and Herz *et al.* (1971) contributed to scientific support of this new type of treatment and gradually decreased the prejudices of hospital-oriented clinicians and other staff.

Comparison with in-patient and out-patient services

To understand its inherent characteristics and qualities, PH should be compared with in-patient and out-patient services. In comparison with in-patient services, PH has the advantages that the disruption to life's normal routine (finances, housemaking, social contacts, hobbies, etc.) is less pronounced. Making the patient the scapegoat is less severe, as is the rejection by family members and other relatives. Contact with children and partner can be continued. Daily interaction with the outside world gives the patient good opportunities to develop skills and to generalize those from the therapeutic environment to the normal living situation (Dibella *et al.*, 1982; Schene, 1985; Piper *et al.*, 1996).

There is also a constant interplay in the way in which the patient and family or support system interact with each other. Because patients have to travel each day, they expect to obtain an active treatment and not just to hang around. The change from in-patient to PH to out-patient can be more gradual. PH is accepted more easily by patients and carers, providing the opportunity to intervene at an earlier stage of the illness or decompensation. The therapeutic climate provides less opportunities for regression, stimulates healthy behaviour and produces less loss of self-esteem (Davidson *et al.*, 1996). Stigmatization of patients might be lower as well as costs.

The disadvantages of PH, in comparison with FTH, for patients are the daily travelling, the fact that they get less structure, support and care, and mostly have no 24-hour availability of staff. They do not have the opportunity to be free of family contacts for a period of time, which in certain cases can be healing. For professionals, the control of aggression and other disturbing behaviours is less easy and therefore more distressing. They have to decide each day anew if patients can go home. Involuntary admissions are not possible.

In comparison with out-patient treatment, PH has the advantage of providing more intensive, more differentiated and mostly multi-disciplinary treatment. Medical diagnostics, assessments, observations and certain therapeutics are given more easily. PH also provides more structure, more support and more contact, and learning opportunities with other patients or consumers. The disadvantages of PH in comparison with out-patient treatment are more stigmatization, more opportunity for regression and pathological behaviour, and more travelling.

Definition

The Task Force on Partial Hospitalization of the American Psychiatric Association (Casarino *et al.*, 1982) was first to define PH as an ambulatory treatment programme that includes the major diagnostic, medical, psychiatric, psychosocial and pre-vocational treatment modalities, designed for patients with serious mental disorders, who require co-ordinated intensive, comprehensive and multi-disciplinary treatment not provided in an out-patient setting.

DiBella *et al.* (1982) defined psychiatric PH more quantitatively as a psychiatric treatment programme of eight or more waking hours per week, designed for improvement of a group of six or more ambulatory patients, provided by two or more multi-disciplinary clinical staff, and consisting of carefully co-ordinated, multi-modality interconnected therapies within a therapeutic milieu. Patients participate regularly in the entire programme, which almost always occurs during at least 2 days per week for at least 3 weeks, with most of the treatment periods of at least 3 hours but less than 24 hours.

Later Block and Lefkovitz (1991) restricted the definition of PH to a time-limited, ambulatory, active treatment programme that offers therapeutically intensive, co-ordinated and structured clinical services within a stable therapeutic milieu. Programmes are designed to serve individuals with significant impairment resulting from a psychiatric, emotional or behavioural disorder. PH is a general term embracing day, evening, night and weekend treatment programmes which employ an integrated, comprehensive schedule of recognized treatment approaches.

Typology of partial hospitalization

In the field of PH, an amalgam of terms and terminology is being used, including day services, day hospital, partial hospital, day centres, day treatment, day care and partial hospitalization. This multitude of terms becomes even more confusing when we realize that in different countries these terms have different meanings. Moreover, the terminology often is employed incorrectly or haphazardly. The confusion has to do with the wish to categorize and characterize PH services for which many criteria could be used, such as target population, type of treatment, duration of treatment or care, staff composition, organizational structure and connection with other mental health services, etc.

Looking at specific target populations (Farndale, 1961), we can distinguish age groups (young children, adolescents, adults, old people), diagnostic categories (Rosie *et al.*, 1995; Bystritsky *et al.*, 1996; Lussier *et al.*, 1997) or combinations such as elderly and infirm old people, mentally defective patients, handicapped persons, young patients with schizophrenia and others.

Considering the connection with the mother institution, we find services that are freestanding and organizationally independent, freestanding but organizationally connected with other mental health services, freestanding on the terrain of a psychiatric or general hospital, units where patients use the same facilities as in-patients, and PH integrated on a psychiatric unit, which also contains in-patient and out-patient services.

In organizational terms, PH services can be connected to the long-term treatment system, to the intensive treatment system and to the District Mental Health Plan. Considering the time of day, a distinction between day treatment, evening treatment, evening and night treatment and week-end treatment can be made (DiBella *et al.*, 1982; Schene 1985; De Hert *et al.*, 1996).

With regard to programmes, we can distinguish short-term, medium-term and long-term services. The therapeutic orientation can be medical psychiatric, psychotherapeutic or rehabilitative. PH has to be distinguished from psychosocial rehabilitation programmes (self-help houses,

Fountain House, therapeutic social clubs and lounge programmes).

Four functions of partial hospitalization

In the UK, a distinction is made between day hospitals and day centres. Day hospitals offer (i) active treatment, including medication and a range of professional interventions (psychological, social, occupational), aimed at people who need more intensive treatment than could be given on an out-patient basis, or (ii) rehabilitation for those for whom day care is a step in the transition process from in-patient treatment towards the community (Shepherd, 1991). Day centres, on the other hand, meet clients' long-term needs for support and social contact, assisting them in adjusting or re-adjusting to the demands of work and trying to relieve the strain on the family.

In the USA, a distinction is made between day hospital, day treatment and day care (Rosie, 1987) as well as between intensive care model, rehabilitation model and chronic care model (Klar *et al.*, 1982). The day hospital/intensive care model provides diagnostic and treatment services for acutely ill patients who would otherwise be treated in traditional psychiatric in-patient units. The typical length of stay is between 4 and 8 weeks.

The day treatment programme/rehabilitation model provides an alternative to out-patient care for patients who have severe impairments in vocational or social performance. These programmes strive for symptom reduction and improved functioning, and have a length of stay of between 3 and 12 months.

The day care centre/chronic care model is indicated for patients who would otherwise require custodial care, for patients who might deteriorate in the community and for patients who require regular treatment but cannot tolerate a more active treatment programme. It has modest expectations of patient improvement, high symptom tolerance and a supportive, practical treatment approach. It offers maintenance care and social programming for individuals who require daily

structure and supervision to prevent relapse. The length of stay is more than 1 year.

Trying to summarize and integrate these classifications, Schene *et al.* (1988) described PH in terms of the distinct functions it could fulfil in the total mental health care system and distinguished:

- alternative to acute in-patient: a medically oriented staff with a high staff:patient ratio offers PH in or close to a general hospital for patients with acute illnesses who would otherwise be treated as in-patients,

- continuation of acute in-patient: transition to out-patient care can be organized on or close to the in-patient unit; staff, patients and treatment resemble those of the first function,

- extension to out-patient care: either for specialized intensive treatment or rehabilitation for patients who do not require in-patient care but who benefit from more intensive care than is possible on an out-patient basis,

- day care or rehabilitation: long-term maintenance or rehabilitation of patients with chronic, debilitating mental disorders.

Evaluative research

The main questions researchers have tried to answer considered the (cost-) effectiveness of PH in comparison with FTH as well as with out-patient treatment. The evaluative research on PH has been reviewed extensively (Herz, 1982; Mason *et al.*, 1982; Schene and Gersons, 1986; Rosie, 1987; Creed *et al.*, 1989a; Tantam and McGrath, 1989; Parker and Knoll, 1990).

Effectiveness of partial versus full-time hospitalization

Acute day hospital treatment as an alternative for in-patient treatment has been studied in randomized controlled trials (RCTs) in the USA (Zwerling and Wilder, 1962, 1964; Herz *et al.*, 1971; Washburn *et al.*, 1976; Sledge *et al.*, 1996), the UK (Dick *et al.*, 1985a,b; Creed *et al.*, 1989b,

1990) and The Netherlands (Kluiter *et al.*, 1992; Schene *et al.*, 1993). Three non-randomized controlled trials give some additional information (Michaux *et al.*, 1972; Fink *et al.*, 1978; Penk *et al.*, 1978).

The aim of most studies was to randomize the patient population admitted to hospital towards FTH or PH in order to find how many patients could be treated by PH just as well as by FTH. However, in most studies, only some of all admitted patients could actually be randomized. Only Zwerling and Kluiter carried out a randomized study on an unselected group of patients referred to FTH. All the other studies suffered from design violation between admission and randomization, mostly because patients were too ill to be randomized. This pre-randomization attrition results in a relationship between the percentage of the admission cohort that could be randomized and the percentage of the population randomized to PH that after randomization had to be admitted and received FTH: the smaller the selection before randomization the higher the percentage of patients who failed in PH and had to be admitted. Zwerling, for instance, randomized 100% of admitted patients and had to admit to FTH 34% of those randomized to PH. For the other studies, the percentages were: 100 and 39.2 (Kluiter), 55 and 12 (Creed), 42 and 12 (Schene), 22 and 0 (Herz), 22 and 0 (Dick), and 15 and 0 (Washburn).

Earlier studies were less stringent and sophisticated in their methodology. Later studies had more differentiated outcome measures, made better descriptions of their patient selection, and also measured family burden, costs and satisfaction with services and calculated the use of medication.

The overall conclusion must be that PH can be a good alternative for 30–40% of patients in need of acute psychiatric admission. For that group, there are no differences between PH and FTH in the reduction of symptoms while there is some tendency for social functioning to have a better outcome in PH, although the differences have disappeared 2 years later. This finding was from the earlier studies in particular, later studies have not been able to replicate these results (Creed

et al., 1990; Kluiter *et al.*, 1992; Schene *et al.*, 1993).

These RCTs also teach us something about contra-indications for PH: patients who could harm themselves or others, patients who fail to care for themselves, patients with no support systems due to their symptomatology, patients who also suffer from a severe addiction disorder, patients with organic disorders and patients in need of somatic nursing care. In those cases, patients have to be admitted to in-patient services first.

Other outcome measures showed that satisfaction with services is equal or somewhat better in PH (Schene *et al.*, 1997). Also family members are more satisfied, while almost all studies have shown no difference in family or care-giver burden. Only Creed *et al.* (1997) found that day hospital patients were less of a burden to their carers at 1 year post-admission. Schene *et al.* (1993), Wiersma *et al.* (1995) and Sledge *et al.* (1996) found no difference in readmissions, while Creed *et al.* (1990) found more readmissions for those treated in FTH.

Apart from those of Herz *et al.* (1971) and Sledge *et al.* (1996), all RCTs found PH to have a longer treatment duration than FTH. This might be related to greater acceptance of PH by patients, more satisfaction and compliance with services, but may be due to the time needed to reach treatment effectiveness as well as Hawthorne effects. Schene *et al.* (1993) mentioned the interaction of treatment length and treatment intensity as a possible causative factor. PH offers a lower intensity, but longer duration type of treatment than FTH. On the other hand, Sledge *et al.* (1996) explained his finding of shorter PH admission by suggesting different clinical decisions about discharges in the day hospital/crisis respite programme as well as patients being treated more effectively in this programme.

Cost-effectiveness of partial versus full-time hospitalization

Three RCTs have also considered costs. Wiersma *et al.* (1995) found over a 2-year period that direct costs (number of in- and day-patients days and out-patient contacts) for PH and FTH were more or less the same. In this study, costs per day for PH and FTH were the same as well as the number of staff needed to run the service. Because patients' compliance and satisfaction with services for both patient and families was better in PH, Wiersma concluded that day treatment can be considered a cost-effective alternative to in-patient treatment.

Sledge *et al.* (1996) compared FTH with a day hospital/crisis respite programme. Over a 10-month period, the experimental condition was $7100 (20%) cheaper than FTH. In particular, the index admission was 43% less expensive due to operating costs, which were twice as high in FTH. Personal costs were equal in both conditions as well as effectiveness. Therefore, Sledge concluded that in his study, FTH was more expensive for two reasons: the length of stay during index admission was 7 days less in PH and operating costs were lower.

Creed *et al.* (1997) assessed costs over 12 months after the date of admission. They found that overall day hospital treatment was £1994 less expensive than FTH for the 30–40% of potential admissions that can be treated in this way. Although day hospital patients were less of a burden to their carers, the latter may bear additional costs.

Acute day hospital care

The percentage of an admissions cohort eligible for PH of course is dependent on other patient, network or support and service characteristics. If, for instance, patients are well integrated into community support systems, this percentage will rise. If the threshold for psychiatric admissions is very high, because of a shortage of beds in a certain region, it will be lower because the condition of admitted patients will be more severe. Residents and junior staff (Washburn *et al.*, 1976; Platt *et al.*, 1980; Kluiter *et al.*, 1992) seem to lower this percentage.

Acute day hospital care seems to have better opportunities, with a well trained and skilled staff with an attitude favouring PH (Herz *et al.*, 1971; Schene, 1992). The service has to be closely connected to in-patient services, having available all diagnostic and treatment facilities necessary for acutely ill psychiatric patients.

Practical issues such as transport from home to service and overnight accommodation or a back-up bed if needed (Gudeman *et al.*, 1983) are also important prerequisites. Additional support at home by, for instance, a community psychiatric nurse, a 24-hour crisis telephone service and the opportunity for outreach to patients in crisis can help to make PH a success for more of the admitted patient group.

Partial hospitalization and beds

In a day hospital functioning as an alternative to in-patient hospitalization, Turner *et al.* (1991) studied the use of an overnight hospitalization or back-up bed. Twenty percent of patients admitted to the day hospital used the back-up bed (47% for one night, 19% for two nights and 34% for three nights). The main reasons were psychotic symptoms (44% of back-up admissions), dangerousness (81%) and extreme agitation (5%). Of all episodes, 73% returned to the day hospital and 27% resulted to full in-patient admission. Only 50% of the back-up bed users were able to complete their day hospitalization, the other 50% received a standard in-patient admission.

To really understand the relationship between the use of FTH, PH and out-patient services, we first have to calculate for a specific catchment area the total number of days that acutely ill patients should spend in a hospital setting because that setting is more effective or protective than out-patient care. Secondly, we have to consider the percentage of the total number of days which could be spent just as safely and effectively in an acute day hospital. Of all patients referred for in-patient treatment, k% will spend their whole admission in FTH, l% will have a combination of x days in FTH and y days in PH (the percentage $x/x + y$ will vary between 1 and 99) and m% will spend their total time in PH (Schene, 1992).

In The Netherlands, acute day hospital treatment over the last few years has become integrated in many open and even some closed psychiatric admission wards (Cohen and Sanders, 1995). It is now called 'admission substitution day treatment'. In-patient places are allowed to be used for day treatment. This means that the budget paid and the number of professional staff are the same for an FTH and that place used as a PH place. In this way, care can be individualized more efficiently.

Effectiveness of partial hospitalization versus out-patient treatment

In RCTs, PH has been studied in comparison with out-patient services for psychotic and non-psychotic patients. Meltzhoff and Blumenthal (1966) found better results for PH for patients with chronic schizophrenia: fewer admissions days, more work and greater independence. Day treatment changed the deterioration of those patients. Guy *et al.* (1969) reported that medication and PH for patients with schizoaffective disorder has advantages in terms of reduction of symptoms. Linn *et al.* (1979) studied 122 male patients with schizophrenia and found a better outcome on symptoms at the end of the 2-year study period and better social functioning during the whole 2-year period. There were no differences in readmissions. Also Weldon *et al.* (1979) showed better functioning and significantly more work or training after 3 months.

Two studies compared out-patient and day hospital care for patients with depression, anxiety and phobia (Tyrer *et al.*, 1987; Dick *et al.*, 1991) and found different results. Tyrer found no differences on symptoms and social functioning, while Dick found better outcome in PH on symptoms, time structuring and socialization, ability to cope and satisfaction.

In summary, PH seems to have advantages over out-patient care for psychotic patients although cost-effectiveness has not been studied. For non-psychotic patients, in particular those with long-standing and severe personality disorders for whom out-patient treatment has been unsuc-

cessful, PH is an effective treatment (Piper *et al.*, 1996). However again no cost-effectiveness studies have been done. Those with less severe neurotic conditions do better with out-patient treatment.

Therapeutic factors

To learn more about therapeutic factors, three studies need to be considered. Hoge *et al.* (1988) studied these factors in a day hospital functioning as an alternative to FTH. Patients and staff mentioned the following therapeutic factors in declining frequency: structure, interpersonal contact, medication, altruism, catharsis, learning, mobilization of family support, connection to community, universality, patient autonomy, successful completion and security. He concluded that it was striking that PH in this setting provides security and structure while simultaneously promoting patient responsibility and autonomy.

Schreer (1988) carried out a comparable study in a private, not-for-profit, short-term psychiatric partial hospital with more affective and less psychotic disorders than the population studied by Hoge. She found interpersonal contact just as important, but feedback on behaviour, universality and learning were more important, while structure, medication, and security were less important.

Davidson *et al.* (1996) studied the social environment of a conventional psychiatric in-patient setting in comparison with a combined day hospital and crisis respite programme. The day hospital programme had higher expectations for patient functioning, a lower tolerance for deviance, more patient choice and allowed for more continuation of patients' ongoing community involvement. The programme had a more stimulating and attractive physical environment and social milieu. It promoted higher levels of patient functioning and activity, increased help with daily living skills and social and recreational resources, and more integration of patients into the community outside the facility.

Discussion and conclusions

From this review, it can be concluded that PH represents a spectrum of mental health services which indeed bridges the wide gap between FTH on the one end and out-patient services on the other. In comparison with FTH, it can certainly have advantages for both patients and carers. However, the percentage of patients admitted for in-patient treatment in hospital who could be admitted directly to PH as an initial alternative seems to be no higher than about 30–40%. For this reason, integrated admission units which offer FTH and PH in a flexible way seem to be the most practical and need-based way of working. Patients treated on those units start to sleep at home as soon as their clinical condition allows them to do so, and the number of nights at home per week can be increased according to their condition.

In our own Programme for Affective Disorders, all admitted patients are screened for PH at admission. If possible, they start PH immediately, if not they start FTH. It is possible that they will be treated in FTH for the whole length of their admission. For most patients, however, a combination of FTH and PH is used during their 8–6 week stay. Therefore, it is possible to have a unit which has a capacity for 22 patients and also has staff for 22 patients at least during the daytime. In reality, it only has 12 beds and outside office hours staff are adapted to that quantity of patients.

If we compare this way of organizing services with the description of the four functions of PH, as an alternative to acute in-patient, continuation of acute in-patient, extension of out-patient care and day care or rehabilitation, the first two functions are combined with in-patient places in one setting. Here the utilization of acute PH must be higher, because Schene *et al.* (1987) found that only 9% of all Dutch PH places were used as an alternative for FTH. Mbaya *et al.* (1998) did a comparable study in the UK where he found a similar level of 13%.

It is not only the clinical condition of patients that determines the utilization of PH. Staff attitudes and skills, hospital policy, staff:patient ratios, structured programming, resources for managing clinical emergencies, distance from home to PH service, attitudes of family members, payment of service and other factors certainly also have an influence. Choosing PH in an early phase and not only when a patient's decompensation is so severe that only FTH is possible, makes PH an important function in a comprehensive system of care. For such short-term PH to be an alternative to FTH, Hoge and Farrell (1987) described five functions: (i) reduction of acute symptoms (first 2 weeks); (ii) decrease of demoralization (weeks 3 and 4); (iii) facilitating community re-entry (weeks 1–4); (iv) education and skill building (weeks 3–4); and (v) connection to community (week 4).

This chapter had shown that the evidence for PH as an alternative for FTH has strong empirical support from RCTs. So far, it is equal to FTH on most outcome measures and probably better in terms of satisfaction. One of the puzzling findings is that the duration of treatment in most studies is longer in PH. The earlier finding that social functioning increased more in PH than in FTH has not been replicated recently. This is still puzzling because the inherent characteristic of PH, the intense interaction between the therapeutic and outside world, has great potential for the training and generalization of skills. Further research to develop this therapeutic factor of PH is needed.

Looking at the third function, extension to out-patient care (or day treatment), the conclusions are less clear. Hoge *et al.* (1992) was of the opinion that this type of PH should be changed into assertive community treatment. Rosie *et al.* (1995) described that this view may be correct for patients with psychotic disorders, but does not hold for patients with personality disorders or severe neurosis. For them, a time-limited 4-month programme had good outcome if it had a close relationship to a highly active out-patient clinic. What the future will bring in this field is not clear. The development and empirical testing of new intensive out-patient treatment for personality disorders and the lack of cost-effectiveness studies comparing PH and out-patient treatment do not make this future look very promising. Further research with RCTs which compare PH and intensive out-patient treatment with a long-term follow-up are needed.

Finally, the fourth function of PH, rehabilitation or day care, is rarely discussed in research terms. It is one of the cornerstones of community support systems, with a strong emphasis on training, support and continuity of care, and lends itself to careful evaluation in the future.

References

Bierer, J. (1951) *The Day Hospital, An Experiment in Social Psychiatry and Syntho-analytic Psychotherapy.* London: H.K. Lewis and Co.

Bierer, J. (1961) Day hospitals, further developments. *International Journal of Social Psychiatry*, 7, 148–151.

Block, B.M. and Lefkovitz, P.M. (1991) *Standards and Guidelines for Partial Hospitalization.* Alexandria, VA: American Association for Partial Hospitalization.

Bosch, G. and Veltin, A. (1983) *Die Tagesklinik als teil der psychiatrischen Versorgung.* Köln: Rheinland-Verlag GmbH.

Brocklehurst, J. (1979) The development and present status of day hospitals. *Age and Ageing*, 8, 76–79.

Bystritsky, A., Muford, P.R., Rosen, R.M., Martin, K.M., Vapnik, T., Borbis, E.E. and Wolson, R.C. (1996) A preliminary study of partial hospital management of severe obsessive–compulsive disorder. *Psychiatric Services*, 47, 170–174.

Cameron, D.E. (1947) The day hospital: an experimental form of hospitalization for psychiatric patients. *Modern Hospital*, 69, 60–62.

Casarino, J.P., Wilner, M. and Maxey, J.T. (1982) American Association for Partial Hospitalization (AAHP) standards and guideline for partial hospitalization. *International Journal of Partial Hospitalization*, 1, 15–21.

Cohen, D. and Sanders, H.E. (1995) Day-program-based treatment in the Amsterdam city center. *International Journal of Social Psychiatry*, 41, 120–131.

Creed, F., Black, D. and Anthony, P. (1989a) Day-hospital and community treatment for acute psychiatric illness; a critical appraisal. *British Journal of Psychiatry*, 154, 300–310.

Creed, F., Anthony, P., Godbert, K. and Huxley, P. (1989b) Treatment of severe psychiatric illness in a day hospital. *British Journal of Psychiatry*, 154, 341–347.

Creed, F., Black, D., Anthony, P., Osborn, M., Thomas, P. and Tomenson, B. (1990) Randomized controlled trial of day versus inpatient psychiatric treatment. *British Medical Journal*, 300, 1033–1037.

Creed, F., Mbaya, P., Lancashire, S., Tomenson, B., Williams, B. and Holme, S. (1997) Cost-effectiveness of day and inpatient psychiatric treatment. *British Medical Journal*, 314, 1381–1385.

Davidson, L., Kraemer Tebes, J., Rakfeldt, J. and Sledge, W.H. (1996) Differences in social environment between inpatient and day hospital-crisis respite settings. *Psychiatric Services*, 47, 714–720.

De Hert, M., Thys, E., Vercruyssen, V. and Peuskens, J. (1996) Partial hospitalization at night: the Brussels Nighthospital. *Psychiatric Services*, 47, 527–528.

DiBella, G., Weitz, G.W., Pogntes Bergen, D. and Yurmark, J.L. (eds) (1982) *Handbook of Partial Hospitalization.* New York: Brunner/Mazel.

Dick, P.H., Ince, A. and Barlow, M. (1985a) Day treatment: suitability and referral procedure. *British Journal of Psychiatry*, 142, 250–253.

Dick, P.H., Cameron, L., Cohen, D., Barlow, M. and Ince, A. (1985b) Day and full time psychiatric treatment: a controlled comparison. *British Journal of Psychiatry*, 147, 246–250.

Dick, P.H., Sweeney, M.L. and Crombie, I.K. (1991) Controlled comparison of day-patient and out-patient treatment for persistent anxiety and depression. *British Journal of Psychiatry*, 158, 24–27.

Dzagharov, M.A. (1937) Experience in organizing a day hospital for mental patients. *Nevropathologi Psikhiatri*, 6, 137–146.

Farndale, J. (1961) *The Day Hospital Movement in Great Brittain.* London: Pergamon Press.

Fink, E.B., Longabaugh, R. and Stout, R. (1978) The paradoxical underutilization of partial hospitalization. *American Journal of Psychiatry*, 135, 713–716.

Gudeman, J.E., Shore, M.F. and Dickey B. (1983) Day hospitalization and an inn instead of inpatient care for psychiatric patients. *New England Journal of Medicine*, 308, 749–753.

Guy, W., Gross, M., Hogarty, G.E. and Dennis, H. (1969) A controlled evaluation of day hospital effectiveness. *Archives of General Psychiatry*, 201, 329–338.

Herz, M.I. (1982) Research overview in day treatment. *International Journal of Partial Hospitalization* 1, 33–45.

Herz, M.I., Endicott, J., Spitzer, R.L. and Mesnikoff, A. (1971) Day versus inpatient hospitalization: a controlled study. *American Journal of Psychiatry*, 127, 1371–1381.

Hoge, M.A. and Farrell, S.P. (1987) Functions of short term partial hospitalization in a comprehensive system of care. *International Journal of Partial Hospitalization*, 4, 177–188.

Hoge, M.A., Farrell, S.P., Munchnel, M.E. and Strauss, J.S. (1988) Therapeutic factors in partial hospitalization. *Psychiatry*, 51, 199–210.

Hoge, M.A., Davidson, L., Leonard Hill, W., Turner, V.E. and Ameli, R. (1992) The promise of partial hospitalization. *Hospital and Community Psychiatry*, 43, 345–354.

Klar, H., Francis, A. and Clarkin, H. (1982) Selection criteria for partial hospitalization. *Hospital and Community Psychiatry*, 33, 929–933.

Kluiter, H., Giel, R., Nienhuis, F.J., Rüphan, M. and Wiersma, D. (1992) Predicting feasibility of day treatment for unselected patients referred for inpatient psychiatric treatment: results of a randomized trial. *American Journal of Psychiatry*, 149, 1199–11205.

Kris, E.B. (1960) Intensive short-term treatment in a day care facility for the prevention of rehospitalization of patients in the community showing recurrence of psychotic symptoms. *Psychiatric Quarterly*, 34, 83–88.

Linn, M.W., Caffey, E.M., Klett, C.J., Hogarty, G.E. and Lamb, H.R. (1979) day treatment and psychotropic drugs in the aftercare of schizophrenic patients. *Archives of General Psychiatry*, 36, 1055–1066.

Lussier, R.G., Steiner, J., Grey, A. and Hansen, C. (1997) Prevalence of dissociative disorders in an acute care day hospital populaton. *Psychiatric Services*, 48, 244–246.

Mason, J., Louks, J., Burmer, G. and Scher, M. (1982) The efficacy of partial hospitalization: a review of recent literature. *International Journal of Partial Hospitalization*, 1, 251–269.

Mbaya, P., Creed, F. and Tomenson, B. (1998) The different uses of day hospitals. *Acta Psychiatrica Scandinavica*, 98, 283–287.

Meltzhoff, J. and Blumenthal, R. (1966) *The Day Treatment Center: Principles, Application and Evaluation*. Springfield, IL: Charles C. Thomas.

Michaux, M.H., Chelst, M.R., Foster, S.A., Prium, R.J. and Dasinger, E.M. (1972) Day- and full-time treatment, a controlled comparison. *Current Therapeutic Research*, 14, 279–292.

Parker, S.P. and Knoll, J.L., III (1990) Partial hospitalization: un update. *American Journal of Psychiatry*, 147, 156–160.

Penk, W.E., Charles, H.L. and Van Hoose, T.A. (1978) Comparative effectiveness of day hospital and inpatient psychiatric treatment. *Journal of Consulting and Clinical Psychology*, 46, 94–101.

Piper, W.E., Rosie, J.S., Joyce, A.S. and Azim, H.F.A. (1996) *Time-limited Day Treatment for Personality Disorders*. Washington, DC: American Psychological Association.

Platt, S.D,. Knights, A.C. and Hirsch, S.R. (1980) Caution and conservatism in the use of a psychiatric day hospital; evidence from a research project that failed. *Psychiatric Research*, 3, 123–132.

Rosie, J.S. (1987) Partial hospitalization: a review of recent literature. *Hospital and Community Psychiatry*, 38, 1291–1299.

Rosie, J.S., Azim, H.F.A., Piper, W.E. and Joyce, A.S. (1995) Effective psychiatric day treatment: historical lessons. *Psychiatric Services*, 46, 1019–1026.

Schene, A.H. (1985) *Psychiatric Partial Hospitalization: An Overview*. Utrecht: Netherlands Center of Mental Health (in Dutch).

Schene, A.H. (1992) Psychiatric partial and full time hospitalization: a comparative study. Utrecht: Thesis, University of Utrecht

Schene, A.H. and Gersons, B.P.R. (1986) Effectiveness and application of partial hospitalization. *Acta Psychiatrica Scandinavica*, 74, 335–340.

Schene, A.H., van Lieshout, P. and Mastboom, J. (1986) Development and current status of partial hospitalization in The Netherlands. *International Journal of Partial Hospitalization*, 3, 237–246.

Schene, A.H., van Lieshout, P. and Mastboom, J. (1988) Different types of partial hospitalization programs: results from a nationwide study. *Acta Psychiatrica Scandinavica*, 75, 515–520.

Schene, A.H., van Wijngaarden, B., Poelijoe, N.W. and Gersons, B.P.R. (1993) The Utrecht comparative study on psychiatric day treatment and inpatient treatment. *Acta Psychiatrica Scandinavica*, 87, 427–436.

Schene, A.H., van Wijngaarden, B., and Gersons, B.P.R. (1997) Partial or full-time hospitalization: patients' preferences. In: Tansella, M. (ed.), *Making Rational Mental Health Services*. Roma: Il Pensiero Scientifico Editore, pp. 145–154.

Schreer, H. (1988) Therapeutic factors in psychiatric day hospital treatment. *International Journal of Partial Hospitalization*, 4, 307–319.

Shepherd, G. (1991) Day treatment and care. In: Bennett, D.H. and Freeman, H.L. (eds), *Community Psychiatry*. London: Churchill Livingstone, pp. 386–414.

Sledge, W.H., Tebes, J., Wolff, N. and Helminiak, T.W. (1996) Day hospital/crisis respite care versus inpatient care. Part II. Service utilization and costs. *American Journal of Psychiatry*, 153, 1074–1083.

Tantam, D. and McGrath, G. (1989) Psychiatric day hospitals—another road to institutionalization? *Social Psychiatry and Psychiatric Epidemiology*, 24, 96–101.

Turner, V.E. and Hoge, M.A. (1991) Overnight hospitalization of acutely ill day hospital patients. *International Journal of Partial Hospotalization*, 7, 23–36.

Tyrer, P., Remington, M. and Alexander J. (1987) The outcome of neurotic disorders after out-patient and day hospital care. *British Journal of Psychiatry*, 151, 57–62.

Washburn, S., Vannicelli, R., Longabaugh, R. and Scheff, B.J. (1976) A controlled comparison of psychiatric daytreatment and inpatient hospitalization. *Journal of Consulting and Clinical Psychology*, 44, 665–675.

Weldon, E., Clarkin, J.E., Hennessy, J.J. and Frances, A. (1979) Day hospital versus outpatient treatment. A controlled study. *Psychiatric Quarterly*, 51, 144–150.

Wiersma, D., Kluiter, H., Nienhuis, F.J., Ruphan, M. and Giel, R. (1995) Costs and benefits of hospital and day treatment with community care of affective and schizophrenic disorders. *British Journal of Psychiatry*, 27 (Suppl.), 52–59.

Zwerling, I. and Wilder, J.F. (1962) Day hospital treatment for acutely psychotic patients. *Current Psychiatric Therapies* 2, 200–210.

Zwerling, I. and Wilder, J.F. (1964) An evaluation of the applicability of the day hospital in treatment for acutely disturbed patients. *Israel Annals of Psychiatry and Related Disciplines* 2, 162–185.

26 | Day care and occupation: structured rehabilitation and recovery programmes and work

Alan Rosen and Karen Barfoot

Introduction

On the whole, real 'rehabilitation' and the 'recovery' process in psychiatry have been chronically hampered rather than helped by health services and society. Harding *et al.* (1992) reviewed studies which separated out the residual effects of the disorder from effects due to institutionalization, socialization into the patient role, the lack of meaningful rehabilitation, side effects of medication, self-fulfilling staff prophecies and their low expectations, and loss of hope.

Anthony (1993) states that what was thought to be a result of the disorder is now thought to be due to the way people are treated by the health system. He notes that stigma, low social status, restricted choices, lack of self-determination and low staff expectations are all contributing factors to chronicity from which the consumer must recover. McGorry (1992) identifies similar restraining variables in the recovery process, while emphasizing the importance to the person's recovery of highly skilled psychosocial therapies, and attending to helping individuals through their developmental stages and in retaining their social relationships in the community.

It usually has taken about a decade or more for senior decision makers to notice that the locus of psychiatric rehabilitation services has shifted from the hospital to the community. While many of their long-term in-patients 'flew the coop', resources and staff allocated to psychiatric rehabilitation often remained locked within psychiatric institutions, largely devoted, with notable exceptions, to long-term human warehousing, and maintenance or minding programmes, often masquerading as rehabilitation. During that period, mental health workers on the ground and voluntary organizations had usually been striving with few staff and resources, to develop a range of active day and evening rehabilitation programmes and work opportunities for individuals with severe mental illnesses in the community. These programmes were sometimes part of the development of 24-hour mobile community-based mental health services, clinically integrated with local acute psychiatric in-patient care (Hoult *et al.*, 1984).

In Australia, a study demonstrated that by 1984, 90% of patients with severe psychiatric disability lived in the community, while 90% of public mental health staff and resources remained within hospitals (Rosen *et al.*, 1987). Consequently, most psychiatric professionals continued for too long to receive their 'rehabilitation' training and experience within the walls of psychiatric hospitals and became socialized into believing they knew what was best ('vocational ownership' as coined by Thornicroft, 1993) for the dwindling population with long-term disability who remained in their care.

At the same time, observations made in studies by Anthony *et al.* (1982) and Bellack (1984) established that repeated attempts at rehabilitation and teaching of new skills while individuals were retained in psychiatric hospitals were often a waste of time, because on discharge these skills did not generalize to the person's place of residence or occupation. Skills needed to be taught in the person's local environment (e.g. their own home) for them to have a chance of becoming self-sufficient (Weir and Rosen, 1989). It was found further that the success of a person's rehabilitation was often contingent on working 'out there' in the community with the person together with their family and/or social support network to reach a common understanding of and approach to their mental illness (Falloon and Talbott, 1982; Falloon *et al.*, 1990). A growing body of clinical research reviewed by Warner (1999) has also established that paid work also substantially improves outcome in schizophrenia, decreasing likelihood of readmission (e.g. Fairweather, 1969) and better functioning, though not necessarily leading to a reduction in symptom severity (Warner, 1994). More recently, studies have focused on the importance of consumer, carer, staff and community mind-sets regarding rehabilitation and recovery (Tooth *et al.*, 1997).

Psychosocial rehabilitation is defined by the WHO (1996) as a process that facilitates the opportunity for individuals who are impaired, disabled or handicapped by a mental disorder to reach their optimum level of independent functioning in the community. It implies both improving individuals' competencies and introducing environmental changes in order to create a life of the best quality possible, for people who continue to experience mental disorder producing a certain level of disability.

In contrast, *recovery* is defined (Anthony, 1993) as a deeply personal, unique process of changing one's attitudes, values, feelings, goals, skills and/or roles. 'It is a way of living a satisfying, hopeful and contributing life even with limitations caused by illness'. It involves 'the development of a new meaning and purpose in one's life as one grows beyond the catastrophic effects of mental illness'. The concept of recovery facilitates empowerment and active participation in treatment and rehabilitation.

Paradigm shifts

Have conceptual shifts regarding psychosocial rehabilitation driven shifts of provision, or vice versa? Arguably it is a reciprocal conversation, as mental health professionals, consumers and carers have discovered many life-enhancing visions and strategies once they are based together in community settings, with opportunities to work in partnership together, as well as with the local community. The major shifts appear to have been:

(i) the shift from stand-alone hospital and outpost community mental health services to administratively and clinically integrated local mental health services, combining both acute and rehabilitation services available on a 24-hour basis both in hospital and in the community (Rosen, 1992).

(ii) The shift of centre of gravity of mental health services for people with severe and long-term disability from hospital to the community, with the funding and staffing following the patients to the community, where most now live and prefer to live. In Australia and New Zealand, both of these shifts have been formally backed with financial incentives via their respective National Mental Health Strategies. In Australia, progress is actively monitored through annually published comparative data reviews, state by state, and qualitatively monitored by periodic formal accreditation by internal audit and external survey with the National Mental Health Standards (Gianfrancesco *et al.*, 1997).

Implied here also is the shift from artificial '*in vitro*' rehabilitation programmes based in institutions, where patients can be mustered at the convenience of professional staff for ease of minding, monitoring and research, dislocated from their families, to '*in vivo*' rehabilitation environments, where individuals prefer to live, work and play, in close proximity to their own families or actual social networks.

(iii) The shift from an overwhelming focus on treating biological symptoms and implied pathology to specific interventions to address the spectrum of biological, psychological, social and cultural sequelae of severe psychiatric disorders. This is the basis of the WHO (1996) definition of psychosocial rehabilitation, tackling functional impairment, disability and handicap, the interaction of that disability with that society, including discrimination and stigma.

(iv) The shift to a focus on individual needs and priorities, with tailor-made unique rehabilitation plans, rather than wholesale group streaming and programming (Crichton, 1989).

(v) The shift to an emphasis of detecting, eliciting, measuring and working on strengths and on noticing and celebrating victories, however incremental, rather than focusing on failures, weaknesses and lapses, which can so easily be internalized as indelible personal flaws (Rosen, 1994).

(vi) The more recent shift from programmes centrally focused on psychosocial rehabilitation to programmes providing support and a fertile foundation for processes of recovery and personal empowerment (Anthony, 1993) requiring the de-colonizing by services of individuals with mental illness and their families (Rosen, 1994).

(vii) The shift from sequestered centre-based community programmes, vulnerable to becoming a ghetto of long-term disability, segregating these individuals from the community to social integration, using local community facilities alongside other members of the community, aiming towards full membership of the local community (Carling, 1995).

(viii) From professionally run facilities to consumer-run and controlled programmes (Segal *et al.*, 1995).

(ix) From perpetual maintenance programmes to always having the explicit expectation of moving to the next stage, and working towards creating the conditions of readiness to assist individuals to make such moves in their own time frame (Strauss, 1989; Harding *et al.*, 1992; Rosen, 1994).

There have been parallel shifts in vocational provision over recent years, from more institutionally based sheltered work facilities to jobs in the real world, from 'play' or pretend work to real work for real pay, from heavily subsidized work programmes to economically competitive 'social firms', from work groups or crews to individual jobs and contracts, from pre-vocational preparation for work to direct placement and support in the person's job of choice in the community (see 'choose–get–keep' model, later), from supported employment to fully independent employment in the competitive workforce, from consumers as casual employees, to consumer-run and owned small business enterprises.

What are 'day care' and 'occupation'?

The title given to us for this chapter was 'Day care and occupation'. Day care is an overly narrow term (e.g. many programmes occur during the evenings, and may not involve supervised care but consumer-run self-help groups). Occupation is a very wide and useful concept, but encompasses a lot more than vocational needs and interventions. The model of occupational performance (Chapparo and Ranka, 1997) defines 'occupations' as the ability to perceive, recall, plan and carry out roles, activities and tasks for the purpose of self-maintenance, productivity, leisure/play and rest in response to demands of the internal and/or external environment. We prefer a wider definition of occupations, which includes role performance in the arenas of social and intimate life as well as work, rest, play and self-care.

Psychosocial rehabilitation programmes should involve interventions to enhance all such occupational roles, including subsets of interventions on work, leisure, relationships, and self-care. We therefore suggest that the more accurate titles for the two overlapping terrains covered by this chapter would be 'Structured rehabilitation and recovery programmes, and work'.

Day and evening care: structured rehabilitation and recovery programmes

Table 26.1 follows the evolution of rehabilitation services towards full community integration. The accompanying text describes associated evidence for the major evolutionary shifts.

From hospital to community rehabilitation programmes

Up to 50 years ago, day hospitals emerged as an alternative to some short- and long-term psychiatric hospital care, but have been criticized on the basis that as clients in day treatment are segregated from the community, participation may induce institutional dependency and impede the development of natural support networks and

Table 26.1 *Structured rehabilitation and recovery programmes*

	Term	Definition	Model
1	Day hospital/day treatment (Torrey *et al.*, 1998a; Almarez-Serrano *et al.*, 1999) Evidence level: III–IV but Cochrane Review is forthcoming	Hospital without beds; or a facility that provides medical review plus a range of activities in recreational, vocational, social and living skills for people requiring intensive short-term support, as an alternative or follow-up to in-patient admission	Targeting those recently discharged or those in crisis who would otherwise require hospitalization
2	Partial hospitalization (Hoge *et al.*, 1992; Falloon and Fadden, 1993) Evidence level: I–III but only in comparison with in-patient care	Day treatment providing comprehensive, multi-disciplinary services for clients with severe mental disorders, striving for symptom reduction and improved functioning over weeks to months Both models 1 and 2 may be more costly than community-based alternatives.	Alternative to short- and long-term in-patient care, alleviating the demand for in-patient services and providing patients with less restrictive and less regressive forms of care. However, the future of models 1 and 2 appears uncertain, as community-based psychosocial rehabilitation and assertive mobile treatment programmes are assuming these functions, so comparative research is needed.
3	Fountain House Clubhouse model (Beard *et al.*, 1982; Crowther *et al.*, 1999; Warner *et al.*, 1999) Evidence level: IV–III	Intentional community designed to create a restorative environment helping individuals achieve or regain the confidence and skills necessary to lead vocationally productive and socially satisfying lives.	The Clubhouse belongs to its members whose input is expected, wanted and needed. Staff are theoretically almost indistinguishable from members.
4	Living Skills Centres (Weir and Rosen, 1989; Falloon and Fadden, 1993) Evidence level: IV–V	Facility that provides a range of activities in living skills with an intense individualized rehabilitation approach aimed at upgrading level of functioning and encouraging use of other community resources.	Rehabilitation resource centre and informal meeting place from which community living experiences are organized with coaching and support.

social integration (Anthony and Liberman, 1986). Day hospitals may also be costly relative to community-based day care alternatives (Falloon and Fadden, 1993).

New York's Fountain House developed the first 'Clubhouse' in 1948, and there are now such Clubhouses in operation all over the world. Under this model, rehabilitation programmes are run conjointly with 'members' co-operating and working alongside paid clinical staff. With an emphasis on transitional employment, the Clubhouse can also provide members with the opportunity for:

- empowerment in social relations;
- expanded social networks;
- an enhanced social environment and improved nutrition (one work group will run the kitchen and put on meals for the members);

Table 26.1 *continued*

Term	Definition	Model
5 Drop-in centres Evidence level: V	Range of social and prevocational activities available on a drop-in basis	May vary in models with use of consumers, professionals and volunteers, staffing and co-ordinating the programme.
6 Consumer-run drop-in centres (Kaufmann et al., 1993) Evidence level: IV	Consumer-run alternative to professional drop-in care to provide friendship and social support	Consumer-providers welcoming those individuals who lack access to family and friends.
7 Self-help centres (Segal *et al.*, 1995) Evidence level: III	Emphasizing mutual reliance and providing mutual assistance and peer support, they are concerned with improving members' lives and helping them to gain skills and resources to achieve stability	Often incorporated as voluntary agencies, and independently managed and staffed by mental health consumers.
8 Neighbourhood centres (Richmond Implementation Unit, 1987) Evidence level: V	Voluntary organizations offering a wide range of leisure activities, day and evening classes, community services and social functions.	Targeting and accessing all local residents. Often tolerant and welcoming but no specific support for psychiatric disability.
9 Community integration programmes (Carling, 1995) Evidence level: V	Aimed at accessing mainstream facilities for individuals living with a mental illness.	Basic belief that all people, including people with a psychiatric disability have a right to full participation in, and membership of the community.
10 Fully independent living (Gianfrancesco *et al.*, 1997) Evidence level: V	Rehabilitation and recovery programme aimed at exiting and/or outliving the need to live with the assistance of such specialized programmes.	Disability programmes should be ongoing while individuals remain in need, but should not necessarily be lifelong. They should provide a mechanism for graduating from such programmes altogether.

- training and assessment in job skills and work functioning (Beard *et al.*, 1982; Warner *et al.*, 1999).

Warner *et al.* (1999) found that when matched with similar patients, Clubhouse users achieved reasonable employment status and good social relationships. Subjective feelings of well-being were improved in the Clubhouse group, as were patterns of service utilization, and treatment costs were lowered.

The Living Skills Centre model (Weir and Rosen, 1989), based usually in a low-key domestic setting in the community, provided a combination of local informal drop-in centre, a base for community activities, for individualized functional goal attainment programmes, for group vocational opportunities or work co-operatives, and psychoeducational multiple family groups. They were usually developed as key components of a locally integrated community and hospital mental health service.

From professionally run to consumer-run programmes

Although day treatment remains a core component of many community programmes around the western world catering for persons with severe mental disorders, many are shifting to a vocational focus, offering supported employment programmes (McCarthy *et al.*, 1998). However, such conversions may entail a social loss for consumers. Torrey *et al.* (1995) found that consumers, staff members and families identified the loss of social opportunities as the primary negative consequence of such changes. Torrey and colleagues (1998b) describe how some community mental health centres consequently have facilitated the development of consumer-run facilities meeting such social support needs.

For those services which have proved to be the most successful, consumers believe that a key to the success has been a focus on supporting recovery. Torrey *et al.* (1998b) defined this as a natural outcome of a shift from a support and maintenance ideology to a recovery ideology. Staff no longer focus so much on protecting consumers

from stress in an effort to prevent relapse, but instead become a resource instilling hope, encouraging positive risk taking, and using their knowledge and experience to help consumers effectively meet their own life goals.

The challenge faces mental health services to facilitate development of consumer-run services. Torrey *et al.* (1998b) found that the following ingredients led to 'active, well attended, consumer run services':

- dynamic consumer leadership;
- public financial support—funding to cover the costs of a non-depressing environment and a paid consumer leader with a competitive salary;
- technical and political support from the state and the community mental health centre—including advice on structuring the corporation, administrative coaching and strong advocacy.

From non-specific minding to individual goal-focused programme

Misconceptions regarding mental health rehabilitation include that the rehabilitation environment should be structured to:

(i)   minimize any pressure of expectation or challenge;

(ii) provide just a backwater perpetual maintenance programme; and/or

(iii) create a vague expectation of gradual improvement just from being in such an environment, without any focus on specific learning goals (Tobin, 1999).

Arguably, there should be no such thing as a 'maintenance' programme. We should always look together for the next specific goal or potential achievement, however incremental, with the client concerned. The expectation of moving on to the next stage of independence should be explicit, but in the clients' own time frame, involving some awareness of the clients sense of 'readiness' (Strauss, 1989; Harding *et al.*, 1992; Rosen, 1994).

Service providers need to develop specific skills relevant to individual needs assessment (from the client's and family's viewpoints) and strategies to improve particular functions (e.g. cognitive, self-care, domestic, social, financial and occupational), not as an end in themselves, but to allow them to resume culturally valued roles in the community (Chadwick *et al.*, 1996; Shepherd, 1998; Tobin, 1999). Planning for eventual exit from the mental health service system should be within the range of expectations for many consumers (Gian-francesco *et al.*, 1997).

From tailor-made rehabilitation to individually focused recovery

For those individuals who have difficulty accessing community facilities, active outreach is necessary, as exemplified by the PACT models described in Table 26.2 (Stein *et al.*, 1980; Test, 1995). Shepherd (1998) argues that "if services are going to work successfully with the most difficult and disabled people, then there needs to be specialist teams, clearly targeted, with small protected caseloads, extended hours of operation and the capacity to deliver intensive support. Such intensive support teams give more emphasis to practical help, social support and facilitating access to mainstream community activities."

Incorporating consumer-run facilities and encouraging their evolution into current methods of practice is a challenge for many mental health professionals.

Deborah Salem (1990) states that it is tempting to try to define a more universal role for consumer-run options, and perhaps even more tempting to bring them under the umbrella of the professional mental health system. The interest of the consumer may be better served by recognizing the self-help movement as a distinct, sometimes complementary, sometimes divergent, force in mental health service provision.

Rather than trying to narrowly define the role of any particular service option, we should encourage the development of multiple points of entry into the human service system and multiple approaches to support and resource mobilization. Assertive outreach programmes, drop-in centres and the range of consumer-run approaches all offer different resource options. Strategies that encourage consumer involvement, ownership and control help to provide diversity of services and to empower the consumer.

From 'vocational programmes' to 'real jobs for real pay'

Table 26.2 and the accompanying text show the historical progression and development of programmes aimed at assisting individuals with psychiatric disability to find meaningful work.

From sheltered work to transitional employment

Innovative approaches to vocational rehabilitation began in the 1950s at Fountain House. Members were encouraged to participate in work units at the Clubhouse as part of their work-ordered day. Fountain House went on to pioneer transitional employment (Beard *et al.*, 1982). Contributions include its focus on the normalizing function of community employment, and giving members a chance to work regardless of employment or psychiatric history (Bond *et al.*, 1997).

Job creation and consumer control

Workers co-operatives employing people with a mental illness began in Italy in the 1970s. Each business consortium employs a mixed workforce of mentally disabled and healthy workers in manufacturing and service enterprises such as hotels, cafes, restaurants, hairdressing salons, furniture workshops and plant nurseries. Enterprises compete with local businesses winning contracts by competitive bid. Different co-operatives use varying amounts of public subsidy. Co-operatives advertise widely and have high community visibility. This model has been developed in other European cities and elsewhere (Warner, 1999).

The co-operatives are based on the concept of self-management by members through democratic decision making. Social integration is achieved

Table 26.2 *From 'vocational programmes' to 'real work for real pay'*

Term	Definition	Model
1 Sheltered workshops (Warner 1994, 1999) Evidence level: IV	Provide structured and sheltered work environment comprised primarily of individuals with disabilities, sometimes still within institutions.	Individuals assessed as requiring a protected and specifically structured environment in a non-competitive, non-integrated setting.
2 Fairweather Lodge (Fairweather, 1969; Warner, 1994) Evidence level: III	Strives towards self-governance within a self-contained society in which participants live, work and socialize together.	Opportunities exist for autonomy and an important role within the society but within a relatively sheltered environment.
3 Clubhouse model Fountain House (Beard *et al.*, 1982; Crowther *et al.*, 1999) Evidence level: III	Programme components are pre-vocational day programme, transitional employment and other psychosocial programmes. Membership is voluntary, programmes are run conjointly with members and paid clinical staff	Initially a social club run by a group of ex-patients with work units providing voluntary services to run the centre. It developed into a vocational programme emphasizing transitional employment. The two house vocational models of 'the work-ordered day' and 'transitional employment' may be less effective than individual job placement and support. This requires more comparative research.
4 Pre-vocational training Evidence level: V	'Train and place': providing work skills training opportunities, individually or in groups, in mental health centre or similar setting, hoping that these skills will transfer to real workplaces.	Training within a specialized setting by health professionals preparing individuals for placement in open employment. Based on the premise that acquired skills are transportable.
5 Social firms and co-operatives (Warner, 1999) Evidence level: IV–V	Non-profit user-employing enterprises which have the dual function of creating integrated work settings for people with mental illness and providing a valuable service or product.	Each business employs a mixed workforce of mentally disabled and healthy workers. Public subsidy amounts vary.
6 Work crew (Campbell, 1989) Evidence level: V	Group model with up to eight individuals sharing the same specially trained supervisor. The crew operates like a small business, with crews moving around the community providing contracted services.	Supported working conditions, crews compete for contracts on the open market. Work demands are graded according to the individual's level of ability.
7 Brokered service model (Bond *et al.*, 1997) Evidence level: V	Clients are referred to vendors of vocational rehabilitation services	Mental health services work in a in a parallel system to vocational services.

Table 26.2 *continued*

	Term	Definition	Model
8	Transitional employment (Barker, 1994) Evidence level: IV–V	Temporary, part time community jobs. Designed to acclimatize clientele to work, increase self-confidence, and help build up resumes. Subsequently, the same jobs are temporarily filled by other clients.	Staff negotiate with community employers for entry level jobs, in which clients are employed on a temporary basis with support and supervision provided, by the programme.
9	Job coach (Warner, 1994; Bond *et al.*, 1997) Evidence level: III	The consumer receives supervision from a mental health centre job coach during the early stages of working.	Consumers are placed in a private business with help provided to adjust to the job. Support and reassurance can also be provided to the employer.
10	Job club (McGurrin, 1994) Evidence level: III–IV	Clients participate in a programme learning job-seeking skills rather than work skills *per se*. The job club provides resources necessary in a job search and use motivational systems to encourage morale and persistence.	Clients are responsible for finding a job but have the assistance of rehabilitation staff. The Job club provides resources necessary for job searches, e.g. phone, desk, secretarial support, job counsellor and fresh job leads.
11	Individual placement and support (Becker et al., 1996; Bond et al., 1997; Bond, 1998; Bond et al., 1998; Crowther et al., 1999) Evidence level: I–II	A specific model of supported employment for consumers with long-term impairment due to severe mental illness. It proves practical assistance in finding and maintaining competitive employment.	Emphasizes integrating vocational services and treatment services. A team approach, and a client-centred philosophy. Employment specialists work closely with case managers and other members of the clinical team.
12	Choose, get and keep (Danley and Anthony, 1987; Bond *et al.*, 1997) Evidence level III–IV	<u>Choose:</u> goal setting, job investigation, decision making <u>Get:</u> placement planning, direct placement, placement support <u>Keep:</u> assessing critical needs, planning required interventions, developing skills and supports.	Has the purpose of helping persons with psychiatric disabilities be satisfied and successful in work environments of their choice with the least possible professional support. This model encourages career planning which typically occurs in pre-placement counselling sessions.
13	PACT (assertive community treatment) model (Stein *et al.*, 1980; Russert and Frey, 1991; Rosen 1992, 1998; Test, 1995) Evidence level: I–III	Comprehensive, community-based programme which integrates clinical and rehabilitative services. Work is viewed as treatment and outcome.	A variety of options are available depending on the consumer's needs including competitive, supportive and pre-vocational. Support is provided on all levels, varying according to need, to both consumer and employer.

through the community placement of socially disadvantaged citizens. This particular experience has its cultural roots in the political and social movement that led to closing the mental hospitals and the resulting legislation for health reform. A work environment is created that fosters a sense of well-being. Such well-being and working on acceptance by the community purportedly results in a sense of belonging and of importance (Di Mascio and Crosetto, 1994).

Real jobs for real pay

Earlier approaches to vocational rehabilitation implied that due to the severity of their handicaps, a considerable percentage of mentally ill people would never be ready to work in normal settings. The supported employment approach, in contrast, assumes that all people, regardless of the severity of their disability, can do meaningful, productive work in normal settings, if that is what they choose to do, and if they are given the necessary supports (Anthony and Blanch, 1987). Supported employment as described by Bond *et al.* (1997) includes the following features:

- A goal of permanent competitive employment
- Minimal screening for employability
- Avoidance of pre-vocational training
- Individualized placement
- Time-unlimited support.

Drake *et al.* (1994 and replicated 1996) found that eliminating day treatment in favour of supported employment could improve integration into the community and produce competitive jobs even amongst persons with severe mental disabilities. Bailey *et al.* (1998) concluded that clients with very lengthy day treatment who expressed interest in employment could succeed in active supported employment programmes.

An integrated approach to supported employment has demonstrated success relative to a brokered service model (Russert and Frey 1991; Bond *et al.*, 1997; Bond, 1998). Clashes in orientation and attitudes between clinicians and vocational specialists serving the same client has long been identified as a major barrier which clients must overcome to attain and maintain employment (Torrey *et al.*, 1998a). Positive outcomes for programmes that followed the assertive community treatment approach of integration of services within multi-disciplinary teams support this principle (Blankertz and Robinson, 1996).

Further studies have shown that direct approaches to finding and attaining employment increase rates of competitive employment more than do gradual, stepwise approaches. Not surprisingly, clients prefer paid employment to programmes that require unpaid pre-vocational training (Bond *et al.*, 1997). Helping people with severe mental illness obtain competitive jobs that correspond to their explicit job preference increases job satisfaction and tenure. Job preferences are more likely to develop or change through searching for a job than through pre-vocational training (Danley and Anthony, 1987; Becker *et al.*, 1996).

Overcoming barriers and disincentives

Although ongoing support is a central tenet of the supported employment model, studies have shown that decreased employment rates occurred around the time of termination of grant support, suggesting that uncertainty about staff availability may affect job tenure. Totally self-directed strategies such as the job club, that require clients to assume most of the responsibility for searching for jobs and making contacts with employers, do not appear to be satisfactory for the large majority of persons with serious mental illness (Bond *et al.*, 1997).

Despite rhetoric about job matching and job preferences, most supported employment job placements are in unskilled entry-level jobs. Many clients still lack experience, credentials, education and training. Studies of job terminations indicate that many clients experience negative job endings (Bond *et al.*, 1997). Stigma, discrimination, lack of training and a sporadic work history may account for the difficulties people with long-term mental illness have in getting and keeping jobs that are stable, permanent and pay enough to provide a safe alternative to disability benefits. Many services are adopting supported education programmes such as the 'choose–get–keep' approach providing assistance, preparation and support to those with psychiatric disabilities who wish to pursue post-secondary education or training (Sullivan *et al.*, 1993; Mowbray *et al.*, 1996).

Warner (1999) states that like everybody else, people with psychiatric disabilities balance several factors to optimize their income. The decision to work is based on three counter-balancing factors:

- the economic return to the individual
- the stress and effort involved
- the satisfaction derived from the work.

The risk of losing pension or benefit entitlements by joining the workforce may present a significant obstacle to many individuals. Warner's findings (1999) suggest two possible social policy innovations to tackle this issue:

- increasing the allowable earned income before reducing the disability pension,
- providing wage subsidies.

Innovative options

As with day care, range and diversity in vocational programmes are essential for quality services to exist. Barker (1994) states "it is critical to remember that persons with psychiatric disabilities are at least as diverse a population as citizens in general. The task of developing community-based employment options must be accomplished within the framework of recognising the target population as individuals with more differences than similarities." She describes the 'wit' factor—whatever it takes, maintaining creativity and flexibility as a standard operating procedure.

Some examples of innovative community-based programmes include Cornucopia in Australia, which is a facility that brings together clinical support and vocational rehabilitation in a consumer-run coffee shop, restaurant and organic nursery. Cornucopia aims to provide a flexible

work situation whose employees receive trade union-negotiated award conditions and rates of pay and have access to further workplace training and a career structure (Newton, 1999).

Many people experienced in helping to develop such service-intensive consumer-run businesses say that they usually involve at least one of the '4fs': *food, floors, flowers and furniture* (P. Sherman, personal communication). However, some consumer enterprises have moved into a wider range of businesses: e.g. a courier service using public transport (Warner, 1999) and a consultancy firm advising on how to optimize consumer participation in public and private organizations (C. Harris, Framework Trust, New Zealand, personal communication). Polak and Warner (1996) describe the proposed development of a consumer-oriented, profit-sharing pharmacy at the Mental Health Centre of Boulder County, creating consumer employment opportunities and generating capital for other consumer-employing businesses.

Akabas (1994) found that the most successful programmes are ones where services are an integral part of the community in which they are based. In particular:

- The programme needs to be responsive to the particular needs of individuals within a particular community rather than attempting to design services around some abstract concept of who the target population will be.
- Programmes need to be designed to build on the strengths, resources, relationships and unique aspects of a particular community. Just as there is no single service package that works for all individuals, there is no single programme model that works for all communities.
- Developing relationships with businesses in the particular community rather than adopting any single marketing approach.

The very working situations and conditions that enhance the employment experience for all persons are those that are effective in fostering successful competitive outcomes for people with a mental illness. A worksite that responds to diversity will encompass accommodation to the specific needs of those with mental health problems as just one more subset of response to the needs of diverse employee populations (Akabas, 1994).

Conclusion

The death of day care and sheltered work?

These shifts do not necessarily indicate that earlier programmes are now completely redundant: they illustrate a widening of the range, providing more latitude for individual choice and needs. As Warner (1999) points out, even within an environment offering many vocational options for people with mental illness, for some individuals with very limited functioning capacity, a sheltered workshop may still be the only feasible workplace.

On the other hand, Warner (1994) considers that developments in community treatment and consumer-run programmes have made most day care and sheltered workplaces more or less obsolete. Such programmes are in essence a transfer of the institutional setting to the community. Day care may offer close observation, daily medication, monitoring and 'a welcome release from an otherwise aimless existence'. However, these aims can be achieved with much greater rehabilitation, recovery and empowerment potential through initiatives with much greater consumer involvement and ownership.

The direction of structured (day and evening) rehabilitation and recovery programmes, and of work-related programmes for individuals with a mental illness, are being determined increasingly by evidence-based reviews, including the forthcoming Cochrane Collaboration reports on Day Hospitalisation (Almarez-Serrano *et al.*, 1999) and vocational programmes (Crowther *et al.*, 1999). At the same time, more rigorous qualitative evidence (including consumer-led research) must be both sought and heeded. As the mental health system realizes the importance of empowerment, the field of vocational rehabilitation must do likewise. Individuals severely affected by mental illness must have:

- Freedom of choice regarding one's individual services.
- A significant role in the operation and decision-making structure of programmes and agencies that provide services.
- Participation in planning, evaluation and decision making on a system-wide level.
- Participation in civic issues on community, city, county, state and federal levels.

(Howie the Harp—Consumer Activist, 1994).

Acknowledgements

Thanks to Sylvia Hands, Magda Rzoska-Krzyszton and Melanie Kammerman for assistance with the literature search and preparation, and Rebecca McCahon and Vivienne Miller for comments on the manuscript.

References

Akabas, S.H. (1994) Workplace responsiveness: key employer characteristics in support of job maintenance for people with mental illness. *Psychosocial Rehabilitation Journal*, 17, 91–101.

Almarez-Serrano, A.M., Marshall, M. and Creed, F. (1999) The Cochrane Library.

Anthony, W.A. (1993) Recovery from mental illness: the guiding vision of the mental health service system in the 1990's. *Psychosocial Rehabilitation Journal*, 16, 11–23.

Anthony, W.A. and Blanch, A (1987) Supported employment for persons who are psychiatrically disabled: an historical and conceptual perspective. *Psychosocial Rehabilitation Journal*, 11, 5–23.

Anthony, W.A. and Liberman, R.P. (1986) The practice of psychiatric rehabilitation: historical conceptual and research base. *Schizophrenia Bulletin*, 12, 542–559.

Anthony, W.A., Cohen, M. and Farkas, M. (1982) A psychiatric rehabilitation programme, can I recognise one if I see one? *Community Mental Health Journal*, 18, 83–95.

Bailey, E.L., Ricketts, S.K., Becker, D.R., Xie,H. and Drake, R.E. (1998) Do long-term day treatment clients benefit from supported employment? *Psychiatric Rehabilitation Journal*, 22, 24–29.

Barker L.T. (1994) Community based models of employment services for people with psychiatric disabilities. *Psychosocial Rehabilitation Journal*, 17, 55–65.

Beard, J.H., Propst, R.N. and Malamud, T.J. (1982) The Fountain House model of psychiatric rehabilitation. *Psychosocial Rehabilitation Journal*, 5, 47–53.

Becker, D.R., Drake, R.E., Farabaugh, A. and Bond, G.R. (1996) Job preferences of clients with severe psychiatric disorders participating in supported employment programmes. *Psychiatric Services*, 47, 1223–1226.

Becker, D.R., Bebout, R.R. and Drake, R.E. (1998) Job preferences of people with severe mental illness: a replication. *Psychiatric Rehabilitation Journal*, 22, 46–50.

Bellack, A.S. (ed.) (1984) *Schizophrenia Treatment, Management and Rehabilitation*. Orlando: Grune and Stratton.

Blankertz, L. and Robinson, S. (1996) Adding vocational focus to mental health rehabilitation. *Psychiatric Services*, 47, 1216–1222.

Bond, G.R. (1998) Principles of the individual placement and support model: empirical support. *Psychiatric Rehabilitation Journal*, 22, 11–23.

Bond, G R. and McDonel, E.C. (1998) Vocational rehabilitation outcomes for persons with psychiatric disabilities: an update. *Journal of Vocational Rehabilitation*, 1, 9–20.

Bond, G.R., Drake, R.E., Mueser, K.T. and Becker, D.R. (1997) An update on supported employment for people with severe mental illness. *Psychiatric Services*, 48, 335–346.

Campbell, J.A. (1989) Employment programmes for people with a psychiatric disability: an overview. *Community Support Network News*, 6, 1–11.

Carling, P.J. (1995) *Return to Community*. New York. The Guilford Press.

Chadwick, P., Birchwood, M. and Trower, P. (1996) *Cognitive Delusions, Voices and Paranoia*. Chichester, UK: Wiley,.

Chapparo, C. and Ranka, S. (1997) *OPM, Occupational Performance Model (Australia)*. Monograph 1. Castle Hill, Australia: Occupational Performance Network.

Crichton, E (1989) Principles and practices in rehabilitation. In: Jacobs. P., Crichton, E. and Visotna, M. (eds), *Practical Approaches To Mental Health Care*. Sydney: Macmillan, pp. 133–156.

Crowther, R. *et al.* (1999) *Vocational Rehabilitation for People with Severe Mental Disorders (Protocol)*. The Cochrane Library.

Danley, K.S. and Anthony, W.A. (1987) The choose–get–keep model: serving severely disabled psychiatrically disabled people. *American Rehabilitation*, 13, 6–9, 27–29.

Di Mascio, A. and Crosetto, P.G. (1994) Work reintegration of the mentally disabled: the experiences of the Nuova Cooperativa. *International Journal of Mental Health*, 23, 61–70.

Drake, R.E., Becker, D.R., Biesanz, J.C., Torrey, W.C. et al. (1994) Rehabilitative day treatment vs. supported employment: l: vocational outcomes. *Community Mental Health Journal*, 30, 519–532.

Drake, R.E., Becker, D.R., Biesanz, J.C., Wyzik, P.F. and Torrey, W.C. (1996) Day treatment vs supported employment for persons with severe mental illness: a replication study. *Psychiatric Services*, 47, 1125–1127.

Fairweather, G.W. (1969) *Community Life for the Mentally Ill*. Chicago: Aldine.

Falloon, I.R.H. and Fadden, G. (1993) *Integrated Mental Health Care: A Comprehensive Community Based Approach*. Cambridge: Cambridge University Press.

Falloon, I.R.H. and Talbot, R. (1982) Achieving the goals of day treatment. *Journal of Nervous and Mental Disease*, 170, 279–285.

Falloon, I.R.H., Shanahan, W., Laporta, M. and Krekorian H.A.R. (1990) Integrated family, general practice and mental health care in the management of schizophrenia. *Journal of the Royal Society of Medicine*, 83–225.

Gianfrancesco P., Miller, V., Rauch A., Rosen, A. and Rotem, W. (1997) *National Standards for Mental Health Services*. Canberra: Australian Health Ministers National Mental Health Working Group.

Harding, C.M., Zubin, J. and Strauss, J.S. (1992) Chronicity in schizophrenia: revised. *American Journal of Psychiatry*, 161, 27–37.

Hoge, M.A., Davidson, L., Hill, L.W., Turner, V.E. and Rezvan, A. (1992) The promise of partial hospitalisation: a reassessment. *Hospital and Community Psychiatry*, 43, 345–353.

Hoult, J., Rosen, A. and Reynolds, I. (1984) Community orientated treatment compared to psychiatric hospital orientated treatment. *Social Science Medicine*, 18, 1005–1010.

Howie the Harp (1994) Empowerment of mental health consumers in vocational rehabilitation. *Psychosocial Rehabilitation Journal*, 17, 83–89.

Kaufmann, C.L., Ward-Colasante, C. and Farmer, J. (1993) Development and evaluation of drop-in centres operated by mental health consumers. *Hospital and Community Psychiatry*, 44, 675–678.

McCarthy, D., Thompson, D. and Olson, S. (1998) Planning a statewide project to convert day treatment to supported employment. *Psychiatric Rehabilitation Journal*, 22, 30–33.

McGorry, P.D. (1992) The concept of recovery and secondary prevention of psychotic disorders. *Australian and New Zealand Journal of Psychiatry*, 26, 3–17

McGurrin, M.C. (1994) An overview of the effectiveness of traditional vocational rehabilitation services in the treatment of longterm mental illness. *Psychosocial Rehabilitation Journal*, 17, 37–54.

Mowbray, C. T., Bybee, D. and Shriner, W. (1996) Characteristics of participants in a supported education program for adults with psychiatric disabilities. *Psychiatric Services*, 47, 1371–1377.

Newton, L. (1999) *Cornucopia—A Community Based Supported Employment Program in Sydney*. Melbourne, Australia: Themhs Conference Proceedings 1999.

Polak, P. and Warner, R. (1996) The economic life of seriously ill people in the community. *Psychiatric Services*, 47, 270–274.

Richmond Implementation Unit (1987) *Glossary of Terms: Adult Mental Health Services*. Sydney, Australia: State Health Publication.

Rosen, A. (1992) Community Psychiatry Services: will they endure. *Current Opinion in Psychiatry*, 5, 257–265.

Rosen, A. (1994) 100% Mabo: de-colonising people with mental illness and their families. *Australian and New Zealand Journal of Family Therapy*, 15, 128–142.

Rosen, A. (1998) *Mobile Intensive Community Management Teams: Beyond Assertive Community Treatment*. York: Sainsbury Centre for Mental Health Summer Conference. Workshop.

Rosen, A., Parker G., Hadzi-Pavlovic D. and Hartley, R. (1987) *Developing Evaluation Strategies for Area Mental Health Services in N.S.W.* Sydney: State Health Publication.

Russert, M.G. and Frey, J.L. (1991) The PACT vocational model: a step into the future. *Psychosocial Rehabilitation Journal*, 14, 7–18.

Salem, D.A. (1990) Community-based services and resources: the significance of choice and diversity. *American Journal of Community Psychology*, 18, 909–915.

Segal, S.P., Silverman, C. and Temkin, T. (1995) Characteristics and service use of long-term members of self-help agencies for mental health clients. *Psychiatric Services*, 46, 269–274.

Shepherd, G. (1998) Models of community care. *Journal of Mental Health*, 7, 165–177.

Strauss, J.S. (1989) Subjective experience of schizophrenia. *Schizophrenia Bulletin*, 15, 179–185.

Stein, L.I., Test, M.A. and Marx, A.J. (1980) Alternative to mental hospital treatment, parts I and II. *Archives of General Psychiatry*, 37, 392–397, 409–412.

Sullivan, A.P., Nicolellis, E.L., Danley, K.S. and MacDonald-Wilson, K. (1993) Choose, get keep: a psychiatric rehabilitation approach to supported education. *Psychosocial Rehabilitation Journal*, 17, 55–68.

Tarrier, N., Yusupoff, L., Kinney, C., McCarthy, E., Gledhill, A., Hadock, G. and Morris, J. (1998) Randomised controlled trial of intensive cognitive behaviour therapy for patients with chronic schizophrenia. *British Medical Journal*, 317, 303–307.

Test, M.A. (1995). Impact of seven years of assertive community treatment. *Presentation at the American Psychiatric Association Institute on Psychiatric Services*. Boston, MA

Thornicroft, G., Ward, P. and James, S. (1993) Care management and mental health, countdown to community care series, *British Medical Journal*, 306, 768–771.

Tobin, M.J. (1999) Rehabilitation in mental illness: what GPs need to know. *Current Therapeutics*, 40, 47–53.

Tooth, B.A., Kalyanansundaram, V. and Glover, H. (1997) Recovery from schizophrenia: a consumer perspective. *Final Report to Health and Human Services Research and Development Grants Program (RADGAC)*.

Torrey, W.C., Becker, D.R. and Drake, R.E. (1995) Rehabilitative day treatment vs. supported employment: II. Consumer, family and staff reactions to a program change. *Psychosocial Rehabilitation Journal*, 18, 67–75.

Torrey, W.C., Bebout, R., Kline, J., Becker, D.R., Alverson, M. and Drake, R.E. (1998a) Practice guidelines for clinicians working in programs providing integrated vocational and clinical services for persons with severe mental disorders. *Psychiatric Rehabilitation Journal*, 21, 388–393.

Torrey, W.C., Mead, S. and Ross, G. (1998b) Addressing the social needs of mental health consumers when day treatment programs convert to supported employment: can consumer-run services play a role? *Psychiatric Rehabilitation Journal*, 22, 73–75.

Warner. R. (1994) *Recovery from Schizophrenia: Psychiatry and the Political Economy*, 2nd edn. London: Routledge.

Warner, R. (1999) Work: opportunities and obstacles. In: Bhugra, D and Holloway, F. (eds), *Rehabilitation Psychiatry: Principles and Practice*. Cambridge: Cambridge University Press.

Warner, R., Huxley, P. and Berg, T. (1999) An evaluation of the impact of clubhouse membership on quality of life and treatment utilisation. *International Journal of Social Psychiatry*, in press.

Weir, W. and Rosen, A. (1989) Living skills centres for people with serious psychiatric disorders. *Australian Occupational Therapy Journal*, 36, 85–91.

World Health Organisation (1996) *Psycho-social Rehabilitation—A Consensus Statement*. Geneva: WHO.

27 | Residential care

Geoff Shepherd and Alison Murray

Introduction

Everyone needs somewhere to live. The provision of an adequate range of good quality accommodation must therefore be at the centre of attempts to develop community-based systems of care. Perhaps it is surprising then that mental health services—and mental health professionals—have taken so little interest in housing issues. For far too long, housing has been seen as 'outside' the mental health system, rather than as integral with it. While the importance of adequate housing may be recognized in principle, in practice relatively little research has been done to assess outcomes in housing systems, to develop and evaluate interventions to improve joint working between mental health services and specialist housing providers, and to understand the factors that make for successful staff and successful leadership within such facilities.

It is the purpose of the present chapter to explore these issues. We will sketch out the historical and policy background, review the current issues, bring together the available research and try to make some practical suggestions as to how to move forward using an 'evidence-based' approach. The context for this is the 'mixed economy' of care that now characterizes housing provision for people with mental health problems in the UK (and in most other countries in northern Europe, Australasia and the USA). This has grown up as institutional care has decreased in size and a range of new providers has entered the field. The 'total institution' may thus have disappeared, but we now have many 'institutions', with many different management authorities, cultures and values. This has disadvantages as well as many obvious benefits. How have we arrived at this point? Before tracing the historical story, let us begin with questions of definition and needs.

Defining terms

The range of residential alternatives is notoriously difficult to classify. One of the most useful attempts is to be found in Lelliott *et al.* (1996). They used a multi-dimensional system based on the availability of different kinds of staff cover, number of beds and staff:resident ratios. This is shown in Table 27.1.

The range moves from acute in-patient wards with constant staffing and relatively high numbers of staff; through high staffed hostels ('24-hour nursed care'); low staffed hostels; staffed care homes with sleeping night staff; and group homes without staff on the premises, but regular visiting. This classification reflects a traditional view of residential care based on a 'sheltered housing' model where the extent of support available from staff *in situ* is seen as one of the predominant defining characteristics. As we shall see, more recent developments in the housing field have tended to emphasize 'supported housing' models (Carling, 1993) where staff are used more flexibly to provide high (or low) levels of support according to fluctuating levels of individual need. This opens up the possibility of using a much greater range of 'ordinary housing' options in a more cost-efficient way compared with traditional hostels and group homes. It is also more consistent with service users' increasing demands for increased privacy and reduced stigma.

Estimating needs

One of the major reasons for wishing to develop agreed and consistent definitions for sheltered and supported housing is to inform the planning process by providing guidelines as to the numbers of different kinds of accommodation required

Table 27.1 *The spectrum of residential care*

Facililty type	Resident places	Night cover	Day cover	Ratio of staff: resident places	% staff with a care qualification
Forensic unit	>6	Waking	Constant	1.3	62%
Acute ward	>6	Waking	Constant	1.3	63%
Long-stay ward	>6	Waking	Constant	0.9	49%
High-staffed hostel	>6	Waking	Constant	0.7	15%
Mid-staffed hostel	>6	Sleep-in	Constant	0.4	14%
Low-staffed hostel	>6	On call/none	Regular	0.2	15%
Group home	<6	On call/none	Visited	0.2	33%
Staffed care home	>6	Sleep-in	Constant	1.0	7%

Based on Lelliott *et al.* (1996).

to meet the needs of a given, local population. In practice, this is extremely difficult to achieve. In any given locality, there are a number of local factors which influence the demand for specialist housing: demography, transport, unemployment, ethnic composition, funding priorities of the Local Authority, attitudes of primary care, effectiveness of specialist mental health services, etc. Some of these can be partially taken into account by sophisticated quantitative modelling (e.g. Glover, 1996), but at the heart of such algorithms remain guesses—albeit sensible and well-informed guesses—about what numbers of different kinds of provisions a given pattern of local morbidity implies.

An additional complicating factor is that one kind of housing or accommodation potentially can 'substitute' for another. Thus, high support hostels may substitute for in-patient beds; flexible, 'high support' community teams may substitute for sheltered housing (or hospital beds); family care with intensive professional support may

substitute for professional support or specialist housing, and so on. Housing needs assessments therefore depend crucially on the range and quality of other local services and cannot be separated from the functioning and dynamics of the total service 'system'. The 'confidence limits' surrounding estimates of different kinds of accommodation needs therefore remain large (Johnson *et al.*, 1996) and the value of general norms is limited.

For all these reasons, it is probably more helpful to begin local planning by conducting a simple inventory of local housing availability to see *who* is currently accommodated (and who is not). If one then surveys levels of disability and case mix in existing provision and adds in information on who is currently excluded from provisions (e.g. the homeless), then this should highlight obvious shortfalls. This should also give a starting point in terms of development priorities. On the basis of national information, shortages in high dependency housing and flexible, intensive community support are the most likely areas of greatest deficiency (Audit Commission, 1998; Department of Health, 1998a).

Historical and policy background

As indicated earlier, the central theme in the story of the development of residential care has been the move from a single provider of hospital care (the NHS) to a multiplicity of independent 'for-profit' and 'not-for-profit' community providers. In 1955, there were more than 155 000 beds in long-stay hospitals in England and Wales; by 1998 this figure had dropped to just 36 000. This dramatic change in overall numbers was accompanied by an equally striking change in the nature of the provider and this is illustrated in Figure 27.1.

As can be seen, in little more than 10 years, from 1986 to 1996, the proportion of specialist accommodation provided by the private and voluntary sector increased from 5% to 52% and the contribution of NHS provision to the total

more than halved (from 91% to 43%). A substantial proportion (23%) of the growth in the private sector has been in private hospitals and nursing homes (mostly nursing homes for the elderly), but there has also been a steady increase in private and voluntary sector residential care for the under 65s.

The policy background that drove these changes was signalled in 1962 in the NHS 'Hospital Plan' (Ministry of Health, 1962). This proposed a reduction by half of the beds in long-stay institutions over the next 10 years. It was based on projections of bed use which turned out to be almost completely wrong, but nevertheless the policy has proved extremely robust and has been pursued actively by successive governments over the last 30 years (see Carrier and Kendall, 1996, for a good historical account of this process). The policy of bed reductions in long-stay hospitals has been accompanied by an increase in acute units in general hospitals and a change in the responsibility for managing and providing residential care towards greater involvement of various non-statutory agencies. Thus, following *Care in the Community* (DHSS, 1981), the

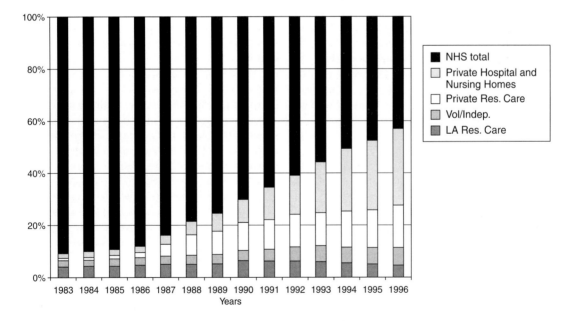

Figure 27.1 *Changing balance of specialist accommodation. [The authors are grateful to Professor Martin Knapp (CEMH, London School of Economics) who supplied the data for this figure.]*

responsibility for managing residential care was shifted from Regional Health Authorities towards local authorities. The *NHS and Community Care Act* (Department of Health, 1990) then enabled agencies other than the NHS and local authorities to become involved in operating and managing residential facilities. Current policy shows no signs of reversing this general direction. The emphasis is now on closer *joint* working between the statutory agencies (e.g. *Partnerships in Action*, Department of Health, 1998b), particularly in terms of joint commissioning of local services, and there is clearly a desire to remove the practical constraints to creating single budgets and 'cross-management' arrangements. We are therefore now no more likely to go back to a single provider for specialist residential care for the mentally ill than we are likely to build a lot of new mental hospitals. So, what are the problems of the present system?

Current issues

In many respects, the move from traditional long-stay hospitals to smaller, independent providers in the community has been very successful. Quality of care for previous long-stay patients is generally better, their functioning is improved, they are more satisfied and costs are no greater than those in hospital—in many cases they are rather less. The research evidence in support of these conclusions will be reviewed later; for the moment, let us focus on some of the operational and management problems that have emerged.

In the first place, there still seems to be an overall shortage in appropriate residential places, particularly for those with the most severe and enduring problems. Given that more than 120 000 long-stay beds have been closed and only around 50 000 new places have been created, perhaps this is not surprising. However, simple 'one-for-one' comparisons are misleading. Most of the patients who were resettled from the old institutions have fared reasonably well, although there are still problems with regard to the regulation and inspection of a dispersed and largely private, or 'semi-private', system. There are also problems

with the ageing nature of this population, and housing schemes which were set up in the context of hospital closure programmes are now having to care for an increasingly elderly and frail population where the original social groupings have broken up through illness or death.

However, the major problems are not with 'old' long-stay patients coming out of hospital, they are with the failure to anticipate the needs of the next generation of potential 'new' long-stay patients now presenting to services. Beds are relatively easy to close: it is much more difficult to ensure that resources are redirected to the development of effective alternatives in the community which are targeted specifically on those who are most likely to be affected by bed reductions. One of the unforeseen consequences of the failure to provide for the next generation of patients with long-term needs has been the accumulation of 'new' long-stay patients in acute admission wards (Lelliott and Wing, 1994) or in the 'revolving door' of repeated admission and unstable adjustment in the community. The failure to develop a comprehensive range of housing alternatives is therefore directly related to the problems of perceived lack of acute in-patient beds. This is particularly severe in some inner city areas (e.g. London; see Johnson *et al.*, 1997). However, the most cost-effective solution may not be to provide more acute beds, but to develop 'beds' of a different kind, both as part of NHS provisions and in the community (Shepherd *et al.*, 1997). As we shall see later, there are various, specialist 'high dependency' housing schemes that have the potential to provide both more effective, and *less expensive*, care than traditional hospital beds for most of those who are now 'blocking' acute beds.

If such alternatives are to be effective, then they clearly must be targeted specifically to those with the greatest needs. The growth of a 'mixed economy' of care and a diverse range of providers has made this difficult. Providers often have been in a situation where they can choose who they will take into a new facility and, not surprisingly, they tend to choose the apparently 'easier' clients. Thus, there is evidence that during the movement of 'old' long-stay patients out of hospital, residential facilities were 'creaming off' the less disabled (Jones, 1993; Holloway and Faulkener, 1994; Shepherd *et al.*, 1996). With the advent of a new generation of very difficult 'new' long-stay patients, who may have co-morbid drug and alcohol problems, histories of violence, contact with the police, difficulties in engagement with services, etc., these tendencies have been exacerbated (Lelliott *et al.*, 1996).

A stereotype has therefore grown up that independent sector providers will not take 'difficult patients'. Conversely, many independent sector providers believe that statutory services simply want to 'dump' difficult cases and fail to give adequate support and follow-up. Both views undoubtedly contain some degree of truth. They underline the need for statutory and non-statutory agencies to work closely together and for each to be clear about what they can reasonably expect of each other and what they need in order to work together effectively to meet a common set of objectives. To achieve this requires more than simple exhortation. It needs careful and skilled, interagency organizational development. Developing and evaluating effective interventions for achieving this have received little attention.

Even if effective local partnerships can be forged, then the problems of negative public attitudes and community resistance still have to be addressed. The public remain generally fearful of those they perceive as being 'mentally ill' and distrustful of policies of 'community care'. However, many also express sympathy, concern and a desire to help. These positive attitudes can be harnessed, providing there is direct contact between local people and those with mental health problems and an opportunity to address fears and anxieties in a structured way. For example, as part of the TAPS study (see below). Wolff *et al.* (1996) evaluated the effectiveness of a community education programme aimed at preparing a new supported housing scheme. They targeted approximately 150 people in a local community and provided information sheets, a video, a public meeting with a 'question-and-answer' session, a barbecue and other social events. Common stereotypes of risk and dangerousness were addressed and the public were reassured that residents would not be simply 'dumped' and left to fend for

themselves. Attitudes before and after the intervention were compared with a control group who were retested over the same time period with no intervention. The experimental group showed a small increase in knowledge concerning mental illness, but a significant reduction in fearful and rejecting attitudes. They were also more likely to make contact with patients in their own homes (28% versus 8%) and for patients to make contact with them. Thus, community education programmes *can* make a difference providing they are clearly focused and involve prolonged contact with those who hold prejudiced attitudes. This is consistent with other research on tackling stigma in schizophrenia (Penn *et al.*, 1994).

Next, we come to the questions of staffing and leadership. The growth of provision by a variety of non-statutory agencies has meant that many more of the staff now involved in delivering care do not have formal mental health training or qualifications. In some ways, this is a positive benefit as 'institutional attitudes' undoubtedly are associated with institutional training and experience. However, it also has disadvantages since staff who feel themselves to be 'untrained' to deal with difficult clinical problems are more likely to be reluctant to accept such individuals (hence contributing to the stereotype of avoiding 'difficult' referrals). It is therefore disappointing that so little attention has been paid to the development and evaluation of staff training programmes for housing and residential care staff. For example, in their survey of the TAPS reprovision schemes, Senn *et al.* (1997) found that almost a quarter offered no training at all, not even in the management of violence or risk.

A notable exception in terms of specific training programmes for staff in the housing field is the work of Phelan and Strathdee (1994). They offered half-day sessions covering basic information on mental illness (signs and symptoms, etc.), interviewing skills, prevention and management of violence, and an exercise aimed at promoting insight and understanding into the experiences of people with mental health problems in terms of their dealing with housing authorities. The results were described as 'very positive' and the authors emphasize the importance of breaking down traditional prejudices and stereotypes among housing department staff.

Part of the reason for the failure to develop and evaluate training programmes for residential care staff undoubtedly is a lack of clarity regarding exactly what skills they require. One potentially important area which has emerged recently is the application of 'Expressed Emotion' (EE) models from the research with family carers (Ball *et al.*, 1992). This holds out exciting possibilities in the residential care field; however, it must be acknowledged that the evaluative research is, at present, very limited.

A similar situation holds regarding the recruitment and selection of staff. It is recognized that staff characteristics are important, but almost no attention has been paid to developing more reliable and valid selection processes. Again, the 'low EE' model may have applicability as a framework for staff selection. Leadership skills are of central importance. The management 'style' of project leaders may have more influence than any other single factor on the quality of care experienced by residents (Shepherd *et al.*, 1996), but how to identify good leaders for residential projects and how to support them effectively are almost entirely unexplored areas. In other fields (e.g. care of the elderly), there are some interesting examples of 'mentoring programmes', with senior, experienced practitioners providing ongoing support and skills development for new project managers, but such programmes are not common in the residential care field. Given all these problems, perhaps it is not surprising that there are so many difficulties in joint working and so many problems in independent sector providers accepting the most difficult and 'challenging' residents. The problems are clear: what we now need are practical, well-researched solutions.

The final problem with the present system of residential care concerns the increasing expectations of residents and their clearly expressed preferences for care. Perhaps it is unfair to label this a 'problem' since what has happened is simply that a new generation of service users has now emerged who have not been socialized into believing that what they must expect in terms of accommodation from mental health services is a 'special' home or hostel, with staff on site to look after their clinical and social needs. The evidence is now very strong that such arrangements are unattractive to a large proportion of those that they are designed to serve. Most users want a much less 'stigmatized' environment, with greater privacy, and staff who are 'on tap' in a flexible way, rather than available 'around the clock' (Keck, 1990; Tanzman, 1993; Owen *et al.*, 1996; Rose and Muijen, 1997). In planning terms, this implies a re-think of housing priorities and a need to move away from traditional group homes and hostels towards more flexible, 'ordinary housing' alternatives. Whether the resulting system will be more effective in terms of producing better clinical and social outcomes and reduced use of hospital admission remains to be demonstrated.

Research evidence—outcomes

So, to the question of outcomes: for obvious reasons, the evaluation of housing schemes is not an area where randomized controlled trials are common. The best controlled trial of long-stay patients leaving hospital is probably the 'Team for the Assessment of Psychiatric Services' (TAPS) study which examined the progress of over 700 patients leaving Friern and Claybury hospitals in north London over a period of more than 5 years (Leff, 1997). Patients were assessed using a variety of symptom and social functioning measures and progress compared with matched controls remaining in hospital. The results showed few differences in terms of positive symptoms, but significant reductions in negative symptoms among the community group. This was paralleled by significant improvements in social functioning, domestic and daily living skills. There was also some evidence of increases in the size and 'normalization' of social networks. Physical health status showed no differences, but the authors note problems of increased mortality (due to physical illness) and the effects of ageing. There were no increases in rates of suicide or crime. In general, levels of satisfaction were much greater for the groups who were resettled, and these differences persisted to 5 years. If all costs were taken into account, care was slightly less expensive for the community group, but increased with increasing levels of disability (Beecham *et al.*, 1997). Uncontrolled follow-up studies of community re-settlement show a very similar picture (Andrews *et al.*, 1990; Segal and Kofler, 1993; Donnelly *et al.*, 1996; Borge *et al.*, 1999).

Regarding outcomes in specialist residential provisions for the 'new' long-stay, the Department of Health has recommended the establishment of '24-hour nursed beds' (NHSE, 1996) which aim to combine high levels of professional supervision with a setting which resembles as much as possible an ordinary home. This concept is very similar to that of a 'ward-in-a-house' or 'hospital hostel' proposed by Bennett (1980) and Young (1991). It is intended that these facilities will fill the gaps highlighted earlier in terms of high dependency accommodation and thereby relieve the pressure on acute beds. The evidence for their effectiveness has been reviewed by Shepherd (1995, 1998). It consists of a mixture of randomized controlled trials, matched controlled trials and uncontrolled follow-ups. The data suggest that such units may be effective in improving the functioning of up to 40% of those referred sufficiently for them to be resettled into the community after an average of 2–3 years. Residents generally make more progress than controls regarding their social functioning, they show increased contact with the community and higher levels of satisfaction. For those who are not resettled, their functioning is maintained more effectively and satisfaction is higher compared with traditional long-stay wards or acute admission units. Overall, costs are generally less than acute beds, but greater than long-stay beds in traditional institutions. Despite these rather positive results, such options may remain unattractive to many potential residents because of the problems mentioned earlier of group living and the 'stigma' of segregated facilities. Such facilities therefore need to be integrated with a comprehensive range of less stigmatized, 'ordinary housing', options in the community, combined with flexible, high support, 'assertive outreach' teams (Mueser *et al.*, 1998).

The outcome evidence for these newer forms of community living is limited and paints a rather mixed picture (Hodgkins *et al.*, 1990; Nelson *et al.*, 1997). In general, the evidence in favour of the *relative* effectiveness of different community residential provisions is weak and there seem to be few differences in terms of clinical functioning, social functioning or readmission rates associated with different forms of sheltered and supported housing. However, it is clear that most residents prefer those facilities that are smaller and offer greater degrees of privacy and independence. Problems of physical ill-health and increased mortality are common for older residents resettled from hospital. For a substantial minority of patients living in the community, fears of loneliness and isolation are a problem and these can reduce their subjective quality of life significantly. On the other hand, those living in close proximity with others who have similar problems may be exposed to additional stresses which can add to their difficulties.

Quality of care and self-reported satisfaction

What is the relationship between quality of care and residents' satisfaction? 'Quality of care' is a complex construct and may be operationalized in a number of different ways. In residential care, the common indicators include: quality of the physical environment; size and degree of individualization of care; choice (e.g. regarding room-mates, meals, etc.); privacy; numbers of rules and restrictions; levels of disturbance among peers; and attractiveness of the local neighbourhood. All these factors have been shown to be associated with measures of self-reported satisfaction ('quality of life'). Since they are more likely to be present in a favourable sense in community settings, this seems to account for the consistent findings of generally higher 'quality of life' in community, as opposed to hospital (Andrews *et al.*, 1990; Lehman *et al.*, 1991; Lewis and Trieman, 1995; Seilheimer and Doyal, 1996; Shepherd *et al.*, 1996). However, the apparent advantages of community living must be interpreted with a little caution.

This is because there are usually sampling biases in most studies of self-reported satisfaction comparing community residents and hospital in-patients. As indicated earlier, community residents are likely to be generally less disabled than those left in hospital. Since there is usually a positive correlation between overall levels of functioning and feelings of satisfaction, it is therefore possible that some of the differences between community and hospital in-patients may be attributable to differences in their physical and mental health, rather than in the quality of the caring environment. This sampling bias may be compounded by problems in gaining the co-operation of the most disabled patients, whether in hospital or in the community (Shepherd *et al.*, 1996; Borge *et al.*, 1999). Once again, community samples are likely to be biased towards those reporting higher levels of satisfaction.

Having said this, the differences between hospital and community samples are very consistent and probably do reflect genuine differences in satisfaction (and quality of care). What gives rise to these differences appears to be apparently small items—access to the kitchen in the evenings, choice over mealtimes, locks on the bathroom door, one's own television, etc. These relatively small differences seem to have a large impact on residents' personal judgements regarding their 'quality of life'.

What about evidence linking 'quality of care' indices to outcomes other than differences in subjective satisfaction or quality of life? Here, the results are less clear-cut. Baker and Douglas (1990) studied the effect of quality of housing environment on community adjustment over a 9-month period in a large sample ($n = 729$) of clients in community support programmes in upstate New York. Clients who were resident in housing rated 'good' or 'fair' showed significant improvements in functioning and no increases in maladaptive behaviour compared with those in housing rated as 'poor'. In a small uncontrolled study, Keck (1990) examined the progress of 20 people moving into apartments which had been selected specifically on the basis of residents' preferences. After 21 months, 16 were still in the same settings and the author concluded that this supported the notion that being responsive to expressed preferences is an important factor in successful residential placement. Middleboe *et al.* (1998) working in Copenhagen studied the progress of 47 patients entering a variety of community residences. After 1 year, they found small improvements in overall symptoms and reduced use of hospitalization. However, as indicated earlier, several studies—particularly those of older residents—note the remarkable stability of symptoms and overall skill levels (see also Segal and Kofler, 1993; Donnelly *et al.*, 1996).

The area where there is probably the strongest evidence for the effectiveness of specific programmes on skills and behaviour is with regard to specialist residential provisions for the 'new' long-stay (Shepherd, 1995, 1998). These tend to show positive gains—including some reductions in violence—compared with controls, and this seems to be associated with the delivery of highly individualized, 'user-centred' programmes (Trieman and Leff, 1996). Such programmes combine structure and support, in the context of frequent, high quality, low 'EE', staff–resident interactions. In order to change behavioural skills (and maintain improvements) specific, individualized programmes of this kind are likely to be most effective.

Social networks and reintegration

One final area of outcome evidence that is worth considering is the effects of residential care on social networks and reintegration. Do residents with severe and enduring mental health problems become a *real* part of the communities in which they live? It has been known for some time that the social networks of people with severe mental health problems tend to be smaller than age-matched, general community samples and more dominated by family and professionals (Sokolovsky *et al.*, 1978). In addition, those with smaller, less supportive networks are at a higher risk of admission, while those with larger networks tend to use a greater range of other services (Becker *et al.*, 1997). These relationships hold even when symptom severity is controlled for (Albert *et al.*, 1998). We noted earlier that care in the community can have benefits in terms of increased social contacts and leisure activities (Borge *et al.*, 1999), and this finding is supported by the studies of Tempier *et al.* (1997) and Middleboe *et al.* (1998). Both found an increase in social networks and social integration. Patients engaged in more leisure and social activities in the community and began to use a greater variety of both professional and non-professional services. The TAPS study found a similar increase in contact with non-mental health services (e.g. church groups, social clubs, etc.) over the first year of follow-up which was maintained up to 5 years. There was also a significant increase in the number of people considered by the patients to be 'friends' at 1 year which was maintained at 5 years. The number of confidants remained steady during the first year and then increased significantly over the next 4 years, suggesting that closer personal relationships ('confidants') take longer to acquire than friends (Leff, 1997). On a less positive note, Goering *et al.* (1992) examined the social network composition of a group ($n = 40$) of residents in two supported housing programmes in Toronto. They found that residents had similar size social networks ($n = 12$) compared with the general population, but that they were more likely to be composed of professionals and other patients and less likely to contain non-mental health 'friends' and family members. The authors note the problems with networks which are too dependent on professionals and the link between the number of professionals in social networks and lower levels of self-esteem.

The literature on social networks and social integration is therefore generally quite positive. Community living does seem to be associated with an increase in network size and engagement with a range of community services, and this may reduce the likelihood of admission. However, the protective value of social networks is likely to depend on a number of qualitative, as well as quantitative, factors. There is also a danger that some kinds of community accommodation may 'isolate' patients from mainstream activities and lead to an over-reliance on professionals and other staff. As with the acquisition of social and domestic skills, social networks will probably

change most if they are targeted specifically (e.g. Thornicroft and Breakey, 1991). This provides an interesting potential new focus for community programmes in the future.

Practical steps forward

(i)   Definitions of residential alternatives must be multi-dimensional and should include a consideration of staff availability (hours of working, etc.), number of beds and staff:resident ratios. They should also reflect user preferences for flexible, 'supported housing' models, rather than traditional group homes and hostels with fixed staffing.

(ii) Local planning should be built on locally collected information about *who* the housing network is serving (and who it is not). It should not rely on 'norms'. Any planning process must also not neglect the needs of those requiring the highest levels of support, whether provided by specialist residential places (e.g. 'hospital hostels') or through the flexible, high support, 'assertive outreach' teams in the community.

(iii) New projects are likely to be undertaken in partnership between statutory agencies and independent sector providers. To make these partnerships work effectively, there needs to be mutual respect and understanding between the agencies regarding their respective roles and responsibilities. They may need help to achieve this.

(iv) Local communities must be prepared for new developments. This includes the provision of information, reassurance and an opportunity to meet some of the users likely to be involved in the project.

(v)   More attention needs to be given to the development and evaluation of joint training initiatives, aimed at improving the knowledge and skills of residential care workers from non-statutory agencies.

(vi) Attention should also be given to staff selection processes and to identify those staff who will be most effective in their interactions with residents. Although the empirical evidence currently is weak, 'Expressed Emotion' (EE) models may provide a useful framework.

(vii) Particularly careful consideration should be given to the desirable attributes of project leaders and to mechanisms for supporting them and helping them develop their leadership skills.

(viii) The outcome evidence suggests that residents resettled from traditional institutions are likely to be functioning better and to be more satisfied than those who remain in hospital, but the long-term quality of care in these settings needs to be monitored. In particular, physical health needs, associated with increased ageing, need to be addressed.

(ix) Regarding the effectiveness of different types of community provision, the evidence is limited. Loneliness and isolation may be problems for some people, but so can stress caused by too close proximity to others with mental health difficulties. There is some evidence that domestic skills and social networks may improve, but they are most likely to change if specifically targeted

(x) The evidence in favour of specialist residential provisions for the 'new' long-stay is generally positive; however, there may be problems with their acceptability to users.

Conclusions

Housing should be at the centre of community psychiatry. In order to achieve meaningful improvements in housing provision, we need to adopt a sophisticated, multi-level approach. Starting with the experience of residents, we need to consider questions of staffing skills and staff–resident interactions and go on to examine 'micro' and 'macro' organizational and management issues. This is a complex area where there are no simple solutions. It is also an area where the 'dynamics' of service systems, as well as the impact (and leadership) of key individuals at all levels, are crucially important. At the heart of these services remain interac-

tions between individuals—understanding these and how to maximize and maintain their potential benefits over time are our biggest challenges. Residential care is certainly an area where 'more research is needed', but we would also make considerable progress *now*, if we could simply implement effectively what we already know.

References

Albert, M., Becker, T., McCrone, P. and Thornicroft, G. (1998) Social networks and mental health service utilisation—a literature review. *International Journal of Social Psychiatry*, 44, 248–266.

Andrews, G., Teesson, M., Stewart,G. and Hoult, J. (1990) Follow-up of community placement of the chronic mentally ill in New South Wales. *Hospital and Community Psychiatry*, 41, 184–188.

Audit Commission (1998) *Home Alone*. London: Audit Commission.

Baker, F. and Douglas, C. (1990) Housing environments and community adjustments of severely mentally ill patients. *Community Mental Health Journal*, 26, 497–505.

Ball, R.A., Moore, E. and Kuipers, L. (1992) Expressed emotion in community care staff. A comparison of patient outcomes in a nine month follow-up of two hostels. *Social Psychiatry and Psychiatric Epidemiology*, 27, 35–39.

Beecham, J., Hallam, A., Knapp, M., Baines, B., Fenyo, A. and Asbury, M. (1997) Costing care in hospital and in the community. In: Leff, J. (ed.), *Care in the Community: Illusion or Reality?* London: Wiley, pp. 93–108.

Becker, T., Thornicroft, G., Leese, M., McCrone, P., Johnson, S., Albert, M. and Turner, D. (1997) Social network and service use among representative cases of psychosis in South London. *British Journal of Psychiatry*, 171, 15–19.

Bennett, D. (1980) The chronic psychiatric patient today. *Journal of the Royal Society of Medicine*, 73, 301–303.

Borge, L., Martinsen, E.W., Ruud, T., Watne, O. and Friis, S. (1999) Quality of life, loneliness and social contact among long-term psychiatric patients. *Psychiatric Services*, 50, 81–84.

Carling, P.J. (1993) Housing and supports for persons with mental illness: emerging approaches to research and practice. *Hospital and Community Psychiatry*, 44, 439–449.

Carrier, J. and Kendall, I. (1996) *Health and the National Health Service*. London: Athlone Press.

DHSS (1981) *Care in the Community*. London: HMSO.

Department of Health (1990) *NHS and Community Care Act*. London: HMSO

Department of Health (1998a) *Modernising Mental Health Services—Safe, Sound and Supportive*. London: HMSO.

Department of Health (1998b) *Partnerships in Action—New Opportunities for Joint Working Between Health and Social Services: A Discussion Document*. London: HMSO.

Donnelly, M., McGilloway, S., Mays, N., Knapp, M., Kavanagh, S., Beecham, J. and Fenyo, A. (1996) Leaving hospital: one and two-year outcomes of long-stay psychiatric patients discharged to the community. *Journal of Mental Health*, 5, 245–255.

Glover, G. (1996) The Mental Illness Needs Index (MINI). In: Thornicroft, G. and Strathdee, G. (eds), *Commissioning Mental Health Services*. London: HMSO.

Goering, P., Durbin, J., Foster, R., Boyles, S., Babiak, T. and Lancee, B. (1992) Social networks of residents in supportive housing. *Community Mental Health Journal*, 28, 199–214.

Hodgkins, S., Cyr M. and Gaston, L. (1990) Impact of supervised apartments on the functioning of mentally disordered adults. *Community Mental Health Journal*, 26, 507–515.

Holloway, F. and Faulkner, A. (1994) Psychiatric hospital re-provision and the long stay patient: clinical outcomes and the user perspective. *Journal of Mental Health*, 3, 241–248.

Johnson, S., Thornicroft, G. and Strathdee, G. (1996) Population-based assessment of needs for services. In: Thornicroft, G. and Strathdee, G. (eds), *Commissioning Mental Health Services*. London: HMSO.

Johnson, S., Ramsay, R., Thornicroft, G., Brooks, L., Lelliot, P., Peck, E. *et al.* (1997) *London's Mental Health. The Report of the Kings Fund Commission*. London: Kings Fund Publishing.

Jones, D. (1993) The TAPS project 11. The selection of patients for re-provision. Evaluating community placement of longstay patients. *British Journal of Psychiatry*, 162 (Suppl.), 36–39.

Keck, J. (1990) Responding to consumer housing preferences: the Toledo experience. *Psychosocial Rehabilitation Journal*, 13, 51–58.

Leff, J. (1997) *Care in the Community: Illusion or Reality?* London: Wiley.

Lehman, A.F., Slaughter, J.G. and Myers, C.P. (1991) Quality of life in alternative residential settings. *Psychiatric Quarterly*, 62, 35–49.

Lelliott P. and Wing, J.A. (1994) National Audit of New Longstay Psychiatric Patients. II Impact on services. *British Journal of Psychiatry*, 165, 170–178.

Lelliott, P., Audini, B., Knapp, M. and Chisholm, D. (1996) The mental health residential care study: classification of facilities and descriptions of residents. *British Journal of Psychiatry*, 169, 39–47.

Lewis, A. and Trieman, N. (1995) The TAPS project 29: residential care provision in north London: a representative sample of ten facilities for mentally ill people. *International Journal of Social Psychiatry*, 41, 257–267.

Middelboe, T., Mackeprang, T., Thalsgaard, A. and Christiansen, P.B. (1998) A housing support programme for the mentally ill: need profile and satisfaction among users. *Acta Psychiatrica Scandinavica*, 98, 321–327.

Ministry of Health (1962) *The Hospital Plan for England and Wales* (Cmnd. 1604). London: HMSO.

Mueser, K., Bond, G., Drake, R. and Resnick, S. (1998) Models of community care for severe mental illness: a review of research on case management. *Schizophrenia Bulletin*, 24, 37–74.

Nelson, G., Brent Hall, G. and Walsh-Bowers, R. (1997) A comparative evaluation of supportive apartments, group homes, and board-and-care homes for psychiatric consumer/survivors. *Journal of Community Psychology*, 25, 167–188.

NHS Executive (1996) *24 Hour Nursed Care for People with Severe and Enduring Mental Illness*. Leeds: NHSE.

Owen, C., Rutherford, V., Jones, M., Wright, C., Tennant, C. and Smallman, A. (1996) Housing accommodation preferences of people with psychiatric disabilities. *Psychiatric Services*, 47, 628–632.

Penn, D., Guyman, K., Daily, T., Spaulding, W.D., Garbin, C.P. and Sullivan, M. (1994) Dispelling the stigma of schizophrenia: what sort of information is best? *Schizophrenia Bulletin*, 20, 567–578.

Phelan, M. and Strathdee, G. (1994) Living in the community: training house officers in mental health. *Journal of Mental Health*, 3, 229–233.

Rose, D. and Muijen, M. (1997) Nursing doubts. *Health Services Journal*, 107, 34–35.

Segal, S.P. and Kofler, P.L. (1993) Sheltered care residences: ten-year personal outcomes. *American Journal of Orthopsychiatry*, 63, 80–91.

Seilheimer, T.A. and Doyal, G.T. (1996) Self-efficacy and consumer satisfaction with housing. *Community Mental Health Journal*, 32, 549–559.

Senn, V., Kendal, R. and Trieman, N. (1997) The TAPS project 38: level of training and its availability to carers within group homes in a London district. *Social Psychiatry and Psychiatric Epidemiology*, 32, 317–322.

Shepherd, G. (1995) The 'ward-in-a-house—residential care for the severely disabled. *Journal of Mental Health*, 31, 53–69.

Shepherd, G. (1998) Social functioning and challenging behaviour. In: Mueser,K.T. and Tarrier,N. (eds), *Social Functioning and Schizophrenia*. New York: Allyn Bacon, pp. 407–423.

Shepherd, G., Muijen, M., Dean, R. and Cooney, M. (1996) Residential care in hospital and in the community—quality of care and quality of life. *British Journal of Psychiatry*, 168, 448–456.

Shepherd, G., Beadsmoore, A., Moore, C., Hardy, P. and Muijen, M. (1997) Relation between bed use, social deprivation, and overall bed availability in acute psychiatric units and alternative residential options: a cross sectional survey, one day census data and staff interviews. *British Medical Journal*, 314, 262–266.

Sokolovsky, J., Cohen, C. and Berger, D. (1978) Personal networks of ex-mental patients in a Manhattan hotel. *Human Organisations*, 37, 5–15.

Tanzman, B. (1993) An overview of surveys of mental health consumers' preferences for housing and support services. *Hospital and Community Psychiatry*, 44, 450–455.

Tempier, R., Mercier, C., Leouffre, P. and Caron, J. (1997) Quality of life and social integration of severely mentally ill patients: a longitudinal study. *Journal of Psychiatry and Neuroscience*, 22, 249–255.

Thornicroft, G. and Breakey, W. (1991) The COSTAR programme: improving social networks of the mentally ill. *British Journal of Psychiatry*, 159, 245–249.

Trieman, N. and Leff, J. (1996) The TAPS project. 36: the most difficult to place long-stay psychiatric in-patients outcome one year after relocation. *British Journal of Psychiatry*, 169, 289–292.

Wolff, G., Pathare, S., Craig T. and Leff, J. (1996) Public education for community care: a new approach. *British Journal of Psychiatry*, 168, 441–447.

Young, R. (1991) *Residential Needs for Severely Disabled Psychiatric Patients—The Case for Hospital Hostels*. London: HMSO.

28 | *In-patient treatment*

George Szmukler and Frank Holloway

Introduction

A striking reduction in hospital beds can be seen as the defining characteristic of mental health services in many western countries in the second half of the 20th century (see Figure 28.1). The process of 'deinstitutionalization' has been driven by a variety of forces. These include the harmful effects of large institutions on patients, as demonstrated by research (Wing and Brown, 1970) and headline-grabbing scandals (Martin, 1984); a movement towards enhancing patients' liberties and quality of life (Peele and Chodoff, 1999); better treatments—drugs, methods of rehabilitation and alternatives to in-patient care for those in crisis; reducing costs, since hospital in-patient costs are very high; evidence that community-based systems of care can result in at least equal outcomes (Kluiter, 1997); and a general social movement which emphasized the 'community' as a positive resource for helping people (Hawks, 1975).

During the deinstitutionalization era, the focus in mental health services has been on methods of community treatment, and a substantial literature has been published about alternatives to in-patient care (see, for example, Marshall and Lockwood, 1998; Joy *et al.*, 1999). As a consequence, in-patient care has, from a practical and research perspective, been neglected despite its continuing importance within the overall spectrum of mental health care and significant changes in its nature. Although much has been written about the problems associated with hospital care (see, for example, Wing and Brown, 1970; Jones and Fowles, 1984; Martin, 1984), we know very little, for example, about what is required to make in-patient treatment effective.

While beds have reduced significantly in number, few people have claimed they are entirely dispensable. Every service has recourse to some hospital beds, especially short-stay beds for the acutely ill (some of which may be designated 'intensive care') and longer-stay 'secure beds' for patients who pose a serious risk to others (usually under the direction of forensic services). Long-stay beds of other types vary greatly across services. One of the most difficult tasks for mental health services is getting the right balance between the number of hospital beds and community services. Miscalculations can have dire consequences for patients, staff and the financial stability of a service.

In this chapter we will:

- Describe the scale and nature of changes in bed provision
- Review the changing functions of in-patient treatment
- Examine determinants of the number of beds required in a mental health service.

Changes in bed provision over time

The scale of bed reductions

Table 28.1 summarizes bed number changes in a number of countries. It has not been possible to use comparable statistics for all, but it will be seen that bed reductions have been striking in most but not all of the countries, that the rates of change have varied and that bed numbers per population varied substantially in the 1990s. Profound changes have occurred especially in the USA and Italy. In California in 1993, there were only 14 state hospital beds per 100 000 population.

In some places, the process has been very rapid over a few years. Between 1994 and 1997, the

Table 28.1 *Examples of historical changes in bed numbers*

Country	Interval	Change in beds	Changes
England and Wales[a]	1956 1995	−74%	154 000 to 42 000 beds (80/100 000)
USA[b]	1955 1994	−88%	339/100 000 to 40/100 000 (State hospital beds)
Italy: Emilia-Romagna[c]	1978 1996	−85%	220/100 000 to 34/100 000
Italy: South Verona[d]	1977 1995	−62%	104/100 000 to 40/100 000
Finland[e]	1980 1993	−64%	420/100 000 to 150/100 000
Germany[f]	1970 1988	−29%	160/100 000 to 113/100 000
Netherlands: Groningen[g]	1976 1990	0%	(adults 20–74 years)
Denmark[h]	1978 1998	−50%	
Japan[i]	1960 1993	+380%	95 067 to 362 963 beds

[a]Davidge *et al.*, 1993; [b]Lamb and Shaner, 1993; [c]Fioritti *et al.*, 1997; [d]Tansella *et al.*, 1998; [e]Korkeila *et al.*, 1998; [f]Rossler and Salize, 1994; [g]Oldehinkel, 1998; [h]Munk-Jorgensen, 1999; [i]Shinfuku *et al.*, 1998.

Veterans Administration system in the USA closed 44% of its beds (Rosenheck and DeLilla, 1999). Especially well documented are changes in Australia's public mental health services between 1993 and 1996 (Commonwealth Department of Health and Family Services, 1998). Overall, there was an 18% reduction in psychiatric beds, with a 31% decrease in stand-alone psychiatric hospitals; in the state of Victoria, psychiatric beds fell by 36%. There were striking funding changes with an overall increase of 55% in community-based spending. However, substantial variation from state to state remained. For example, in 1996, Victoria had 27 beds per 100 000 population whereas Tasmania had 52.3. Variation is a subject we shall return to.

In some countries, the process of deinstitutionalization has been slower or has not occurred at all. In Japan, beds increased in numbers between 1960 and 1993 from 95 067 to 362 963 (Shinfuku *et al.*, 1998). Oldehinkel (1998) reported that between 1976 and 1990, in the Groningen region

of The Netherlands, the number of in-patients per day for adults aged 20–74 years did not change significantly: it even increased slightly between 1983 and 1990.

Variations between services in the number of beds are noteworthy. We have already mentioned several examples. Goldberg and Thornicroft (1998) report beds per capita for 11 world cities. Bed numbers were about twice as high in Verona and Sydney as in Madison, Wisconsin (which had ~25 hospital beds per 100 000 population); three times as high in London; five times as high in Baltimore, USA; eight times as high in Copenhagen; and about 10 times as high in Amsterdam, The Netherlands and Kobe, Japan. In the VA system, where there are now 22 Integrated Service Networks, the number of mental health beds per 1000 veterans varies fourfold (Rosenheck and DeLilla, 1999).

Understanding the marked variation in hospital beds between countries and over time requires appreciation of the service context. Published reports are difficult to compare because of differences in definition of both numerator (beds) and denominator (populations). National statistics rarely differentiate between different kinds of hospital beds: this is important because spectacular declines in bed numbers within the mental hospital system may be traded-off by more modest increases in other forms of residential care. Further difficulties of interpretation occur in countries where there is a substantial private sector, or a plethora of providers, both public and private.

Long-stay beds are easier to close than acute beds, and their closure has less of an impact on the overall mental health system, at least in the short term. The marked bed reductions observed in many countries have been associated with parallel increases in (much cheaper) non-hospital alternative facilities, such as group homes, hostels and nursing homes for those with chronic handicaps. For example, in England, the steep reduction in hospital bed numbers since 1982 has been almost matched by an increase in alternative residential options—private, local authority and non-statutory (Davidge et al., 1993). Some have termed this process 'trans-institutionalization', and in the UK and USA it has been associated with a decline in state-run provision in favour of the private sector operating within a mixed economy of care.

Associated changes

A reduction in hospital beds has been associated with decreased *lengths of stay* and usually an increase in the *number of admissions*, the majority of which are readmissions rather than first contacts. In England and Wales, admissions rose from 190 389 to 213 240 between 1984 and 1996. In Madison, Wisconsin (the home of assertive community treatment), the number of admissions almost doubled between 1981 and 1996 while the mean length of stay dropped from 39 days to 14 days (Le Count, 1998). In the VA system in the USA, following reorganization in 1995, average length of stay fell by 20%, but readmissions increased. However, in South Verona, Italy, admissions remained fairly constant (Tansella et al., 1991, 1998). In Finland, between 1990 and 1993, during a rapid phase of deinstitutionalization that saw a 35% reduction in patients in hospital, the annual rate of admissions remained stable (at a relatively high rate of 490 per 100 000 population), although readmissions comprised an increasing proportion of total admissions (Korkeila et al., 1998).

Variations also apply to *involuntary admissions*. In England and Wales, the number of compulsory admissions almost doubled between 1984 and 1996 (Wall et al., 1999). There was also an increase in the number of patients admitted voluntarily who were placed on an order when they wished to leave (Szmukler et al., 1998). However, an increase in involuntary hospitalization is not an inevitable consequence of reduced bed numbers and thus an increased threshold of disturbance for admission. Large bed reductions have occurred in association with a fall rather than a rise in compulsory admissions—Emilia-Romagna, Italy, by 35% in a decade (Fioritti et al., 1997), and Finland, by 14% in 3 years (Korkeila et al., 1998) are examples. Social policy and a fear that community care results in increased risks of harm to the public may be more significant in determining the use of compulsory powers (Szmukler et al., 1998). There is substantial variation in recourse to compulsory admission, even within similar populations. The Nordic countries are an example, with a sevenfold variation in compulsory admissions that is only explained to a minor degree by social variables (Hansson et al., 1999). Urban Stockholm had five times the rate of compulsory admissions as an urban area of Copenhagen.

The changing functions of in-patient care

The traditional psychiatric hospital served many functions. As a total institution offering long-term custodial care of patients with continuing disability, it provided for the basic needs of its residents for food, shelter, clothing and a minimal income (Thornicroft and Bebbington, 1989) and offered some opportunities for occupation, leisure, social interaction and (furtively) sexual expression. It is now clear that for people with continuing care needs occurring in the context of long-term severe mental illnesses these needs can largely be met satisfactorily outside the hospital (Leff, 1997). However, even in the era of community care, in-patient provision forms a significant, and expensive, component of any comprehensive mental health service.

The mental hospital also served a range of functions that might be termed 'clinical'. These included crisis intervention; assessment or reassessment of diagnosis; the development and institution of a treatment plan; respite (for patient and carer); removal of the patient from a stressful environment; protection of the patient from exploitation; and protection of the public from dangerous or deviant behaviour, in either the long or short term (Bachrach, 1976; Talbott and Glick, 1986). Developments in community mental health services show how each of these functions can be undertaken without automatic recourse to admission. However, even enthusiastic proponents of assertive community treatment (PACT), which has an explicit aim of the avoidance of hospital admission (Stein and Test, 1980), acknowledge that there are limits. Allness and Knoedler (1998), in a manual for PACT teams, set out criteria for short-term in-patient treatment where PACT crisis intervention will not immediately reduce risk:

- Suicidal or homicidal ideation or behaviour
- Serious self-neglect or risk of physical harm (due to, for example, confusion, disorganized thinking)
- Mixed mental illness and acute drug intoxication requiring a brief period of medical care
- Adjustment of medication where concern for medical complications, side effects, risk of symptomatic exacerbation requires medical supervision
- Serious physical co-morbidity
- Incapacity of the PACT team to provide safe community management because of workload.

These criteria accord reasonably well with the reported reasons for admission identified by Flannigan *et al.* (1994) in a prospective study carried out in inner London. Reasons fell into two clusters: challenging behaviours (violence, suicidality) and social/preventive factors (relief for carers, removal from stress, prevention of psychosocial harm).

The effective management of an in-patient episode requires identification of the reasons for admission, thorough assessment of the problems presented by the patient (and to the patient by their home environment), the development of a set of treatment aims and objectives, and early consideration of discharge plans (Ramsay and Holloway, 1998). This process should, as far as possible, involve the patient, carers and the whole in-patient multi-disciplinary team. Nursing staff, who have the primary responsibility for the maintenance of a safe and therapeutic environment within the in-patient setting, should produce a care plan. Treatment will address a range of needs: safety of the patient and others; emotional support; structuring time and activity; reduction of distressing symptoms; detoxification; and physical health problems (Allness and Knoedler, 1998). It will include specific interventions (e.g. medication, occupational therapy, psychological therapies, addressing patients' practical problems) (Ramsay and Holloway, 1998) as well as the non-specific effect of removal from a stressful environment to one that is (one hopes) less stressful and more supportive. Some units, generally serving very large catchment areas, deploy highly specialized skills to specific patient groups, such as people with eating disorders and mothers with puerperal illnesses. Interestingly, patients identify the supportive relationships that they build up with staff as the major therapeutic ingredient of hospital admission (Lieberman and Strauss, 1986).

Only a small proportion of admitted patients remain in hospital for prolonged periods, and it is generally agreed that an acute ward is an inappropriate setting for stays over a few months duration (Bridges *et al.*, 1994). However, 'new long-stay' patients may accumulate (discussed below). Long-stay patients were, in the past, managed within large mental hospitals. In contemporary services, they will be found in acute wards, specialist long-term care units (not all based on a hospital site) and a range of secure hospital provision (Holloway *et al.*, 1999). Patients who require treatment within a secure setting in the medium or long term generally will have committed serious offences or be presenting severely socially unacceptable behaviours. Depending on the local service configuration and attitudes to risk, people with identical characteristics of behavioural disturbance and severe social handicap can be found within forensic psychiatry services, in long-stay hospital care in settings that do not offer a high degree of security, and rotating through the 'revolving door' in and out of acute wards.

The effects of bed reduction

Advances in community treatment and the process of deinstitutionalization have radically changed the acute in-patient unit in ways that have rarely been recorded systematically but have been experienced vividly by patients and practitioners. Patrick *et al.* (1989) observed the effect of bed reductions on an inner urban mental health service. As bed numbers decreased, the threshold for admission became higher, the morbidity of in-patients increased and the ward environment became less acceptable for patients. The authors surmised that an observed increase in the number of compulsorily detained patients was due to the increasingly disturbed and disturbing environment of the in-patient unit, which made the decreasing proportion of patients with affective disorders reluctant to stay while exacerbating the behavioural disturbance of patients with psychoses.

In the UK, there has been a strong demand, supported by government, for single-sex wards to ensure the safety of female patients. A similar pattern of increased morbidity and disturbance on in-patient wards was observed in a study of 'down-sizing' mental hospitals in Massachusetts, USA (Fisher *et al.*, 1996). The desirable development of community alternatives to hospital care, although it diverts many patients to alternative settings, leaves a residual group who present a wide variety of behavioural problems, risks and clinical and social needs.

Factors influencing the number of beds in a mental health service

Deciding how many beds are appropriate for a mental health service is exceedingly complex. Much is determined by the local specifics and the whole system in which beds are embedded. While recognizing that any divisions within the system of influences is largely arbitrary, for ease of exposition we will examine four groups of factors:

- socio-demographic
- ideology and policy
- system control factors
- local custom and convention.

Socio-demographic variables

A number of studies have found bed use to be highly correlated with socio-demographic variables, generally those taken to represent social deprivation. We present some examples. Thornicroft (1991) reviewed a range of social variables with an established relationship to psychiatric morbidity. These include lower social class; male gender; single marital status; ethnic group; aspects of domicile such as living alone, in overcrowded circumstances or in a neighbourhood with a large transitory population; and inner cities with high population densities and poverty. For the Southeast Thames region of England, he showed that individual census variables could account for up to 71% of the variance in admission rates, while in combination this could increase to 95%. A similar study of service utilization between 1986 and 1990 in Victoria, Australia, again found that measures linked to social deprivation and isolation strongly predicted admission episodes and bed days (Burgess *et al.*, 1992). The variation explained was 70–80% in urban areas and 35–48% in rural areas. The indicators were remarkably stable over the 5 years. A measure of service accessibility was also included—proximity to the in-patient facility. This accounted for a significant but small amount of variation, 4–8%, more in rural areas. A more sophisticated measure of accessibility might have explained even more of the rural variation.

In England, two indices have been developed to predict needs for mental health care, both relating to admissions to hospital. The MINI (Glover *et al.*, 1998) and the York formulae (Smith *et al.*, 1996) are again based on census data, different for each, but reflecting poverty and social conditions (e.g. marital status, rates of permanent sickness, no car, unemployment, household not self-contained, type of lodgings, dependants without a carer, proportion of persons born in the New Commonwealth). The York index attempts to take into account the geographical accessibility of beds since nearby services may inflate utilization. However, this model may not be appropriate for psychiatric beds where access to beds may not be related to distance but to historical ties. The MINI accounts for 20–74% of variation between health authorities. The York index accounts for about 40% at a district level and is used by the National Health Service as the basis for distributing money for psychiatric services between health authorities. Lower explained variabilities are to be expected when applying equations prospectively to new areas on which their predictive capacities have not been maximized.

When a formula is used as the basis of allocation of resources, a key issue is how much it should favour deprived areas. There is evidence that inner London, for example, is relatively deprived of in-patient and other resources, even with current redistribution (Goldberg and Thornicroft, 1998). Judgements are made more complex still by evidence that more severe mental illness is selectively more concentrated in deprived areas. Glover *et al.* (1999) suggest that comparing English Health Authorities, the most 'morbid' have about twice the prevalence of primary care level mental illness of the least 'morbid'. For secondary care, the ratio is between 2.2:1 and 4:1. For services for mentally disordered offenders, it is in excess of 20:1. By comparison, the York index predicts a ratio of need of about 3:1 between highest and lowest at a district level in England (Smith *et al.*, 1996).

Attempts have been made to translate deprivation indices into bed requirements. The MINI incorporates estimates of the level of facilities required in a geographical area based on where it lies within the range of the country's health districts from the most needy to the least based on the MINI key social indices (Glover, 1996). The limits of the estimated range of facilities are based on actual service utilization as well as expert judgement based on reviews of research studies by Wing (1992) and Strathdee and Thornicroft (1992). An instrument such as the MINI provides a 'first estimate' of how resources should be apportioned for in-patient care. For example, the 1-year period prevalence of admissions (persons likely to spend some time in hospital in a year) as predicted by the MINI ranges across district health authorities in England from 140 per 100 000 population in Huntingdon, Cambridgeshire, to 468 per 100 000 population in Bloomsbury and Islington in London.

The available models for predicting need for in-patient care are inherently limited. The demand for and utilization of beds clearly will be influenced by supply, which will be determined historically. Bed need will also be influenced by factors affecting length of stay, such as case complexity and the local spectrum of social care provision. Glover (1996) points out sources of error in MINI predictions. Local factors, such as clusters of highly disabled resettled patients or an influx of refugees, may determine the distribution of need in ways the model could not anticipate. Even if the model successfully predicts the number of admissions, associated costs may vary separately if care costs are unusually high in some districts. Revision of the MINI was required following an in-depth study of London's mental health services which showed that in the most morbid parts of the capital, the level of need substantially exceeded highest previous estimates (Ramsay *et al.*, 1997). Table 28.2 shows predicted residential requirements for general adult mental health services according to the estimates discussed above. Details of underlying assumptions for the 1996 PRiSM revisions are given in Ramsay *et al.* (1997). It is important to note that the estimate for any category assumes that *all* the other

Table 28.2 *Estimated need and actual provision of general adult mental health services (aged 15–64 only), in-patient and residential care, places per 250 000 population*

Category of service	Range Wing 1992[a]	Strathdee and Thornicroft 1992[a]	PRiSM 1996[b]
1. Medium secure unit	1–10	1–10	5–30
2. Intensive care unit/ local secure unit	5–15	5–10	5–20
3. Acute ward	50–150	50–150	50–175
4. 24-hour nurse-staffed units/hostel wards/staff awake at night	25–75	40–150 for categories 4 and 5 together	12–50
5. 24-hour non-nurse-staffed hostels/ night staff sleep-in	40–110		50–300
6. Day staffed hostels	25–75	30–120	15–60
7. Lower support accommodation[c]	n/a	48–100	30–120

[a]Wing (1992) estimates include old age assessment places, and the Strathdee and Thornicroft figures apply only to general adult service for those aged 16–65.

[b]PRiSM (1996) estimated need levels based upon: London actual values, and an expected fourfold variation of need from least to most deprived parts of England, for most categories of service, with a far greater variation in medium secure beds, and NHS Executive (1996) guidance of an average of 25 places in 24-hour nurse staffed accommodation per 250 000.

All estimates given assume that each category of service exists in the given appropriate range of volume.

[c]Includes respite beds and supported self-contained flats. As not all agencies gave information on these categories, these estimates should be regarded as conservative.

From Ramsay *et al.* (1997).

categories of service are provided for at an appropriate level.

Ideology and policy

The rate of decrease in bed numbers in England and Wales has been remarkably smooth since the peak year of 1954, well before mental hospital closure was articulated as government policy (Fig. 28.1). However, the most striking reductions of hospital beds that have occurred have followed governments and health departments pronouncing this as a major intention. Where there is a will to reduce beds, this usually will be achieved. The pace of change varies according to controls and sanctions imposed. Precipitate changes are more likely to occur where funders have the financial control and political will to pursue their goals. Change is unlikely to occur when, as has historically been the case in Japan, there are perverse financial incentives on providers to fill beds and there is no societal consensus in favour of deinstitutionalization. In the USA, the legal system has been a powerful force in promoting rapid bed closures in response to challenges raised in the courts by the mental patients' rights movement (Brown, 1981). Geller *et al.* (1990a,b) provide a case study of the impact of a legal decision that patients have the right to be treated in the least restrictive setting appropriate to their needs. This led to all residents of Northampton State Hospital, Massachusetts, being discharged over a 10-year period.

Change will be influenced by the prevailing ideology of key actors. By 'ideology', we mean a system of beliefs or values resting to a greater or lesser degree on an evidence base. Italy in the late 1970s provides an excellent example at a national level of an ideologically inspired major change in mental health services resulting from radical legislation, Law No. 180, which blocked admissions to public mental hospitals. There was in most regions a subsequent steep reduction in admissions and a substantial reduction in bed numbers. Hospitalization was to be regarded as an exceptional intervention, to be used only if community treatment was not feasible or had failed (Mosher and Burti, 1994). Factors contributing to such radical change included: a general climate of libertarianism; charismatic professional advocates centred around Dr Franco Basaglia in Gorizia; a particular balance of party political power; and the threat of a referendum which, if successful, would have led to a repeal of existing mental health legislation leaving no legal basis for the operation of mental health services.

Less dramatic but equally effective changes have occurred in Australia, the results of which have been described above. A critical step was the creation of a National Mental Health Strategy adopted by all state health ministers in 1992. Previously states had pursued their own independent policies with respect to public mental health provision. The strategy was clear in its intent, focused on a shift from institutional to community care, received strong political endorsement and was supported by a budget to promote change. A large proportion of this budget was 'reform and incentive funding' to foster restructuring of mental health services in line with Strategy objectives. There are few national policy areas in Australia which have been subject to an equivalent level of reporting and accountability as required under the National Mental Health Strategy (Commonwealth Department of Health and Family Services, 1998). On a smaller scale, but again showing striking changes, has been the reorganization of the Veterans Administration System in the USA (Rosenheck and Horvath, 1998). A clear strategy and budgetary control seem again to have been key.

When aims remain general and a specific strategy is lacking, major changes in bed use are less likely. Pijl *et al.* (2000) report that in The Netherlands, the government expected local mental health services to make innovations in community service provision in the absence of forceful measures such as reducing budgets of large mental hospitals. Between 1989 and 1997, community services expanded significantly, the number of patients treated under 'intensive community care' increased threefold and the total number of patients treated by services increased by 15%. However, in-patient days declined very slowly.

Sometimes, although the stated policy may be to increase community care while reducing reliance on in-patient services, political pressures and subsequent policy may act in the opposite direction. In the UK, government in the 1990s became very sensitive to claims that community care has 'failed'. Such claims have been fuelled particularly by highly publicized homicides by persons with a history of contact with mental health services. In 1994, the Department of Health published 'discharge guidance' focusing on risk (Department of Health, 1994a) and in the same year introduced a 'supervision register' aimed at providing close community monitoring of 'risky' individuals (Department of Health, 1994b). As a consequence, in many services, lengths of in-patient stay have risen and, in a climate of 'moral panic', bed numbers within long-stay medium and low secure provision are expanding rapidly.

One is often struck by another aspect of ideologically driven change—the role of 'product champions'. These charismatic leaders influence government policy as well as local service providers. They often are also inspirational leaders of their own clinical teams. 'Ideologies' exist at a local level, where they may influence the extent to which attempts at reducing bed use are successful. As an example of this process, Rosenheck and Neale (1998) found that the degree to which intensive case management was effective across a number of VA sites depended on the level of preexisting community focus of the local service.

System control factors

In this section, we consider control of the *overall* system of services as well as two subsystem components: *inflow* control factors and *outflow* control factors.

A helpful view of factors operating across the whole system is given by Thornicroft and Tansella in their account of the 'Mental Health Matrix' (Thornicroft and Tansella, 1999). This model shows how changes in 'inputs' or 'processes' at a regional or national level, for example, affect local service changes and eventually patient outcomes. A change in social policy may have dramatic effects on local services, especially if the change is driven by a panic reaction to a highly publicized but rare event and ignores system factors. Eisenberg, in his preface to the 'Mental Health Matrix', gives an excellent example. A mentally ill Cuban refugee passenger on the Staten Island ferry in New York killed two passengers and wounded nine others in 1986. When it was learnt that he had been seen 4 days earlier by a psychiatric resident but not admitted, a striking chain of events ensued. A constellation of relevant system factors relating to the provision of public beds and the system of insurance were ignored. Instead, fearful responses were provoked from the public as well as professionals, professional standards were criticized and there was a 50% increase in patients brought to emergency rooms together with a large increase in admissions. A similar sequence occurs regularly in England because of the introduction of a policy instituting mandatory independent inquiries following every homicide by a person in contact within the previous 2 years with mental health services.

Managed care is an attempt to control key elements of the whole system in order to control variation in clinical practice and contain costs: a range of mechanisms are put in place by the funders and contractually enforced on the providers. These include prior authorization procedures, treatment protocols, maximum reimbursable lengths of stay and utilization review. The impact of managed care on the quality of care is uncertain, is a subject of very active research and is likely to evolve over time. Gittleman (1998) provides a brief overview of the history and current practices of managed mental health care for the international reader.

At a local level, control of admission to, and discharge from, hospital by the same team that is responsible for treatment of the same patients in the community may have a profound effect on bed usage. The 'Daily Living Programme' involved a randomized controlled trial of home-based treatment of acutely ill patients at the Maudsley Hospital in London. A follow-up study showed that as long as the community team controlled admission and discharge decisions, bed use was significantly reduced. When control was lost, differences in bed use between the community team patients and the controls disappeared (Marks *et al.*, 1994). Even when a single team is responsible across the whole range of services in a sector, control may still break down when the system is effectively unable to operate as a sectorized one. This may occur when, because all local beds are occupied, patients requiring admission are admitted to other hospitals, often at some distance from the geographical sector, and fall under the care of a new team. Discharge can thus become easily delayed. If 'overflow' beds are in the private sector, the incentive for early discharge is likely to be less (Tyrer *et al.*, 1998). These delays place further pressure on the system, resulting in even more patients being placed outside the area.

Other factors to be considered at this level include how well money is transferred from in-patient to community services, and how well health and social agencies, governmental as well as non-governmental, can work together to meet the needs of vulnerable patients in the community. The provision of a spectrum of residential care is critical in determining the number of patients located in acute hospital beds because appropriate alternatives such as 24-hour low-intensity nursed care are missing (Ramsay *et al.*, 1997; Shepherd, 1998).

Inflow factors

It is easy to forget that admission and readmission to hospital remain common for patients with severe mental illnesses. Kavanagh *et al.* (1995) estimated that in 1995 at any one time 14% of persons suffering from schizophrenia in the UK were in hospital, with a slightly higher percentage in specialist-supported accommodation. Daniels *et al.* (1998) used the Tasmanian mental health register in Australia to study the 5-year pattern of rehospitalization for all patients admitted to public in-patient facilities with a primary diagnosis of schizophrenia, bipolar disorder or depression. Seventy one percent of patients with schizophrenia were readmitted, 59% with bipolar disorder and 48% for depression. Even in highly developed community services, admission is a common event. Almost 30% of patients with schizophrenia in contact with the Verona service were admitted in the course of a year (Gater *et al.*, 1995). A comparison of Victoria, Australia and Groningen, The Netherlands suggests that for patients with schizophrenia, the relative risk of readmission to hospital may not differ between community-orientated and hospital-orientated services, but that the number of days spent in hospital is less for the former (Sytema and Burgess, 1999).

Control over admission decision making has been emphasized by assertive community treatment programmes. The PACT model places the community team in the gate-keeper role (Stein and Test, 1980). However, for gate-keeping to be fully effective, alternatives to in-patient care are required. Diversion to 'home treatment' by assertive community treatment teams has been shown to reduce hospital bed days despite the fact that a substantial proportion of patients will need admission at some point (Joy *et al.*, 1999). Assertive community treatment reduces admissions and in-patient days for those who were previously high bed users (Marshall and Lockwood, 1998; Meuser *et al.*, 1998). Acute day hospital treatment, with (Sledge *et al.*, 1996) or without (Creed, 1990, 1997) supplementary crisis accommodation has been shown to reduce admissions for patients at low risk. The role of respite accommodation and crisis houses is yet to be researched extensively. Uncontrolled studies show that the approach may have promise (Hawthorne *et al.*, 1999)

A variation on the gate-keeping theme is an interesting experiment involving a capitation demonstration programme for high bed users that integrates clinical and fiscal structures (Baron *et al.*, 1998). The lead agency assuming responsibility for community care is given an all-inclusive budget from which it must also pay for all health needs, including in-patient care. The financial incentive to avoid admission coupled with an unusual freedom to develop innovative responses to crises may lead to significant reductions in hospital in-patient care.

The reduction in size of in-patient units has in itself a significant impact on the ability to manage admissions within the unit. Admissions, on a day to day basis, occur unpredictably—some days there are few, on others there are many. A Poisson distribution predicts that the variability in admissions is a function of the $\sqrt{n}$ where n is the mean number of expected admissions. Five dispersed individual units of 20 beds with a mean number of admissions of four per week each, (95% confidence interval for admissions = $4 \pm 2\sqrt{4}$; i.e. 0–8) will buffer the variation less well locally than a single large unit of 100 beds with a mean number of admissions of 20 per week (95% confidence interval for admissions = $20 \pm 2\sqrt{20}$; i.e. 11–29), perhaps resulting in patients needing to be sent to distant hospitals with a further disruption in the continuity of care.

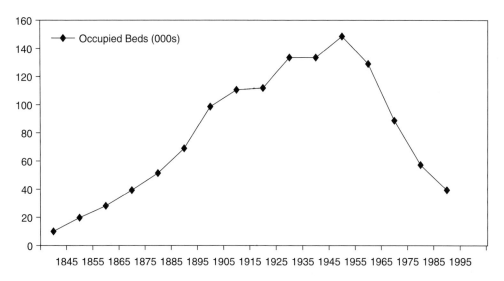

Figure 28.1 *Mental illness hospitals: occupied beds in England and Wales 1845–1995 (based on Davidge et al., 1993)*

Outflow factors

Although there is some literature on the decision to admit patients to hospital, no systematic information has been collected on the decision to discharge. Surveys of in-patients in acute beds, in England at least, consistently have found that despite bed occupancy rates of well over 100%, around 30% of patients are placed inappropriately on acute wards (see, for example, Ramsay *et al.*, 1997; Shepherd *et al.*, 1997). The causes generally lie not so much with 'inflow' but with 'outflow'. Residential options, more appropriate than acute in-patient care, are unavailable or can only be accessed after delays.

Few falling within the difficult to place group belong to the historic '*old long-stay*', that is patients who a decade or more ago had been in hospital for over a year (often for very many years, 20 or more). The evidence is good that these patients can be resettled largely successfully in supported accommodation in the community, given adequate resources. For example, over 700 long-stay patients from two London mental hospitals destined for closure were followed carefully over more than a decade as their care was reprovided in a range of community settings

(Leff, 1997). Five years after discharge, adverse outcomes in terms of vagrancy, crime or suicide were few, while there were significant improvements in 'negative symptoms', social networks and use of community services (Leff *et al.*, 1994; Trieman *et al.*, 1999). Almost 40% of patients required readmission at some point, and 30% of all admissions were long term (> 6 months). However, at 5 years follow-up, only 10% were in-patients. Similarly successful resettlement of long-stay patients has been reported elsewhere (Andrews *et al.*, 1990; Rothbard *et al.*, 1999).

It is the next generation of long-stay patients, the '*new long-stay*' (NLS), who highlight difficulties in placement and who account for a large proportion of patients inappropriately placed on acute wards. A national study in England estimated that there were six per 100 000 with a length of stay over 3 years (Lelliott *et al.*, 1994), but the prevalence was much higher in an inner London area (Holloway *et al.*, 1999). The latter study showed that the number of NLS patients was strongly determined by the availability of rehabilitation and continuing care beds. Between 1993 and 1995, the numbers had reduced from 26.7 per 100 000 to 16.7 per 100 000 following a concerted policy of placement in the community.

Patients difficult to discharge were those with 'challenging' behaviours—violence, non-compliance with medication and absconding. This raises the issue of the need for beds providing medium or low security, whose estimation (17% of NLS in Shepherd *et al.*, 1997) is complicated by the degree to which risk is tolerable in a particular community. Shortfalls in specialized rehabilitation places and 24-hour nursed care in community-based residences are especially important for the NLS (Johnson *et al.*, 1997; Shepherd *et al.*, 1997).

There is another new generation of chronically ill patients variously described as *the 'new chronic'* or *'revolving door'* patient. Lamb and Shaner (1993) describe this group as not having been "institutionalised to passivity" and therefore, unlike the old long-stay, they are not prepared "to do what they are told or go where they are told". They do not see themselves as ill, do not wish to engage with services, and when they are admitted to hospital, they do not stay long, either because of bed pressures or because they press to leave as soon as possible. They may end up homeless or 'criminalized'. The revolving door cycle might be broken by intermediate or long-term hospitalization. Only then might appropriately supported community care become acceptable.

Does a policy of shortening admissions contribute to the 'revolving door' phenomenon by increasing readmissions? Perhaps surprisingly, a clear answer cannot be given. Looking at data at a regional or national level, one usually finds a reduction in beds, a reduction in length of stay and usually an increase in admissions, including proportionally more readmissions. We have cited national evidence for these trends above. However, controlled studies of planned reductions in length of hospital stay have usually, but not always, failed to show increased readmission rates for patients allocated to shorter stays. For example, a rigorous systematic review by Johnstone and Zolese (1999) identified five randomized trials involving a total of 628 patients with severe mental illness. Unfortunately the most recent study, the only one not to be carried out in the USA, was published over 20 years ago. The average length of stay for patients allocated to short stay ranged from 10.8 to 25.0 days (which approximates to contemporary practice in the USA and UK). For conventional stays, it ranged from 28 to 94 days. There was no difference in readmission rates in these experimental studies at 1 or 2 years. Short-stay patients were also more likely to be discharged on time, and no more likely to later default from care.

Recent 'before and after' studies where reduced lengths of stay have been introduced in large patient populations have provided mixed results, with unchanged readmissions being observed in some (Edward-Chandran *et al.*, 1996; Thomas *et al.*, 1996; Lyons *et al.*, 1997) but an increase being found in others (Wickizer and Lessler 1998). Interestingly, Lyons *et al.* (1997) found that the success of the previous hospital intervention in terms of clinical status at discharge, rated using standardized instruments, did not predict readmission within a managed care environment. It was predicted by patient characteristics at initial presentation, notably social impairment, symptom severity and past history.

One way in which the epidemiological data might be reconciled with findings from smaller research studies turns on a group of patients who have high readmission rates, but who are too small in number to produce group differences, or who might have been excluded from such studies. This is illustrated in a study by Appleby *et al.* (1996). In a quasi-experimental design, readmissions were compared for three matched groups of patients treated in separate units with different mean lengths of stay. An analysis based on the units with different lengths of stay showed no differences in outcome. However, a second analysis examined all patients irrespective of their unit assignment. In-patients treated for 30 days or less relapsed sooner than those with stays longer than 30 days. A group of primarily young males with schizophrenia, an early age of onset and multiple previous admissions was at greater risk of relapse with short admissions. A previous study by the same group found that 40% of all admissions were accounted for by 15% of patients. Thomas *et al.* (1996) also found in a study of 1363 admissions to a university affiliated in-patient psychiatric unit that reducing length of stay from 20 days to 6 days did not change overall readmission rates. However, rates did increase for a subgroup of patients with psychotic disorders. This group resembles the *'new chronic'* group of patients discussed above.

There is clearly much still to be learnt concerning optimal lengths of in-patient stay for different groups of patients. As lengths of stay have reduced, readmission rates have not increased for a large proportion of patients. For an important minority, however, they have, and we are struggling to find the right interventions to help them. Extended admissions for some patients may in the long-term be the most effective, both clinically and in terms of cost (Edell *et al.*, 1990). Controlled studies clearly are called for.

On a related issue, we find that the literature demonstrates a striking lack of clarity behind the purpose of psychiatric admission and the way in which the process is conducted. There are few examples of the contrary. Jayaram *et al.* (1996) describe methods they used to create a short-stay service. These include screening and use of assessment tools at the outset, increasing the seniority of those making decisions, enhanced 24-hour communication between staff, twice daily rounds, proactive and skilled nursing staff able to institute care plans without delay, early involvement of carers, early discharge planning, rapid progression of patients through a series of in-patient privileges, targeting specific symptoms or behaviours and 'step-down' systems. Similar principles were used by Schneider and Ross (1996) in an 'ultra-short hospitalization unit. Evaluation of such 'care pathway' approaches is urgently required.

Custom and convention

We have already commented on national and regional variations. The same occurs at a local level. We offer a few examples. The median lengths of stay for six acute wards in Nottingham, England under the control of separate sector teams ranged from 19 to 35 days (Croudace *et al.*, 1998). This could not be accounted for by patient differences, indicating that sector teams differed in their management strategies. Similar findings occurred in a Nordic comparison of first hospi-

talizations of patients in seven hospitals (Oiesvold *et al.*, 1999); median length of stays varied three-fold and could not be accounted for by clinical or social differences, nor by hospital resources.

A detailed analysis of differences in the care of highly comparable groups of high severity patients (derived from a detailed case-mix classification) across 16 sites in Australia showed a threefold variation in length of stay (10.7–30.0 days) and a similar variation in the amount of one-to-one clinical time dedicated to individual patients (Buckingham *et al.*, 1998). Since detailed information was available for each site, it was possible to control for the overall complexity and volume of cases treated at each site. No relationship between complexity of cases seen at a site and length of stay was evident. The authors concluded that 'provider factors' are critical, some of which may be structural (e.g. types of service available, overall resources) while others may be under the control of individual clinicians (e.g. differences in clinical practices). To these may be added local history and belief systems.

Conclusion: the evolving role of in-patient care

In-patient care is, from a research perspective, the Cinderella of contemporary mental health services. Its evolving role can only be understood as a component of a complex system of care. Despite the successful closure of the traditional long-stay mental hospitals, it seems undeniable that, even in the most highly evolved system of community care, some in-patient beds are required. Utilization of hospital beds will depend on a complex interaction between supply (as historically determined) and demand. Demand will reflect professional behaviours, societal expectations of care and control of the mentally ill and acceptance of their return to the community, the local epidemiology of mental illness and the availability of alternative forms of psychiatric provision. If, in a publicly funded system attempting to respond to need, adequate bed provision is not made, service costs can, paradoxically, escalate.

The current policy climate is seeking to eliminate variations in clinical practice and service utilization using the practices of managed care in the USA, and, in the UK, a National Service Framework for Mental Health and the introduction of 'clinical governance'. Reducing variations will be difficult as long as we do not clearly understand their underlying causes (Gilbody and House, 1999). The Italian and Australian experience have both, in different ways, shown that major systemic change can be introduced successfully: but a change strategy should be incremental, evidence-based and adequately resourced.

References

Allness, D.J. and Knoedler, W.H. (1998) *The PACT Model of Community-based Treatment for Persons with Severe and Persistent Mental Illnesses. A Manual for PACT Start-up.* Arlington, VA: NAMI.

Andrews, G., Teesson, M., Stewart, G. and Hoult, J. (1990) Follow-up of community placement of the chronic mentally ill in New South Wales. *Hospital Community Psychiatry*, 41, 184–188.

Appleby L., Luchins D.J., Desai P.N., Gibbons R.D., Janicak P.G. and Marks R. (1996) Length of inpatient stay and recidivism among patients with schizophrenia. *Psychiatric Services*, 47, 985–990.

Bachrach, L. (1976) *Deinstitutionalisation: An Analytical Review and Sociological Perspective.* Rockville, MD: US Department of Health, Education and Welfare, NIMH.

Baron, S.T., Agus, D., Osher, F. and Brown D. (1998) The city of Baltimore, USA: the Baltimore experience. In: Goldberg, D. and Thornicroft, G. (eds), *Mental Health in our Future Cities.* Maudsley Monograph 42. Hove: Psychology Press, pp. 57–76.

Bridges, K., Huxley, P. and Oliver, J. (1994) Psychiatric rehabilitation: redefined for the 1990s. *International Journal of Social Psychiatry*, 40, 1–16.

Brown, P. (1981) The mental patients' rights movement and mental health institutional change. *International Journal of Health Services*, 11, 523–540.

Buckingham, B., Burgess, P., Solomon, S., Pirkis, J. and Eager, K. (1998) *Developing a Casemix Classification for Mental Health Services.* Canberra, Australia: Commonwealth Department of Health and Family Services.

Burgess, P.M., Joyce, C.M., Pattison, P.E. and Finch, S.J. (1992) Social indicators and the prediction of psychiatric inpatient service utilisation. *Social Psychiatry and Psychiatric Epidemiology*, 27, 83–94.

Commonwealth Department of Health and Family Services (1998) *National Mental Health Report 1996.* Canberra, Australia: Commonwealth Department of Health and Family Services

Creed, F., Black, D., Anthony, P., Osborn, M., Thomas, P. and Tomenson, B. (1990) Randomised controlled trial of day patient versus inpatient psychiatric treatment. *British Medical Journal*, 300, 1033–1037.

Creed, F., Mbaya, P., Lancahire, S. *et al.* (1997) Cost effectiveness of day and inpatient psychiatric treatment: results of a randomised controlled trial. *British Medical Journal*, 314, 1381–1385.

Croudace, T., Beck, A., Singh, S. and Harrison, G. (1998) Profiling activity in acute psychiatric services. *Journal of Mental Health*, 7, 49–57.

Daniels, B.A., Kirkby, K.C., Hay, D.A. *et al.* (1998) Predictability of rehospitalisation over 5 years for schizophrenia, bipolar disorder and depression. *Australian and New Zealand Journal of Psychiatry*, 32, 281–286.

Davidge, M., Elias, S., Hayes, B. *et al.* (1993) *Survey of English Mental Illness Hospitals.* Birmingham: Inter-Authority Comparisons and Consultancy, Health Services Management Centre, University of Birmingham.

Department of Health (1994a) *Discharge Guidance.* HSG(94)27. London: Department of Health.

Department of Health (1994b) *The Supervision Register.* HSG(94)5. London: Department of Health.

Edell, W.S., Hoffman, R.E., DiPietro, S.A. and Harcherik, D.F. (1990) Effects of long-term psychiatric hospitalization for young, treatment-refractory patients. *Hospital and Community Psychiatry*, 41, 780–785.

Edward-Chandran, T., Malcolm, D.E. and Bowen, R.C. (1996) Reduction of length of stay in an acute care psychiatric unit [published erratum appears in *Canadian Journal of Psychiatry*, 1996 Jun; 41(5): 319] [see comments]. *Canadian Journal of Psychiatry*, 41, 49–51.

Fioritti, A., Lo, R.L. and Melega, V. (1997) Reform said or done? The case of Emilia-Romagna within the Italian psychiatric context [see comments]. *American Journal of Psychiatry*, 154, 94–98.

Fisher, W.H., Simon, L., Geller, J.L. *et al.* (1996) Case mix in the 'downsizing' state hospital. *Psychiatric Services*, 47, 255–262.

Flannigan, C.B., Glover, G.R., Wing, J.K. *et al.* (1994) Inner London collaborative audit of admission in two health districts. III: reasons for acute admission to psychiatric wards. *British Journal of Psychiatry*, 165, 750–759.

Gater, R., Amaddeo, F., Tansella, M., Jackson, G. and Goldberg, D. (1995) A comparison of community-based care for schizophrenia in south Verona and south Manchester. *British Journal of Psychiatry*, 166, 344–352.

Geller, J.L., Fisher, W.H., Wirth-Cauchon, J.L. and Simon, L.J. (1990a) Second-generation deinstitutionalisation, I: the impact of Brewster v. Dukakis on state hospital case mix. *American Journal of Psychiatry*, 147, 982–987.

Geller, J.L., Fisher, W.H., Simon, L.J. and Wirth-Cauchon, J.L. (1990b) Second-generation deinstitutionalisation, II: the impact of Brewster v. Dukakis on correlates of community and hospital utilization. *American Journal of Psychiatry*, 147, 988–993.

Gilbody, S. and House, A. (1999) Variations in psychiatric practice. Neither unacceptable nor unavoidable, only under-researched. *British Journal of Psychiatry*, 175, 303–305.

Gittleman, M. (1998) Public and private managed care. *International Journal of Mental Health*, 27, 3–17.

Glover, G.R. (1996) The mental illness needs index (MINI). In: Thornicroft, G. and Strathdee, G. (eds), *Commissioning Mental Health Services*. London: HMSO.

Glover, G.R., Robin, E., Emami, J. and Arabscheibani, G.R. (1998) A needs index for mental health care. *Social Psychiatry and Psychiatric Epidemiology*, 33, 89–96.

Glover, G.R., Leese, M. and McCrone, P. (1999). More severe mental illness is more concentrated in deprived areas. *British Journal of Psychiatry*, 175, 544–548.

Goldberg, D. and Thornicroft, G. (1998) Overview and emerging themes. In: Goldberg, D. and Thornicroft, G. (eds), *Mental Health in our Future Cities. Maudsley Monograph 42*. Hove: Psychology Press, pp. 269–282.

Hansson, L., Muus, S., Saarento, O., Vinding, H.R., Gostas, G., Sandlund, M., Zandren, T. and Oiesvold, T. (1999) The Nordic comparative study on sectorized psychiatry: rates of compulsory care and use of compulsory admissions during a 1-year follow-up. *Social Psychiatry and Psychiatric Epidemiology*, 34, 99–104.

Hawks, D. (1975) Community care: an analysis of assumptions. *British Journal of Psychiatry*, 127, 276–285

Hawthorne, W.B., Green, E.E., Lohr, J.B. *et al.* (1999) Comparison of outcomes of acute care in short-term residential treatment and psychiatric hospital settings. *Psychiatric Services*, 50, 401–406.

Holloway, F., Wykes, T., Petch, E. and Lewis-Cole, K. (1999) The new long stay in an inner city service: a tale of two cohorts. *International Journal of Social Psychiatry*, 45, 93–103.

Jayaram, G., Tien, A.Y., Sullivan, P. and Gwon, H. (1996) Elements of a successful short-stay inpatient psychiatric service. *Psychiatric Services*, 47, 407–412.

Johnstone, P. and Zolese, G. (1999) Systematic review of the effectiveness of planned short hospital stays for mental health care. *British Medical Journal*, 318, 1387–1390.

Jones, K. and Fowles, A.J. (1984) *Ideas on Institutions*. London: Routledge and Kegan Paul.

Joy, C.B., Adams, C.E. and Rice, K. (1999) Crisis intervention for those with severe mental illnesses (Cochrane Review). *The Cochrane Library*, Issue 4. Oxford: Update Software.

Kavanagh, S., Opit, L., Knapp, M. and Beecham, J. (1995) Schizophrenia: shifting the balance of care. *Social Psychiatry and Psychiatric Epidemiology*, 30, 206–212.

Kluiter, H. (1997) Inpatient treatment and care arrangements to replace or avoid it—searching for an evidence-based balance. *Current Opinion in Psychiatry*, 13, 333–341.

Korkeila, J.A., Lehtinen, V., Tuori, T. and Helenius, H. (1998) Patterns of psychiatric hospital service use in Finland: a national register study of hospital discharges in the early 1990s. *Social Psychiatry and Psychiatric Epidemiology*, 33, 218–223.

Lamb, H.R. and Shaner, R. (1993) When there are almost no state hospital beds left. *Hospital and Community Psychiatry*, 44, 973–976.

Le Count, D. (1998) The city of Madison, USA: the Madison model, keeping the focus of treatment in the community. In: Goldberg, D. and Thornicroft, G. (eds), *Mental Health in our Future Cities. Maudsley Monograph 42*. Hove: Psychology Press, pp. 147–172.

Leff, J. (ed.) (1997) *Care in the Community—Illusion or Reality?* Chichester: Wiley

Leff, J., Thornicroft, G., Coxhead, N. and Crawford, C. (1994) The TAPS project. 22: a five-year follow-up of long-stay psychiatric patients discharged to the community. *British Journal of Psychiatry*, (Suppl.), 13–17.

Lelliott, P., Wing, J. and Clifford, P. (1994) A national audit of new long-stay psychiatric patients. I: method and description of the cohort [see comments]. *British Journal of Psychiatry*, 165, 160–169.

Lieberman, P. and Strauss, J.S. (1986) Brief hospitalization: what are its effects? *American Journal of Psychiatry*, 143, 1557–1562.

Lyons, J.S., O'Mahoney, M.T., Miller, S.I., Neme, J., Kabat, J. and Miller, F. (1997) Predicting readmission to the psychiatric hospital in a managed care environment: implications for quality indicators [see comments]. *American Journal of Psychiatry*, 154, 337–340.

Marks, I.M., Connolly, J., Muijen, M., Audini, B., McNamee, G. and Lawrence, R.E. (1994) Home-based versus hospital-based care for people with serious mental illness [see comments]. *British Journal of Psychiatry*, 165, 179–194.

Marshall, M. and Lockwood, A. (1998) Assertive community treatment for people with severe mental disorders (Cochrane Review). In: *The Cochrane Library*, Issue 4.

Martin, J.P. (1984) *Hospitals in Trouble*. Oxford: Blackwell.

Mosher, L. and Burti, L. (1994) *Community Mental Health: A Practical Guide*. New York, W.W. Norton & Co.

Mueser, K., Bond, G., Drake, R. *et al.* (1998) Models of community care for severe mental illness: a review of research on case management . *Schizophrenia Bulletin*, 24, 37–74.

Oiesvold, T., Saarento, O., Sytema, S., Christiansen, L., Gostas, G., Lonnerberg, O., Muus, S., Sandlund, M. and Hansson, L. (1999) The Nordic Comparative Study on Sectorized Psychiatry—length of in-patient stay. *Acta Psychiatrica Scandinavica*, 100, 220–228.

Oldehinkel, A.J. (1998) Time trends in mental health care utilization in a Dutch area, 1976–1990. *Social Psychiatry and Psychiatric Epidemiology*, 33, 181–185.

Patrick, M., Higgitt, A., Holloway, F. and Silverman, M. (1989) Changes in an inner city psychiatric inpatient service following bed losses: a follow-up of the East Lambeth 1986 Survey. *Health Trends*, 21, 121–123.

Peele, R. and Chodoff, P. (1999) The ethics of involuntary treatment and deinstitutionalization. In: Bloch, S., Chodoff, P. and Green, S. (eds), *Psychiatric Ethics*, 3rd edn. Oxford: Oxford University Press, pp. 423–440.

Pijl, Y.J., Kluiter, H., Wiersma D. (2000) Calculated change in Dutch mental health care. *Social Psychiatry and Psychiatric Epidemiology*, in press.

Ramsay, R. and Holloway, F. (1998) Mental health services. In: Stein, G. and Wilkinson, G. (eds), *General Psychiatry. College Seminars in Psychiatry.* London: Gaskell, pp 1274–1333.

Ramsay, R., Thornicroft, G., Johnson S., Brooks L. and Glover, G. (1997) Levels of inpatient and residential provision throughout London. In: Johnson, S., Ramsay, R., Thornicroft G. *et al.* (eds), *London's Mental Health: The Report to the King's Fund London Commission*. London: King's Fund Publishing, pp. 193–219.

Rosenheck, R. and DiLella, D. (1999) *Department of Veterans Affairs National Mental Health Program Performance Monitoring System: Fiscal Year 1998 Report*. West Haven CT: Northeast Program Evaluation Centre.

Rosenheck, R. and Horvath, T. (1998) The impact of VA reorganization on patterns of mental health care. *Psychiatric Services*, 49, 53.

Rosenheck, R. and Neale, M. (1998) Intersite variation in the impact of intensive psychiatric community care on hospital use. *American Journal of Ortho-psychiatry*, 68, 191–200.

Rossler, W. and Salize, H.J. (1994) Longitudinal statistics of mental health care in Germany. *Social Psychiatry and Psychiatric Epidemiology*, 29, 112–118.

Rothbard, A.B., Kuno, E., Schinnar, A.P., Hadley, T.R. and Turk, R. (1999) Service utilization and cost of community care for discharged state hospital patients: a 3-year follow-up study. *American Journal of Psychiatry*, 156, 920–927.

Schneider, S.E. and Ross, I.M. (1996) Ultra-short hospitalization for severely mentally ill patients. *Psychiatric Services*, 47, 137–138.

Shepherd, G. (1998) System failure? The problems of reductions in long-stay beds in the UK. *Epidemiologia e Psichiatria Sociale*, 7, 127–134.

Shepherd, G., Beadsmoore, A., Moore, C., Hardy, P. and Muijen, M. (1997) Relation between bed use, social deprivation, and overall bed availability in acute adult psychiatric units, and alternative residential options: a cross sectional survey, one day census data, and staff interviews [see comments]. *British Medical Journal*, 314, 262–266.

Shinfuku, N., Sugawara, S. and Yanaka, T. (1998) Mental health in the city of Kobe, Japan. In: Goldberg, D. and Thornicroft, G. (eds), *Mental Health in our Future Cities. Maudsley Monograph 42*. Hove: Psychology Press, pp.125–146.

Sledge, W.H., Tebes, J., Rakfeldt, J., Davidson, L., Lyons, L. and Druss, B. (1996) Day hospital/crisis respite care versus inpatient care, part I: clinical outcomes. *American Journal of Psychiatry*, 153, 1065–1073.

Smith, P, Sheldon, T.A. and Martin, S. (1996) An index of need for psychiatric services based on in-patient utilisation. *British Journal of Psychiatry*, 169, 308–316

Stein, L. and Test, M.A. (1980) Alternative to mental hospital treatment. *Archives of General Psychiatry*, 37, 392–397.

Strathdee, G. and Thornicroft, G. (1992) Community sectors for needs led mental health services. In: Thornicroft, G, Brewin, C. and Wing, J.K. (eds), *Measuring Mental Health Needs*. London: Gaskell, pp. 513–533.

Sytema, S. and Burgess, P. (1999) Continuity of care and readmission in two service systems: a comparative Victorian and Groningen case-register study. *Acta Psychiatrica Scandinavica*, 100, 212–219.

Szmukler, G., Thornicroft, G., Holloway, F. and Bowden, P. (1999) Homicides and community care: the evidence. *British Journal of Psychiatry*, 174, 564–565.

Talbott, J. and Glick, I.D. (1986) The inpatient care of the chronically mentally ill. *Schizophrenia Bulletin*, 12, 129–140.

Tansella, M., Balestrieri, G., Meneghelli, G. and Micciolo, R. (1991) Trends in provision of psychiatric care 1979–1988. *Psychological Medicine. Monograph Supplement*, 19, 5–16.

Tansella, M., Amaddeo, F., Burti, L., Garzotto, N. and Ruggerim M. (1998) Community-based mental health care in Verona, Italy. In: Goldberg, D. and Thornicroft, G. (eds), *Mental Health in our Future Cities. Maudsley Monograph 42*. Hove: Psychology Press, pp. 239–262.

Thomas, M.R., Rosenberg, S.A., Giese, A.A., Fryer, G.E., Dubovsky, S.L. and Shore, J.H. (1996) Shortening length of stay without increasing recidivism on a university- affiliated inpatient unit. *Psychiatric Services*, 47, 996–998.

Thornicroft, G. (1991) Social deprivation and rates of treated mental disorder. Developing statistical models to predict psychiatric service utilisation. *British Journal of Psychiatry*, 158, 475–484.

Thornicroft, G. and Bebbington, P. (1989) Deinstitutionalisation—from hospital closure to service development. *British Journal of Psychiatry*, 155, 739–753.

Thornicroft, G. and Tansella. M. (1999) *The Mental Health Matrix: A Manual to Improve Services*. Cambridge: Cambridge University Press.

Trieman, N., Leff, J. and Glover, G. (1999) Outcome of long stay psychiatric patients resettled in the community: prospective cohort study. *British Medical Journal*, 319, 13–16.

Tyrer, P., Evans, K., Gandhi, N., Lamont, A., Harrison-Read, P. and Johnson, T. (1998) Randomised controlled trial of two models of care for discharged psychiatric patients [see comments]. *British Medical Journal*, 316, 106–109.

Wall, S., Hotopf, M., Wessely, S. and Churchill, R. (1999) Trends in the use of the Mental Health Act: England, 1984–96. *British Medical Journal*, 318, 1520–1521.

Wickizer, T.M. and Lessler, D. (1998) Do treatment restrictions imposed by utilization management increase the likelihood of readmission for psychiatric patients? *Medical Care*, 36, 844–850.

Wing, J.K. (1992) *Epidemiologically-based Needs Assessment: Review of Research on Psychiatric Disorders*. London: Department of Health.

Wing, J.K. and Brown, G.W. (1970) *Institutionalism and Schizophrenia*. London: Cambridge University Press.

29 | *Forensic services*
Paul Bowden

Introduction

Forensic psychiatry is a relatively new and developing specialty. This chapter is written from a British perspective; the scope and details of practice and the relationship with the legal system may differ significantly from those in other countries. However, it would be surprising if there were not underlying common principles likely to find useful applicability elsewhere.

The origins of forensic psychiatry

The first annual meeting of the Royal College of Psychiatrists on Friday 19th November 1971 confirmed 'section' status for child psychiatry, psychotherapy and mental deficiency as it had existed under the Royal Medico-Psychological Association. Item 5 on the business agenda was 'Formation of a Forensic Psychiatry Specialist Section'; it was proposed by Dr Patrick McGrath (Robert Bluglass, personal communication). In January 1973, *News and Notes*, the supplement to that month's *British Journal of Psychiatry*, contained reference to the specialist section's (acting) representative for forensic psychiatry, Dr McGrath, then medical superintendent at Broadmoor hospital. Three months later, the result of the section elections appeared in *News and Notes*: Dr McGrath became chairman and the secretary's post was unfilled. Executive committee members comprised: three from the Bethlem and Maudsley hospitals/Institute of Psychiatry; two from English prisons; two from Scotland; and four from the new English forensic psychiatry posts.

Under the title ''Norms' for medical staffing of a forensic psychiatry service within the National Health Service in England and Wales' *News and Notes* for June 1975 contained a definition of forensic psychiatry which had been prepared by the forensic section and approved by the College's council. The definition was prefaced by both the doubtful observation that the field of forensic psychiatry had been practised in prisons and Special Hospitals for more than a century, and the observation that since 1967 eight joint appointments had been made. (Here 'joint' refers to appointments funded and held by individuals based equally in both the NHS and prisons.)

"Forensic psychiatry is the application of the principles of general psychiatry to that part of the population which comes into direct contact with legal processes either in criminal or civil actions. (Surely, it should have continued: '. . . as a result of mental disorder'). Forensic psychiatrists are also concerned with the management of behaviour disorder in settings where management is difficult and specialised methods of treatment may be required. There are four main branches . . .: (Special Hospitals, regional national health service hospitals, the prison medical service, and universities) . . . there is a need for a body of specialists in this work to run special units and out-patients clinics and to take a lead in the development of forensic psychiatry and in education and research. There is also a need for a variety of different kinds of base to train forensic psychiatrists for work in various arms of the speciality" (pp. 5–10).

Almost two decades later, the well-received textbook *Basic Forensic Psychiatry* (Faulk, 1994) contained a definition of its subject which reflected its author's work as a regional joint appointee who saw a need to draw limits.

"'Forensic' means pertaining to, connected with, or used in, courts of law. A forensic psychiatrist's work may be said to start with the preparation of psychiatric reports for the court on the mental state of offenders suspected of having a mental abnormality. (Although strictly an 'offender' is a person convicted of a crime). The psychiatrist will then be expected to provide or arrange treatment for the mentally abnormal offender where appropriate. Other psychiatrists, and other professionals seeing the sort of patient the forensic psychiatrist is looking after, will refer similar patients who may not have actually reached the court or broken the law. (Some psychiatrists do some of this work and others take a special interest in it). The term 'forensic psychiatrist' is used to describe those for whom this is their principal work" (p. 1).

It seems that Faulk acknowledged the existence of individuals in whom there is a link (which may be tenuous) between their offence behaviour (which may be undetected) and their mental disorder (which may be obscure), but he ignores those in whom there is no connection and where the association is one of chance. For its part, the glossary of the Reed report (Department of Health and Home Office, 1992) provides a model of tautological minimalism.

"Mentally disordered offender. A mentally disordered person who has broken the law. In identifying broad service needs, this term is sometimes used to include mentally disordered people who are alleged to have broken the law" (p. 115).

The joint appointments referred to in the 1975 *News and Notes* definition were the fruit of the Gwynne report (Home Office, 1964) which examined the prison medical service and concluded that joint appointments would result in closer links between prison medicine and the NHS. The initiative was not a success, and after several years it was accepted that the prison aspect of the appointments was largely unworkable. However, driven by wholly unanticipated events, the NHS limb would provide a springboard for other developments. Although both the Royal Commission on the Law Relating to Mental Illness and Mental Deficiency (House of Commons, 1957) and the Emery report (Ministry of Health, 1961) had recommended regionally based secure forensic developments, little if anything happened until the arrest in 1971 of the St Albans poisoner, Graham Young, who was charged with murders and other serious offences while on conditional discharge from Broadmoor hospital (Bowden, 1996).

Graham Young appeared in court 4 days after the Royal College of Psychiatrists first annual meeting; vested interests were to ensure that things would never be the same. Three Young-inspired bodies reported in a way which was to provide both financial and ideological bases for change: the Aarvold report on the supervision of psychiatric patients subject to special restrictions (Department of Health and Social Security and the Home Office, 1973); the DHSS in-house Glancy report (Department of Health and Social Security, 1974); and the prestigious Butler reports (Home Office and Department of Health and Social Security, 1974, 1975). Scotland was excluded from the planned developments in forensic psychiatry on the grounds that its 'unreformed' psychiatric hospitals and a well-endowed maximum secure hospital at Carstairs meant that change was unnecessary.

It was in this climate that the June 1975 *News and Notes* 'Norms' paper appeared. It argued that the DHSS should recognize a separate 'forensic administrative category' comprising those psychiatrists who exercized their skills in a forensic setting, overwhelmingly that of antisocial activity. The paper also gave information from a census: the eight joint appointees were in Durham, Birmingham, Leeds, London, Winchester, Bristol, Manchester and Liverpool. There were seven senior trainee posts and two un-established (i.e. personal) academic positions, both at the Institute of Psychiatry. The Portman Clinic was mentioned, as was the prison medical service; there were 17 consultant psychiatrists at the, then, three Special Hospitals; and an unknown number of 'doctors' assessing children and adolescents for courts and social service departments. Rather disparaging remarks were made about consultants in general psychiatry who did forensic work.

'Norms' had a vision. It was that the forensic psychiatrist should advise, train and take responsibility for assessments or therapies as joint appointees (in prisons and the NHS), in Special Hospitals, universities or the Home Office. It was envisaged that the new units, recommended by the Glancy and Butler reports, would be short- or medium-stay assessment and treatment centres. "The amount of reporting and treatment activity will be intense, and will be associated with out-patient clinics and work in a forensic psychiatry service based on the unit". The forensic psychiatrist was not to spend the whole of his professional life in the new, and old, institutions: "It is also anticipated that forensic consultants will have commitments in general psychiatric hospitals". Contracts were to suit local needs: ". . . others (will have) more sessions in the community services".

Although 'Norms' recognized that general psychiatrists would continue to do much of the forensic work in the community, it failed to address the issue of *what community and general psychiatric hospital forensic psychiatry* would be done by generalists, and what by the new 'administrative category' of forensic specialists. It left those who were in a position of exercizing choice, to do just that.

The second Butler report (Home Office and Department of Health and Social Security, 1975) made reference to the management of mentally disordered offenders (MDOs) *outside institutions*. It emphasized the need for improved communication between hospitals and those responsible for the management of discharged patients in the community. [The probation service had complained that following Graham Young's discharge from Broadmoor, information regarding his offences as a child had been kept from the service, and see Petch and Bradley (1997) for a summary of the significance of failures of communication in subsequent homicide inquiries.] Chapter 8 of the report has a section (8.9) which deals with 'Specialisation in the after-care of mentally disordered offenders'. It envisaged the 'important' part which forensic psychiatric services would play in aftercare: providing places for social workers in initial generic training, and contributing to in-service training and post-qualification specialist training. Given the changes which have occurred in the relevant services over the last two decades, the recommendations seem utopian and obsolete: ". . . (all) social workers and probation officers (would be) given opportunities by in-service training to acquire the specialist knowledge and expertise necessary to enable them to approach the particularly difficult cases of mentally dis-

ordered offenders with confidence" (p.125). There would be some psychiatric follow-up, but: "Responsibility for the after-care of discharged hospital offender patients should be given to the person who can bring most to the case . . . regardless of whether he or she belongs to the local authority social service department or the probation and after-care service" (p. 130). "Forensic psychiatric services . . . should be . . . integrated with the existing hospital and community mental health services. The main emphasis should be on community care and out-patient work (p.264) . . . Area psychiatric hospitals will continue to have an important role to play in the treatment of forensic patients" (p. 265).

Institutional development

Following the government's acceptance of the majority of the Butler report's recommendations for service development (the same was not true of the legal reforms which were canvassed widely), there was to be no market place competition for funds; regional developments were to be financed directly by the exchequer with new moneys. In the mid-1980s, there were 14 statutory regional health authorities in England. Their functions were, *inter alia*, the co-ordination of strategic plans; resource allocation; ensuring that expenditure is kept within cash limits; and determining the extent and provision of specialist services (Gostin, 1986). Charged with planning regional secure unit (RSU) developments, the regions were often devoid of informed advice and did not know how to spend the new revenue; in others, a health service trades union blocked plans for change; elsewhere, wards were converted and retitled 'interim' RSUs. More ambitious plans slowly emerged: a single large unit (e.g. Birmingham); a number of smaller units located at different points (e.g. South East Thames); and a mixture of both (e.g. South West Thames). Where developments did occur, they met skill shortages and financial constraints. The early RSU developments led no further; there was little integration with general psychiatry, which was itself moving into the community.

Forensic psychiatry's early development was a result of the most direct form of positive discrimination; it had not occurred as a result of either prioritization or competition in the sense that those processes usually serve to direct service development. In many NHS regions, the 1980s brought an isolation of forensic psychiatry in its RSU ghettos. Where there were advances, they were into areas where the position of forensic psychiatry was least challenged: in prisons and the Special Hospitals, and with services such as probation. Not only had forensic psychiatry failed to find a role in the new order, it had little sense of, or sympathy with, what generic community teams were trying to create and the principles of care which underpinned their work. The relationship between general and forensic psychiatry moved from non-understanding to acrimony, a situation made worse by the pay lead which forensic nurses received (it had been negotiated as the price paid for trades union support of the RSU programme).

Once the RSUs were full, and with very limited patient turnover, forensic staff were in the business of rejecting most referrals, although old allegiances were honoured and transfer requests from prisons and Special Hospitals were prioritized. The independent ('private') sector expanded rapidly but it remained outside mainstream psychiatry, compounded patients' isolation and was difficult to monitor. Regional RSUs chose who they took, and when, and their staff had good reason not to be involved in the struggles which were going on elsewhere. Forensic psychiatry's only acknowledgement that it must put its house in order was a phoney (and continuing) debate about whether it should operate a 'parallel' or 'integrated' model of care. Here 'parallel' implied a duplication of those services provided by general psychiatry, targeted at only the forensic population (a population identified by forensic specialists themselves). Once deemed 'forensic', the patient would be managed by dedicated, and often well-endowed, specialist services. The parallel model ignored both the arbitrary and self-serving nature of the forensic/general dichotomy, and the facts that needs, and status, change over time. For its part, the integrated model failed because of the reluctance of both services to accept what was sometimes seen as 'planned patient dumping' in the form of recategorization and transfer from one service to another, and a shortage of staff to maintain the elitism of the forensic service.

A role in the community?

The *National Health Service and Community Care Act 1990* attempted to clarify the separate responsibilities of health and social services, and Health Circular (90)23/Local Authority Letter (90)11 was designed to ensure that in future patients treated in the community received the health and social care they needed. For the reasons outlined above, forensic services insulated themselves from these developments. Also in 1990, an efficiency scrutiny of the prison medical service proposed that health care should be contracted into prisons, predominantly from the NHS, and Home Office Circular 66/90 [and NHS Management Executive Letter (90)168] promoted court diversion as a means of ensuring that mentally disordered offenders (MDOs) did not get caught up unnecessarily in the criminal justice system. These initiatives were complemented by a review of suicide and self-harm in prisons (Chief Inspector of Prisons, 1990).

In November 1992, the *Review of Health and Social Services for Mentally Disordered Offenders and Others Requiring Similar Services* (Department of Health and Home Office, the Reed report) was published. "Since the 1970s, forensic psychiatry has come to be seen as a speciality in its own right. There are now over seventy consultants, compared to just two, thirty years ago" (para. 2.8). One advisory group dealt with community matters and its report was prefaced with a cliché: "In line with current policy, MDOs should, wherever possible, receive care and treatment from health and social services rather than in the criminal justice system" (para.11.1). The community advisory group made recommendations in four main areas: diversion and discontinuance (of prosecution); community services; families, carers and users; and strategic issues.

The Reed report outlined the steps that needed to be taken if diversion and discontinuance were to be achieved. There needed to be effective local arrangements between the police, health and social services, and probation, an example being in the use of section 136 Mental Health Act 1983 (which refers to powers for the removal to a place of safety of individuals who are in a public place and are believed to suffer from mental disorder). Probation services should be involved before MDOs are charged with offences, and psychiatrists should be available to advise the prosecuting authority (the Crown Prosecution Service) and arrange access to treatment. Some bail hostels should specialize in providing services to MDOs, and: "There should be nation-wide provision of court psychiatrist or similar schemes for assessment and diversion of mentally disordered offenders" (para. 11.10). The recommendations for MDO community service provision mirrored the principles applicable to all services and emphasized that patients should be cared for:

- with regard to the quality of care and proper attention to the needs of individuals;
- as far as possible, in the community, rather than institutional settings;
- under conditions of no greater security than is justified by the degree of danger they present to themselves or to others;
- in such a way as to maximize rehabilitation and their chances of sustaining an independent life;
- as near as possible to their own homes and families if they have them (para.3.3).

It should be self-evident that these are ideals rather than principles; few are achievable. (An example is court diversion, which proved impossible to implement because of an absence of secure intensive care beds to which would-be offenders could be diverted. The scheme is now mostly one of court liaison, with, paradoxically, diversion being to places in remand prisons.) Services for MDOs should be planned and developed as part of community mental health services generally, and smooth the transfer of care from hospitals and prisons to the community through the application of the Care Programme Approach (CPA, paras 11.12 and 11.16). The absence of common boundaries means that co-ordination between agencies involved with MDOs is essential (para.11.19), with core teams being available at any time of day or night to ensure that patients are being assessed and treated appropriately (paras 11.20 and 11.22). Service users, carers and families should be involved in treatment decisions, and their needs and views be taken into account (paras 11.26–27). With regard to strategic issues, the Reed report recommended the commissioning of a national study for the needs of MDOs in the community (para. 11.28); service provision should reflect continuing local multi-agency needs assessment (para.11.29), with quality and effectiveness checks (para. 11.30). Lastly, ways should be sought to earmark funds for MDO services (para.11.34).

At the same time, the needs of another 'community' with a serious over-representation of persons with mental illness has been recognized. *Psychiatric morbidity among prisoners* is very high. A survey in 1997 by the Office for National Statistics on behalf of the Department of Health in England Wales (Singleton *et al.*, 1998) provided information about the prevalence of psychiatric problems among male and female, remand and sentenced prisoners. In the 12 months before entering prison, about 20% of male prisoners, both remand and sentenced, had received help or treatment for a mental or emotional problem. The proportions among female prisoners was double, 40%. The prevalence of personality disorder was up to 78% in male remand prisoners and 50% for females. Functional psychosis, determined by clinical interview, was found in 7% of male sentenced, 10% male remand and 14% of female prisoners. Neurotic disorders were found in 40, 59 and 76% of the corresponding groups. Previous suicide attempts were also common. Histories of substance abuse were extremely common, with over 50% probably having been drug dependent in the year prior to prison entry. Important questions concerning the most appropriate organization of mental health services to meet these needs remain unanswered. For example, to what extent should mentally ill prisoners be seen as 'community' patients to be looked after by local community mental health teams?

Working together

It is nearly 30 years since forensic psychiatry received institutional recognition. The way in which the speciality has contributed to the work of community mental health teams has depended on the precedents of both history and policy, on the geographical disposition of secure services and special treatment facilities, the socio-demographic characteristics of the client population, and the vagaries of personalities and ambitions. More recently, as risk-to-others has become a common criterion for access to generic services, it is not surprising that forensic psychiatry should be called on increasingly for more than good advice. Underpinning any forensic contribution is the principal of the dedicated caseload, the first coherent proposal for which came in a statutory post-homicide inquiry (the Clunis report, Richie *et al.*, 1994). A dedicated caseload has three characteristics: an upper limit on the number of cases managed; smaller caseloads; and targeted high-risk groups. Like the nurses pay lead referred to earlier, there is a downside to the principal: it is difficult to justify smaller caseloads in the face of colleagues who benefit from no similar luxury, and the absence of a valid ability to predict risk. What research evidence there is tends to support the view that dedicated case management provides a quality service which has little other effect on outcome measures. For example, Solomon and Draine (1995) in the USA studied 200 jail discharges. They were men who had been receiving mental health services in prison, and on discharge they were allocated randomly to one of three groups: an assertive community treatment model (with a very wide remit); forensic specialist case management; or usual referral to a community mental health centre. Final analysis failed to show a difference in psychological or clinical outcomes for 1 year for the two case management service models as compared with the usual services.

Central to any joint working between forensic and generic teams is clarity about roles and responsibilities. Other than in exceptional circumstances, professionals managing a case should belong to one clinical team. We need only to consider the example of aftercare arrangements under the *Code of Practice* (Department of Health and Welsh Office, 1999) to appreciate the dangers of neglecting this area. The Care Programme Approach applies to all patients receiving treatment and care whether or not they are admitted to hospital and irrespective of legal status. Whether served by a generic or specialist team, the formulation of a care plan (including an element of risk assessment and management), the appointment of a keyworker and the execution of responsible medical officer (RMO) responsibilities [defined in section 34 (1) (a) Mental Health Act 1983 as the registered medical practitioner in charge of the treatment of the patient who is liable to be detained, and including in this context care plan audit and consideration of supervised discharge, paras 27.5 and 27.6] could only be undertaken by a single team. That members of forensic teams should contribute to the management of some patients through joint (or co-) working seems highly appropriate but, again, responsibilities need to be clearly defined, even to the extent of deciding on the ownership of unwanted (or unhelpful) advice.

Forensic services deal with a population some of whose characteristics [e.g. maleness, over-representation of some ethnic groups, co-morbidity (dual diagnosis), non-compliance, restricted legal status, and, social instability and deprivation] are seen less frequently by generic teams; it follows that the former should have special experience in some areas. For those working in specialist services, a concentration of risk factors in the client population brings with it a particular requirement for stable and close working relationships, with clear communication and information sharing. Teams should have the capacity to respond quickly to requests for advice and they should be paradigms of efficient information recording and processing. While intrusive and assertive care is the norm, some patients find it intolerable, and a flexible approach to case management is essential. Familiarity with the work of complementary services (e.g. the police, prison, probation, court, prosecution) is achieved by formal liaison with those organizations. It also seems important that forensic services should provide in-house treatment programmes for their 'bread-and-butter' clientele (sex offenders, those with dual diagnoses, the angry, the non-compliant) and to which generic teams can refer patients.

Whittle and Scally (1998) described a model of forensic community care which they were involved in developing in South-east London. The service was funded by the responsible Health Commission and it lent towards an integrated (rather than parallel) approach. "The team promotes community-focused links with other services through co-working, which involves liaison, consultation and provision of support to psychiatric teams as they manage their patients, rather than a system of transferring clinical responsibility for patients to the forensic outreach team". A small number of patients were keyworked by forensic services and those patients were admitted to a forensic unit if that was necessary; community psychiatrists retained responsibility for admitting co-worked patients to community in-patient beds. The forensic community team also provided prison and court liaison, training programmes (e.g. in risk management), risk management assessments and a forum for case conferences where advice is sought urgently.

References

Bowden, P. (1996) Graham Young (1947–90): the St Albans poisoner. His life and times. *Criminal Behaviour and Mental Health* (Suppl.), 17–24.

Chief Inspector of Prisons (1990) *Report of a Review of Suicide and Self-harm in Prison Establishments.* London: HMSO.

Department of Health and Home Office (1992) *Review of Health and Social Services for Mentally Disordered Offenders and Others Requiring Similar Services.* (Cm. 2088, the Reed Report). London: HMSO.

Department of Health and Social Security (1974) *Revised Report of the Working Party on Security in NHS Psychiatric Hospitals.* (The Glancy report). London: DHSS.

Ministry of Health (1961) *Special Hospitals: Report of a Working Party.* (The Emery Report). London: HMSO.

Department of Health and Social Security and the Home Office (1973) *Report on the Review of Procedures for the Discharge and Supervision of Psychiatric Patients Subject to Special Restrictions.* (Cm. 5191, the Aarvold Report). London: HMSO.

Department of Health and Welsh Office (1999) *Code of Practice. Mental Health Act 1983.* London: HMSO.

Faulk, M (1994) *Basic Forensic Psychiatry*, 2nd. edn. Oxford: Blackwell.

Gostin, L. (1986) *Mental Health Services—Law and Practice.* Shaw: London.

Home Office (1964) *Report of the Working Party on the Prison Medical Service.* (The Gwynne report). London: HMSO.

Home Office and Department of Health and Social Security (1974) *Interim Report of the Committee on Mentally Abnormal Offenders.* (Cm. 5698). London: HMSO.

Home Office and Department of Health and Social Security (1975) *Report of the Committee on Mentally Abnormal Offenders.* (Cm. 6244, the Butler Report). London: HMSO.

House of Commons (1957) *Report of the Royal Commission on the Law Relating to Mental Illness and Mental Deficiency.* (Cm.169). London: HMSO.

Petch, E. and Bradley, C. (1997) Learning the lessons from homicide inquiries: adding insult to injury? *Journal of Forensic Psychiatry*, 8, 161–84.

Ritchie, J., Dick, D. and Lingham, R. (1994) *Report of the Inquiry into the Care and Treatment of Christopher Clunis.* London: HMSO.

Royal College of Psychiatrists (1973a) *British Journal of Psychiatry, News and Notes*, January, p. 2.

Royal College of Psychiatrists (1973b) *British Journal of Psychiatry, News and Notes*, April, p. 2.

Royal College of Psychiatrists (1975) *British Journal of Psychiatry, News and Notes*, June, pp. 5–10.

Singleton, N., Melzer, H. and Gatward, R. (1998) *Psychiatric Morbidity Among Prisoners in England and Wales.* London: HMSO.

Solomon, P. and Draine, J. (1995) One-year outcomes of a randomised trial of case management with seriously mentally ill clients leaving jail. *Evaluation Review*, 19, 256–273.

Drug and alcohol services

M. Susan Ridgely and Sonia Johnson

Introduction

Research literature on the co-occurrence of mental and substance abuse disorders suggests that substance abuse among people with mental illness, especially severe mental illness, is a profound problem with service and funding implications. As was emphasized in a recent paper aimed at raising awareness of the issue in the UK, "the interaction of substance use and severe mental illness can provide an explosive mixture and this dual diagnosis population will probably present the biggest single challenge for our mental health services in the future" (Gournay *et al.*, 1997). Reviews of the UK and US literature over the last two decades suggest that the presence of co-occurring disorders is almost the rule rather than the exception among persons seeking mental health and substance abuse treatment in US public sector specialty facilities (Ridgely *et al.*, 1986; Galanter *et al.*, 1988; Smith and Hucker, 1994) and that the problem is not being addressed adequately. These reviews also suggest that people with co-occurring disorders, although they have complex clinical needs, are more likely to be refused admission or discharged prematurely from specialty facilities in both the mental health and substance abuse sectors, which makes them particularly vulnerable to homelessness, criminalization and other social problems.

One reason that the clinical problem of co-occurring disorders remains unaddressed in many US communities is that the problem extends beyond the clinical realm—involving organizational, financial and philosophical barriers that are often as intractable as the illnesses themselves. In the USA, mental health and substance abuse systems have developed almost completely independently of one another and, where there has

been overlay, it has been characterized by distrust, antagonism and competition for scarce resources. Philosophical differences, different training and credentialing of practitioners (especially the differential focus on professional credentials in the mental health field), and stereotyped attitudes fuelled by poor communication and lack of respect for the competency of practitioners in the other field have exacerbated the problems (Ridgely *et al.*, 1990). Within these fields, preconceived notions about the effectiveness of specific treatment approaches are rarely challenged, and little solid empirical evidence on successful treatment of co-occurring disorders exists. Gournay and colleagues indicate that this state of affairs in the USA is mirrored in Britain where substance abuse services often are organizationally and financially separate from mainstream mental health services (Gournay *et al.*, 1997), although generally organization and financing for mental health and substance abuse services is not as fragmented in the UK as in the USA. These systems failures have resulted in inefficient use of existing treatment resources and often put the mentally ill person in the unenviable position of having to co-ordinate their own care across strict institutional boundaries, possibly with the aid of a case manager or care-giver, but more often on their own.

In this chapter, we will first discuss co-occurring substance abuse disorders, mainly from a *US perspective*. Developments there generally have antedated those elsewhere. We will then examine their relevance in a *European context*. We shall use the term '*co-occurring substance abuse*' to refer to the co-occurrence of a mental disorder and substance abuse, although, as discussed later, different terms are used in different places and contexts.

Co-occurring substance abuse from a US perspective

There is a growing recognition of the problem of co-occurring disorders as evidenced by an increasing literature over the past two decades, reflecting a first generation of research into the epidemiology, aetiology and treatment of co-occurring disorders. Whether this attention in the literature will be reflected in changes in local service programmes remains an open question. While much has been written in the USA over the past two decades, and there is much 'lip service' to the problem at national, state and local levels, there is little evidence of significant changes. Knowing what to do clinically does not seem to be sufficient to change the status quo. Strategies focused on addressing the barriers to care appear to be necessary to enhance the delivery of appropriate treatment. A number of national demonstration programmes in the USA have addressed the fragmentation of systems of care serving vulnerable populations, and evaluations of those efforts hold some clues to how local communities can reorganize services to address the challenge of treating co-occurring disorders within existing resources. As consensus begins to develop around appropriate treatment interventions for people with co-occurring disorders, agreement about how to address system problems will probably also evolve. Whether the political will to make those changes accompanies the developing clinical consensus is an open question.

Prior to addressing issues of epidemiology, treatment and systems change, it is important to define what is meant by co-occurring disorders or 'dual diagnosis.' The term 'dual diagnosis' is a short hand descriptor for the co-occurrence of mental and substance abuse disorders, but a variety of terms (including dual disorders, co-morbidity, co-occurring disorders, mentally ill/chemical abusers, substance abusing mentally ill, psychiatrically impaired substance abuser) have been used to describe what is a diagnostically and functionally heterogeneous population with a variety of clinical needs.

In keeping with the prioritization of services to the most severely disabled in the last two decades, much of the attention in the dual diagnosis area has been on severe mental illness. Severe mental illness is generally defined as including DSM diagnoses of schizophrenia, other psychoses, bipolar disorder and major depression. Regardless of diagnosis, mental illness is considered severe when it is enduring enough to cause lasting disability and recurrent contact with mental health care systems. The prioritization in the mental health field of severe mental illness is not due to their numbers in the general population. In fact, as we will discuss in the section on prevalence of co-occurring disorders, schizophrenia and other severe mental disorders are not nearly as prevalent as anxiety and depressive disorders. However, the prevalence of co-occurring substance abuse disorders is higher in schizophrenia and bipolar disorder than in anxiety and depressive disorders (Regier *et al.*, 1990). In addition, people with severe mental illnesses account for a much higher percentage of the mental health costs than their numbers would imply. A recent analysis of the prominence of people with severe mental illness (with and without health insurance) found that 2.2% of mentally ill people accounted for 33% of the public sector costs of mental health care in the USA in 1990 (Frank and McGuire, 1996). Costs of care for these individuals was $17.9 billion in 1990.

Substance abuse is generally defined as including DSM diagnoses of substance abuse or substance dependence, including abuse or dependence on alcohol or any other drug, whether it be an illicit drug (e.g. heroin and cocaine), a prescription drug (e.g. valium and other benzodiazepines) or an over-the-counter drug. However, in the case of people with severe mental illness, attention has also been paid to the problem of recreational or binge use of alcohol and other drugs. This concern is based on the clinical observation that small amounts of substances (posing little hazard normally) can have devastating effects on people with psychoses (Ridgely *et al.*, 1986; Drake *et al.*, 1990), including increased psychopathology, poor quality of life or repeated and ineffective episodes of mental health treatment. Regardless of level of severity of substance abuse, evidence suggests that it is unlikely to remit spontaneously without treatment (Drake *et al.*, 1996) and predicts poor prognosis in mental health treatment.

It is also worth noting that people with co-occurring severe mental illness and substance abuse disorders also have high rates of physical health disorders with little evidence of detection of those disorders, appropriate treatment or collaboration across the mental health–physical health divide. People with severe mental illness in the USA die at rates 1.5–3 times higher than matched general population samples (Black *et al.*, 1985). It is estimated that 10–12% of people with schizophrenia commit suicide (Miles, 1977), but causes of death include a full range of disorders including cardiovascular disease, circulatory, respiratory, digestive and genitourinary illnesses (Corten *et al.*, 1991; Newman and Bland, 1991). In addition, there is evidence of increased human immunodeficiency virus (HIV) risk among people with severe mental illness and substance abuse disorders, especially women (Krakow *et al.*, 1998).

Many people with mental illnesses seek and receive their care exclusively through the primary health care system (Shapiro *et al.*, 1984; Gournay *et al.*, 1997). Needs may be addressed inadequately by primary care physicians as evidence suggests they often do not detect mental and addictive disorders. In the Medical Outcomes Study, RAND investigators used an integrated economic and clinical evaluation approach to study the health care of patients with chronic conditions. Within the sample, only one half of patients with high psychological distress or with depressive disorder were recognized by their primary care physicians as distressed at the time of an office visit (Wells *et al.*, 1989; Ford, 1994), and an even lower percentage of those with substance abuse disorders were recognized. Even when recognized, appropriate treatments often were not provided (Wells *et al.*, 1996). Additionally, the data suggest that poor people who primarily use the specialty mental health or substance abuse systems for their care, at least in the USA, can expect to have their co-occurring physical health needs unrecognized.

Aetiology

A variety of explanations have been offered for the high prevalence of co-occurring substance abuse disorders in people with severe mental illnesses. In a comprehensive review, Mueser and his colleagues sort the major theories into four types of models and review the empirical evidence supporting each. The four types of models are: common factor models (that high rates of co-morbidity are the result of risk factors shared across both severe mental illness and substance abuse disorders); secondary substance abuse models (that severe mental illness increases a person's chances of developing substance abuse disorder); secondary psychiatric disorders models (that substance abuse precipitates severe mental illness in people who would not otherwise develop severe mental illness); and bi-directional models (that either severe mental illness or substance abuse disorder can increase a person's vulnerability to developing the other disorder) (Mueser *et al.*, 1998b). Cautioning that different models may account for co-morbidity in different patients and that some of the models have not been examined systematically, Mueser concludes,

"The research provides modest support for two etiological models in particular, the [antisocial personality disorder] model (a common factor model) and the supersensitivity model (a secondary [substance use disorder] model). On the other hand, there is little evidence for the common factor model of shared genetic vulnerability to [substance use disorder] and [severe mental illness]. Among psychosocial risk factor models, the self medication model has received the least empirical support . . ." (Mueser *et al.*, 1998a, p. 727).

According to Mueser and his colleagues, the antisocial personality disorder model hypothesizes that antisocial personality disorder is a common factor that contributes to the increased rate of substance abuse in people with severe mental illness, based on empirical evidence that links antisocial personality disorder and substance abuse and other empirical evidence that links antisocial personality disorder and severe mental illness. The supersensitivity model hypothesizes that the biological vulnerability of severe mental illness leads to a supersensitivity to substances that precipitates the onset of a substance abuse disorder. Mueser supports this hypothesis with research suggesting that people with severe mental illnesses are less capable of using alcohol or drugs in even moderate amounts without significant consequences (Drake and Wallach, 1993).

Evidence of range of prevalence of such disorders

Over the past two decades in the USA there have been a number of studies describing extremely high rates of co-occurrence of severe mental illness and substance abuse disorders—as high as 75–90% in some treated samples (see, for example, Hall *et al.*, 1978; Safer, 1987; Drake *et al.*, 1990). As a group, these studies of treated prevalence have suffered from a number of methodological problems including lack of uniformity in defining dual disorder, variation in instrumentation and data sources for establishing diagnoses, and sampling bias (Sacks *et al.*, 1997), making generalization to the community population difficult. Notwithstanding the methodological problems, clinical experience of treatment agencies, especially in the public sector, suggests that they may be facing a disproportionately large number of people with co-occurring disorders.

Two general population studies conducted in the USA provide perhaps the best data available on the prevalence of co-occurring disorders both in the general community population (treated and untreated) and in selected institutional settings (e.g. long-term mental hospitals, nursing homes and correctional facilities). The first, the Epidemiologic Catchment Area (ECA) study, estimated the true prevalence rates of specific mental and substance abuse disorders in the general community and specific institutional populations (Regier *et al.*, 1990). According to the ECA,

"Estimated U.S. population lifetime prevalence rates were 22.5% for any mental disorder, 13.5% for alcohol dependence/abuse, and 6.1% for drug dependence/ abuse. Among those with a mental disorder, the odds ratio of having some addictive disorder was 2.7%, with

a lifetime prevalence of about 29% (including an overlapping 22% with an alcohol and 15% with another drug disorder). For those with either an alcohol or drug disorder, the odds of having the other addictive disorder were seven times greater than in the rest of the population. Among those with an alcohol disorder, 37% had a comorbid mental disorder. The highest mental-addictive disorder comorbidity rate was found for those with drug (other than alcohol) disorders, among whom more than half (53%) were found to have a mental disorder with an odds ratio of 4.5" (Regier *et al.*, 1990, p. 2511)

The ECA also found that people treated in specialty mental health and substance abuse clinical settings had significantly higher odds of having co-morbid disorders. Among the institutionalized sample, co-morbidity of severe mental disorder and addiction was highest in the prison population (90% among people with antisocial personality, schizophrenia and bipolar disorders) (Regier *et al.*, 1990). Figure 30.1 presents the lifetime prevalence of co-morbid disorders in graphic form.

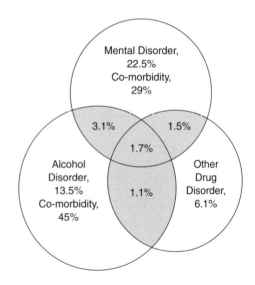

Figure 30.1 *Lifetime prevalence of co-morbid mental and addictive disorders in the USA, combined community and institutional five-site Epidemiologic Catchment Area data, standardized to the US population. From Regier et al. (1990)*

Regier *et al.* emphasize the importance of their data to mental health professionals,

"For mental health professionals, it is also important to recognise the high rate of substance abuse disorders among those with severe mental disorders. Almost 20% of individuals with mental disorders who come to a specialty [mental health] treatment setting will have a current diagnosis of a substance abuse disorder, and 29% of all persons with mental disorders have a lifetime diagnosis of a substance abuse disorder. For schizophrenia, the lifetime rate of substance dependence/abuse is 47%; for bipolar disorder, the rate increases to 56%" (Regier *et al.*, 1990, p. 2517).

The second important study is the National Comorbidity Survey (NCS). The NCS estimates are based on a nationally representative stratified, multi-stage area probability study of people aged 15–54 years in the non-institutionalized population of the USA (*n* = 8098) (Kessler *et al.*, 1996). There were a small number of individuals with psychosis in the sample but there was an extremely high co-occurrence of psychosis with the other mental disorders (e.g. mood disorders, anxiety disorders and antisocial personality disorders). According to the NCS, 50.9% of people with one or more lifetime diagnoses of mental disorders also have a lifetime history of at least one addictive disorder, and 41–65% of respondents with a lifetime addictive disorder also have a lifetime history of a mental disorder (Kessler *et al.*, 1996).

The rates of co-occurrence found in the NCS are higher than those found in the ECA (51% in the NCS and 38% in the ECA), as are the overall rates of the prevalence of individual disorders. The differences may be explained by differences in the study designs (e.g. a nationally representative sample versus five local samples, the inclusion of institutional samples in the ECA, differences in the age ranges, differences in the diagnostic instruments used, etc.) (Kessler *et al.*, 1996). The data in Europe are of lesser quality, but there may be significant differences in frequency as well as types of drug abuse. We will consider these later.

Two key issues of interest to the broader society

Two possible impacts of substance abuse on mental disorders have particular salience for the larger society, in addition to being of interest to practitioners: (i) does substance abuse create or contribute to violence among people with mental illness? and (ii) does substance abuse increase the costs of care for people with mental illness—either by increasing the costs of publicly financed care or by increasing the contribution which taxpayers make to underwriting the costs of their health insurance?

First, there is a public perception that mental illness and violence are closely correlated—that mentally ill people are more violent than the general population. The earlier research has been inconsistent and methodological problems (such as use of weak markers for occurrence of violence) have 'compromised' the studies (Steadman *et al.*, 1998). Recent data from the MacArthur Violence Risk Assessment Study provide a new look at the rates of violence among people discharged from acute psychiatric in-patient facilities and compare those rates with the rates of violence among the general population in the same neighbourhoods.

Evidence from the study of 1136 patients in three US cities suggests that whether patients abuse alcohol or drugs is key to understanding whether they will be violent:

"Substance abuse symptoms significantly raised the rate of violence in both the patient and comparison groups, and a higher portion of patients than others in their neighbourhoods reported symptoms of substance abuse" (Steadman *et al.*, 1998, p. 393).

Diagnosis matters—patients discharged with a diagnosis of schizophrenia or depression are less likely to be violent than people with a diagnosis of substance abuse and a personality disorder (see Table 30.1). Steadman and colleagues also report that the targets of violence are more often family members and friends, and that the violence takes place more often at home rather than in public places (Steadman *et al.*, 1998).

Table 30.1 *Year aggregate prevalence of violence*

Major mental disorder/ no substance abuse	17.9%
Major mental disorder/ substance abuse	31.1%
Other mental disorder[a]/ substance abuse	43.0%

[a]Other mental disorder includes personality disorder, adjustment disorder and suicidality.

From Steadman *et al.* (1998).

As to the issue of whether substance abuse increases the costs of psychiatric care, there is evidence from two recent studies in the USA that co-occurring substance abuse substantially increases the costs of treatment. In the USA, Dickey and Azeni (1996) examined the public sector costs of psychiatric treatment for people with severe mental illness and substance abuse problems. Dickey found that "psychiatrically disabled substance abusers" had psychiatric treatment costs that were 60% higher than those of non-abusers. (see Table 30.2). Most of the cost differences were the result of a higher use of acute in-patient treatment.

Costs also appear to be higher among the employed population and their dependents who are insured through commercial health insurance plans. Using private health insurance claims in the USA, Garnick *et al.* (1996) evaluated the costs of coverage for co-occurring disorders under commercial insurance. Garnick's findings suggest that patients with dual diagnoses incur high total health care charges. Annual charges for patients with co-occurring mental and substance abuse disorders ranged from $9723 (compared with $3672 for mental disorder alone) in one firm to $18 888 (compared with $4679 for mental disorder alone) in another. These charges were also significantly higher than charges for people diagnosed for substance abuse disorders alone. Major depressive disorder was the most frequent diagnosis among these claims.

Evidence of efficacy, effectiveness and costs of treatments

There is a developing consensus in the USA that the integration of mental health and substance abuse services is necessary to achieve good outcomes (Ridgely *et al.*, 1987; Minkoff, 1989; Carey, 1989; Osher and Kofoed, 1989; Kline *et al.*, 1991; Ridgely, 1991). This consensus is drawn from clinical experience, anecdotal accounts and from a first generation of research on integrated treatment using models that have emerged in the last two decades. While the models employ different programmatic approaches, they all emphasize the provision of intensive treatments for both disorders within one integrated programme.

Table 30.2 *Age- and sex-adjusted mean annual psychiatric treatment expenditures among mentally ill Medicaid beneficiaries, by substance abuse status*

Diagnosis	No substance abuse (n = 10 509)	With treated substance abuse (n = 1493)	With untreated substance abuse (n = 4393)
Schizophrenia	$12 350	$23 169	$19 568
Major affective disorder	$4686	$10 049	$9836
Other psychosis	$3455	$6722	$5440

From Dickey and Azeni (1996).

There are several recent reviews of programme models or approaches developed specifically to treat people with severe mental illnesses and co-occurring substance abuse disorders (e.g. Sacks *et al.*, 1997; Bellack and Gearson, 1998; Drake *et al.*, 1998b). Each of the programme models has its roots in either mental health or substance abuse treatment, and each has been modified in some way to address the particular clinical needs of people with severe mental illness. An illustrative (though not exhaustive) list includes:

- *Assertive community treatment (ACT) or intensive case management (ICM)*. The rationale for the use of ACT in dual diagnosis treatment is similar to the rationale outlined by Test and Stein who originally developed the multi-disciplinary treatment team model to divert admissions from public mental hospitals by providing intensive community treatment (Test, 1991). ACT or ICM improves engagement and compliance with treatment by focusing on the basic life needs of clients (food, shelter, subsistence) and by delivering services *in vivo* where client learning is more generalizable. Dual diagnosis ACT, a modified version of the original model developed in Madison, Wisconsin, adds a substance abuse treatment approach as a part of the ACT or ICM intervention. ACT or ICM models for treating people with severe mental illness and co-occurring substance abuse disorders have been studied in two recent cost-effectiveness studies (Jerrell 1994; Drake *et al.*, 1996, 1998a; Jerrell *et al.*, 1996) with generally positive but somewhat mixed results (see discussion below).

- *Behavioural skills training*. The rationale for using behavioural skills training in this context is similar to that outlined by Liberman and his colleagues when they developed the Social and Independent Living Skills (SILS) Training Program at UCLA and the Brentwood VA Medical Center. The goal of the programme is to provide rehabilitation services to individuals with Axis I disorders to 'gradually shape the patient's behaviour by reinforcing successive approximations of the appropriate skill'.

Behavioural skills training employs 'behavioural learning techniques' such as practising skills, role playing, feedback, homework assignments and positive reinforcement to achieve its effect. Relapse prevention (Niagram *et al.*, 1992; Ziedonis and Fisher, 1994) is another of the skills-based interventions that employ these strategies. A modification of the SILS approach has been studied in a cost-effectiveness trial (Jerrell and Ridgely, 1995), with behavioural skills training showing the most positive effects when compared with the other psychosocial interventions studied.

- *Modified self-help approaches*. Literature about the effectiveness of self-help groups such as Alcoholics Anonymous (AA) is sparse, but empirical findings do suggest that more active AA attendance during and following treatment is positively associated with better drinking outcomes (Bebbington, 1976). Obvious advantages of AA include the fact that it is readily available in almost all US communities, often on a daily basis, and costs nothing to attend. The main disadvantage has been that many people with severe mental disorders feel as if they do not 'fit' in traditional AA groups. Those who have 'modified' AA and other self-help programmes have either employed a training approach to teach clients to use AA appropriately and to support the development of sponsor relationships (Ridgely and Jerrell, 1996), or created dual diagnosis self-help groups attended exclusively by people with severe mental illness. The modified AA programme studied by Jerrell and Ridgely (1995) produced some positive effects on the participating clients over time, although in the study design the AA model was the 'usual care' or comparison condition.

- *Motivational enhancement therapy*. MET, originally developed by Miller and Rollnick (1991), "assumes people are ambivalent about change and must work toward their own decision concerning substance use reduction" (Bellack and Gearson, 1998). The process focuses on breaking down denial by using non-confrontational techniques to help the person make the connections between their own substance use and their lack of attainment of their own life goals (Carey, 1996). The 'harm reduction' approach is intuitively appealing to clinicians who have struggled with the lack of 'fit' of these clients in abstinence-oriented programmes. MET has been evaluated as a treatment for alcohol problems but not as a treatment for dual diagnosis. However, several of the other programme models have adapted motivational interviewing as a part of their interventions (e.g. Mueser and Noordsy, 1996; Ridgely and Jerrell, 1996; Drake *et al.*, 1998a).

- *Modified therapeutic community (TC)*. According to Sacks and his colleagues (1997), the TC model is focused not only on substance use but on affecting a global change in lifestyle, "The TC views drug use as a disorder of the whole person, reflecting problems in conduct, attitudes, moods, values and emotional management. Treatment focuses on drug abstinence and social and psychological change. It requires a multi-dimensional effort, involving intensive self-help in a residential setting." Only recently has the TC model been modified to address the special needs of people with severe mental disorders—prior experience had suggested that people with severe mental illness did not do well when exposed to the aggressively confrontative atmosphere of the original TC model. Sacks and colleagues report that at least one US National Institute of Drug Abuse study has compared the retention rates of people with dual diagnoses in modified versus traditional TCs (findings in favour of better retention in modified TCs) and that there is at least one study reporting favourable outcomes from modified TC treatment of a group of homeless men when compared with a community residence control group (Rahav *et al.*, 1995).

Possibly the closest to a comprehensive review of the treatment effectiveness literature in the USA was published recently by Drake *et al.* (1998b), in which they concluded:

"We reviewed 36 research studies on the effectiveness of integrated treatment for dually diagnosed patients. Studies of adding dual-disorders groups to traditional services, studies of intensive integrated treatment in controlled settings, and studies of demonstration projects have thus far yielded disappointing results. On the other hand, 10 recent studies of comprehensive integrated, outpatient treatment programs provide encouraging evidence regarding the potential of these programs to engage dually diagnosed patients in services and to help them reduce substance abuse and attain remission. Outcomes related to hospital use, psychiatric symptoms, and other domains are less consistent."

The 'most encouraging evidence' cited by Drake *et al.* comes from studies of a limited number of the models, including their own studies on the ACT model implemented in rural New England (Drake *et al.*, 1998a) and the behavioral skills training model, ICM and modified AA approaches implemented in northern California (Jerrell and Ridgely, 1995). These projects are important in that they employed the most sophisticated research designs, the interventions were implemented in 'real world' clinical settings in public sector agencies (as contrasted to enriched demonstration programmes) and the researchers evaluated the costs, effectiveness and implementation of the programmes.

In a large, urban public mental health system, Jerrell *et al.* (Jerrell *et al.*, 1994; Jerrell and Ridgely, 1995; Jerrell, 1996) used a quasi-experimental design to evaluate the cost-effectiveness of specialized interventions for people with severe mental illness and co-occurring substance abuse disorders. (The study has been described as quasi-experimental because ~50% of clients were clinician assigned from existing caseloads and ~50% of clients were assigned randomly to the interventions.) The three psychosocial interventions were: behavioural skills training, ICM and the twelve-step (AA) recovery model. The final sample consisted of 132 clients (75% male, 70% white, 76% diagnosed with schizophrenia, 48% had been hospitalized in the 6 months prior to study entry). Clients were followed for 24 months. Differential effectiveness was evident, with clients in the behavioural skills group demonstrating the most positive and significant differences in psychosocial functioning, role functioning and symptomatology (mental illness and alcohol and drug abuse) compared with the twelve-step recovery programme. However, the ICM intervention also resulted in several positive changes in psychosocial outcomes (global life satisfaction and mental health but not alcohol and drug abuse symptoms) at 12 and 18 months. In addition, the treatment costs for intensive acute and subacute mental health services were lower for the behavioural skills group than for the other two interventions. Supportive services costs were also lower for the ICM intervention.

This study suggests that the behavioural skills training intervention may be superior to either ICM or modified self-help approaches. The investigators reported extensively on the challenges associated with implementing a demonstration programme in the 'real world', reporting on several factors that might explain decrements in anticipated programme effects, including 'delivery errors' (Rossi and Freeman, 1993) such as variations in the extent to which the programmes were implemented 'robustly'. In an analysis of 'robustness' of implementation (based on qualitative data collected in an implementation analysis), the investigators reported that the quality of the implementation did have an effect on consumer functioning and service costs (Jerrell and Ridgely, 1999).

In contrast, Drake and colleagues (Clark *et al.*, 1998; Drake *et al.*, 1998a) used an experimental design to study individuals with severe mental illness and co-occurring disorders across predominantly rural New Hampshire. The clients were assigned randomly to ACT or to standard case management and followed for 3 years. The final experimental group sample consisted of 203 individuals (75% male, 96% white, 53% diagnosed with schizophrenia). According to the investigators, "ACT patients showed greater improvements on some measures of substance abuse and quality of life but the two groups were equivalent on most of the outcome measures, including stable community days, hospital days, psychiatric symptoms and remission of substance use disorder" (Drake *et al.*, 1998a). The analysis of costs indicated that there were no significant differences in

cost-effectiveness over the entire 3-year period, although ACT was significantly more efficient than standard case management during the final year of the study (Clark *et al.*, 1998). The investigators report that the study was limited by "treatment diffusion (i.e. the standard case management condition increased service intensity and dual disorders services by linking with other services to resemble the ACT condition), by the variability of ACT implementation, and by the use of a relatively intensive case management condition for the usual services control group" (Drake *et al.*, 1998a). In a formal analysis of programme 'fidelity' ("faithful implementation of, and adherence to, the ACT model"), the investigators found that for some (although not all) important client outcomes, fidelity to the model clearly mattered (McHugo *et al.*, 1999). For example, high fidelity was associated with reductions in substance use.

These two studies are important precisely because there have been so few controlled trials of treatment for this population and some disagreement exists about the weight to be given to the existing evidence in support of specialized integrated interventions. In a recent empirical review, the influential UK Cochrane Collaborative concluded, "there is no clear evidence supporting an advantage of any type of substance misuse programme for those with serious mental illness over the value of standard care. No one programme is clearly superior to another" (Ley *et al.*, 1999). In contrast, Drake and his colleagues, while acknowledging the significant limitations of most of the research to date, have argued that the weight of the evidence is in favour of integrated treatment (Drake *et al.*, 1998b).

Perhaps the best way to draw together the threads of these two reviews is to suggest that, in light of the high prevalence and negative consequences of substance abuse among people with schizophrenia, the evidence suggests that routine screening and assessment of substance abuse is clearly warranted; that offering and attempting to engage people with dual diagnoses in some kind of treatment that focuses on reducing use and abuse of substances is appropriate; and that, without presuming the superiority of one particular model of treatment over another, there are programme features that these models share that may be associated with effectiveness, including providing interventions that are assertive and community based, are comprehensive and longitudinal, that include specific mental health and substance abuse interventions, and that approach treatment in stages or phases (Ridgely *et al.*, 1987; Drake *et al.*, 1998b). Even advocates must admit, however, that findings from existing studies, while 'encouraging', do not provide compelling evidence of the cost-effectiveness of integrated treatment at this point.

Evidence from systems change demonstrations

As was mentioned early in this chapter, knowing what to do by way of specialized programming is insufficient to address the problem of dual diagnosis. Often the systems barriers are as intractable as the chronic illnesses themselves. A number of national demonstration programmes in the USA, funded by the federal government and private philanthropic foundations, have addressed the fragmentation of systems of care serving vulnerable populations. The Robert Wood Johnson (RWJ) Foundation Program on Chronic Mental Illness (Goldman *et al.*, 1990; Ridgely *et al.*, 1996), the National Institute on Alcohol Abuse and Alcoholism (NIAAA) Community Demonstration Grant Projects for Alcohol and Drug Abuse Treatment of Homeless Individuals (Orwin *et al.*, 1994), and the US Center for Mental Health Services (CMHS) Access to Community Care and Effective Services and Supports (ACCESS) Program (Morrissey *et al.*, 1997) are three examples. While none of these programmes were focused on people with dual diagnoses *per se*, each of the target populations included large numbers of people with severe mental illness and co-occurring substance abuse disorders.

The findings from these studies of systems change and service interventions suggest a number of important lessons.

(i)   Large multi-site demonstrations have confirmed the feasibility of implementing comprehensive systems of care for vulnerable populations with dual disorders.

(ii)   The local communities involved have used a number of integration strategies to achieve their goals, including developing locally based 'authorities' with administrative and clinical authority and control over all relevant financial resources dedicated to the care of the target population, using interagency agreements to facilitate interagency co-operation, using interagency teams of clinicians for service provision, developing 'coalitions' of provider agencies and pooling resources of multiple agencies to achieve a common agenda.

(iii) Empirical data suggest that at least some of the experimental interventions are effective in improving clients' lives—while other demonstrations have shown that it is possible to improve access, provide more appropriate services and improve satisfaction but not affect clients' outcomes.

(iv)   Successful implementation of innovative approaches to clinical care or service co-ordination requires extensive programme planning, model development and start up time, especially when integrating services provided by diverse agencies across different sectors and with different agency 'cultures'.

(v)   Gaps in non-clinical services (e.g. the lack of safe, affordable housing and jobs offering decent wages) must be addressed whether or not they are a specific focus of the demonstration.

(vi)   Integrating systems of care and improving co-ordination of services does not necessarily reduce the overall costs of care.

These demonstrations and others prove that systems change alone will not necessarily translate into improvements in symptoms and quality of life *unless* systems improvements also result in improved access to *high quality services of known therapeutic impact*. For example, investigators were able to demonstrate in the RWJ Program that systems had improved and there were large-scale expansions of case management services (designed to improve access and co-ordination of care). However, client outcome studies failed to find improvements. The lesson is that clinically appropriate services must accompany systems improvement (Ridgely *et al.*, 1996).

Other lessons learned in these multi-site evaluations are lessons for researchers aiming to do effectiveness studies in the 'real world'. Analysis of the NIAAA demonstration findings suggests that a number of design factors may have been responsible for the absence of differential effects between the experimental and comparison groups. These threats to the integrity of evaluations include: (i) selection bias, differential attrition across groups and low statistical power; (ii) lack of sufficient intervention intensity to give interventions a 'fair test'; (iii) lack of distinctions between experimental and control groups or the blurring of differences over time; (iv) initiating data collection for the outcome studies before the interventions have had time to 'mature'; (5) contextual factors in the local community; and (vi) measurement issues (Ridgely and Willenbring, 1992; Orwin *et al.*, 1994).

The interface between general adult services and substance abuse services: European perspectives

Until the early 1990s, there was almost no published research from Europe regarding 'dual diagnosis', the favoured term, and little evidence of any service development targeting this combination of problems. This gap recently has begun to be filled, and the beginnings of an evidence base regarding prevalence and social and clinical correlates in European countries are now available. Clinicians and service planners also appear to be in the early stages of developing innovative interventions, although as yet the literature contains very few evaluations of such services.

In the following, we will summarize the current state of European evidence on co-occurring substance abuse by addressing the following questions:

- Are rates of co-occurring substance abuse and associated problems as high in Europe as in the USA?
- How are individuals with co-occurring substance abuse currently managed by services in European countries?
- To what extent are lessons from US experiences in co-occurring substance abuse treatment applicable in European countries?
- What strategies could be used to incorporate co-occurring substance abuse interventions into sectorized community mental health service systems?

Are rates of co-occurring substance abuse and associated problems as high in Europe as in the USA?

Table 30.3 summarizes the findings from some key European studies of the prevalence of co-occurring substance abuse. Whereas at the beginning of the 1990s evidence regarding substance abuse among populations with severe mental illness in European countries was almost completely lacking, a few pieces of the jigsaw are now in place. Gaps are still prominent: many of the studies relate to samples in service settings which may not be representative of the local population of people with severe mental illness, methods of case ascertainment vary widely and samples are often small.

However, two general observations can be made. First, several studies suggest that rates of substance abuse among people with severe mental illness may be substantial, at least in some European countries, though the figures are rarely as high as those reported in the USA. Secondly, prevalence and patterns of drug use probably vary, and, in particular, use of amphetamines and other stimulants does not seem to be as prominent as in North American samples (e.g. Mueser *et al.*, 1990), while opiate use appears to feature more prominently. These findings also indicate a need for researchers in each country to carry out their own local surveys of patterns and prevalence of co-occurring substance abuse: it cannot be

Table 30.3 Co-morbid serious mental illness and substance abuse in European studies

Authors	Area	Sample	Findings
Duke et al. (1994)	UK (inner London)	Community sample of people with schizophrenia	Problem drinking in 22%
Menezes et al. (1996a,b)	UK (inner London)	People with psychosis in contact with local services	Evidence of alcohol or drug misuse in 36% Main substances used: alcohol and cannabis
Cantwell et al. (1999)	UK (Nottingham)	First-episode psychosis	One year prevalence of alcohol misuse: 12% One year prevalence of drug misuse: 20%
Farrell et al. (1998)	UK (national survey)	'Institutional' sample of severely mentally ill	Alcohol dependence in 6% of people with schizophrenia, 8% people with affective psychosis, 5% general population
Hambrecht and Häfner (1996)	Germany (Mannheim)	First-episode psychosis	Alcohol misuse disorders: 24%, drug misuse: 14%. Main substances: alcohol, cannabis, hallucinogens, cocaine
Soyka et al. (1993)	Germany (Munich)	Admissions to hospital with schizophrenia	Lifetime prevalence of substance misuse disorders: University clinic admissions: 22%, state hospital 43%. Main substances: alcohol, cannabis, stimulants
Lambert et al. (1997)	Germany (Hamburg)	Severely mentally ill in contact with services	Substance choices: alcohol and cannabis predominant substances used. Some evidence of opiate use, little of stimulant use.
Krausz et al. (1996)	Germany (Hamburg)	People with schizophrenia, in contact with a clinic	Some evidence of lifetime history of substance misuse in 47%
Arias Horcajadas et al. (1997)	Spain	Out-patients with schizophrenia	Cannabis dependence (current or past): 22%, alcohol dependence: 11%, cocaine dependence: 9%, opioid dependence: 7%.

Table 30.3 *continued*

Authors	Area	Sample	Findings
Fernandez and Marquina (1995)	Spain (Madrid)	Attenders of vocational rehabilitation programme	Harmful consequences of alcohol use: 27%, of cannabis use: 10%, of combination including opiates:10%
Cassano *et al.* (1998)	Italy (Pisa)	Hospital admissions	Substance misuse or dependence: 12%
Civitarese *et al.* (1996)	Italy (Pavia) schizophrenia	Hospital admissions with area service during 2-year period)	Low rates of alcohol and drug misuse (17 detected among consecutive admissions to catchment
Verdoux *et al.* (1996)	France (Nantes)	Day and in-patient service users	Lifetime prevalence of substance misuse: 25% among people with schizophrenia or bipolar disorder. Alcohol and cannabis main substances, followed by opiates.
Launay *et al.* (1998)	France (Ile de France)	Community mental health team patients	Substance choice: alcohol and cannabis predominant, some opiate use, little evidence of stimulant use
Modestin *et al.* (1997)	Switzerland	In-patients with any psychiatric disorder	32% using alcohol three or more times a week. 27% using illicit drugs three or more times a week

assumed that findings from the major USA studies will be mirrored elsewhere.

As in the USA, the costs of care are likely to be increased by co-occurring substance abuse. In the UK, Menezes *et al.* (1996) looked at differences in service use among people with serious mental illness alone and those with co-occurring substance abuse. Although differences in numbers of admissions to in-patient care were not substantial, people with co-occurring substance abuse spent 1.8 times as many days in the hospital and used emergency psychiatric services 1.3 times as much as non-abusers. Given that in-patient and emergency services are among the most costly to provide, these differences are significant in their cost implications.

How are individuals with co-occurring substance abuse currently managed by services in European countries?

Little evidence is available regarding either current patterns of service use or of service innovations in European countries. Reviews (e.g. Verdoux *et al.*, 1990; Smith and Hucker, 1993; Krausz *et al.*, 1996; Weaver *et al.*, 1999), however, indicate that researchers, clinicians and service planners generally see current service configurations as ill equipped to manage co-occurring substance abuse. High levels of in-patient and emergency service use (Soyka *et al.*, 1993; Menezes *et al.*, 1996; Launay *et al.*, 1998) may also indicate a struggle to engage and manage these individuals successfully in the community. Problems that have been identified in the European literature in the management of people with co-occurring substance abuse resemble those identified by North American authors and include:

- *Problems with joint management by both substance abuse and general mental health services:* continuity of care and engagement are already difficult for this group, and these may be exacerbated if two services are involved.

- *Problems with treatment by general mental health services:* workers in the community mental health teams may lack training in helping people with substance abuse. It may be seen as

difficult behaviour rather than as a disabling problem for which treatment is needed.

- *Problems with treatment by substance abuse services:* staff in substance abuse services may lack confidence in working with individuals with psychoses (especially if positive symptoms are present) and may feel that such clients are beyond their remit. Conventional substance abuse treatments may be inappropriate for individuals with severe mental illnesses, especially where the approach is relatively confrontational, where there are strict limits on tolerance of relapse, or where the emotional temperature in treatment sessions tends to run high.

Thus a service response is needed which provides a greater integration between substance abuse and mental health services than is currently available. At least in some countries it appears that the quest for effective ways of doing this has begun. Models resemble those described by us earlier. For example, from Switzerland, Moggi *et al.* (1996) report on a transitional in-patient facility with elements of modified therapeutic community and behavioural skills training. Patients stay 4–9 months, until they are ready for longer term placement in residential or day rehabilitation services. The authors report some basic data regarding 42 patients admitted to the facility, finding some evidence of improvements in positive symptoms, anxiety, depression and hostility, but no indications of reduction in negative symptoms or, following discharge, in substance use. Wuensch (1998) describes a centre in Hamburg devoted to in-patient rehabilitation of people with schizophrenia or affective psychosis combined with substance problems. Length of stay was generally 12–14 months, with a programme based on individual and group therapy, a substantial programme of work rehabilitation and occupational therapy, and work with families. By 1997, 172 patients had been admitted, of whom around half were abusing alcohol and/or cannabis, whilst the other half were heroin users. Premature discharge was a significant problem, with almost 50% stopping treatment prematurely in the first 2 years of the programme, and most discharges taking place for 'disciplinary' reasons.

In the UK, descriptions or evaluations of model services for co-occurring substance abuse have not as yet been published in peer-reviewed journals. However, sources such as non-peer-reviewed publications and local and national health services web sites demonstrate that the increasing pre-occupation with the problem of dual diagnosis among clinicians and service planners is giving rise to a variety of local initiatives in both voluntary (e.g. Boyd, 1999; Penfold, 1999) and statutory sectors. However, evaluations in Europe lag behind those in the USA, and the reports mentioned describe approaches but not their effectiveness.

To what extent are lessons from US experiences in co-occurring substance abuse treatment applicable in European countries?

It is obvious from the above that so far US experience in developing and evaluating innovative services has been much more extensive than in Europe. Should European policy makers, service planners and clinicians then look first to the USA in seeking to meet the needs of this group?

There are a number of reasons for hesitation. *First*, while many of the innovative US models are of great interest, as we have seen, the question of how best to manage co-occurring substance abuse cannot be said to have been resolved in North America. Our earlier discussions indicate that outcomes from the most apparently successful models tend at best to be 'promising'. *Second*, not every European country has as radical a separation between mental health and substance abuse treatment systems as exists in the USA. Thus in the UK there are many workers who have some basic training in both areas, so that the obstacles to developing good clinical practice for these clients within existing service structures may not be so great. *Third*, recent service planning in European countries, including the UK, France and Italy, has been based principally on a sectorized model, with an emphasis on generic community mental health teams providing a full range of services to the population with severe mental illness of a small geographical catchment area.

Such teams have advantages in community-based working, and specialist dual diagnosis teams serving larger catchment areas may be less able to achieve close integration with other services in their catchment areas, such as primary care and social services. *Finally*, the variation in patterns and probably social contexts of substance abuse between countries means that the same intervention strategies may not necessarily be appropriate in each country. For example, opiate use among patients with severe mental illness appears more prominent in some European countries than in the USA.

While the evaluations of co-occurring treatment interventions cited earlier rarely employed such techniques, the scope for US teams to engage clients in treatment through 'coercive' methods is probably more extensive than in Europe. Discharges from hospital conditional on acceptance of treatment, involuntary out-patient commitment and the representative payeeships which allow mental health professionals to take control of the finances of those clients who are known to be spending state benefits on drugs and alcohol (Ries and Dyck, 1997) provide opportunities for greater control in the USA. Such methods are not available currently in many European countries, nor would they necessarily find wide acceptance among professionals.

What strategies could be used to incorporate co-occurring substance abuse intervention into sectorized community mental health service systems?

This section refers primarily to options in European countries such as the UK, France and Italy where the predominant model of service delivery for people with severe mental illness is by a community-based multi-disciplinary team for the population of a small geographical sector. Service models for co-occurring substance abuse should fit with, and build on, the strengths of the existing system. Potential strategies include the following.

Developing closer links between mental health and substance abuse services

Perhaps the simplest model, this might be approached by linking a substance abuse worker to each sector mental health team, facilitating referrals and joint discussions, by attaching community mental health team workers to the substance abuse specialist teams, or by setting up mechanisms for joint assessments and reviews of clients. A limitation of this model is that it does not readily allow both types of care to be delivered by the same keyworker, desirable at least for difficult to engage patients. Furthermore, the techniques most effective for substance abuse among those with severe mental illness may not be the same as those that work best in mainstream substance abuse services. Also, the problems encountered may be different. For example, problems arising from cannabis use are probably more frequent among severely mentally ill populations than in specialist drug abuse services.

Providing training and supervision in substance abuse techniques for all sector community mental health staff

This could lead to a large number of professionals being well equipped to manage problems of co-occurring substance abuse wherever they present in the community mental health services, desirable in view of the high prevalence of these problems. However, in hard-pressed services, it may be difficult, at least initially, to find resources to provide the necessary intensive training and supervision to all.

Attaching specialist co-occurring substance abuse keyworkers to community mental health teams

Selected individuals within each team could become co-occurring substance abuse specialists, receiving intensive training and supervision and taking on a caseload largely of these clients. Such specialists could also provide advice and supervision to the rest of the team. Potential problems

are 'burn-out' from having large numbers of 'difficult' clients on a caseload, and isolation from being the only drug abuse specialist within a team. Small caseloads, appropriate pay and being valued as specialists might alleviate these. So might plentiful training and supervision and opportunities to meet with specialist workers from other teams. Another possibility would be to train two or three staff per sector team as specialist keyworkers, dividing the team's dual diagnosis caseload between them.

Developing specialist co-occurring substance abuse teams

Apparently successful US model services described above have taken the form of specialist teams with a caseload consisting entirely of people with co-occurring substance abuse. High levels of expertise in managing co-occurring substance abuse are likely to develop within such a team and workers are well placed to support one another. However, the advantages associated with sectorized care for a small geographical area may be lost.

Developing co-occurring substance abuse interventions within other forms of specialist team

Specialist assertive outreach teams currently are favoured in UK central policy planning as a promising means of providing effective care for individuals who are difficult to engage, frequently admitted and who often have histories of offending and of homelessness (Sainsbury Centre, 1998), although robust evidence on the effectiveness of such teams in a UK context is not yet available. The proportion of individuals with co-occurring substance abuse on the caseloads of such teams is likely to be high and they are a group for whom management by separate addictions and mental illness services is particularly problematical. Thus development of the skills of workers in these teams in managing co-occurring substance abuse seems especially important. Given the propensity of individuals with co-occurring substance abuse to present in crisis, similar considerations apply to specialist crisis teams or home treatment teams. Teams for people who are homeless and mentally ill also have a high proportion of such clients on their caseloads.

Little evidence is available on how many people with co-occurring severe mental illness and substance misuse are at present in contact mainly with substance abuse services. These services also encounter many individuals who meet criteria for broader definitions of 'dual diagnosis' such as having co-occurring non-psychotic disorders like anxiety and depression. There is a need for research and service developments focused on this group, for example enhancing the availability of psychological interventions for depression and anxiety within the substance abuse services. High rates of co-occurring personality disorder and substance abuse are likely to be encountered within both mental health and substance abuse services, but the most effective treatment strategies have been little researched.

Perhaps subgroups among those with co-occurring substance abuse may be best served by different models, so that a combination of the above strategies may be appropriate. Thus there may be a group who are relatively compliant with services and whose needs might be met by improving links between substance abuse services and community mental health teams. For a further less compliant group, but whose substance abuse is not as yet severe, training community mental health team workers to detect substance abuse and acquire basic management skills may be appropriate. Specialist co-occurring substance abuse teams or specialist workers within assertive outreach teams could be reserved for the most challenging clients—those with high levels of need for intervention both for substance abuse and for clinical and social problems arising from severe mental illness.

Conclusions: implications of research evidence for service models

There now exists a 'first generation' of research, largely from the USA, on integrated treatment for people with severe mental illness and co-occurring substance abuse disorders. However, those who review the literature are often advocates of a particular approach to treatment, raising questions about bias. As our discussion indicates, the broader service context may also be crucial. In Europe, both the patterns of co-occurring substance abuse and the service context may differ significantly from the USA. Attempts are being made to learn from US experiences while trying to develop models consistent with local service configurations.

Generally, we need additional high quality research on treatment for co-occurring disorders—research that avoids the methodological problems that have hampered earlier studies. We need to ask more sophisticated questions of the research—not "is it effective?" but, rather, "what is effective for whom, under what circumstances and at what cost?" Unfortunately, the cost of some intensive treatment models may make their widespread implementation cost-prohibitive.

The research suggests, if anything, that it is too early to stop innovating. We need to develop and test new approaches to delivering care and modify and retest some of the more promising models that failed to show an impact because of problems in the design of the original research.

Finally, the research provides significant evidence that doing nothing about substance abuse among people being treated for mental disorders is a losing strategy—both clinically and financially. Breaking down the historical barriers, improving systems of care and developing new and better programmes to address the needs of people with co-occurring disorders will not only benefit the dually diagnosed, but also has the potential to improve services generally for all people who have mental health and substance abuse problems.

References

Arias Horcajadas, F., Padin Calo, J.J. and Fernandez Gonzalez, M.A. (1997) Consumo y dependencia de drogas en la esquizofrenia. *Actas Luso-Espa(olas de Neurologia y Ciencias Afines*, 25, 379–389.

Bebbington, P. (1976) The efficacy of Alcoholics Anonymous: the elusiveness of hard data. *British Journal of Psychiatry*, 128, 163–188.

Bellack, A.S. and Gearson, J.S. (1998) Substance abuse treatment for people with schizophrenia. *Addictive Behaviors*, 23, 749–766.

Black, D.W., Warrack, G. and Winokur, G. (1985) Excess mortality among psychiatric patients: the Iowa record-linkage study. *Journal of the American Medical Association*, 253, 58–61.

Boyd, D. (1999) Multiple needs and multiple gaps. *Addiction Today*, March/April issue.

Carey, K. (1989) Emerging treatment guidelines for mentally ill chemical abusers. *Hospital and Community Psychiatry*, 40, 341–349.

Carey, K. (1996) Substance use reduction in the context of outpatient psychiatric treatment: a collaborative, motivational, harm reduction approach. *Community Mental Health Journal*, 32, 291–306.

Cassano, C.B., Pini, S., Saettoni, M. *et al.* (1998) Occurrence and clinical correlates of psychiatric comorbidity in patients with psychotic disorders. *Journal of Clinical Psychiatry*, 59, 60–68.

Civitarese, G.C., Pozzi, L. and Papale, L. (1996) Abuso di sostanze e schizofrenia tra i pazienti di un servizio di diagnosi e cura. *Rivista di Psichiatria*, 31, 143–151.

Clark, R.E., Teague, G.B. , Ricketts, S.K., Bush, P.W., Xie, H., McGuire, T., Drake, R.E., McHugo, G.J., Keller, A.M. and Zubkoff, M. (1998) Cost-effectiveness of assertive community treatment versus standard case management for persons with co-occurring severe mental illness and substance use disorders. *Health Services Research*, 33, 1285–1308.

Corten, P., Ribourdouille, M. and Dramaix, M. (1991) Premature death among outpatients at a community mental health center. *Hospital and Community Psychiatry*, 42, 1248–1251.

Dickey, B. and Azeni, H. (1996) Persons with dual diagnoses of substance abuse and major mental illness: their excess costs of psychiatric care. *American Journal of Public Health*, 86, 973–977.

Drake, R.E. and Wallach, M.A. (1993). Moderate drinking among people with severe mental illness. *Hospital and Community Psychiatry*, 44, 780–782.

Drake, R.E., Osher, F.C. and Noordsy, D.L. (1990) Diagnosis of alcohol use disorders in schizophrenia. *Schizophrenia Bulletin*, 16, 57–67.

Drake, R.E., Mueser, K.T., Clark, R.E. and Wallach, M. (1996) The course, treatment and outcome of substance disorder in persons with severe mental illness. *American Journal of Orthopsychiatry*, 66, 42–51.

Drake, R.E., McHugo, G.J., Clark, R. E., Teague, G. B. Xie, H., Miles, K. and Ackerson, T. (1998a) Assertive community treatment for patients with co-occurring severe mental illness and substance use disorder: a clinical trial. *American Journal of Orthopsychiatry*, 68, 201–215.

Drake, R.E., Mercer-McFadden, C., Mueser, K.T., McHugo, G. and Bond, G. (1998b) A review of integrated mental health and substance abuse treatment for patients with dual disorders. *Schizophrenia Bulletin*, 24, 589–608

Duke, P., Pantellis, C. and Barnes, T. (1994) South Westminster Schizophrenia Survey: alcohol use and its relationship to symptoms, tardive dyskinesia and illness onset. *British Journal of Psychiatry*, 164, 630–636.

Farrell, M., Howes, S., Taylor, C. *et al.* (1998) Substance misuse and psychiatric comorbidity: an overview of the OPCS national psychiatric morbidity survey. *Addictive Behaviors*, 23, 909–918.

Fernandez Fernandez, J.A. and Marquina Planchadell, M.M. (1995) El uso de drogas en personas con problemas psiquiatricos cronicos. *Psicothema*, 7, 557–567.

Ford, D.E. (1994) Recognition and under-recognition of mental disorders in adult primary care. In: Miranda, J., Hohmann, A.A., Attkisson, C.C. and Larson, D.B. (eds). *Mental Disorders in Primary Care*. San Francisco: Jossey-Bass Publishers, pp. 186–205.

Frank, R. and McGuire, T. (1996) Introduction to the economics of mental health payment systems. In: Levin, B.L. and Petrila, J. (eds), *Mental Health Services: A Public Health Perspective*. New York: Oxford University Press, pp. 23–37.

Galanter, M., Casteneda, R. and Ferman, J. (1988) Substance abuse among general psychiatric patients: place of presentation, diagnosis and treatment. *American Journal of Drug and Alcohol Abuse*, 14, 211–235.

Garnick, D.W., Hendricks, A.M., Drainoni, M., Horgan, C. and Comstock, C. (1996) Private sector coverage of people with dual diagnoses. *Journal of Mental Health Administration*, 23, 317–328.

Goldman, H.H., Morrissey, J.P. and Ridgely, M.S. (1994) Evaluating the RWJ Foundation Program on Chronic Mental Illness. *Milbank Quarterly*, 72, 37–47.

Gournay, K., Sandford, T., Johnson, S. and Thornicroft, G. (1997) Dual diagnosis of severe mental health problems and substance abuse/dependence: a major priority for mental health nursing. *Journal of Psychiatric and Mental Health Nursing*, 4, 89–95.

Hall, R.C.W., Popkin, M,K., Stickney, S.K. and Gardner, E.R. (1978) Covert outpatient drug abuse. *Journal of Nervous and Mental Disease*, 166, 343–348.

Hambrecht, M. and Häfner, H. (1996) Fòhren Alkohol und Drogenmi(brauch zur Schizophrenie? *Nervenarzt*, 67, 36–45.

Jerrell, J.M. (1996) Cost effective treatment for persons with dual disorders. In: Drake, R.E. and Minkoff, K. (eds), *New Directions for Mental Health Services 70: Dual Diagnosis of Major Mental Illness and Substance Disorder: Volume 2 Recent Research and Clinical Implications*. San Francisco: Jossey-Bass Publishers.

Jerrell, J.M. and Ridgely, M. S. (1995) Comparative effectiveness of three approaches to serving people with severe mental illness and substance abuse disorders. *Journal of Nervous and Mental Disease*, 183, 566–576.

Jerrell, J.M. and Ridgely, M.S. (1999) Impact of robustness of program implementation on outcomes of clients in dual diagnosis programs. *Psychiatric Services*, 50, 109–112.

Jerrell, J.M., Hu, T. and Ridgely, M.S. (1994) Cost-effectiveness of substance disorder interventions for the severely mentally ill. *Journal of Mental Health Administration*, 21, 281–295.

Kessler, R.C., Nelson, C.B., McGonagle, K.A., Edlund, M.J., Frank, R.G.and Leaf, P.J. (1996) The epidemiology of co-occurring addictive and mental disorders: implications for prevention and service utilization. *American Journal of Orthopsychiatry*, 66, 17–31.

Kline, J., Harris, M., Bebout, R. and Drake, R.E. (1991) Contrasting integrated and linkage models of treatment for homeless, dually diagnosed adults. In: Drake, R.E. and Minkoff, K. (eds), *New Directions for Mental Health Services 50: Dual Diagnosis of Major Mental Illness and Substance Disorder*. San Francisco: Jossey-Bass Publishers, pp. 95–106.

Krakow, D.S., Galanter, M., Dermatis, H. and Westreich, L.M. (1998) HIV risk factors in dually diagnosed patients. *American Journal of Addictions*, 7, 74–80.

Krausz, M., Mass, R., Haasen, C. et al. (1996) Psychopathology in patients with schizophrenia and substance abuse: a comparative clinical study. *Psychopathology*, 29, 95–103.

Lambert, M., Haasen, C., Mass, R. et al. (1997) Konsummuster und Konsummotivation des Suchtmittelgebrauchs bei schizophrenen Patienten. *Psychiatrische Praxis*, 27, 185–189.

Launay, C., Petitjean, F., Perdereau, F. and Antoine, D. (1998) Conduites toxicomaniaques chez les malades mentaux: une enquête en Ile-de-France. *Annales Medico-Psychologiques*, 156, 482–486.

Ley, A., Jeffrey, D.P., McLaren, S. and Siegfried, N. (1999) Treatment programmes for people with both severe mental illness and substance misuse (Cochrane Review). In *The Cochrane Library*, Issue 2. Oxford: Update Software.

McHugo, G.J., Drake, R.E., Teague, G.B. and Xie, H. (1999) Fidelity to assertive community treatment and client outcomes in the New Hampshire dual disorders study. *Psychiatric Services*, 50, 818–824.

Menezes, P.R., Johnson, S., Thornicroft, G., Marshall, J., Prosser, D., Bebbington, P. and Kuipers, E. (1996) Drug and alcohol problems among people with severe mental illness in south London. *British Journal of Psychiatry*, 168, 612–619.

Menezes, P., Johnson, S., Thornicroft, G. et al. (1996) Drug and alcohol problems among individuals with severe mental illness in South London. *British Journal of Psychiatry*, 169, 334–337.

Miles, C. (1977) Conditions predisposing to suicide. *Journal of Nervous and Mental Disease*, 164, 231–246.

Miller, W.R. and Rollnick, S. (1991) *Motivational Interviewing: preparing people to change addictive behaviour*. New York: Guildford.

Minkoff, K. (1989) An integrated treatment model for dual diagnosis of psychosis and addiction. *Hospital and Community Psychiatry*, 40, 1031–1036.

Modestin, J., Nussbaumer, C., Angst, D., Scheidegger, P. and Hell, D. (1997) Use of potentially abusive psychotropic substances in psychiatric inpatients. *European Archives of Psychiatry and Clinical Neurosciences*, 247, 146–153.

Moggi, F., Hirsbrunner, H.-P., Wittig, R. et al. (1996) Stationäre Behandlung von Patienten mit Doppeldiagnosen. *Verhaltenstherapie*, 6, 201–209.

Morrissey, J.P., Calloway, M., Johnson, M. and Ullman, M. (1997) Service system performance and integration: a baseline profile of the ACCESS Demonstration Sites. *Psychiatric Services*, 47, 374–380.

Mueser, K.T. and Noordsy, D. (1996) Group treatment for dually diagnosed clients. In: Drake, R.E. and Minkoff, K. (eds), *New Directions for Mental Health Services 70: Dual Diagnosis of Major Mental Illness and Substance Disorder: Volume 2 Recent Research and Clinical Implications*. San Francisco: Jossey-Bass Publishers, pp. 33–51.

Mueser, K.T., Yarnold, P.R., Levinson, M.E. et al. (1990) Prevalence of substance abuse in schizophrenia: demographic and clinical correlates. *Schizophrenia Bulletin*, 16, 31–56.

Mueser, K.T., Drake, R.E. and Wallach, M.A. (1998a) Dual diagnosis: a review of etiological theories. *Addictive Behaviors*, 23, 717–734.

Mueser, K.T., Drake. R.E. and Noordsy, D. (1998b) Integrated mental health and substance abuse treatment for severe psychiatric disorders. *Journal of Practical Psychiatry and Behavioral Health*, 4, 129–139.

Newman, S.C. and Bland, R.C. (1991) Mortality in a cohort of patients with schizophrenia: a record linkage study. *Canadian Journal of Psychiatry*, 36, 239–245.

Niagram, R., Schottenfeld, R. and Kosten, T.R. (1992) Treatment of dual diagnosis patients: a relapse prevention group approach. *Journal of Substance Abuse Treatment*, 9, 305–309.

Orwin, R., Goldman, H.H., Sonnefeld, L.J., Ridgely, M.S., Smith, N.G., Garrison-Mogren, R., O'Neill, E. and Sherman, A. (1994) Alcohol and drug treatment of homeless persons: results from the NIAAA Community Demonstration Program. *Journal of Health Care for the Poor and Underserved*, 5, 326–352.

Osher, F.C. and Kofoed, L.L. (1989) Treatment of patients with psychiatric and psychoactive substance abuse disorders. *Hospital and Community Psychiatry*, 40, 1025–1030.

Penfold, F. (1999) Dual diagnosis within mental health. Abstract describing a programme funded by the NHS Executive. http://www.doh.gov.uk/swro/proj209. htm.

Rahav, M., Rivera, J.J., Nuttbrock, L., Ng-Mak, D., Sturz, E., Link, B., Struening, E., Pepper, B. and Gross, G. (1995) Characteristics and treatment of homeless, mentally ill chemical-abusing men. *Journal of Psychoactive Drugs*, 21, 93–103.

Regier, D.A., Farmer, M.E., Rae, D.S., Locke, B.Z., Keith, S.J., Judd, L.L. and Goodwin, F.K. (1990) Comorbidity of mental disorders with alcohol and other drug abuse: results from the Epidemiologic Catchment Area (ECA) study. *Journal of the American Medical Association*, 264, 2511–2518.

Ridgely, M.S. (1991).Creating integrated programs for severely mentally ill persons with substance use disorders. In: Drake, R.E. and Minkoff, K. (eds), *New Directions for Mental Health Services 50: Dual Diagnosis of Major Mental Illness and Substance Disorder*. San Francisco: Jossey-Bass Publishers, pp. 29–41.

Ridgely, M.S. and Jerrell, J.M. (1996) Analysis of three interventions for substance abuse treatment of severely mentally ill people. *Community Mental Health Journal*, 32, 561–572.

Ridgely, M.S. and Willenbring, M. (1992) Application of case management to drug abuse treatment. In: Sager, R. (ed.), *Progress and Issues in Case Management*. Washington, DC: NIDA Research Monograph, US Government Printing Office, pp.12–33.

Ridgely, M.S., Goldman, H.H. and Talbott, J.A. (1986) *Chronically Mentally Ill Young Adults with Substance Abuse Problems: A Review of the Literature and Creation of a Research Agenda*. Baltimore, MD: University of Maryland, Department of Psychiatry, Mental Health Policy Studies Program.

Ridgely, M.S., Osher, F.C. and Talbott, J.A. (1987) *Chronically Mentally Ill Young Adults with Substance Abuse Problems: Treatment and Training Issues*. Baltimore, MD: University of Maryland, Department of Psychiatry, Mental Health Policy Studies Program.

Ridgely, M.S., Goldman, H.H. and Willenbring, M. (1990) Barriers to the care of persons with dual diagnoses: organizational and financing issues. *Schizophrenia Bulletin*, 16, 123–132

Ridgely, M.S., Morrissey, J.P., Paulson, R.I., Goldman, H.H. and Calloway, M.O. (1996) Characteristics and activities of case managers in the RWJ Foundation Program on Chronic Mental Illness. *Psychiatric Services*, 47, 737–743.

Ries, R.K. and Dyck, D.G. (1997) Representative payee practices of community mental health centers in Washington State. *Psychiatric Services*, 48, 811–814.

Rossi, P. and Freeman, H. (1993). *Evaluation: A Systematic Approach*. Newbury Park, CA: Sage, pp. 187–191.

Sacks, S., Sacks, J., DeLeon, G., Bernhardt, A.I. and Staines, G.L. (1997) Modified therapeutic community for mentally ill chemical abusers: background; influences; program description; preliminary findings. *Substance Use and Misuse*, 32, 1217–1259.

Safer, D.J. (1987) Substance abuse by young adult chronic patients. *Hospital and Community Psychiatry*, 38, 511–514.

Sainsbury Centre (1998) *Keys to Engagement*. London: Sainsbury Centre for Mental Health.

Sanford, T. (1995) Drug use is increasing. *Nursing Standard*, 9, 16–17.

Shapiro, S., Skinner, E.A., Kessler, L.G., Von Korff, M., German, P., Tischler, G.L., Leaf, P.J., Benham, L., Cottler, L. and Regier, D.A. (1984) Utilization of health and mental health services: three Epidemiologic Catchment Area sites. *Archives of General Psychiatry*, 41, 971–982.

Smith, J. and Hucker, S. (1993) Dual diagnosis patients: substance abuse by the severely mentally ill. *British Journal of Hospital Medicine*, 50, 650–654.

Smith, J. and Hucker, S. (1994) Schizophrenia and substance abuse. *British Journal of Psychiatry*, 165, 13–21.

Soyka, M. , Albus, M., Kathmann, M. *et al.* (1993) Prevalence of alcohol and drug abuse in schizophrenic in-patients. *European Archives of Psychiatry and Clinical Neurosciences*, 242, 362–372.

Steadman, H.J., Mulvey, E.P., Monahan, J., Robbins, P., Appelbaum, P., Grisso, T., Roth, L. and Silver, E. (1998) Violence by people discharged from acute psychiatric inpatient facilities and others in the same neighborhoods. *Archives of General Psychiatry*, 55, 393–401.

Test, M.A. (1991) The training in community living model: delivering treatment and rehabilitation through a CTT. In: Liberman, R. (ed.), *Handbook of Psychiatric Rehabilitation*. New York: Pergamon Press, pp. 153–170.

Verdoux, H., Mury, M., Besançon, G. and Bourgeois, M. (1996) Etude comparative des conduites toxicomaniaques dans les trouble bipolaires, schizophréniques et schizoaffectifs. *L'Encéphale*, 22, 95–101.

Weaver, T., Renton, R., Stimson, G. and Tyrer, P. (1999) Severe mental illness and substance misuse. 318, 137–138.

Wells, K.B., Hays, R.D., Burnam, M.A., Rogers, W., Greenfield, S. and Ware, J.E. (1989) Detection of depressive disorder for patients receiving prepaid or fee-for-service care: results from the Medical Outcomes Study. *Journal of the American Medical Association*, 262, 3298–3302.

Wells, K.B., Sturm, R., Sherbourne, C.D. and Meredith, L.S. (1996) *Caring for Depression*. Cambridge, MA: Harvard University Press.

Wuensch, St. (1998) Therapeutic interventions and course of treatment for patients wth psychosis and drug abuse. *International Journal of Mental Health*, 26, 83–90.

Ziedonis, D.M. and Fisher, W. (1994) Assessment and treatment of comorbid substance abuse individuals with schizophrenia. *Psychiatric Annals*, 24, 447–493.

31 | Psychotherapies

Jeremy Holmes

Psychotherapy and community psychiatry

Community psychiatry roots psychiatry in its historical, social and political context. Nowhere is this more evident than in the changing meanings of its key words and phrases. While community psychiatry's founding fathers can be traced back to the Quaker reformers of the early 19th century, the modern era as we know it in Britain began with the Northfield experiments towards the end of the second world war (Harrison, 1999). Here a group of psychiatrists, mostly psychoanalytically trained, disrupted the traditional medical and military hierarchy with the introduction of a more democratic, open organization of care for traumatized soldiers—mental illness was the enemy, and doctors and patients, officers and men, were to fight side by side to defeat it. While Northfield was short-lived, its intellectual impact was considerable, and many of its officers—Maxwell-Jones, Foulkes and Main—became associated in the post-war years with the development of therapeutic communities, run along Northfield lines.

In the 1950s, community psychiatry was synonymous with therapeutic community and, by implication, with psychotherapeutic as opposed to administrative or narrowly biomedical approaches to psychiatric treatment. The idea was to transform the anti-therapeutic mores of the mental hospital—sequestered, static, rigid—into a place where psychological growth and development could take place, and from which the mentally ill would eventually emerge once more to rejoin the wider community, free from stigma and constraint. The therapeutic community defined itself in opposition to the traditional mental hospital. Patients were to be encouraged to be active rather than passive: therapeutic work,

domestic self-sufficiency, and involvement of patients in the day to day practical and political running of the community were some of the means by which this was to be achieved. A collaborative atmosphere with more fluid boundaries between staff and patients was encouraged. Expression rather than suppression of feelings was valued, through the use of various forms of psychotherapy, especially creative therapies such as art therapy, music therapy and psychodrama. Above all a 'culture of enquiry' (Main, 1989) was fostered, in which the community itself became a 'living–learning' environment (Pullen, 1999), where, through large and small groups and individual therapy, patients came to understand themselves and their difficulties better.

At this stage then, psychotherapy and community psychiatry were inextricably linked. The leaders of the community psychiatry movement were mostly psychoanalytically trained. Psychotherapy and community psychiatry tended to be opposed to the use of medication in the management of mental illness, and both held to a utopian vision of care for the mentally ill transformed through the use of humane, psychotherapeutically informed communities, acting as models for the reform of other ossified social institutions. The predominant psychotherapeutic ideology was psychodynamic, 'behaviourism' being viewed with the same suspicion as psychotropic medication—as sinister means of social control rather than valid therapeutic tools.

Today, all this has changed. A complex set of social, political and technological forces—which include the advent of more effective psychotropic medication, the push to save money in public services and a general mistrust of institutions and the rise of individualism—has seen a recession of the therapeutic community movement, paralleling the decline of the mental hospital generally as a required antithesis to the therapeutic community. Today, rather than creating a 'good' alternative to the 'bad' traditional institution, community psychiatry tries to do away with the institution all together, basing itself in the 'natural' community—however fragmented—as opposed to the fragile artefact of the therapeutic community. Community psychiatry is psychiatry *in* the community as it exists, rather than an aspirational community *of* psychiatry and its patients. While there have been great gains in this change, there have also, I shall argue, been substantial losses, one of which has been the disengagement of psychotherapy and community psychiatry, to the detriment of both.

Nevertheless, aspects of therapeutic community ideology continue to inform community psychiatry practice. Patient autonomy and activity is inherent in the attempt to help the mentally ill live independent lives in the community. There is a strong emphasis on destigmatization. Mental health professionals and patients aspire to a collaborative relationship rather than one based on privilege and hierarchy. On the other hand, with the loss of the community as a container for disturbance and difficulty, there is a greater reliance on medication and a move to a functionalist approach in which risk assessment and control take precedence over the expressive slant and the search for meaning which characterized the therapeutic community. Despite its opposition to the traditional mental hospital, contemporary community psychiatry is more firmly based on a 'medical model' than the therapeutic community which, with its psychoanalytical roots, tended to see mental disorders from a developmental rather than illness perspective.

In parallel with this evolution of community psychiatry, and subject to similar social and economic forces, psychotherapy has over the past half century also undergone a quiet revolution in its meanings and practice. Psychological therapy can no longer be equated exclusively with psychoanalysis. A substantial research literature establishing the efficacy of psychotherapy now exists (Roth and Fonagy, 1996). A pluralistic discipline is emerging in which cognitive behavioural therapies, systemic and family treatments, psycho-analytical psychotherapy, and a number of eclectic therapies drawing on all three traditions, have emerged in response to the demand for targeted, evidence-based, replicable psychological treatments that meet the need of the wide variety of psychiatric difficulties which present themselves to mental health services. These developments have taken place within the autonomous disciplines of psychotherapy and psychology, often somewhat separate from the mainstream of acute and community psychiatry.

From their earlier confluence, psychotherapy and community psychiatry have thus evolved along separate pathways. The purpose of this chapter is to look at ways in which they impact on one another and how more intimate relationships between them can begin to be forged. I start with some general remarks about points of divergence and overlap between psychotherapy and community psychiatry, go on to look at referral patterns, examine some of the evidence for the relevance of psychotherapeutic treatments in community psychiatry and, finally, consider administrative and managerial arrangements that exist, or might exist, between the two disciplines.

General considerations

Conceptual space

Firstly, the terms community psychiatry and psychotherapy occupy rather different conceptual space. Community psychiatry currently defines itself as a mode of delivery of psychiatric services. As the editors of this volume put it: "the central emphasis is upon the *delivery* of psychiatric services in ways which are oriented towards local communities" (my italics). Psychotherapy, in contrast, is a mode of treatment, part of the psychiatric treatment triad whose other members are psychopharmacology and social engineering. Psychotherapy concerns itself primarily with *what* is delivered, community psychiatry with *where* and *how* that delivery takes place.

Location of treatment

Two significant aspects flow from this, one practical the other theoretical. At a practical level, psychotherapy traditionally is office based, while much of community psychiatry takes place in patients' homes, or in locations such as drop-in centres, day centres and so on. Delivering psychotherapy in the community can entail considerable modifications in standard technique. It is one thing to undertake a family therapy session in an out-patient department, with all the paraphernalia of one-way screen, video camera and a supporting team to guide the therapist. It is quite another to go into the patient's home and contend with the TV, the family dog and the boiling kettle and to remain true to the therapeutic task.

At a deeper level, psychodynamic understanding would suggest that the location of treatment may have a profound influence on the meaning and impact of therapeutic interventions. Meeting in the patient's home may help with engagement and to enhance the therapist's awareness of the psychosocial context, but equally can reduce the impact of therapeutic interventions, reinforcing the temptation to turn therapy into cosy chats, and diminishing the opportunities for focused containment and challenge. There are of course important differences between different therapeutic modalities here—to oversimplify, analytic therapists expect the patient to come to the therapist, whereas in more cognitive behavioural orientations, the therapist is more prepared to go out to meet the patient.

Behaviour therapists have always had a community orientation, and are familiar with accompanying their agoraphobic patients into supermarkets, visiting graveyards of loved ones during guided grief therapy, or setting up home-based response-prevention programmes in cases of obsessive–compulsive disorder (OCD). In contrast, psychoanalytic psychotherapy, whether individual, group or in a therapeutic community, emphasizes the importance of firm boundaries, and the need to offer the patient uninterrupted time and space, providing a holding environment—or secure base—within which painful emotions can be safely explored, all of which are achieved more easily within the relative anonymity and neutrality of an office than in the patient's home. Therapeutic reticence is essentially a technical procedure designed to maximize patient projection and transference, and to foster appropriate regression. If the therapist is too 'real' or transparent—although too much rigidity and opacity can also be counter-therapeutic—as inevitably is the case in home-based treatments, this process may be impeded, thereby subverting a vital part of standard psychoanalytical techniques.

Change versus support

A related point, and one where community psychiatry and psychotherapy are potentially at variance, concerns the question of change versus support as aims of intervention. Analytic therapists justify office-based practice on the grounds that it is a test of the patient's motivation for change; going out to the patient can be a recipe for collusion and supporting the status quo, and can undermine autonomy. In general, the aims of psychotherapy are to produce significant behavioural and intrapsychic change, and the justification for the intensity and relatively high costs of some psychotherapeutic interventions lies in their potential for a radical alteration in the quality of life and pattern of service utilization of its subjects. Cost–benefit studies of psychotherapy are still in their infancy, but what evidence there is does seem to suggest that the high costs of psychotherapy are indeed offset by improved clinical outcomes and diminished dependency on services as compared with 'standard care', which usually represents a version of community psychiatry (see below, Chisholm, 1998). Supportive psychotherapy has an important place in community psychiatry—indeed most non-pharmacological interventions in community psychiatry could come under that heading—but needs to be differentiated from formal psychotherapeutic modalities of treatment which are the core contribution of psychotherapy.

Balance between individual need and population need

Medical practice can be characterized as guided by either public health or physician–patient ideologies. Community psychiatry lies at the public health end of the spectrum, and expects to deploy resources in ways that equitably benefit the population as a whole, including groups traditionally excluded—whether by gender, class, educational level, language or ethnicity. Psychotherapy traditionally has occupied the opposite end of the polarity, offering total commitment and high levels of intensity to help the individual patient as she or he presents, but paying little heed to those unable or unwilling to come forward for help, however deserving they may be. Practical consequences flow from this dichotomy. There is a dose–effect relationship in psychotherapy, and on the whole the longer the treatment the greater the benefit, although this effect does attenuate after around 40 sessions (Orlinsky *et al.*, 1994). Psychotherapy departments agonize therefore about getting the right balance between providing brief therapy for the many, with the possibility of relapse, and more prolonged and intense treatments for the few, with the inevitable accumulation of waiting lists and unmet need.

A further point concerns the so-called 'YAVIS' problem in psychotherapy—the tendency for 'young, attractive, verbal, intelligent and successful' individuals to be over-represented among those referred for therapy, and apparently to benefit from it, compared with the less well educated, those with lower levels of achievement or attainment, and those from ethnic minorities. At worst, this is a characature and slur on psychotherapy—standard fare in most British departments are highly disturbed, ill, borderline individuals who are often the victims of multiple disadvantage and abuse. Nevertheless psychotherapy outreach is in its infancy, and targeted psychotherapy programmes for the disadvantaged or for ethnic minorities are relatively rare, and in general have not yet been well evaluated (Sue *et al.*, 1994).

Efficacy and effectiveness

All medical practice is underpinned by some sort of belief system or ideology, and this is perhaps particularly true of psychiatry. The traditional mental hospital relied on tradition, medical authority and charismatic leadership to justify many of its practices. Contemporary community psychiatry subjects its beliefs to the scrutiny of research and evaluation, and aspires to 'evidence-based practice'. If psychotherapy is to make a significant contribution to the work of the community psychiatry team, it too must be shown to be efficacious. Here the distinction between efficacy, i.e. whether a particular treatment can be shown to work in a research setting, and effectiveness, i.e. whether it works in the reality of day to day clinical practice, is a key issue. Narrowing the gap between research and practice is essential if psychotherapy is to play a major role in the practice of community psychiatry. As we shall see, many of the conditions with which community psychiatry concerns itself have proved themselves susceptible to psychological therapies, but these need to be delivered by trained skilful therapists, and to be tailored to the particular difficulties and diagnosis of the patient. Many community psychiatry workers see themselves as offering psychotherapy to their clients, but this is often unsystematic, unevaluated, unsupervized, unsustained or overextended, and may bear little relationship to psychotherapy as defined in research protocols. Finding systematic administrative and educational ways in which to translate 'laboratory' findings about psychotherapy into clinic practice—of moving from efficacy to effectiveness—is a major challenge for both disciplines.

Cost-effectiveness

The egalitarian thrust of community psychiatry means that resources should be used wisely for the benefit of all sufferers of mental illness. Psychotherapy services are comparatively expensive: a course of cognitive therapy for depression, for example, is several fold more costly than the prescription of tricyclic antidepressants. If psychotherapy is to justify its presence within the spectrum of community psychiatry services, it must be demonstrably cost-effective. Recent health economic studies of psychotherapy suggest that it represents good value for money. Comparing psychotherapy with 'standard care' (i.e. community keyworking, drug prescription and in-patient care when needed) in schizophrenia, depression, bipolar disorder and antisocial personality disorder, the overall cost of therapy was no greater than standard care, due to greatly reduced service utilization in the treatment groups who consumed fewer psychotropic drugs, consulted their GPs less often, had fewer days in hospital and reduced their dependency on benefits (Chisholm, 1998). Since clinical outcome in patients receiving therapy was much better than for those getting standard care, this constitutes a powerful argument for its cost-effectiveness. Unfortunately, this only applies when a comprehensive view of costing is taken—psychotherapy departments remain vulnerable at times of economic stringency. For this to be resisted, there has to be a political and ideological commitment on the part of politicians and health administrators—and community psychiatrists—to psychological therapies, comparable with the fervour shown by pharmaceutical companies in championing their products.

Education and training

Psychotherapy currently is practised by four types of practitioners within the mental health system: medical psychotherapists, i.e. psychiatrists who have undergone specialist training in psychotherapy, predominantly analytic, but increasingly cognitive behavioural and systemic; clinical psychologists who, in addition to basic training, may have specialized in a particular psychotherapeutic modality, often cognitive behavioural; generic mental health workers such as psychiatrists and community nurses who offer supportive psychotherapy as part of their routine practice; and non-medical (formerly 'lay') psychotherapists for whom psychotherapy is a primary profession, and who have done specific training in psychotherapy in a university (e.g. in Art Therapy) or private institution such as the Institute of Group Analysis.

The varying contributions of the different professions was clarified in a recent British government report which distinguished between three types of psychotherapy practice (NHS Executive, 1996): 'Type A', psychotherapy as part of a package of therapeutic measures, often delivered by generic workers; 'Type B', client-focused therapy in which the therapist, usually a psychologist, draws eclectically on a number of different models, tailoring them to the client's requirements; and 'Type C', formal psychotherapy practised according to standard models, and often practised in psychotherapy departments or psychological treatment units, often headed by a medical psychotherapist. The psychotherapy department has a responsibility for ensuring good integration and collaboration between this variety of psychotherapy practitioners, and to provide appropriate training to help interested community psychiatry workers improve their skills.

Patterns of referral

If psychological therapies are integral to the practice ot community psychiatry, where, in what 'dose', by whom and at which level of the community psychiatry system should they be delivered? These are easy questions to pose, but evidence-based solutions are harder to come by.

Psychological therapies in primary care

As in much of medicine, the principle of triage provides a good basis for deciding how resources (always insufficient) should be allocated. In general, it seems sensible for people with circumscribed, well-defined psychological difficulties of relatively short duration to be treated within the primary care setting. At the other end of the severity spectrum, those with long-term relatively static illnesses who have reached maximal levels of functioning can also often be well contained at the primary care level. Primary care physicians themselves provide much psychological support for their patients, and there is an established tradition of peer group supervision of this work, based on the work of the pioneering psychoanalyst

Michael Balint. Prevention is an important community psychiatry principle and much of the work of health visitors in helping with mother–infant bonding and monitoring childrens' emotional development comes into this category (Cicchetti *et al.*, 1999).

Psychological therapy in primary care generally is delivered either by practice counsellors or by attached workers from secondary care such as psychologists or community psychiatric nurses (CPNs). There has been much debate about the efficacy of counselling in general practice (e.g. King *et al.*, 1994). In general, it seems likely that non-specific 'Rogerian'-type counselling is likely to produce less benefit than structured, problem-solving therapies (Catalan *et al.*, 1991), although, as with all psychotherapy research, there may be a methodological bias in favour of those whose methods and goals are more easily defined, to the disadvantage of therapies whose value to the patient may be equal, or greater, but whose effects are more subtle and complex to measure. Many studies confirm that structured interventions can improve symptoms, lessen dependency on psychotropic medication and reduce consultation rates (e.g. Corney, 1990).

Referral 'on' from primary care rests mainly in the hands of the GP. In theory, she will choose those patients with more complex and/or risky problems and in whom there is a reasonable chance that more intensive psychological therapies will produce benefit. In practice, the decision to refer may be influenced by arbitrary factors such as the articulateness or pushiness of the patient, or 'compassion fatigue' on the part of the physician. Regular contact with members of the secondary care team—based for example around a lunchtime meeting with a Consultant Psychotherapist or Psychologist—may help foster more rational referral patterns.

Psychological therapies at the level of secondary care

The bulk of Type A, and much Type B therapy goes on in secondary care, mainly in community mental health centres (CMHCs), day hospitals and day centres, and to a lesser extent in acute in-patient facilities. Therapies offered usually include counselling, various forms of structured groups ranging from art or music therapy, anxiety management and self-esteem, gender-specific groups—for example for abuse survivors in women, and men with problems of aggression—and groups for carers of those suffering from long-term mental illness. In general, these therapies are carried out by members of the mental health team, often with a nursing or occupational therapy background. Only a minority will have undergone further psychotherapy training, and the quality and extent of supervision is variable. Mental health workers trained in specific therapies relevant to the needs of the long-term mentally ill such as nurses capable of delivering family interventions or cognitive therapy in schizophrenia remain relatively scarce (Brooker *et al.*, 1994).

Assessment at the point of entry to the community mental health team (CMHT) is usually carried out by senior members of the team, often in pairs. The decision to refer for specialist psychological therapies will usually be taken at that point. As with the visiting consultant in general practice, a close working relationship between the CMHT and the Psychological Therapy Unit (PTU) will facilitate smooth and appropriate referrals, especially if a member of the PTU spends defined sessions in the CMHT for assessment, case discussion and supervision.

Acute in-patient units are an integral part of community psychiatry: their functions include assessment, diagnosis, investigation, containment and respite. There is a movement towards greater traffic between community- and hospital-based mental health workers, but an unfortunate consequence of the success of community psychiatry has been a relative undervaluing of in-patient units, which at worst are barren uninviting unstimulating environments. Psychotherapy departments can play an important part in reversing this trend, with a revival of therapeutic community principles, especially the culture of enquiry which can emerge from a programme of regular groups for both patients and staff.

Access to specialist psychotherapy facilities

Some psychotherapy and psychology departments take referrals directly from primary care, others act as purely tertiary services and accept referrals only via CMHTs operating a 'single point of entry system'. Skilled assessment by a senior member of the PTU team is a key contribution to the workings of community psychiatry (Mace, 1995). While not all patients referred for psychotherapy prove suitable for Type B or C treatment, an assessment interview often can clarify and formulate patients' psychopathology in a way that will enable the keyworker or GP to continue working supportively with them.

A core contribution of the PTU to the work of the CMHT lies in taking on difficult cases requiring longer term intensive therapy delivered by therapists with special skills. Popular prejudice that PTUs 'cherry pick' less ill cases is not born out by research (Amies, 1996). In particular, PTUs have a key role in consultation with, and the assessment and treatment of patients suffering from severe personality disorder. This is an area of active research and development, and there is much debate about the most appropriate methods and delivery of treatment (see below).

Some severely ill patients may need further referral to supradistrict or supraregional units offering specialized in-patient or day-patient therapy for specific disorders such as severe OCD, sexual perversion, eating disorders, or borderline or dyssocial personality disorder. Here too the gate-keeping function is best held by the PTU which can offer the weight of specialist expertise behind requests for these comparatively costly, but increasingly validated specialized treatments (Gabbard, 1997).

Psychological therapies: the evidence base

There is an extensive literature on the efficacy of psychotherapy in the main psychiatric disorders (Roth and Fonagy, 1996). A comprehensive review would be out of place here, but I shall pick out some salient findings relevant to this chapter's theme.

Psychotherapy and schizophrenia

Contemporary community psychiatry stands or falls by its capacity to improve outcomes and patient and carer satisfaction in people suffering from schizophrenia. Four main psychotherapeutic approaches have been studied: individual psychoanalytic therapy; family interventions; cognitive behavioural methods; and supportive therapy as part of early interventions programmes. In most studies, psychological treatments have been delivered in parallel with psychotropic medication.

Early work was bedevilled by lack of diagnostic precision, and the fact that psychoanalytic writers tend to use terms such as 'psychotic' much more loosely than psychiatrists. Pioneering work by Searles, Fromm-Reichman and Sullivan in the USA of psychoanalytic therapy with schizophrenia, while contributing to knowledge of its phenomenology, has been largely discredited (Goldstein, 1991). Drop-out rates tend to be high, and in some cases expressive therapy may lead to deterioration (Mueser and Berenbaum, 1990), presumably by exposing the patient to an atmosphere of high emotional intensity. Few, if any, psychotherapy departments nowadays would see psychoanalytic psychotherapy as the primary treatment of choice for patients suffering from an unequivocal diagnosis of schizophrenia, although modified psychoanalytic approaches may be due for a comeback (see Alanen, 1999), and short-lived psychotic episodes occur in borderline personality disorder, which, in contrast, is treated routinely in such departments. Personal therapy (Hogarty *et al.*, 1997) brings a psychoanalytic commitment to a long-term empathic relationship with the patient based on affect regulation, together with attention to drug compliance, crisis management and environmental stabilization.

There is an extensive literature documenting the effectiveness of various forms of family intervention in schizophrenia (Kuipers and Bebbington, 1988; Mari de Jesus and Steiner, 1994), with marked reductions in relapse rates and improved social functioning emerging in most studies in a variety of cultural and national settings. Such work, to be effective, is quite labour intensive: most programmes involved specially trained workers intervening over prolonged periods at frequent intervals. Non-compliance is fairly high, and not all families agree to enter treatment (Tarrier, 1991). However, Brooker *et al.* (1994) showed that a naturalistic design in which family interventions were delivered by nursing staff also produced significant benefit, suggesting that, given the will and leadership, this approach can be translated into routine clinical practice. Similar results are reported by Barrowclough *et al.* (1999).

Pioneering work in several UK centres has shown that cognitive behavioural therapy combined with psychotropic medication can reduce the intensity and distressing nature of positive symptoms, and relieve negative symptoms in chronic schizophrenia (Kuipers *et al.*, 1997; Tarrier *et al.*, 1998). Again, intensity is quite high—twice weekly sessions extending over a 6-month period delivered by psychologists with special training, but improvements are maintained at 1-year follow-up (Turkington and Siddle, 1998).

Evidence that family and cognitive behavioural interventions can play a significant part in improving the clinical course of schizophrenia presents a major challenge for the practice and organization of community psychiatry. The evidence suggests that research findings can be translated into routine clinical practice, but for this to happen appropriate training, supervision and clinical time need to be made available for mental health workers. Psychotherapy departments could play a major part in ensuring that these specialized psychological therapies are delivered and sustained, although so far this has not been part of their traditional role.

Several research studies have used a three-way design comparing active psychotherapeutic interventions, supportive counselling or befriending, and standard care (Tarrier *et al.*, 1999). Although specific therapy is clearly superior in most measures, supportive psychotherapy/befriending also tends to do well compared with routine care, suggesting that 'non-specific factors' are as important as the particular psychotherapeutic techniques used. Other studies also suggest that a long-term sustained relationship with a therapist or keyworker can help to stabilize the illness and may improve outcomes. Early intervention programmes in psychosis which contain a significant psychotherapeutic component sustained over time show promise in reducing distress and time spent in hospital (Martindale *et al.*, 1999). There are significant national differences in the extent to which psychotherapeutic resources are available for the treatment of schizophrenia. Here the UK, while at the leading edge in research, tends to lag behind when it comes to offering psychotherapeutic programmes as part of everyday community psychiatry practice, with Scandinavian countries especially advanced in this respect (Alanen *et al.*, 1999). Enhanced investment in psychotherapy departments as part of a comprehensive community psychiatry service might go some way towards redressing this.

Affective disorders

There is a substantial literature on the impact of various forms of psychotherapy in depression. Cognitive behavioural therapy (CBT) (Hollon *et al.*, 1992), interpersonal therapy (IPT) (Elkin, 1994), marital therapy (Leff *et al.*, 1999) and brief dynamic psychotherapy (Shapiro *et al.*, 1995) have all been shown to produce significant benefit—with effects at least as powerful as antidepressant medication. IPT and CBT have been shown to be helpful in relapse prevention, with 'sleeper' effects even after therapy has come to an end (Kupfer *et al.*, 1992). Medication is of course easier and cheaper to prescribe than psychotherapy. Psychotherapeutic treatments tend to be reserved for patients who fail to respond to, or comply with, antidepressants, or where there are significant personality factors which have been shown to confound the response to medication. Such patients, however, form the bulk of those referred for secondary care in community psychiatry, and here too, as with schizophrenia, there is a significant gap between research findings and routine clinical practice. For example, Scott (1992) pioneered a modified CBT package combined with medication for patients suffering from severe and chronic depression, such as might be referred to a CMHT, comparing this with standard CBT. Although the numbers were small, she found that such 'tailored' treatment produced significantly better outcomes, suggesting that effective interventions for patients suffering with depression need well-trained and supervised therapists, a situation honoured more in the breach than the observance.

Studies of psychotherapeutic approaches to patients suffering from bipolar disorders are sparse. Again, Scott (1995) has shown that a CBT approach can improve psychological adjustment and compliance with mood-stabilizing drugs, and Clarkin *et al.* (1990) in an exploratory study showed that family intervention improved functioning and reduced hospital admissions in females, but not males, as compared with a group receiving standard care. The significance and clinical implications of this gender difference are unclear.

Personality disorder

Patients with severe personality disorder (SPD; a poor prognosis group which draw largely from Cluster B in DSM-IV) provide a powerful test of the concepts and practices of contemporary community psychiatry. SPD impacts adversely on the prognosis of co-morbid conditions such as depression (Shea *et al.*, 1992); these patients have a high incidence of deliberate self-harm (DSH), substance abuse, eating disorders and forensic difficulties (Zimmerman and Coryel, 1990); they form a significant proportion of psychiatric in-patients; and their 'burden' is felt by community mental health workers to an extent disproportionate to their numbers (Montgomery and Holmes, 2000). The majority of SPD sufferers have experienced sexual, physical or emotional trauma and/or neglect in childhood; they tend to impact on multiple agencies, fail to fit neatly into the care programme approach and create professional chaos despair and rage in ways which mirror the state of their inner world.

A key issue concerns the 'treatability' or otherwise of this very heterogeneous group of patients.

Good evidence about effective therapeutic strategies is sparse, and the methodological problems of such research are formidable (Bateman and Fonagy, 2000). An uncontrolled study showed good results with a year of twice weekly analytic psychotherapy (Stevenson and Meares, 1992). In one of the few randoized controlled trials, Linehan (Linehan *et al.*, 1993), using dialectical behaviour therapy (DBT; an eclectic therapy drawing on CBT and Zen Buddhism) showed that a three times a week therapy that included weekly individual and group sessions and telephone contact extended over the course of a year reduced hospital admission and episodes of DSH in the treatment group compared with controls. A year of therapy at the Henderson Hospital (an in-patient therapeutic community dedicated to the treatment of Cluster B patients) reduced the number of personality disorders in the treatment group compared with controls (Dolan *et al.*, 1997). A recent randomized controlled trial in a psychotherapeutic day hospital showed reductions in BDI scores, episodes of DSH and hospital admissions in the treatment group (Bateman and Fonagy, 1999).

Successful treatment strategies with these patients combine a coherent therapeutic philosophy, good supervision and support for the therapists, firm boundaries and realistic expectations of outcome (Bateman and Fonagy, 2000). These objectives are not easy to achieve in the dispersed arrangements which often characterize community psychiatry. Containment of anxiety is a crucial aspect of the management of patients with SPD, and this can only be done effectively on a collective rather than an individual basis. Institutions, for all their faults, provided a 'secure base' for patients and mental health workers alike. On the other hand, prolonged in-patient treatment of these patients is often problematic and can lead to regression, staff splitting and poor outcomes (Holmes, 1999). Psychotherapeutic day hospitals, or an out-patient dedicated personality disorder service with highly motivated and trained staff, can provide a containing function, although its effectiveness in routine clinical practice has yet to be demonstrated. Awareness of the difficult interpersonal dynamics characteristic of these patients, and knowledge of ways to contain the anxiety they inevitably create, can be a key contribution of a psychotherapy unit.

Conclusions: the relationship between community psychiatry and a PTU

As argued at the outset of this chapter, the history of community psychiatry is one of movement from a passionate treatment philosophy centring on psychotherapeutic approaches, to a more ideologically neutral framework within which mental health services are delivered. While much has been gained in terms of equity of access, patient satisfaction and autonomy compared with institutional psychiatry, and the development of an evidence base for treatment, contemporary community psychiatry is problematic in may ways. The pressure on community staff is great, and staff burnout is common; the skill base of community workers is often not commensurate with expectations; the containment of anxiety, whether clinically or politically, is difficult; and there is a credibility gap between showcase highly resourced and researched models, and routine practice.

In all these areas, a PTU or Psychotherapy Department can play a significant part. It can offer staff support, supervision to CMHTs and in-patient wards, and act as a tertiary resource for the treatment of difficult cases. It has an important role in staff training in psychological treatments for patients with severe mental disorders, for example CBT techniques in psychosis. It can take a lead in the provision of services for special groups of patients such as those with eating disorders or SPD. To do this, it needs to retain its own separate identity within the mental health service, while at the same time working closely with community psychiatry facilities. This 'hub and spokes' arrangement avoids the danger of a sequestered isolationist posture for psychotherapy, while enabling it to retain its unique identity and core values (Holmes, 1998).

Throughout this chapter, I have suggested that without a substantial psychotherapy contribution, community psychiatry as a universal model for delivery of mental health services struggles to realize many of its aspirations, and to sustain them over time. Contemporary community psychiatry grew out of therapeutic communities, which in turn were the brain child of psychotherapy; there is now an urgent need to reintegrate these two strands. For this to happen, psychotherapy will have to abandon many of its traditional assumptions and practices. It will have to be prepared to work with difficult patients with major psychiatric diagnoses, and models of therapy will have to be modified to meet the needs of these patients. Staff support and training will have to become a top priority. Psychotherapy will have to become more eclectic, more multi-disciplinary, and to find ways of working with hitherto excluded groups. At the same time, community psychiatry will need to recognize the importance of psychological therapy skills as part of routine work, and to find ways of translating the neglected values of therapeutic community into contemporary practice.

References

Alanen, Y. (1999) The Finnish model for the treatment of schizophrenia and related psychoses. In: Martindale, B. *et al.* (eds), *Outcome Studies of Psychological Treatments of Psychotic Conditions.* London: Gaskell, pp. 76–77.

Amies, P. (1996) Psychotherapy patients: are they the 'worried well'? *Psychiatric Bulletin*, 20, 153–156.

Barrowclough, C., Tarrier, N., Lewis, S. *et al.* (1999) Randomised controlled effectiveness trial of a needs-based psychosocial intervention service for carers of people with schizophrenia. *British Journal of Psychiatry*, 174, 505–511.

Bateman, A. and Fonagy, P. (1999) The effectiveness of partial hospitalisation in the treatment of borderline personality disorder—a randomized controlled trial. *American Journal of Psychiatry*, 156, 1563–1569.

Bateman, A. and Fonagy, P. (2000) The effectiveness of psychotherapeutic treatment of personality disorder: a review. *British Journal of Psychiatry*, 177, 138–143.

Brooker, C., Falloon, I., Butterworth, A. *et al.* (1994) The outcome of training community psychiatric nurses to deliver psychosocial interventions. *British Journal of Psychiatry*, 165, 222–230.

Catalan, J., Gath, D. Anastasiades, P. *et al.* (1991) Evaluation of a brief psychological treatment for emotional disorders in primary care. *Psychological Medicine*, 21, 1013–1018.

Chicchetti, D., Toth, S. and Rososch, F. (1999) The efficacy of toddler–parent psychotherapy to increase attachment security in offspring of depressed mothers. *Attachment and Human Development*, 1, 34–66.

Chisholm, D. (1998) Costs and outcomes of the psychotherapeutic approaches to the treatment of mental disorders. *Mental Health Research Review*, 5, 53–55.

Clarkin, J., Glick, I., Haas, G. *et al.* (1990) A randomized clinical trial of inpatient family intervention. *Journal of Affective Disorders*, 18, 17–28.

Corney R. (1990) Counselling in general practice: does it work? *Journal of the Royal Society of Medicine*, 83, 253–257.

Dolan, B., Warren, F. and Norton, K. (1997) Change in borderline symptoms one year after therapeutic community treatment for severe personality disorder. *British Journal of Psychiatry*, 171, 272–279.

Elkin, I. (1994) The NIMH treatment of depression collaborative research programme: where we began and where we are. In: Bergin, A. and Garfield, S. (eds), *Handbook of Psychotherapy and Behaviour Change*, 4th edn. Chichester: Wiley, p. 201.

Gabbard, G. (1997) Borderline personality disorder and rational managed care policy. *Psychoanalytic Inquiry*, 27, 17–28.

Goldstein, M. (1991) Psychosocial (nonpharmacological) treatments for schizophrenia. *Review of Psychiatry*, 10, 116–135.

Harrison, T. (1999) A momentous experiment: strange meetings at Norfield. In: Haig R. and Campling, P. (eds), *Therapeutic Communities: Past, Present and Future*. London: Jessica Kingsley, p. 56.

Hogarty, G., Kornblith, S., Greenwald, D., DiBarry, SA., Ulrich, R., Carter, M. and Flesher, S. (1997) Three-year trials of personal therapy among schizophrenic patients living with or independent of family, 1: description of study and effects on relapse rates. *American Journal of Psychiatry*, 54, 1504–1513.

Hollon, S., Durubeis, R., Evans, M. *et al.* (1992) Cognitive therapy and pharmacotherapy for depression: singly or in combination? *Archives of General Psychiatry*, 49, 774–781.

Holmes, J. (1998) The psychotherapy department and the community mental health team. *Psychiatric Bulletin*, 22, 54–58.

Holmes, J. (1999) Psychodynamic approaches to the management and treatment of severe personality disorder in general psychiatric settings. *CPD Psychiatry*, 1, 53–67.

King, M., Broster, G., Lloyd, M. *et al.* (1994) Controlled trials in the evaluation of counselling in general practice. *British Journal of General Practice*, 44, 229–232.

Kuipers, L. and Bebbington. P. (1988) Expressed emotion research in schizophrenia: theoretical and clinical implications. *Psychological Medicine*, 18, 893–909.

Kuipers, E., Garety, P., Fowler, D. *et al.* (1997) The London–East Anglia randomized controlled trial of cognitive behavioural therapy for psychoses. *British Journal of Psychiatry*, 171, 319–327.

Kupfer, D., Frank, E., Perel, J. *et al.* (1992) Five year outcome for maintenance therapies in recurrent depression. *Archives of General Psychiatry*, 49, 769–773.

Leff, J., Verneals, S., Brewin, C. *et al.* (2000) The London depression intervention trial: an RCT of anti-depressants versus couple therapy in the treatment and maintenance of depressed people with a partner: clinical outcome and costs. *British Journal of Psychiatry*, 177, 95–100.

Linehan, M., Heard, H. and Armstrong, H. (1993) Naturalistic follow-up of a behavioural treatment for chronically parasuicidal borderline patients. *Archives of General Psychiatry*, 50, 971–974.

Mace, C. (1995) (ed.) *The Art and Science of Psychotherapy Assessment*. London: Routledge.

Main, T. (1989) *The Ailment and Other Essays*. London: Free Association.

Mari de Jesus, J. and Strainer, J. (1994) An overview of family interventions and relapse in schizophrenia: meta-analysis of research findings. *Psychological Medicine*, 24, 565–578.

Martindale, B., Margison, F. and Bateman, A. (eds) (1999) *Outcome Studies of Psychological Treatments of Psychotic Conditions*. London: Gaskell.

Montgommery, C., Holmes, J. and Lloyd, K. (2000) The burden of personality disorder: a district based survey. *International Journal of Social Psychiatry*, 46, 164–169.

Mueser, K. and Berenbaum, H. (1990) Psychodynamic treatment of schizophrenia; is there a future? *Psychological Medicine*, 20, 253–262.

NHSE (1996) *NHS Psychotherapy Services in England*. London: HMSO.

Orlinsky, D., Grawe, K. and Parks, B. (1994) Process and outcome in psychotherapy—noch einmal. In: Bergin, A. and Garfield, S. (eds), *Handbook of Psychotherapy and Behaviour Change*, 4th edn. Chichester: Wiley, pp. 98–130.

Pullen, G. (1999) Schizophrenia: hospital communities for the severely disturbed. In: Haig, R. and Campling, P. (eds), *Therapeutic Communities: Past, Present and Future*. London: Jessica Kingsley, pp. 47–61.

Roth, A. and Fonagy, P. (1996) *What Works for Whom?* London: Guilford.

Scott, J. (1992) Chronic depression: can cognitive therapy succeed when other treatments fail? *Behavioural Psychotherapy*, 20, 25–36.

Scott, J. (1995) Psychotherapy for bipolar disorder: an unmet need? *British Journal of Psychiatry*, 167, 581–588.

Shapiro, D., Rees, A., Barkham, M. *et al.* (1995) Effect of treatment duration and severity of depression on the maintenance of gains following cognitive behavioural and psychodynamic interpersonal psychotherapy. *Journal of Counselling and Clinical Psychology*, 63, 378–387.

Shea, M., Pilkonis, P., Beckham, E. *et al.* (1992) Personality disorders and treatment of depression collaborative programme. *American Journal of Psychiatry*, 147, 711–718.

Stevenson, J. and Meares, R. (1992) An outcome study for patients with borderline personality disorder. *American Journal of Psychiatry*, 149, 358–362.

Sue, S., Zane, N. and Young, K. (1994) Research on psychotherapy with culturally diverse populations. In: Bergin, A. and Garfield, S. (eds), *Handbook of Psychotherapy and Behaviour Change*, 4th edn. Chichester: Wiley, pp. 396–429.

Tarrier, N. (1991) Some aspects of family intervention programmes in schizophrenia. 1: adherence to intervention programmes. *British Journal of Psychiatry*, 159, 475–480.

Tarrier, N. Tusupoff, L., Kinney, E.. *et al.* (1998) A randomised controlled trial of intensive cognitive behavioural therapy for chronic schizophrenia. *British Medical Journal*, 317, 3030–307.

Tarrier, N.. Wittkowski, C., Kinney, E. *et al.* (1999) Durability of the effects of cognitive-behavioural therapy in the treatment of chronic schizophrenia: 12 month follow-up. *British Journal of Psychiatry*, 174, 500–504.

Turkington, D. and Siddle, P (1998) Cognitive behavioural therapy in the treatment of schizophrenia. *Advances in Psychiatric Treatment*, 4, 242–254.

Zimmerman, M. and Coryell, W. (1990) Diagnosing personality disorders within the community: comparison of self-report and interview measures. *Archives of General Psychiatry*, 47, 527–538.

32 | Services for older adults

Sube Banerjee

Introduction

It can be argued that some of the most coherent examples of community psychiatry are to be found in the practice of old age psychiatry. As a discipline, it defined itself from the first as having a primary community focus, insisting on the importance of home-based assessment and care (Arie and Issacs, 1978). More recently, the World Health Organization (WHO) consensus statement on psychiatry for the elderly has affirmed that assessments should be carried out in the patient's home (Wertheimer, 1997). Unlike many principles, these appear to be the reality of clinical practice in old age psychiatry, with nine out of 10 referrals seen at home rather than in out-patient clinics (Wattis *et al.*, 1981).

Old age psychiatry has developed from un-differentiated adult psychiatry and to an extent in reaction to general psychiatry's former asylum and in-patient focus. Old age psychiatry is a young speciality and was designed *a priori* to be patient and community centred rather than hospital based. However, its development and differentiation have been based not only on ideology and the specific unmet needs of the elderly (Lewis, 1946), but also on a practical need to overcome institutional age-related prejudice within psychiatry (Murphy and Banerjee, 1993).

From the very beginnings of old age psychiatry, the special needs of the elderly, including a pattern of multiple pathology and complex co-morbidity of physical and mental health with social care needs, were identified as requiring multi-disciplinary working and effective joint working with carers, primary health care, geriatric medicine and social services (Arie, 1971; Royal College of Psychiatrists and British Geriatric Society, 1979; Wertheimer, 1997). Wider health and social care policy imperatives have worked with these ideological and patient-based reasons for the development of specific services for the elderly.

Worldwide population ageing has generated concerns about the economic ability of social systems and health care services to meet the needs of the elderly (Organisation for Economic Co-operation and Development, 1988; WHO, 1991). This is as active an issue in the developing world, where countries are projected to experience a massive increase in the numbers of older people both in relative and absolute terms (Kalache, 1991; Prince, 1997), as it is in the more developed world. The demographic projections in the UK, as in much of the developed world, are for an increase in the oldest old (those over 75 years and those over 85 years) who have the highest levels of physical and psychiatric morbidity and therefore the greatest need. Particular concern has been focused in the developed world on the funding of long-term care for the elderly, with dementia being a major determinant of need for this type of care. In the UK, around 3.6% of gross domestic product is spent on long-term care at present (Bone, 1995), with some projecting that this may need to rise to 10.8% in the next 30 years (Nuttall *et al.*, 1994).

In terms of service activity in psychiatry, older people are an important group. People over the age of 65 make up around a third of all mental health activity in the UK in terms of admissions, readmissions and community contacts (Philpot and Banerjee, 1998). However, the profile of disorder and needs does differ from that in younger age groups. The challenges presented by dementia and co-morbid physical illness and disability require particular professional skills and services need to be able to deal with the complex mix of social, psychological, physical and biological factors found in the elderly mentally ill.

Table 32.1 *Reifler's (1997) criteria for the development of old age psychiatry and services for the elderly mentally ill*

Stage	Development of old age psychiatry	Development of services for the elderly mentally ill
1	No formal criteria for designation of old age psychiatrists, self-designation	Only very basic services, usually in general psychiatric facilities
2	Certification process for old age psychiatry accepted by professional community	Separate/specialized programmes beginning to be established including long-term care and community-based projects
3	National need for old age psychiatrists established with mechanisms to accomplish this	Full range of long-term, hospital- and community-based programmes in many parts of the country
4	Full complement of accredited old age psychiatrists meeting the needs of the country	Entire spectrum of services for the elderly mentally ill exists throughout the country with access for all in need

International developments in old age psychiatry

As discussed above, old age psychiatry is a relatively young discipline but the needs of older people and demographic ageing are internationally pervasive. The international development of old age psychiatry has been rapid from its origins in the UK in the 1950s (Kay, 1999; Rabins, 1999). The International Psychogeriatric Association now has members in 55 countries. However, the stage of development of services for older adults varies markedly across the world. Reifler (1997) has developed a four-stage model for the development of old age psychiatry and services for the elderly mentally ill from a comparative observational study of services in Ireland, the UK and the USA, and has applied this in an international study (Reifler, 1998). These criteria are helpful in gauging the progress of services and are presented in Table 32.1.

In his initial study, Reifler (1997) contrasted the remuneration-dependent hospital- or physician's office-based practice of the USA with the community-based services and multi-disciplinary working observed in the UK. The differing methods of payment for consultants mean that there is no disincentive to holding multi-disciplinary team meetings and working in the community in the UK compared with the USA. In addition, the UK system allows for responsibility for a defined area to be vested in an individual team which is not the case in the USA. This may result in a more comprehensive knowledge of local resources and the ability to plan services rationally. He concluded that the major strength of the US system is the ability to set up high quality entrepreneurial programmes of care and that the main weakness is that there is no single body with responsibility for service planning and delivery, leading to unco-ordinated and uneven services. The UK's main strengths were the uniformity and comprehensiveness of the services provided, with the main weaknesses being in inadequate long-term care and overtaxed personnel. Using his scale, he rated the USA as being at stage 2 for development of the profession and stage 3 for services, while the UK was at stage 3 for both.

In a subsequent international survey (Reifler *et al.*, 1998), 12 countries met the minimum standard set of stage 2 for development of the profession and services (in rank order of scores: UK, USA, Finland, Canada, Sweden, Switzerland, Hong Kong, Australia, Germany, New Zealand, Israel and Norway), with a further six reaching this limit for service development alone (The Netherlands, Japan, Denmark, Italy, France and Korea). The authors concluded that there is reason for encouragement in much of the developed world but that much of the world, both developed and developing, appears unready to meet the challenge of mental health in the context of population ageing.

The precise nature of service delivery depends on the nature, level and organization of any area or country's health, social and welfare services, legislation and familial social structure. These necessarily vary from country to country and there is insufficient space in this chapter to present the organization and development of old age psychiatric services across the world. However, the needs of older people with mental health problems and the fundamental issues which determine service delivery are remarkably constant. For the remainder of this chapter, the main focus will therefore be on evidence derived from services in the UK. This should allow for a consideration of universal issues in community service provision even if filtered though the particular health and social constructs of the UK.

Service organization

The first comprehensive old age psychiatric service to be established was probably that working from Goodmayes Hospital in east London (Arie, 1970). The underpinning principles upon which this service was based included:

- ease of accessibility;
- flexibility;
- assessments being made at the patients home; and
- management of the patient in close co-operation with GPs and other interested parties.

This model of service, with its comprehensiveness and strong community focus, remains the basis for old age psychiatric services provided in the UK and, through the evangelism of Professor Tom Arie and his many trainees, in a large number of other countries.

It is UK policy that all areas should have a specialist old age psychiatry service, and data held by the Royal College of Psychiatrists' faculty of old age psychiatry suggest that this is now the case. These posts are also generally filled by doctors working full time in old age psychiatry rather than those whose time is split between old age and general psychiatry (Banerjee *et al.*, 1993). However, there remain posts which are poorly resourced with unsustainably large catchment areas and workloads (Jolley and Benbow, 1997). In 1996, 20% of old age psychiatric consultant posts in South London were either vacant or filled by a locum (Philpot and Banerjee, 1997). Recent Royal College of Psychiatrists' guidelines suggest that consultants should generally have a catchment area of around 10 000 people over the age of 65 years, a reduction from the previous recommendation of 22 000 (The Royal College of Psychiatrists, 1989, 1992). These norms appear to be based on 'contemporary standards of provision' rather than systematic needs assessment (Cooper, 1991).

Attempts have been made to develop algorithms which can be applied to the socio-demographic structure of a given area in order to generate an assessment of that population's need for services. These can now be based on increasingly definitive estimations of the age- and gender-specific prevalence and incidence rates of disorders and health conditions in a given population, such as dementia, depression and disability (e.g. Melzer *et al.*, 1997, 1999). One element that has hampered the implementation of such needs assessments has been the lack of consensus on the criteria for access to differing levels and types of care and therefore the proportion of cases of disorder requiring, for example, primary, secondary or long-term care.

Services necessarily vary in response to the organization and service provision of local authority social services and the voluntary and private sectors. While all will include community assessment and treatment and some form of day care, models of service delivery in community of age psychiatry vary markedly. There is, to date, a lack of comparative evaluation (in terms of effectiveness and cost) of these different models of care, but their existence presents opportunities for natural experiments to determine their relative effectiveness.

Community assessment and treatment in old age psychiatry

With the particular ideological and clinical spurs to development discussed above, old age psychiatry has developed some of the most comprehensive and innovative examples of true multidisciplinary working in the whole of psychiatry (Banerjee, 2000). These include the 'Guy's model' of open access generic team working (Coles *et al.*, 1991; Collighan *et al.*, 1993; Brown *et al.*, 1996). This model requires the development of shared generic skills in assessment and teamworking to complement specialist professional and personal skills. Some of the most contentious issues in old age psychiatric service provision are to be found in the way that community teams work, with open access to services and the role of the consultant in initial assessment particularly debated (Dening, 1992).

The degree of openness of access to community old age psychiatric services is subject to considerable variation. A closed system, with referrals made to the consultant and only accepted from GPs and other hospital consultants, may be particularly problematic for the elderly given their multiple service contacts, especially with social and voluntary services and residential care, and the important role of informal carers. Objections to opening out access come from old age psychiatrists and GPs. For old age psychiatrists, requiring that all referrals are channelled though patients' GPs may be seen as a way of managing demand for service and preventing inappropriate referrals. However, GPs may object to the diminution of their gate-keeper role and the potential for them to be unaware of clinically important interactions with mental health services. The introduction of financial implications to service activity is a further complication. There is little evidence with which to weigh these competing concerns, but Macdonald *et al.* (1994) evaluating the effect of establishing an entirely open referral system in Lewisham reported that this did not lead to services becoming overwhelmed or to inappropriate referrals.

The only team member common to in-patient and community old age psychiatric services is often the consultant. Community teams vary from those consisting only of community psychiatric nurses (CPNs) with other professional input by internal referral, to those including the full-time involvement of other professionals including social workers, occupational therapists, psychologists, physiotherapists, case managers and speech therapists (Rosenvinge, 1994; Wattis, 1994).

The traditional model of old age psychiatric service delivery combines first assessment either at home following a GP request for a consultant domicilary visit (DV) or, more rarely, in an out-patient clinic. Follow-up may then be by further consultant home visits, out-patient attendance or CPN follow-up. Out-patient assessment and follow-up may be a particularly problematic in elderly populations for reasons which include:

- it may be impossible to assess the patient's true level of functioning without seeing them in their own homes;

- the need to assess risk in the patient's own environment;

- the value of being able to inspect the home;

- difficulties or unwillingness of patients to attend clinics due to disability, cognitive impairment or lack of insight;

- transporting elderly people with dementia to unfamiliar surroundings may exacerbate disorientation and behavioural disturbance and so compromise the assessment;

- decreased access to information (e.g. medicine bottles and district nursing or social service notes) and informants such as neighbours.

For these reasons, many services have almost entirely done away with hospital-based, clinic- or GP practice-based out-patient assessment and follow-up, or reserve it for highly selected groups of patients.

The traditionalist view of initial assessment is that these should only be carried out by doctors. This is usually asserted on the basis of doctors being the only professional group with the requisite diagnostic skills, and GPs expecting and wanting a medical opinion. This is often supported by asking whether you would want your mother/grandmother to be assessed by a nurse or a doctor. The likelihood of this choice being in reality between a junior doctor with only a few months of appropriate experience or a CPN with years of work in the area is seldom developed adequately. There certainly does not appear to be any empirical evidence to support the view of the necessary primacy of doctors.

The activity of the team and outcome of patients treated by community teams using the 'Guy's model' have been evaluated in some detail (Brown *et al.*, 1996). The 'Guy's model' is based upon the premise that with appropriate induction, training and supervision, a team member of any professional background can make an accurate initial assessment which will allow for a diagnosis and management plan to be formulated by the multi-disciplinary team as a whole. This assumption has been the subject of careful research which demonstrates that non-doctor team members are as accurate as medical team members in assigning psychiatric diagnoses (Collighan *et al.*, 1993) and formulating treatment plans (Lindesay *et al.*, 1996) for those on whom they have completed new assessments. Experience in the specialty rather than professional background appears to be of most importance. This has led some to the conclusion that first assessments can be made safely and effectively by appropriately trained professionals other than doctors (Herzberg, 1995).

However the service is organized, treatment and monitoring are carried out predominantly in patients' homes, and countrywide this is carried out most commonly by CPNs (Wattis, 1994). Multi-disciplinary working is at the core of community old age psychiatry and is required by the complex interplay of physical, psychiatric, social and psychological factors (Rosenvinge, 1994). In addition, increasingly there is the need to take account of issues of culture and ethnicity (Rait and Burns, 1997; Silveira and Ebrahim, 1998).

One indication of the reality of community assessment in old age psychiatry is given by the finding that less than 5% of admissions to in-patient beds were completed without prior community assessment (Wattis *et al.*, 1981) and that two-thirds of new referrals to old age psychiatric services result in community treatment rather than admission (Wattis, 1988).

Unfortunately, there is little research investigating the individual or comparative efficacy, effectiveness or cost-effectiveness of differing models of community old age psychiatric service provision. Again the 'Guys model' is a partial exception in that there is evidence of its effectiveness in the treatment of depression in the frail elderly at home (Banerjee *et al.*, 1996). Of course this lack of evidence does not mean that other forms of service provision are not effective. However, old age psychiatric services increasingly require a firm evidence base to inform the decisions of service planners and funders in a competitive environment (Banerjee and Dickinson, 1997). There is therefore a clear need for research to evaluating the clinical and relative cost-effectiveness of differing models of service provision.

Dementia assessment and care

As might be expected, having dementia is strongly associated with use of community health and social services including old age psychiatry (Philp *et al.*, 1995). Around half of all referrals to old age psychiatric community services are of people with dementia, and they are more dependent and require greater levels of community services than other referrals (Bedford *et al.*, 1996). Dementia care is necessarily a co-operative venture between health and social services and informal carers. Community old age psychiatry is a small, but important, element of this. The services that a person with dementia and their carers receive vary greatly by geography and where one enters the system (Mountain, 1998). It has been argued that the most efficient way of addressing these inequalities in care would be for the establishment of a single dementia service pooling health and social care budgets and functions (Anderson, 1999). However, services at present rely on local service configuration and interagency working.

The interface between primary health care and old age psychiatric services with respect to people with dementia is clouded by the lack of generally agreed criteria for referral. This has resulted in a lack of clarity about what can and should be done by and in primary care, and what requires, and is the responsibility of, old age psychiatry (Downs, 1996). There is a need for locally agreed criteria and guidelines for the diagnosis and management of people which dementia, including information about non-medical resources (Glosser *et al.*, 1985). There is marked variation in GPs' skills in diagnosing and managing dementia (O'Connor *et al.*, 1988; Philp and Young, 1988). Without the identification of the dementia, it is difficult to instigate an appropriate management plan for the patient and his or her informal carers (O'Connor *et al.*, 1993). A further area of concern is the potentially inappropriate prescribing of sedative medication including antipsychotics to those in community and residential care with and without dementia which is associated with negative outcomes including increased cognitive decline (McShane *et al.*, 1997).

Those people with dementia referred to old age psychiatry include those where: the diagnosis is difficult; there is associated psychopathology such as depression or psychosis; there is dangerous or severely disturbed behaviour such as violence, wandering or sexual disinhibition; there is severe carer strain; and where other agencies such as social services have asked the GP to request an assessment for their own needs. Downs (1996) reviewing the role of the GP in dementia diagnosis and care stressed that dementia may not be a simple diagnosis to make in primary care and that GPs have little training in managing the problems associated with dementia. She concluded that

"GPs need to be provided with sufficient information, training and support to fulfil their role in the detection and management of dementia". There is clearly a central role for community old age psychiatric services in helping to meet these information needs, and in transferring skills to the primary care team as a whole (including practice nurses and district nurses).

The majority of the care for people with dementia is provided by informal carers, usually spouses or other family members. Whether or not these carers are co-resident with the person with dementia, they have high levels of psychological strain and carer burden. Referral may be prompted by such strain, and the old age psychiatric team has an important role in assessing and meeting carer needs in co-operation with social services. There is some evidence that, unless systematized, community team assessments of carer stress may be inaccurate (Melzer *et al.*, 1996). The same study suggested that there are positive gains in terms of more accurate needs assessment and service delivery if carers are actively included in service monitoring, and that such involvement was feasible.

Anti-dementia medication

The pathway from dementia to diagnosis and active management has been highlighted by the introduction of the potential for pharmacological treatment. It is an unusual situation in health care for medication to be introduced in a condition where there has been no previous drug treatment. However, this is the case with the anti-dementia drugs such as donepezil and rivastigmine which have been licensed recently in the UK. These anti-cholinesterase inhibitors have modest efficacy in improving cognitive function in some individuals with mild to moderate Alzheimer's disease and have a benign side-effect profile when compared with other potential compounds such as tacrine (Rogers and Friedhoff, 1996; Corey-Bloom *et al.*, 1998; Rogers *et al.*, 1998).

The impact of these compounds and those which will follow them in the near future is likely to be profound in terms of service activity and cost

(Allen, 1999), potential overall long-term cost savings notwithstanding (Knapp *et al.*, 1998). At present, only around 10% of people with dementia come into contact with old age psychiatry services at any time in their illness (Holmes *et al.*, 1995); however, the large majority are in active contact with primary health and social services and so are accessible for referral for treatment (Gordon *et al.*, 1997). Governmental and other guidelines suggest that such treatment should be initiated only by specialists such as old age psychiatrists, neurologists and geriatricians (Harvey, 1999). Currently demand has been managed by health purchasers denying or limiting funding for these drugs and services continuing to act reactively. With increasing publicity and the accumulation of further evidence, these strategies will become increasingly untenable and this will lead to an important increase in the workload of specialist services in completing the detailed assessments needed to decide whether to initiate treatment and to monitor response.

This is a profound challenge for both service providers and commissioners (Kelly *et al.*, 1997; Johnson, 1999). It is likely that other un-met social and health care need in people with dementia would also be uncovered requiring further resources. Present resources could not meet the potential drug and non-drug (increased referrals, assessments, investigations and follow-up appointments) costs. For old age psychiatric services to take on a role in the provision of such drugs needs careful consideration, but may be unavoidable. The option of refusing to play a part is likely to be undesirable from the aspect of delivering high quality patient care and also the continuing development of old age psychiatry as a specialty.

Management of depression in the community

Over the past 15 years, there has been a concerted research effort to describe and quantify the burden of depression in the elderly. Using instruments of known and acceptable validity and reli-

ability, the prevalence of clinically significant depression in the elderly in the UK population over the age of 65 is between 12.6% in Liverpool (Copeland *et al.*, 1987) and 15.9% in London (Livingston *et al.*, 1990). These are defined as depressions which would warrant intervention.

The prevalence of depression is higher in primary care attenders and in secondary care contacts (both in- and out-patients). The prevalence of depression in clients of local authority home care services is twice (26%) that in the community in general, including a fourfold excess of the most serious types (Banerjee, 1993; Banerjee and Macdonald, 1996). In residential care of all kinds, there is a high proportion of dementia, but there have also been consistent reports that up to 50% of residents have significant problems with depression (Ames, 1991).

Only between 10 and 15% of these people with depression, no matter what their source, seem to be receiving anything in the way of active treatment for their depression (Banerjee and Macdonald, 1996; Livingston *et al.*, 1997), with the prescription of potentially harmful benzodiazepines more common. Only 10–20% appear to be referred to psychiatric services at any time during their lives. The reason for this lack of appropriate action is unclear; some implicating low GP recognition (Crawford *et al.*, 1998) and some a lack of action when depression is found (Macdonald, 1986). Whatever the mechanism, there is a clear discontinuity on the path from contact, through recognition to action (Banerjee, 1998).

Unlike younger age groups, the elderly with depression have multiple service contacts. They are maintained in the community by a complex matrix of self-care, informal care, social service care and health care (primary and secondary). They very often have multiple medical and social problems which interact. In this complexity lie the challenges and the opportunities for developing effective care for the elderly with depression. The systems of service delivery in place can be said to be failing older people with depression. There are clear discontinuities along the path from disorder to recognition to treatment in all these settings. There is a need to understand these barriers to care better so as to formulate policy, service and clinical management plans to overcome them.

Depression in older black and other ethnic minority group populations is relatively under-researched. However, the syndrome appears to be at least as prevalent in black groups and methods of case ascertainment seem culture fair (Abas *et al.*, 1998). This is an area of increasing importance which needs further research.

The evidence base for the treatment of depression in the elderly is growing but has large gaps at present, especially where evidence of effectiveness in real populations is needed rather than efficacy in the highly selected groups enrolled into drug trials (Banerjee and Dickinson, 1997).

Without specific intervention, the natural history of depression in the elderly at home is fairly bleak, with only 37% of community-dwelling older people recovering in a 1-year period (Prince *et al.*, 1998), and less (25% in 6 months) in disabled groups (Banerjee *et al.*, 1996). However, in the community at large, there is evidence that people screened as depressed can be engaged successfully and acceptably and treated by an old age psychiatric community nurse, though the effectiveness of this strategy might have been improved by greater liaison with GPs (Waterraus *et al.*, 1994; Blanchard *et al.*, 1995).

For elderly home care recipients, the evidence of effectiveness is even clearer. This is of interest in itself, but also because the demonstration of good outcome in what is considered a group with a poor treatment response (the elderly with high disablement) suggests that in less ill groups an equally successful outcome might be possible. Banerjee *et al.* (1996) screened home care clients in Lewisham and carried out a randomized control trial (RCT) of the effectiveness of an old age psychiatric community team compared with normal GP care, on those identified to be depressed. Sixty percent of the intervention group recovered at 6-month follow-up compared with only 25% of the control group. The intervention had high acceptability; it was formulated individually but involved maximization of physical and social function and care and very often the prescription of antidepressants. In addition to this, the study also demonstrated that a simple screening tool could feasibly be incorporated into home helps' contact with clients and be completed successfully in 75% of the caseload (Banerjee *et al.*, 1998)

There is an important and pressing need to extend our evidence base in this area. It is only with good quality evidence that appropriate and effective policy and clinical interventions can be formulated. In addition, high quality, believable, applicable evidence and interventions are needed if clinical behaviour is to be changed. Therefore, interventions need to be formulated and developed for use in and by primary and social care (with secondary health care support) and tested in wider, more generalizable, populations for their clinical and economic effectiveness.

Treatment choice in older populations

The best quality evidence of whether an intervention works comes from multiple well conducted RCTs, whose results can be summarized by systematic review and meta-analysis as advocated by the Cochrane Collaboration. However, the clinical usefulness of these reviews depends on the RCTs available, in particular their generalizability to clinical caseloads. 'Scientific' RCTs investigate the effect of the intervention in ideal circumstances; while 'practical' RCTs seek to investigate whether it works in real clinical settings. 'Scientific' trials therefore differ from 'practical' trials in (i) the degree to which they impose exclusion criteria for recruitment; and (ii) the extent of mismatch between how the intervention is delivered in the study and how it could possibly be given in the real world. Unfortunately, what studies there are in older populations tend to be 'scientific' rather than 'practical' producing data on the intervention's efficacy (its effect in ideal conditions) rather than its effectiveness (its effect under more normal clinical circumstances in terms of patients and services).

'Scientific' trials are designed to produce the maximum effect size and so require fewer subjects than an equivalent 'practical' trial, but may take time to recruit subjects due to multiple exclusions. Part of their attraction to drug companies and researchers alike lies in this maximization of effect; such trials are more likely to deliver a positive finding. In contrast, 'practical' studies have to be larger and have lower effect sizes, and may also be more complex to conduct and analyse. The populations in 'practical' trials may also be more likely to have severe incidental adverse events, such as death, since they are not selected on the basis of being 'supernormal' (i.e. more healthy or higher functioning than the average patient with the disorder) as is the case in many 'scientific' trials. Severe adverse events are very problematic in evaluations of new drugs, since, while they may be entirely unconnected with the intervention, they are unlikely to be sufficiently common to ensure that they will assort equally across the intervention and control groups. They can therefore compromise trials by chance. The companies who conduct these trials may therefore wish to exclude those with a greater likelihood of such events (e.g. the ill, the disabled, those with co-morbid physical disorder, those who are on other medication) from trials. Unfortunately, it is just such excluded cases who form the bulk of clinical populations in old age psychiatry.

A striking example of the extent of the effect of exclusion criteria on recruitment to an RCT for depression has been described by Yastrubetskaya and colleagues (1997). In a phase III trial of a new antidepressant in an Australian centre, 188 patients were screened and 171 (91%) of them met the inclusion criteria of having sufficiently severe depression for the trial. However, when the RCT's multiple exclusion criteria were applied to this real-world sample of people with depression, only eight (5%) could be included in the trial. A further finding highlighting the gap between the RCT protocol and clinical practice is the report that at least 70% of the sample required and received antidepressant treatment. It is clear that data from the trial might not have been applicable to those excluded. The practice of exclusions removing study populations from clinical groups is not confined to depression, it can also be identified in recent studies of the drug treatment of Alzheimer's disease (Rogers *et al.*, 1996).

Another conundrum is set when seeking evidence of what class of antidepressant or antipsychotic might be best suited to the treatment of depression or psychosis in the elderly. Much of the data we have on antidepressant use come from younger age groups. Gerson and colleagues (1988) estimated that up to 1986 only 189 people aged 65 or older had been included in drug trials of compounds other than amitriptyline or imipramine. This has increased with time, with 1059 subjects identified up to 1991(Anstey and Brodaty, 1995), and further trials have been conducted since then. However, the effect of the subject selection process for trials discussed above is likely to result in study populations which differ systematically from clinical populations and the elderly population as a whole in terms of physical health, disability and socio-economic resources. All of these factors may have an important impact on the outcome of treatment and the cost–benefit equation for differing treatments.

With respect to depression, the consensus holds that tricyclic antidepressants (TCAs) and serotonin-specific reuptake inhibitors (SSRIs) have generally similar efficacy. In addition, there appear to be only modest improvements in compliance, with no evidence of increased cost-effectiveness, when SSRIs are compared with TCAs (Hotopf *et al.*, 1996). However, these data are generally derived from supernormal and younger populations. It may be that the cost–benefit equation for choice of class of antidepressant is very different for a frail elderly population than that for a younger fitter one. In particular, physical co-morbidity, polypharmacy, decreased functional reserve, a propensity to falls and cognitive impairment might favour the use of SSRIs over TCAs and atypical antipsychotics over older antipsychotics in terms of side effect tolerance, discontinuation of therapy and clinician willingness to initiate therapy. However, the present state of the evidence base means that such considerations are a matter for conjecture rather than the weighing of evidence. For such data to be made available, there needs to be the willingness to fund large-scale effectiveness studies, incorporating good quality economic and quality of life evaluation, on clinically relevant frail elderly populations.

Other emerging health technologies

Other emerging technologies including telemedicine may have a particular part to play in enabling older people with disability and dementia to remain safely in the community (Fisk, 1997). One example is electronic tracking for the location of people with dementia who wander and become lost. Such behaviour is often dangerous and a cause of institutionalization (McShane, 1994). Preliminary studies have suggested limited feasibility and utility of such approaches, but their impact is yet to be fully realized (McShane *et al.*, 1998).

However, new technologies of whatever sort which enable people with severe dementia and challenging behaviour to remain in the community rather than move into residential care are likely to result in increased demands on community services of all types including old age psychiatry. In addition, it is important to note that increasing complexity in the man-made environment can also disable older people either because they do not have the funds to access technological advances or because they are unable to use the new technology for reasons of physical or cognitive impairment (Sartorius, 1997).

Younger people with dementia

Younger people with dementia (usually defined as those under 65 years) are generally cared for by old age psychiatric services without specialization though their diagnosis often will have involved contact with a neurologist (Barber, 1997). One of the difficulties in providing specialized care is the low numbers of younger people with dementia in any particular area, and national initiatives such as the CANDID telephone helpline set up by The National Hospital for Neurology and Neurosurgery may be particularly appropriate for such rare disorders (Harvey *et al.*, 1998).

Memory clinics

The role of memory clinics in the diagnosis and treatment of dementia is unclear. They are most usually run by old age psychiatric services and form a specialized part of their community assessment service. However, while they have grown in number, they remain a relatively uncommon element of service provision, with only 20 identified in the British Isles in 1993 (Wright and Lindesay, 1995). They also often have a predominantly diagnostic and pharmacological focus, so failing to take advantage of the potential for early psychosocial intervention (Moniz-Cook and Woods, 1997).

Day care

Day care is an important element of community care for older people with mental health problems and may be provided by social services, the voluntary sector or by health services. Although many mental health services include high cost old age psychiatric day hospitals, there appears to be no good evidence to inform whether purchasing a day hospital is a reasonable use of scarce resources.

The available data when scrutinized seem to consist largely of assertion and anecdote (Ball, 1993; Fasey, 1994; Howard, 1994), with a few small-scale and not definitive exceptions (Collier and Baldwin, 1999). What is clear however is that the cost–benefit equation is likely to be least compelling for those day hospitals with relatively high costs and low throughput. It also seems important to ensure that day hospitals are not duplicating a service that could be provided at no cost (at least to health services) or a lower cost by social service or voluntary sector day centres (such as meals, company and social support).

Consultant domicilary visits (DVs)

Old age psychiatry stresses the importance and value of home assessment and treatment (Fottrell, 1989). While all DVs are home assessments, not all home assessments are DVs. The difference lies in the fee that is payable to the consultant for a GP-requested DV. No such fee is payable to any other member of the multi-disciplinary team and no fee is payable if the consultant chooses to see a patient at home. The routine use of DVs has been described as "costly and ... offensive to other members of the multidisciplinary team" (Baldwin, 1998) and has been the subject of debate (Orrell and Katona, 1998). It has also been suggested that they may be requested by a GP in order to by-pass waiting lists and that as GPs learn that all patients will be seen at home in any case, they ask for them less (Baldwin, 1998). GP-requested DVs do appear to be a way of accessing a rapid response from old age psychiatry services, with most urgent requests being completed within 2 days and routine requests within a week (Hardy-Thompson *et al.*, 1992; Tullett *et al.*, 1997).

The evidence for the cost-effectiveness of home-based assessments is sparse, with only one small audit of a single service suggesting that home-based and out-patient-based consultations were similar in overall cost (Shah, 1997). Indeed, the issue of where the cost for DVs may fall may be of importance with the report that the establishment of GP fundholding statistically significantly reduced GP requests for old age psychiatric DVs (Fear and Cattell, 1994).

Stress and burn-out

Consultants in old age psychiatry have been reported to work long hours with little time for recreation, personal study and research (Benbow *et al.*, 1993). Major stresses identified include over a half of consultants reporting overwork and at least 30% stresses from: management issues, a lack of resources, personal stress and a lack of time (Benbow and Jolly, 1997). A high proportion of time is spent in community work either in direct contact with patients and their carers or working with and in support of their community teams (Jolley and Benbow, 1997).

The particular characteristics of working as an old age psychiatrist have been suggested as potentially contributing to staff burn-out (Benbow, 1998). This is likely to be equally important for other members of the multi-disciplinary team working with older people in general (Anstrom *et al.*, 1991), and with people with cognitive

impairment in particular (Novak and Chappell, 1994) identified as particular stresses in nursing staff.

Liaison old age psychiatry

The general hospital can be considered part of the community served by old age psychiatric teams, and the large majority of acute hospital in-patients are over the age of 65 years. Psychiatric liaison and consultation for this group commonly is provided by old age psychiatric services rather than generic liaison psychiatry services (Benbow, 1994).

Given the numbers of older people in acute hospitals who have problems with dementia, delirium and behavioural disturbance as well as those who require placement, this can be a heavy load on the medical elements of the community team (Ramsey *et al.*, 1991). For example, liaison referrals made up between 36 and 51% of all referrals to the central Manchester service between 1985 and 1990, prompting the establishment of a nurse-based liaison service (Collinson and Benbow, 1998). The acceptability and effectiveness of such innovative schemes require further study.

Interface with general adult psychiatry

Last but certainly not least comes the consideration of the interface between old age and general adult psychiatry. Despite the important links and synergies with primary care and social services described above, old age psychiatry shares most with general adult psychiatry. Frustration in this relationship has led some to suggest that old age psychiatry should become part of geriatric medicine, or community heath services, or fuse with social services. These frustrations have often been resource-driven with a perception that services for older people are at a disadvantage when in competition for funds with services for younger adults. In addition to this, there is great variation in how lines of clinical responsibility are drawn between the two specialities. These include who provides services for 'graduates' (people with functional disorder under the care of general adult services who reach their 65th birthday), and people with non-progressive brain disorder, as well as definitions of which younger patients and graduates would benefit from specialist old age psychiatric care.

These frictions are partly based on the different nature of risk and danger in the elderly mentally ill compared with younger groups (i.e. greater risk of neglect, abuse and self-harm rather than harm to others in older adults). It is therefore easy to lose track of the important elements of service provision that are shared by old age and adult general psychiatry. These include shared training and paradigms of disorder and treatment. A comprehensive community mental health service requires specialist old age psychiatry as well as general adult services. These need to work together co-operatively and effectively if the mental health needs of the adult population as a whole are to be met. Moves towards joint mental health and social services should not necessitate the separation of old age psychiatry from other psychiatric services. If this were to be the case, then this would open up the possibility of the very sorts of failures in communication and lack of clarity in lines of responsibility which the introduction of interagency working aims to reduce.

References

Abas, M., Phillips, C., Carter J *et al.* (1998) Culturally sensitive validation of screening questionnaires for depression in older African-Caribbean people living in South London. *British Journal of Psychiatry*, 173, 249–254.

Allen, H. (1999) Anti-dementia drugs. *International Journal of Geriatric Psychiatry*, 14, 239–243.

Ames, D. (1991) Epidemiological studies of depression among the elderly in residential and nursing homes. *International Journal of Geriatric Psychiatry*, 6, 347–354

Anderson, D.N. (1999) Dementia care in the UK—a single service for all. *International Journal of Geriatric Psychiatry*, 14, 1–2.

Anstrom, S., Waxman, H.M., Nilsson, M. *et al.* (1991) Wish to transfer to other jobs among long-term care workers. *Aging*, 3, 247–256.

Anstey, K. and Brodaty, H. (1995) Antidepressants and the elderly: double blind trials 1987–1992. *International Journal of Geriatric Psychiatry*, 10, 265–279.

Arie, T. (1970) The first year of the Goodmayes psychiatric service for old people. *Lancet*, ii, 1175–1182.

Arie, T. (1971) Morale and planning of psychogeriatric services. *British Medical Journal*, iii, 166–170.

Arie, T. and Issacs, A.D. (1978) The development of psychiatric services for the elderly in Britain. In: Issacs, A.D. and Post, F. (eds), *Studies in Geriatric Psychiatry*. Chichester: Wiley, pp. 241–261.

Baldwin, R.C. (1998) Re: editorial—consultant home visits. *International Journal of Geriatric Psychiatry*, 13, 820.

Ball, C. (1993) The future of day care in old age psychiatry. *Psychiatric Bulletin*, 17, 427–428.

Banerjee, S. (1993) Prevalence and recognition rates of psychiatric disorder in the elderly clients of a community care service. *International Journal of Geriatric Psychiatry*, 8, 125–131.

Banerjee, S. (1998) The needs of special groups: the elderly. *International Review of Psychiatry*, 10, 130–133.

Banerjee, S. (2000) Models of mental health care for the elderly. In: Gregoire, A.(ed.), *Serious Adult Mental Illness*. London: Greenwich Medical Media, pp. 243–256.

Banerjee, S. and Dickinson, E. (1997) Evidence based health care in old age psychiatry. *International Journal of Psychiatry in Medicine*, 27, 283–292.

Banerjee, S. and Macdonald, A. (1996) Mental disorder in an elderly home care population: associations with health and social service use. *British Journal of Psychiatry*, 168, 750–756.

Banerjee, S., Lindesay, J. and Murphy, E. (1993) Psychogeriatricians and general practitioners—a national survey. *Psychiatric Bulletin*, 17, 592–594.

Banerjee, S., Shamash, K., Macdonald, A. *et al.* (1996) Randomised controlled trial of effect of intervention by psychogeriatric team on depression in frail elderly people at home. *British Medical Journal*, 313, 1058–1061.

Banerjee, S., Shamash, K., Macdonald, A. *et al.* (1998) The use of the SelfCARE(D) as a screening tool for depression in the clients of local authority home care services. *International Journal of Geriatric Psychiatry*, 13, 695–699.

Barber, R. (1997) A survey of services for younger people with dementia. *International Journal of Geriatric Psychiatry*, 12, 951–954.

Bedford, S., Melzer, D., Dening, T. *et al.* (1996) What becomes of people with dementia referred to community psychogeriatric teams? *International Journal of Geriatric Psychiatry*, 11, 1051–1056.

Benbow, S.M. (1994) Liaison services for elderly people. In: Benjamin, S., House, A. and Jenkins, P. (eds), *Liaison Psychiatry Defining Needs and Planning Services*. London: Gaskell, pp. 34–44.

Benbow, S.M. (1998) Burnout: current knowledge and relevance to old age psychiatry. *International Journal of Geriatric Psychiatry*, 13, 520–526.

Benbow, S.M. and Jolley, D. (1997) Old age psychiatrists: what do they find stressful? *International Journal of Geriatric Psychiatry*, 12, 879–882.

Benbow, S.M., Jolley, D. and Leonard, I.J. (1993) All work? A day in the life of geriatric psychiatrists. *International Journal of Geriatric Psychiatry*, 8, 1019–1022.

Blanchard, M.R., Waterraus, A. and Mann, A (1995) The effect of primary care nurse intervention upon older people screened as depressed. *International Journal of Geriatric Psychiatry*, 10, 289–298.

Bone, M. (1995) *Trends in Dependency Among Older People in England*. London: OPCS.

Brown, P., Challis, D. and von Abendorff, R. (1996) The work of a community mental health team for the elderly: caseload, contact history and outcomes. *International Journal of Geriatric Psychiatry*, 11, 29–39.

Coles, R.J., von Abendorff, R. and Herzberg, J.L. (1991) The impact of a new community mental health team on an inner city psychogeriatric service. *International Journal of Geriatric Psychiatry*, 6, 31–39.

Collier, E.H., and Baldwin, R.C. (1999) The day hospital debate – a contribution. *International Journal of Geriatric Psychiatry*, 14, 587–591.

Collighan, G., Macdonald, A., Herzberg, J. *et al.* (1993) An evaluation of the multidisciplinary approach to psychiatric diagnosis in elderly people. *British Medical Journal*, 306, 821–824.

Collinson, Y. and Benbow, S.M. (1998) The role of an old age psychiatry consultation liaison nurse. *International Journal of Geriatric Psychiatry*, 13, 159–163.

Cooper, B. (1991) Principles of service provision in old age psychiatry. In: Jacoby, R. and Oppenheimer, C. (eds), *Psychiatry for the Elderly*. Oxford: Oxford University Press, pp. 357–375.

Copeland, J.R.M., Dewey, M.E., Wood, N. *et al.* (1987) Range of mental illness among the elderly in the community prevalence in Liverpool using the GMS-AGECAT package. *British Journal of Psychiatry*, 150, 815–823.

Corey-Bloom, J., Anand, R., Veach, J. *et al.* (1998) A randomised trial evaluating the efficacy and safety of ENA 713 (rivastigmine), a new acetylcholinesterase inhibitor, in patients with mild to moderately severe Alzheimer's disease. *International Journal of Geriatric Psychopharmacology*, 1, 55–65.

Crawford, M.J., Prince, M., Menezes, P. *et al.* (1998) The recognition and treatment of depression in older people in primary care. *International Journal of Geriatric Psychiatry*, 13, 172–176.

Dening, T. (1992) Community psychiatry of old age: a UK perspective. *International Journal of Geriatric Psychiatry*, 7, 757–766.

Downs, M.G. (1996) The role of general practice and the primary care team in dementia diagnosis and management. *International Journal of Geriatric Psychiatry*, 11, 937–942.

Fasey, C. (1994) The day hospital in old age psychiatry; the case against. *International Journal of Geriatric Psychiatry*, 9, 519–523.

Fear, C.F. and Cattell, H.R. (1994) Fund-holding general practices and old age psychiatry. *Psychiatric Bulletin*, 18, 263–265.

Fisk, M.J. (1997) Telemedicine, new technologies and care management. *International Journal of Geriatric Psychiatry*, 12, 1057–1059.

Fottrell, E. (1989) A personal view of psychogeriatric domicilliary visits. *Geriatric Medicine*, 2, 22–25.

Gerson, S.C., Plotkin, D.A. and Jarvik, L.F. (1988) Antidepressant drug studies, 1964 to 1986: empirical evidence for aging patients. *Journal of Clinical Psychopharmacology*, 8, 311–322.

Glosser, G., Wexler, D. and Balmelli, M. (1985) Physicians and families' perspectives on the medical management of dementia. *Journal of the American Geriatrics Society*, 33, 383–391.

Gordon, D.S., Carter, H. and Scott, S. (1997) Profiling care needs of the population with dementia: a survey in central Scotland. *International Journal of Geriatric Psychiatry*, 12, 753–759.

Hardy-Thompson, C., Orrell, M.W. and Bergmann, K. (1992) Evaluating a psychogeriatric domicilliary service: views of general practitioners. *British Medical Journal*, 304, 421–422.

Harvey, R. (1999) A review and commentary on a sample of 15 UK guidelines for the drug treatment of Alzheimer's disease. *International Journal of Geriatric Psychiatry*, 14, 249–256.

Harvey, R.J., Roques, P.K., Fox, N.C. *et al.* (1998) CANDID—counselling and diagnosis in dementia: a national telemedicine service supporting the care of younger people with dementia. *International Journal of Geriatric Psychiatry*, 13, 381–388.

Herzberg, J. (1995) Can multidisciplinary teams carry out competent and safe psychogeriatric assessments in the community? *International Journal of Geriatric Psychiatry*, 10, 173–177.

Holmes, C., Cooper, B. and Levy, R. (1995) Dementia known to mental health services: first findings of a case register for a defined elderly population. *International Journal of Geriatric Psychiatry*, 10, 875–881.

Hotopf, M., Lewis, G. and Normand, C. (1996) Are SSRIs a cost effective alternative to tricyclics? *British Journal of Psychiatry*, 168, 404–409.

Howard, R. (1994) Day hospitals: the case in favour. *International Journal of Geriatric Psychiatry*, 9, 525–529.

Johnson, R. (1999) New drugs for dementia: a commissioning nightmare? *International Journal of Geriatric Psychiatry*, 14, 257–260.

Jolley, D.J. and Benbow, S.M. (1997) The everyday work of geriatric psychiatrists. *International Journal of Geriatric Psychiatry*, 12, 109–13.

Kalache, A. (1991) Ageing is a Third World problem too. *International Journal of Geriatric Psychiatry*, 6, 617–618.

Kay, D.W. (1999) Geriatric psychiatry in the 1950s and 1960s; recollections. *International Psychogeriatrics*, 11, 363–366.

Kelly, C.A., Harvey, R. and Cayton, H. (1997) Treatment of Alzheimer's disease raises clinical and ethical issues. *British Medical Journal*, 314, 693–694.

Knapp, M., Wilkinson, D. and Wrigglesworth, R. (1998) The economic consequences of Alzheimer's disease in the context of new drug developments. *International Journal of Geriatric Psychiatry*, 13, 531–543.

Lewis, A. (1946) Ageing and senility: a major problem of psychiatry. *Journal of Mental Science*, 92, 150–170.

Lindesay, J., Herzberg, J., Collighan, G. et al. (1996) Treatment decisions following assessment by multi-disciplinary psychogeriatric teams. *Psychiatric Bulletin*, 20, 78–81.

Livingston, G., Hawkins, A., Graham, N. et al. (1990) The Gospel Oak Study: prevalence rates of dementia, depression and activity limitation among elderly residents in inner London. *Psychological Medicine*, 20, 137–146.

Livingston, G., Manela, M. and Katona. C. (1997) Cost of community care for older people. *British Journal of Psychiatry*, 171, 56–69.

Macdonald, A.J.D. (1986) Do general practitioners 'miss' depression in elderly patients? *British Medical Journal*, 292, 1365–1368.

Macdonald, A., Goddard, C. and Poynton, A. (1994) Impact of 'open access' to specialist services, the case of community psychogeriatrics. *International Journal of Geriatric Psychiatry*, 9, 709–714.

McShane, R., Hope, T. and Wilkinson, J. (1994) Tracking patients who wander: ethics and the new technology. *Lancet*, 343, 1274.

McShane, R., Keen, J., Gedling, K., Fairbairn, C., Jacoby, R. and Hope, T. (1997) Do neuroleptic drugs hasten cognitive decline in dementia? Prospective study with necropsy follow up. *British Medical Journal*, 314, 266–270.

McShane, R., Gedling, K., Kenward, B. et al. (1998) The feasibility of electronic tracking devices in dementia: a telephone survey and case series. *International Journal of Geriatric Psychiatry*, 13, 556–563.

Melzer, D., Bedford, S., Dening, T. et al. (1996) Carers and the monitoring of psychogeriatric community teams. *International Journal of Geriatric Psychiatry*, 11, 1057–1061.

Melzer, D., Ely, M. and Brayne, C. (1997) Cognitive impairment in elderly people: population based estimate of the future in England, Scotland and Wales. *British Medical Journal*, 315, 462.

Melzer, D., McWilliams, B., Brayne, C., Johnson, T. and Bond, J. (1999) Profile of disability in elderly people: estimates from a population study. *British Medical Journal*, 318, 1108–1111.

Moniz-Cook, E. and Woods, R.T. (1997) The role of memory clinics and psychosocial intervention in the early stages of dementia. *International Journal of Geriatric Psychiatry*, 12, 1143–1145.

Mountain, G. (1998) The delivery of community mental health services to older people. *The Mental Health Review*, 3, 7–15.

Murphy, E. and Banerjee, S. (1993) The organisation of old-age psychiatry services. *Reviews in Clinical Gerontology*, 3, 367–378.

Novak, M. and Chappell, N.L. (1994) Nursing assistant burnout and the cognitively impaired elderly. *International Journal of Aging and Human Development*, 39, 105–120.

Nuttall, S.R., Blackwood, R.J.L., Bussell, B.M.H., Cliff, J.P., Cornall, M.J., Cowley, A. et al. (1994) Financing long term care in Great Britain. *Journal of the Institute of Actuaries*, 121, 1–53.

O'Connor, D.W., Pollitt, P.A., Hyde, J.B. et al. (1988) Do general practitioners miss dementia in elderly patients? *British Medical Journal*, 247, 1107–1110.

O'Connor, D.W., Fertig, A., Grande, M.J. et al. (1993) Dementia in general practice: the practical consequences of a more positive approach to diagnosis. *British Journal of General Practice*, 43, 185–188.

Organisation for Economic Co-operation and Development (1988) *Ageing Population: The Social Policy Implications*. Paris: OECD.

Orrell, M. and Katona, C. (1998) Do consultant home visits have a future in old age psychiatry? *International Journal of Geriatric Psychiatry*, 13, 355–357.

Philp, I. and Young, J. (1988) Audit of support given to lay carers of the demented elderly by members of the primary health care team. *Journal of the Royal College of General Practitioners*, 38, 153–155.

Philp, I., McKee, K.J. and Ballinger, B.R. (1995) Community care for demented and non-demented elderly people: a comparison study of financial burden, service use, and unmet needs in family supporters. *British Medical Journal*, 310, 1503–1506.

Philpot, M. and Banerjee, S. (1997) Mental health services for older people in London. In: Johnson, S., Ramsey, R., Thornicroft G. *et al.* (eds), *London's Mental Health*. London: King's Fund, pp. 46–62.

Prince, M. (1997) The need for research on dementia in developing countries. *Tropical Medicine and International Health*, 2, 993–1000.

Prince, M.J., Harwood, R.H., Thomas, A. *et al.* (1998) A prospective population-based cohort study of the effects of disablement and social milieu on the onset and maintenance of late-life depression. The Gospel Oak Project VII. *Psychological Medicine*, 28, 337–350.

Rabins, P.V. (1999) The history of psychogeriatrics in the United States. *International Psychogeriatrics*, 11, 371–373.

Rait, G. and Burns, A. (1997) Appreciating background and culture: the South Asian elderly and mental health. *International Journal of Geriatric Psychiatry*, 12, 973–977.

Ramsey, R., Wright, P., Katz, A. *et al.*7 (1991) The detection of psychiatric morbidity and its effects on outcome in acute elderly medical admissions. *International Journal of Geriatric Psychiatry*, 6, 861–866.

Reifler, B.V. (1997) The practice of geriatric psychiatry in three countries: observations of an American in the British Isles. *International Journal of Geriatric Psychiatry*, 12, 795–807.

Reifler, B.V. and Cohen, W. (1998) Practice of geriatric psychiatry and mental health services for the elderly: results of an international survey. *International Psychogeriatrics*, 10, 351–357.

Rogers, S.L. and Friedhoff, L.T. (1996) The efficacy and safety of donepezil in patients with Alzheimer's disease: results of a US multicentre, randomised, double-blind, placebo-controlled trial. *Dementia*, 7, 293–303.

Rogers, S.L., Farlow, M.R., Mohs, R. *et al.* (1998) A 24 week double-blind, placebo-controlled trial of donepezil in patients with Alzheimer's disease. *Neurology*, 50, 136–145.

Rosenvinge, H. (1994) The multi-disciplinary team. In: Copeland, J.R.M., Abou-Saleh, M.T. and Blazer, D.G. (eds), *Principles and Practice of Geriatric Psychiatry*. Chichester: Wiley, pp. 887–890.

Royal College of Psychiatrists (1989) Guidelines for regional advisors on consultant posts in old age psychiatry. *Psychiatric Bulletin*, 11, 240–242.

Royal College of Psychiatrists (1992) *Mental Health of the Nation: The Contribution of Psychiatry*. London: Royal College of Psychiatrists

Royal College of Psychiatrists and British Geriatric Society (1979) Guidelines for collaboration between geriatric physicians and psychiatrists in the care of the elderly. *Bulletin of the Royal College of Psychiatrists*, 1, 168–169.

Sartorius, N. (1997) Mental health care for the elderly. *International Journal of Geriatric Psychiatry*, 12, 430–435.

Shah, A. (1997) Cost comparison of out-patient and home-based geriatric psychiatry consultations in one service. *Aging and Mental Health*, 1, 372–376.

Silveira, E.R.T. and Ebrahim, S. (1998) Social determinants of psychiatric morbidity and well-being in immigrant elders and whites in east London. *International Journal of Geriatric Psychiatry*, 13, 801–812.

Tullett, D.C., Orrell, M.W., Kalkat, G.S. *et al.* (1997) Domicilliary visits in old age psychiatry: expectation and practice. *Primary Care Psychiatry*, 3, 195–198.

Waterraus, A., Blanchard, M. and Mann, A. (1994) Community psychiatric nurses for the elderly: well tolerated, few side-effects and effective in the treatment of depression. *Journal of Clinical Nursing*, 3, 299–306.

Wattis, J. (1988) Geographical variation in the provision of psychiatric services for old people. *Age and Ageing*, 17, 171–180.

Wattis, J. (1994) The pattern of psychogeriatric services. In: *Principles and Practice of Geriatric Psychiatry*. Copeland, J.R.M., Abou-Saleh, M.T. and Blazer, D.G. (eds), Chichester: Wiley, pp. 879–883.

Wattis, J., Wattis, L. and Arie, T. (1981) Psychogeriatrics: a national survey of a new branch of psychiatry. *British Medical Journal*, 282, 1529–1533.

Wertheimer, J. (1997) Psychiatry of the elderly: a consensus statement. *International Journal of Geriatric Psychiatry*, 12, 430–435.

World Health Organisation (1991) *World Health Statistics Annual 1990*. Geneva: WHO.

Wright, N. and Lindesay, J. (1995) A survey of memory clinics in the British Isles. *International Journal of Geriatric Psychiatry*, 10, 379–385.

Yastrubetskaya, O., Chiu, E. and O'Connell, S. (1997) Is good clinical research practice for clinical trials good clinical practice? *International Journal of Geriatric Psychiatry*, 12, 227–231.

33 | Community mental health services for adults with learning disabilities

Nick Bouras and Geraldine Holt

Introduction

The term 'learning disabilities' has been used in the UK in recent years instead of mental retardation or mental handicap. It does not reflect the meaning of the term as defined in the classification systems of DSM-IV and ICD-10, but is synonymous with mental retardation and mental handicap. Learning disabilities is used in this chapter in this latter context.

Psychiatric disorders are more prevalent in people with learning disabilities than in the general population, and are a primary reason for failure to adapt to community living. In the past several decades, the pattern of service delivery for people with learning disabilities has changed dramatically. Presently, the overwhelming majority live in the community and are expected to use generic medical and mental health services.

This chapter reviews the development of community care for adults with learning disabilities. The needs for those with mental health problems are highlighted and a conceptual framework of services is proposed. The diagnosis of learning disabilities requires the finding of a significantly subaverage level of intellectual functioning, (i.e. an IQ of <70 on a standardized test), a significant impairment of adaptive functioning and onset in childhood. Thus, the term learning disabilities refers not to a single disorder but to a group of heterogeneous conditions. Its prevalence is estimated at about 1% of the population, and of these about 85% fall within the mild range of learning disabilities (IQ >55) (McLaren and Bryson, 1987;

Fryers, 1993). The prevalence varies in different age groups, the highest being at school age.

Psychiatric disorders frequently co-exist with learning disabilities, with the prevalence estimated at 30–75% (Borthwick-Duffy, 1994). Virtually all categories of mental illness have been reported in this population. Learning disabilities frequently co-exist with psychiatric disorders. These are essentially the same as in the general population, but poor language skills and life circumstances can modify their presentation and a diagnosis might hinge more heavily upon observable behavioural signs.

The current philosophy underpinning services for people with learning disabilities is the 'normalization principle' (Wolfensberger, 1969, 1991): "making available to the mentally retarded patterns and conditions of everyday life which are as close as possible to the norms and patterns of the mainstream of society". Thus, normalization does not imply making people with learning disabilities 'normal', but enabling them to live in as normal conditions as possible.

From the institution to community care

The cornerstone of the marked changes in the provision of services for people with learning disabilities in the last 40 years has been deinstitutionalization, or resettlement, with the development of community care and support systems. The use of institutional care from 1981 to 1991 showed great variability (Hatton *et al.*, 1995) ranging from 3.1/10 000 to 9.7/10 000 among four Scandinavian countries; from 4.7/10 000 to 20.9/10 000 among eight countries in the European Community; from 6.1/10 000 to 13.8/10 000 among three Eastern European countries and 4.5/10 000 in the USA. Rates of annual decrease in the use of institutions were from −1.6% to −5.9% in Scandinavia, from +0.4% to −5.0% in the European Community, +0.6% in Eastern Europe and −3.3% in the USA.

These changes were paralleled in the UK where there has been a major reduction in institutional provision and an analogous increase in community-based services for people with learning disabilities. Between 1983 and 1995, deinstitutionalization accelerated, residential settings reduced considerably in size, the range of day activities diversified, mainstream education was available to more children with learning disabilities, respite care became largely community based and the availability of domiciliary support increased significantly (Perry *et al.*, 1998).

The hospital population of people with learning disabilities in the UK was reduced by 28% over the same period of time (Emerson and Hatton, 1995). By the end of the 20th century, at least 10 000 more people will have been resettled. Residential places vary considerably over the UK, only 2.4% living in settings for less than five, and 13.5% living in settings for between five and nine people, which represents nearly 52% of total facilities (Emerson and Hatton, 1998).

Reforms in the UK and elsewhere have been driven by a desire to replace services which produced poor quality outcomes and represented inadequate value for money with services that are more effective and of high quality. Such alternative services, however, have not necessarily been cheaper to provide. Indeed, evidence suggests that care in the community is at least as expensive as traditionally available institutional provision (Felce, 1994). However, in a recent study, Beecham *et al.* (1997) suggested that care in the community for people with learning disabilities in Northern Ireland was reasonably cost-effective when compared with long-term hospital care. The average cost of community care for the replacement of seven long-stay hospitals with community-based care was less expensive than hospital services. For only 10 people with learning disabilities out of 192 of their sample, the cost of community care exceeded the average costs of long-stay in-patient care. They pointed out, however, that further expenditure on community care for people with learning disabilities would be necessary to enhance their quality of life (Beecham *et al.*, 1997). No information was given of the mental health needs of their sample.

There is a wealth of literature that has demonstrated that institutional closure can be achieved with a variety of positive outcomes for those residents concerned (Haney, 1998; Allen, 1989), although it is evident that there may be considerable differences in observed results (Emerson and Hatton, 1995). Kon and Bouras (1997) followed up 74 people from a long-stay institution 1 and 5 years after their resettlement. They found that the frequency of psychiatric diagnosis and behavioural problems remained fairly consistent over the 5-year period, but there was a marked increase in their utilization of local health and mental health services.

However, research examining people with learning disabilities resettled into community establishments provides evidence that without very careful planning it is possible for the environment to deteriorate, for the residents to become understimulated and withdrawn and for psychiatric and behavioural problems to become more overt (Wing, 1989). Linaker and Nottestad (1998) reported that 109 individuals in Norway who were resettled in the community showed an increase in their physical and psychiatric/behavioural problems over a period of 12 years follow-up (1987–1995).

Psychiatric disorders may be an important, even a primary, factor limiting functioning of persons with learning disabilities, their quality of life and their adaptation to community life (Reiss, 1994). People with learning disabilities and behavioural or mental health problems have repeatedly been identified as those being most at risk of institutional admission (Emerson, 1995). Effective support and treatment services must be developed which reduce the historical dependency on institutions particularly at times of crisis and to avoid the creation of new long-stay populations, which will inhibit closure.

Mental health care

In the past, people with learning disabilities who developed severe behavioural disorders and/or recognized psychiatric illnesses were often removed from the learning disabilities system to psychiatric hospitals. As institutional beds were closed, people with learning disabilities and psychiatric disorders were moved to less restrictive environments, or remained longer with their families. There was an assumption that the mental health problems shown by people with learning disabilities were exaggerated as a consequence of institutional lifestyles and that they would diminish substantially when large-scale community care programmes had been put in place.

However, a significant number of people with learning disabilities, despite progress in care delivery systems, have continued to pose major management difficulties. Progress in standardized assessment methods has revealed that psychiatric disorders frequently are underdiagnosed in this population, and that in some cases aggressive behaviour is associated with a mental illness. This has implications for services.

Having a formal diagnosis of a psychiatric disorder, rather than a non-specific description of a 'behaviour disorder', is important for people with learning disabilities. A diagnosis may lead to a specific treatment. It is also important for planning services and research purposes. The issue of classification of mental illness in people with learning disabilities remains problematic, although the International Classification of Diseases 10, (ICD-10) has begun to address this through its publication of the supplement, the ICD-10 Guide for Mental Retardation (WHO, 1996).

Non-medical professionals working with persons with learning disabilities frequently use the term 'behaviour disorder'. It has no generally accepted definition and commonly is meant to refer to disruptive behaviours that pose problems for the care-givers. Persons with learning disabil-

ities are often referred for assessment specifically to discriminate whether they have a 'behaviour disorder' or a psychiatric disorder. Some care-givers feel that the former should be treated with behavioural modification and the latter with psychopharmacological interventions. However, such a dichotomy is simplistic. In virtually every psychiatric disorder there may be behavioural manifestations that are learned, conditioned by environmental factors or under voluntary control.

With the progress of resettlement programmes, the term 'behaviour problems' was replaced by that of 'challenging behaviours'. It originated as a service concept to identify people with learning disabilities and an additional behavioural disorder, and allocate service resources accordingly (Emerson, 1995). It also attempted ideologically to shift the emphasis of the problem away from the individual and onto the service. However, it is now often used as a clinical diagnosis, and worse still, this 'diagnosis' is used in an attempt to absolve certain service providers of responsibility for the management of such an individual.

In line with the principle of normalization, some proposed that psychiatric problems in people with learning disabilities could be catered for adequately within mainstream mental health services. However, services are needed from both the learning disabilities network and the mental health system. Community-based programmes to provide comprehensive services were not available and problems became apparent (Bouras and Szymanski, 1997).

In the USA, the administrators of Federal government programmes needed to distinguish whether the primary problem of this client group was mental retardation or mental illness, because the services were funded from separate sources (Russell, 1997). Those who had mental retardation as their primary problem were entitled to services provided by mental retardation services organized in 'developmental centres'. Where the diagnosis was primarily of mental illness, community mental health centres were designated as the appropriate providers of psychiatric services.

Frank Menolascino introduced the concept of 'dual diagnosis' as a better alternative (Reiss, 1994). He proposed that services should be provided according to need rather than primary diagnosis, and be delivered in the context of two or more co-existing disabilities, allowing for more appropriate treatment and support.

In the UK, there was a mounting pressure of opinion that a significant number of people with learning disabilities had very complex mental health and/or challenging needs and required specialist support. The expectation that mainstream mental health services could respond to the needs of people with learning disabilities often proved unrealistic. First, the complex behaviour problems of people with severe learning disabilities could not be managed by generic psychiatric services. Mainstream psychiatric services lacked the expertise, training and skills necessary for the assessment and treatment of such a heterogeneous group of people. Secondly, no attempt was made to negotiate the associated service issues and problems between mental health and learning disabilities service providers. There was a lack of clear operational policies or service agreements; only vague definitions of who was entitled to access which service; professional rivalries were common; and budgets constrained. The funding implications for such a shift of service responsibility were never addressed adequately (Bouras *et al.*, 1994).

The American Psychiatric Association (1991) recommended improvements in specialist professional standards, including changing attitudes, generic and specialist professional expertise, and a spectrum of possible service models based on interdisciplinary collaboration. No substantial progress has been noted and there are few specialist training programmes in the USA for psychiatrists. In the UK, training issues have been addressed in a more systematic way through the Royal College of Psychiatrists and other professional bodies (Day, 1998). There is a Faculty of the College specializing in the psychiatry of learning disabilities. Knowledge of this field is required of all psychiatrists in training, and many do a clinical placement. For those wishing to specialize in the psychiatry of learning disabilities, specific training requirements must be fulfilled.

Service responses

The challenge to those commissioning services and those working in the learning disabilities and mental health fields has been to provide appropriate services in the community. Policy guidance in the UK has been broad and open to wide interpretation. The Department of Health (1989) noted that specialist facilities and services may be required for those who were also mentally ill, had behaviour problems or who offended. At a later stage, the Department of Health (1992) recommended that people with learning disabilities should use ordinary health services whenever possible. However, it was recognized that sometimes support would be needed for a person to access these, and that additionally sometimes specialist services would be needed. The Reed Report (Department of Health, 1994) highlighted the relative lack of facilities for mentally disordered offenders with learning disabilities and recommended that a range of services should be available with appropriate levels of security.

There have therefore been a number of service models proposed. Different districts have developed different service models depending on local circumstances (Gravestock and Bouras, 1997). Some services centre around residential, usually hospital, provision perhaps with outreach work, whilst others are more community based, sometimes with access to in-patient facilities (Bouras and Holt, 2000). Approximately two-thirds of NHS Trusts that have completed resettlement have retained some long-stay beds (some for people with enduring mental illness or challenging behaviour), and the majority provide assessment and treatment beds in either specialist units or general psychiatric units (Bailey and Cooper, 1998).

The main focus of service delivery in the community in the UK has been the Community Learning Disabilities Team. These teams have a multi-disciplinary composition and a multi-purpose function, ranging from resettlement programmes to developing services, advocating for the rights of people with learning disabilities, and also providing a clinical service. As it has become obvious that more clinical input was needed, particularly for those with challenging behaviour and/or psychiatric disorders, some services now receive additional resources from psychologists and challenging needs workers. They are known as Community Support Teams (CSTs) or Challenging Behaviour Teams. Most include a consultant psychiatrist specializing in learning disabilities who may be restricted to a largely advisory role, having very few other available clinical resources for treatment interventions.

The publication of the Mansell report in the UK (Department of Health, 1993) offered impetus for the development of CSTs for people with severe learning disabilities and severe challenging behaviours. Emphasis was given to community and locally based services to support good mainstream practice. The major objective was to improve the competence and capacity of services to manage severely disruptive behaviours. This model of CSTs for people with learning disabilities has been applied widely in the UK. Several innovative projects and services have been developed and positive outcomes have already been reported (Allen, 1998; Allen and Felce, 1998).

These developments, however, have had very little influence on the interface between learning disabilities and mainstream psychiatric services. The increasing problems of people with mild learning disabilities and mental illness, the fact that some individuals have very difficult and complex challenging needs, and the increasing evidence that there is an interaction between biological and environmental factors remain major service issues (Hillery, 1998; Bouras and Holt, 2000).

Specialist mental health services

The model of CSTs for people with learning disabilities and challenging behaviour has not been suitable for those people with mild learning disabilities and psychiatric disorders, who as already stated represent the vast majority of those with learning disabilities. This has important service implications as the majority of people with learning disabilities referred for psychiatric assessment have mild cognitive disabilities (Borthwick-

Duffy and Eyman, 1990; Bouras and Drummond, 1992; Crews *et al.*, 1994). Recent studies have indicated that mild cognitive impairment and psychiatric disorder may not be explained entirely by social or educational factors, but by additional independent variables implying some form of common biological cause (Doody *et al.*, 1998; Robertson and Murphy, 1998).

With the closure of institutions for people with learning disabilities together with those for serious mental illness but without learning disabilities, generic psychiatric services have come under increasing pressure. New ways of supporting people with mental health needs in the community have been developed. Admission is generally reserved for those in greatest need of assessment, containment and treatment. Such services may provide a hostile environment for people with mild learning disabilities and those falling in the borderline area of cognitive impairment, some of whom may also offend. They may be bullied and distressed by their fellow patients. Staff may feel that they lack the necessary skills and resources to meet their needs.

In the USA and other countries, where there is an overall lack of specialist services for people with learning disabilities, there are considerable adverse consequences (Davidson *et al.*, 1998; Jacobson, 1998). The prevailing view is that people with learning disabilities and concomitant psychiatric disorders have often been underserved or treated inappropriately because of inter-organizational barriers, leading to unnecessary hospitalization and lengthy delays in community placement. To overcome these barriers, Patterson *et al.* (1995) reported the development of a collaborative system of care between the community mental health centre and the learning disabilities agencies in Washington State that led to a more efficient service over a 2-year period and also reduced interagency tensions.

Driessen *et al.* (1997) reported that in a geographically defined area of The Netherlands, the rate of contact with mental health care facilities in a sample of 465 individuals with learning disabilities was 10%, of whom 3% received psychiatric in-patient treatment. Individuals who were older with mild learning disabilities and were living alone tended to be the highest users of psychiatric services. They speculated that in view of their findings, individuals with severe learning disabilities living in a relatively protected residential environment with trained staff were less likely to need psychiatric services, whereas those with higher levels of functioning are more likely to encounter psychological problems, especially as they grow older.

However, Raitasuo *et al.* (1999a) found in a prospective study of 122 admissions to a special psychiatric unit in Finland that the typical inpatient was a young man with mild learning disabilities and a diagnosis of psychosis, who had lived in several residential places. In another study from the same unit, reduction of psychotic symptoms was reported for a sample of 40 people with mild learning disabilities following psychiatric admission and in-patient treatment (Raitasuo *et al.*, 1999b). Similar results were reported from the evaluation of 64 people with mild learning disabilities admitted to the Mental Impairment Evaluation and Treatment Service in London; 84.2% were improved and discharged to a community placement, although only 17.5% had been admitted from the community (Xenitidis *et al.*, 1999). One criticism of these studies might be their short time scale. It remains to be seen whether clients will maintain their improvement. However, it is known that psychiatric patients are vulnerable to relapses and readmissions, and people with learning disabilities cannot be an exception.

As generic mental health services have been unable to meet the mental health needs of people with mild learning disabilities, an increasing number of private facilities have opened in the UK in an effort to fill the gap. Encouraged by the introduction of the 'internal market' in the early 1990s, some NHS Trusts also developed in-patient assessment and treatment units while replacing some of their institutional-based services, so attracting extra funds from other districts.

In the UK, large sums have been spent by social and health services in buying psychiatric services from private specialist units. In recent years, there has been an increased number of secure and medium secure units for people with mild learning disabilities who are usually detained under a forensic section of the Mental Health Act. Unfortunately, often these new facilities are a long way from a person's home, family, supporters and friends which makes retaining links difficult and planning for a return home a more remote possibility. The implications for the local services are also detrimental because they are deprived of the funds necessary to develop the required services.

In London, 37% of people with learning disabilities originating from a district are living outside it and 49% of those people have some form of mental health need/challenging behaviour (Piachaud, 1999). Even if local solutions continue to be developed, it will be some years before the current geographical dispersion will be resolved.

In an attempt to overcome some of these problems, a model of community-based specialist mental health services for people with learning disabilities has been in operation in two London boroughs over the last 15 years (Bouras *et al.*, 1994). The Community Specialist Mental Health Service for people with learning disabilities uses all the facilities of the generic mental health service including acute and medium-stay in-patient beds and a variety of community resources. The strong clinical interaction between clinical psychologists, psychiatrists, community psychiatric nurses and specialists in functional analysis enables a wide range of mental health needs and/or challenging behaviours to be addressed in people with severe to mild learning disabilities using varying approaches and therapeutic interventions. These methods can be applied in various settings, including the individual's home, usual environment, out-patient clinic and, if necessary, as an in-patient. It is part of the generic mental health services, as are other specialist services, e.g. old age mental health, child mental health, etc., and is funded jointly by learning disabilities and mental health services.

Of 424 consecutive new referrals to the Community Specialist Mental Health Service, the mean age was 32.9 years (SD ± 13.4), 60% were men and 40% were women. Mild learning disabilities were recorded for 60%, moderate for 25% and severe for 15% (Bouras and Holt, 2000). Admission was required for 47 (11%) to generic psychiatric wards of the local adult mental health services. These patients were slightly older (mean age 36.8 years, SD ± 14.1) than those treated in the community (mean age 32.6 years, SD ± 13.5) (Bouras and Holt, 2000). Most (86%) had mild learning disabilities, 12% had moderate and there was only one client with severe learning disabilities. Of those admitted, 87% fulfilled the criteria for a DSM-III-R psychiatric diagnosis compared with 39% of those who received a community intervention. The majority (45%) of the admitted clients suffered from psychotic disorder, 15% from depressive disorder and 9% from personality disorder. Physical aggression was present in 50% of the admitted clients, significantly more than in the non-admitted clients (30%) (Bouras and Holt, 2000). Physical aggression, whether related to psychiatric diagnosis, as in our service, or not (Davidson *et al.*, 1994), seems to be an important factor for determining admission.

The model of Community Specialist Mental Health Services has most of the advantages of the residential units without being tied to buildings and it is distinctly different from the residential model based in the grounds of an institution described by Day (1994). It also has limitations. Generic services have experienced increasing pressure on beds for acute admissions, so that their facilities may offer a hostile environment for vulnerable people, as discussed earlier. In particular, they are unsuitable for people with severe learning disability, or for those who require a long period of admission or secure accommodation.

To address these issues, the Community Specialist Mental Health Service is to be strengthened by the development of a specialist in-patient admission unit (as an extension of the generic mental health admission service), community houses with specialist support and a centre providing training, research and development in 'dual diagnosis'. Admissions for assessment and treatment of psychiatric disorders still remain a serious problem for both learning disabilities and mental health services. The prevalence data of psychiatric disorders among people with learning disabilities would predict higher psychiatric in-patient care utilization. In Sweden, Gustaffson

(1997), however, found a lower frequency of psychiatric care utilization by this client group as compared with the general population. People with mild learning disabilities had longer periods of admission, regardless of living arrangements or diagnosis.

A national debate was sparked recently in The Netherlands by the failure to find suitable care for a teenage girl with mild learning disabilities after a newspaper revealed that she had been kept in restraints in a psychiatric unit for several weeks (Sheldon, 1999). The problem had arisen because of the lack of in-patient psychiatric facilities for people with learning disabilities and psychiatric disorders. In addition to problems with psychiatric admissions, other areas that have been neglected are residential and other community support services such as daytime activities and employment opportunities for people with learning disabilities and mental health needs. Most existing community facilities do not have the expertise to support people with learning disabilities who have complex needs. Staff find working with people with learning disabilities and mental health problems stressful. Giving them skills in this area so that, with support, they can manage people with challenging behaviour and mental illness enables them to find this work more rewarding. The most basic and vital role of support staff in this context is the awareness that a person with learning disabilities may suffer a mental illness, as we all may. They need to be aware of the range of therapeutic options that might be helpful, including environmental changes, behavioural strategies, psychotherapeutic techniques, drugs, etc. A fuller knowledge and consideration of this topic will help to dispel myths and prejudices, for example that medication is to be avoided at all costs, or that its use signifies that staff have in some way failed the client.

Specific knowledge about some disorders will provide insights into why and how interventions must be tailored around someone's strengths and needs (e.g. someone with autistic spectrum disorder may hit himself when his routine is changed). The intervention chosen may be to provide a timetable which the staff and client follow. Flexible training materials, which can be used by staff groups in their own settings, are now available. The training package in the Mental Health of Learning Disabilities (Bouras and Holt, 1997) has been developed along these lines, with materials provided to run a series of workshops encouraging active participation in individual and group activities, some based on information provided and some based on participants' experience. A handbook (Holt and Bouras, 1997a) for reference and further reading accompanies the package for use by workshop facilitators and others if they wish. A video, Making Links (Holt and Bouras, 1997b), complements the package.

Further changes

The emphasis on a community-based, non-institutional service model has meant that deficiencies in the system are much more overt, and clear action has to be taken to address them. Community services cannot rely on the structures and 'safety' of long-stay hospitals to contain their problems or mask poor quality. They also require that specialist staff working in them are clear about their function and competent in their skills (Holt and Joyce, 1999).

The Royal College of Psychiatrists Council Report 'Meeting the Mental Health Needs of People with Learning Disability' (1996) recommended the development of specialist mental health teams to ensure co-ordinated services and effective liaison and integration with other agencies. It seems that even this report has not facilitated the interface between learning disabilities and mainstream mental health services. Nor has the increasing tendency to 'joint commissioning' of services by health and social services together appeared to have had any positive effect. This can be understood within the context of a paradox in the organization of learning disabilities services. Learning disabilities services, with very few exceptions, continue to commission and provide specialist mental health services separately, in isolation from mainstream mental health services. Although this structure might be appro-

priate where there remain long-stay NHS facilities or hospital-based specialized units, it is not workable in community-based learning disabilities services, which are usually small organizations.

At the time of writing, new changes are pending in the UK with the introduction of GP-based Primary Care Groups. These groups, made up of several general practices, will purchase services for a defined population, probably of 100 000–200 000 people. The potential effect on learning disabilities services is not known. There also seem to be important reconfigurations of services underway in several areas. Perhaps this is an opportunity for improving the interface between specialist learning disabilities mental health and mainstream mental health services. A recent publication by the NHS Executive offers a comprehensive overview of services for people with learning disabilities services including mental health services (NHS Executive, 1998). This might act as a platform for action by commissioners and providers of services. Unfortunately, it is unlikely to attract the interest of mainstream mental health services, which will see the problem as only relating to learning disabilities services. As long as the mental health problems of people with learning disabilities are not addressed at a policy level by all those concerned with psychiatric services, very little progress can be expected.

Towards a conceptual framework

A conceptual framework for mental health services for people with learning disabilities is important and needs to be developed. The principles of a matrix model suggested for adult mental health services by Tansella and Thornicroft (1998) can be applied to mental health in learning disabilities services. This model has two dimensions: a geographical, which refers to three levels (country/region, local and patient) and a temporal, which refers to three phases (input, processes and outcomes). Using these two dimensions, a matrix is constructed that focuses on critical issues for mental health services. Such a system could be useful at an organizational level and assist clinicians, commissioners and providers of services and researchers in designing, monitoring and evaluating services. The mental health issues relating to people with learning disabilities are multi-faceted and need to be seen within an understandable framework such as that provided by the matrix system (Moss *et al.*, 2000).

Using the matrix system for a person with learning disabilities and a psychiatric disorder, the reduction of symptoms would not only be related to the quality of treatment, but also to the availability of specialist services and to the expenditure on service and service eligibility criteria at a national level. A research programme based on this conceptual framework is being carried out in five European countries as part of the BIOMED II programme of the European Commission. This project examines the applicability of the proposed matrix model in the participant countries (Holt *et al.*, 2000).

Conclusion

After several years of community care for people with learning disabilities, a national assessment is required to clarify the direction of service developments, and to identify strengths and weakness. Goals must be set for service provision, and to improve service quality and value for money (Perry *et al.*, 1998). Standard setting (such as National Service Frameworks) will provide guidance. (National Service Frameworks have been developed in the UK for a number of health areas. They set out standards for services to achieve.) Such an exercise should estimate the service and resource implications of the mental health problems and/or challenging behaviour for the wide range of people with learning disabilities (severe to mild including those falling in the borderline area).

There is also a need for high quality research to be conducted in the area of mental health in learning disabilities (Moss *et al.*, 1997). Some topics of particular interest include the interaction of biological and environmental factors in the aetiology of mental health problems, the recognition of mental illness in the community, treatment methods (including psychopharmacology and psychological treatments such as cognitive behavioural treatments) and service evaluations.

References

Allen, D. (1989) The effects of deinstitutionalisation on people with mental handicaps. A review. *Mental Handicap Research*, 2, 18–37.

Allen, D. (1998) Changes in admissions to a hospital for people with intellectual disabilities following the development of alternative community services. *Journal of Applied Research in Intellectual Disabilities*, 11, 156–165.

Allen, D. and Felce, D. (1998) Service responses to challenging behaviour. In: Bouras, N. (ed.), *Psychiatric and Behavioural Disorders in Developmental Disabilities and Mental Retardation*. Cambridge: Cambridge University Press, pp. 279–294.

American Psychiatric Association (1991) *Psychiatric Services to Adult Mentally Retarded and Developmentally Disabled Persons: Task Force Report 30.* Washington, DC: American Psychiatric Association.

Bailey, N. and Cooper, S.-A. (1998) NHS beds for people with learning disabilities. *Psychiatric Bulletin*, 22, 69–72.

Beecham, J., Knapp, M., McGilloway, S., Donnelly, M., Kavanagh, S., Fenyo, A. and Mays, N. (1997) The cost-effectiveness of community care for adults with learning disabilities leaving long-stay hospital in Northern Ireland. *Journal of Intellectual Disability Research*, 41, 30–41.

Borthwick-Duffy, S.A. (1994) Epidemiology and prevalence of psychopathology in people with mental retardation. *Journal of Consulting and Clinical Psychology*, 62, 17–27.

Borthwick-Duffy, S.A. and Eyman, R.K. (1990) Who are the dually diagnosed? *American Journal of Mental Retardation*, 94, 586–595.

Bouras, N. and Drummond, C. (1992) Behaviour and psychiatric disorders of people with mental handicaps, living in the community. *Journal of Intellectual Disability Research*, 36, 349–357.

Bouras, N. and Holt, G. (eds) (1997) *Mental Health in Learning Disability Training Package*, 2nd edn. Brighton: Pavilion Publishing.

Bouras, N. and Holt, G. (2000) The planning and provision of psychiatric services for people with mental retardation. In: Lopez-Ibor Jr, J.J. and Andreasen, C. (eds), *The New Oxford Textbook of Psychiatry*. Oxford: Oxford University Press.

Bouras, N. and Szymanski, L. (1997) Services for people with mental retardation and psychiatric disorders: US–UK comparative overview. *International Journal of Social Psychiatry*, 43, 64–71.

Bouras, N., Brooks, D. and Drummond, C. (1994) Community psychiatric services for people with mental retardation. In: Bouras, N. (ed.), *Mental Health in Mental Retardation*. Cambridge: Cambridge University Press, pp. 293–299.

Crews, W.D., Jr, Bonaventura, S. and Rowe, F. (1994) Dual diagnosis prevalence of psychiatric disorders in a large state residential facility for individuals with mental retardation. *American Journal of Mental Retardation*, 98, 724–731.

Davidson, P.W., Cain, N.N., Sloane-Reeves, J.E., Van Speybroech, A., Segel, J., Gutkin, J., Quijano. L.E. and Kramer, B.M. (1994) Characteristics of community-based individuals with mental retardation and aggressive behavioral disorders. *American Journal on Mental Retardation*, 98, 704–716.

Davidson, P., Morris, D. and Cain, N. (1998) Community services for people with dual diagnosis and psychiatric or severe behaviour disorders. In: Bouras, N. (ed.), *Psychiatric and Behavioural Disorders in Developmental Disabilities and Mental Retardation*. Cambridge: Cambridge University Press, pp. 359–372.

Day, K. (1994) Psychiatric services in mental retardation: generic of specialised provision? In: Bouras, N. (ed.), *Mental Health in Mental Retardation*. Cambridge: Cambridge University Press, pp. 275–292..

Day, K. (1998) Professional training in the psychiatry of mental retardation in the United Kingdom. In: Bouras, N. (ed.), *Psychiatric and Behavioural Disorders in Developmental Disabilities and Mental Retardation*. Cambridge: CambridgeUniversity Press, pp. 439–457.

Department of Health (1989) *Needs and Responses: Services for Adults with Mental Handicap Who are Mentally Ill, Who Have Behaviour Problems and Who Offend*. London: HMSO.

Department of Health (1992) *Health Services for People with Learning Disabilities (Mental Handicap)*. HSG (92)42. London: HMSO.

Department of Health (1993) *Challenging Behaviours and/or Mental Health Needs of People with Learning Disabilities. (Mansell Report)*. HMSO. London

Department of Health (1994) Official working group on services for people with special needs. Chairman: J. Reed. *Review of Health and Social Services for Mentally Disordered Offenders and Others Requiring Similar Services, Vol. 7, People with Learning Disabilities (Mental Handicap) or with Autism*. London: HMSO.

Doody, G.A., Johnstone, E.C., Sanderson, T.L., Cunningham Owens, D.G. and Muir, W.J. (1998) 'Pfopfschizophrenie' revisited. *British Journal of Psychiatry*, 173, 145–153.

Dreissen, G., DuMoulin, M., Haveman, M.J. and van Os, J. (1997) Persons with intellectual disability receiving psychiatric treatment. *Journal of Intellectual Disability Research*, 41, 512–518.

Emerson, E. (1995) *Challenging Behaviour. Analysis and Intervention in People with Learning Difficulties*. Cambridge: Cambridge University Press, pp. 4–10.

Emerson, E. and Hatton, C. (1995) *Moving Out. Relocation from Hospital to Community*. London: HMSO.

Emerson, E. and Hatton, C. (1998) Residential provision for people with intellectual disabilities in England, Wales and Scotland. *Journal of Applied Research in Intellectual Disabilities*, 1, 1–14.

Felce, D. (1994) Costs, quality and staffing in services for people with severe learning disabilities. *Journal of Mental Health*, 3, 495–506.

Fryers, T. (1993) Epidemiological thinking in mental retardation: issues in taxonomy and population frequency. *International Review of Research in Mental Retardation*, 19, 97–133.

Gravestock, S. and Bouras, N. (1997) Survey of services for adults with learning disabilities. *Psychiatric Bulletin*, 21, 197–199.

Gustafsson, C. (1997) The prevalence of people with intellectual disability admitted to general hospital psychiatric units. *Journal of Intellectual Disability Research*, 41, 519–526.

Haney, J.I. (1998) Empirical support for deistitutionalisation. In: Heal, L.W. *et al.* (eds), *Integration of Developmentally Disabled Individuals into Community*. Baltimore, MD: Paul H. Brooks, pp. 123–144.

Hatton, C., Emerson, E. and Kiernan, C. (1995) People in institutions in Europe. *Mental Retardation*, 33, 132.

Hillery, J. (1998) Integrating models of challenging behaviour. *Journal of Intellectual Disability Research*, 42, 325–327.

Holt, G. and Bouras, N. (eds) (1997a) *Mental Health in Learning Disabilities: Handbook*, 2nd edn. Brighton: Pavilion Publishing.

Holt, G. and Bouras, N. (eds) (1997b) *Making Links*. Brighton: Pavilion Publishing.

Holt, G. and Joyce, J. (1999) Mental health and challenging behaviour services. *Tizard Learning Disabilities Review*, 4(2), 6–13.

Holt, G., Costello, H., Bouras, N., Diareme, S., Hillery, H., Moss, S., Salvador, L., Tsiantis, J., Weber, G. and Dimitrakaki C. (2000): BIOMED-MEROPE Project: service provision for adults with mental retardation: a european commission. *Journal of Intellectual Disability Research*, 44, 520–534.

Jacobson, J. (1998) Dual diagnosis services: history, progress and perspectives. In: Bouras, N. (ed.), *Psychiatric and Behavioural Disorders in Developmental Disabilities and Mental Retardation*. Cambridge: Cambridge University Press, pp. 327–358.

Kon, Y. and Bouras, N. (1997) Psychiatric follow-up and health services utilisation for people with learning disabilities. *British Journal of Developmental Disabilities*, 84, 20–26.

Linaker, O.M. and Nottestad, J.A. (1998) Health and health services for the mentally retarded before and after the reform. *Tidsskirft for Den Norske Laegeforening*, 118, 357–361.

McLaren, J. and Bryson, S E. (1987) Review of recent epidemiological studies of mental retardation: prevalence, associated disorders, and etiology. *American Journal of Mental Retardation*, 92, 243–254.

Moss, S., Emerson, E., Bouras, N. and Holland, A. (1997) Mental disorders and problematic behaviours in people with intellectual disability: future directions for research. *Journal of Intellectual Disability Research*, 41, 440–447.

Moss, S., Bouras, N. and Holt, G. (2000). Mental health services for people with intellectual disabilities: a conceptual framework. *Journal of Intellectual Disability Research*, 44, 97–107.

NHS Executive (1998) *Signposts for Success in Commissioning and Providing Health Services for People with Learning Disabilities*. Wetherby: Department of Health.

Patterson, T., Higgins, M. and Dyck, D.G. (1995) A collaborative approach to reduce hospitalization of developmentally disabled clients with mental illness. *Psychiatric Services*, 48, 243–247.

Perry, J., Beyer, S., Felce, D. and Todd, S. (1998) Strategic service change: development of core services in Wales, 1983–1995. *Journal of Applied Research in Intellectual Disabilities*, 11, 15–33.

Piachaud, J. (1999) Mental health in learning disabilities services issues. *Tizard Learning Disabilities Review*, 4(2), 47–48.

Raitasuo, S., Taiminen and Salokangas, R.K.R. (1999a) Characteristics of persons with intellectual disability admitted to psychiatric inpatient treatment. *Journal of Intellectual Disabilities Research*, in press.

Raitasuo, S., Taiminen and Salokangas, R.K.R. (1999b) The inpatient care and it's outcome in a specialist psychiatric unit for intellectually disabled persons. *Journal of Intellectual Disabilities Research*, in press.

Reiss, S. (1994) *Handbook of Challenging Behavior: Mental Health Aspects of Mental Retardation*. Worthington, OH: IDS Publishing Co., pp. 4–5.

Russell, O. (1997) Historical overview: concepts and concerns. In: *Seminars in the Psychiatry of Learning Disabilities*. London: Gaskell, pp. 1–15.

Robertson, D and Murphy, D. (1998) Brain imaging and behaviour. In: Bouras, N. (ed.), *Psychiatric and Behavioural Disorders in Developmental Disabilities and Mental Retardation*. Cambridge: Cambridge University Press, pp. 49–70.

Royal College of Psychiatrists (1996) *Meeting the Mental Health Needs of Adults with Mild Learning Disabilities*. London: Royal College of Psychiatrists.

Sheldon, T. (1999) Dutch crisis in care of learning disabilities. *British Medical Journal*, 318, 78.

Van Os, J., Jones, P., Lewis, G. and Murray, R.M. (1997) Development risk factors for affective disorder in a general population birth cohort. *Archives of General Psychiatry*, 54, 625–631.

Tansella, M. and Thornicroft, G. (1998) A conceptual framework for mental health services: the matrix model. *Psychological Medicine*, 28, 503–508.

Wing, L. (1989) *Hospital Closure and the Resettlement of Residents*. Aldershot: Avebury.

Wolfensberger, W. (1969) The original nature of our institutional models. In: Kugel, R. and Wolfensberger, W. (eds), *Changing Patterns in Residential Services for the Mentally Retarded*. Washington, DC: President's Committee on Mental Retardation.

Wolfensberger, W. (1991) Reflections on a lifetime in human services and mental retardation. *Mental Retardation*, 29, 1–16.

World Health Organisation (1996) ICD-10 Guide for mental retardation. Geneva.

Xenitidis, I.K., Henry, J., Russell, A. J., Ward, A. and Murphy, D.G.M. (1999) An inpatient treatment model for adults with mild intellectual disabilities and challenging behaviour. *Journal of Intellectual Disabilities Research*, in press.

34 | *Primary care*

David Goldberg, Anthony Mann and Andre Tylee

Introduction

In the early days of community psychiatry, it was once suggested that GPs would largely concern themselves with mood disorders and social problems, in contrast to those in the community psychiatric services, who would be dealing with the severe mental illnesses (Bennett, 1973). This dichotomy is not true; psychiatric disorders in primary care can be both severe and persisting, and a substantial proportion of those with severe mental illnesses can be dealt with by the primary care team (OPCS, 1995; Goldberg and Gournay, 1998). In this chapter, we emphasize present conditions in the UK, but it must be appreciated that conditions elsewhere in the world vary widely (Üstün and Sartorius, 1995). However, in the developing world, it has been World Health Organization policy for some time to treat severe as well as common mental disorders in primary care (WHO, 1975), so perhaps in this respect the developed world is catching up with developing countries.

The National Morbidity Survey indicated that 16% of the UK population, between 16 and 64 in any one week, suffers from a neurotic disorder, consisting of mixed anxious depression (7.7%), various anxiety states (5%), pure depressive episodes (2.1%) and obsessive–compulsive disorder (1.2%) (OPCS, 1995). A further 4% suffer from alcohol dependence in a given year, 2.2% from drug dependence and 0.4% from a psychosis. At least 95% of the population is registered with a GP and over 60% will consult each year. Thus, the GP and the primary care team will be exposed to much psychiatric morbidity during consultations.

The World Health Organization collaborative study of psychiatric disorders in general medical settings gives an indication of the rates of mental disorders amongst consecutive attenders (Üstün and Sartorius, 1995). Six general practices in central Manchester contributed the UK data to this international project. The interviews showed that 26% of attenders in Manchester had at least one psychiatric disorder diagnosed, according to ICD-10 criteria. The estimated prevalence of these diagnoses were: current depression 16.9%; neurasthenia 9.7%; and generalized anxiety disorder 7.1%. Dysthymia, hypochondriasis, agoraphobia and panic disorder were also present in between 0.5 and 4% of attenders. In addition to these rates among adults, 23% of children who were consecutive attenders aged between 7 and 12 years were diagnosed with psychiatric morbidity consisting, in approximately equal parts, of emotional, conduct or mixed disorders (Garralda and Bailey, 1986). One-third of adolescents have a psychiatric disorder. Most children and adolescents who present with physical symptoms and concurrent psychiatric disorders go unrecognized (Garralda, 1994). The situation in the 15 cities studied by the WHO varied a good deal: in South America (Rio de Janeiro and Santiago de Chile), prevalence rates were very high, while in Shanghai and Nagasaki they were much lower than the world average.

These psychological disorders are associated with considerable disability: indeed, in the WHO study the disability due to psychological disorders exceeded that due to physical illness. This level of disability was similar to that obtained if the patient's own self-report was used as the measure. There was no symptom threshold where disability rapidly increased: instead, disability increases in a linear fashion with the number of symptoms a patient has, and also varies with time as symptoms come and go (Ormel *et al.*, 1993).

Longitudinal studies in primary care are relatively rare, particularly those that consider the whole range of psychiatric morbidity. Mann *et al.* (1981) reported a 1-year follow-up of a 100 patients with diagnosed neurotic disorders and found that 48% still met case criteria after 1 year. Over the follow-up period, 24% recovered early, 52% had run an intermittent course, while 25% had shown persistent symptoms throughout the whole follow-up period.

Relating psychological morbidity in primary care to that seen in specialist care

The Goldberg–Huxley model relates morbidity in primary care to that in the community on the one hand, and that seen by the mental health services on the other. It consists of five levels, each of which are separated from the next by a filter, and it is illustrated in Table 34.1. At each level, we show the annual period prevalence for all mental disorders in Manchester, UK. Comparable figures have been calculated for Groningen, The Netherlands and Seattle, USA (Goldberg, 1995).

It can be seen that rates among consecutive attenders are only slightly less than those found in the community, indicating that most of those with psychological disorders will consult their family doctor in the course of a year. Thus, the first filter (that which determines medical consultation) is fairly permeable. However, the consultation may be for some complaint unrelated to their disorder, or for a somatic symptom which is itself part of the psychological disorder.

Five levels and four filters (from Goldberg and Huxley, 1992)

Level 1   **The community**
All adults who experience an episode of mental disorder in the course of 1 year, satisfying research criteria

260–315/1000/year

First filter

[Illness behaviour]
Level 2   **Primary care attenders (total)**
All adults who experience an episode of mental disorder and seek help from a primary care physician

230/1000/year

Second filter

[Ability to detect disorder]
Level 3   **Primary care attenders (detected: 'conspicuous psychiatric morbidity')**
All adults who are considered mentally disordered by their primary care physician

101.5/1000/year

Third filter

[Referral to mental illness services]
Level 4   **Mental illness services (total)**
All adults treated by the mental illness services during the course of a year

23.5/1000/year

Fourth filter

[Admission to psychiatric beds]
Level 5   **Mental illness services (hospitalized)**
5.71/1000/year

The second filter is passed when the GP recognizes a mental health problem in the patient—although this will often be without a precise ICD-10 diagnosis. At level three, after the second filter, the prevalence rate has fallen, so that on average British GPs identify about 10% of the population registered with them as psychologically disturbed in the course of a year. Those recognized by the GP make up the 'conspicuous' morbidity; in fact, just under half of that estimated to be present in the waiting room population by a two-stage case finding procedure. The undetected morbidity constitutes the 'hidden' psychiatric morbidity in the practice. These undetected patients continue to consult, but an outsider's inspection of notes, prescriptions or even discussion with the relevant doctor will not identify them as patients with psychiatric morbidity. The conspicuous morbidity is that returned in the Morbidity Statistics and is, thus, lower than the true level of morbidity in general practice. Data from the WHO study indicates that these 'undetected illnesses' are on average less severe than those detected by GPs, and have a somewhat better outlook than those detected. The data do not support the view that failure to detect these less severe disorders has serious long-term consequences for the patient (Goldberg *et al.*, 1998).

In the UK, the GP acts as a 'gate-keeper' to mental health care, and the proportion of cases referred to the mental health services is measured by the permeability of the third filter. The figures for Manchester, UK shown in Table 34.1 have been replicated in Groningen, The Netherlands and Seattle, USA (Goldberg, 1995). While rates in the community are fairly similar across the three cities, the ability of patients to go directly to see mental health professionals in Seattle (thus eliminating the third filter) results in a lower rate in general practice, but a higher rate for those seen by mental health professionals.

Mental disorders in primary care compared with those seen by the mental health team

Patients usually present a mixture of physical, psychological and social symptoms, expressed in any order, although somatic symptoms are usually first. Some symptoms are mentioned repeatedly and some are mentioned only in passing. Symptoms left to the end may be the most important of all. Symptoms may not fit a psychiatrist's taxonomy (e.g. 'I feel anyhow'). In primary care, patients often have several concurrent problems of a medical, psychological and social nature. The main problem with the ICD-10 or DSM-IV classifications used by psychiatrists is that they were devised to describe a very different consulting population, they are needlessly complicated and they do not lead directly to management. Most psychologically distressed patients show symptoms of both anxiety and depression. Conventional psychiatric taxonomy deals with this by declaring that these patients are 'co-morbid' for two disorders—most usually major depressive episode and generalized anxiety disorder. GPs themselves rarely emphasize the distinction between the two groups of symptoms, and there appears to be no evidence that any adverse consequences follow this neglect. For the GP, the diagnostic task can be one of separating the symptoms of depression and anxiety from those of an accompanying physical illness, or of probing for psychiatric morbidity in patients, where apparent physical symptoms do not have an organic cause. The WHO has prepared a primary care version of the mental disorders section of the ICD-10, which consists of just 24 conditions which have a reasonably high prevalence in primary care, together with detailed advice on their management—both pharmacological and psychological (Üstün *et al.*, 1995; WHO, 1996). The classification has been customized for the use of local groups of GPs, by also including information about local voluntary agencies and self-help groups to whom the primary care staff can turn in times of need. The ICD-10-PHC classification contains advice on essential information to be given to the patient and the patient's family, for advice to be given to the patient, for the availability of effective drug treatments and the indications for specialist referral. Clearly, these vary from country to country, and WHO allow the primary care staff and mental health professionals to customize the classification to suit conditions in each country.

A preliminary assessment in the UK shows that the system is associated with an increased use of psychological interventions by GPs, although no change in the prescription of antidepressants (Upton *et al.*, 1999). However, British GPs are similar to American GPs in usually prescribing antidepressants rather than benzodiazepines for depressed patients: elsewhere in the world—for example Athens or Verona—depressed patients are most likely to be treated with sedatives.

Computerized self-treatment packages have also been developed for common conditions, and some have been shown to be as effective as treatment by a live clinician (Marks, 1999). They are important because even in developed countries there is a severe shortage of staff able to deliver effective psychological treatments for common mental disorders, and it is likely that there will be still further developments in years to come.

In contrast, most of the patients seen by specialist mental health services have more severe disorders, notably schizophrenias, bipolar illness, dementias and substance abuse. Patients with unipolar depressive disorders are only referred if they have failed to respond to treatment offered in primary care, or if there is thought to be a severe risk of suicide.

Relationships between GPs and psychiatrists

What GPs expect of psychiatrists

GPs expect psychiatrists to possess and exhibit specialized skills not possessed by the primary health care team (PHCT) of assessment and management and to be available when appropriately needed. Because of sheer numbers (in England and Wales there are 12 times as many GPs as psychiatrists), the GP must protect this valuable resource by not overloading it with inappropriate referrals and by obtaining and maintaining certain assessment and management skills that can be used in primary care as well as sharing the care of certain patients whose care is led by secondary care. The GP expects the psychiatrist to provide in-patient care when needed (e.g. in cases of serious self-neglect, suicide intent, etc.) and day-patient facilities to provide a place of care, respite and safety when needed. They can also expect the psychiatrist to use diagnostic facilities and investigations (e.g. scans) as needed and to provide highly specialized treatments when indicated (e.g. ECT). Less frequently, occasions may occur when the GP needs respite from particular doctor–patient relationships for the longer term good (e.g. so-called 'heart-sink' patients). Referral is also sometimes a result of pressure by the relatives or patient.

Access to specialist assessment when appropriate is paramount for a primary care service. GPs are usually not trained in specialist assessment, and therefore to match need to services a psychiatrist, community psychiatric nurse (CPN) or psychologist from the community mental health team (CMHTs) can perform this function —often in a primary care setting or the patient's home. Other CMHTs operate an out-patient clinic (which may be shifted into the surgery). Often 'true consultancy' is being sought by the GP whereby the GP may receive advice only. Other practices operate a joint consultation system whereby the specialist and generalist see the patient together and formulate a plan.

Psychiatric clinics in primary care

In the early 1980s, Strathdee and Williams (1984) described 'the silent growth of a new service', since 19% of English psychiatrists were found to be carrying out various kinds of clinics in primary care. The following year, Pullen and Yellowlees found that half of Scottish psychiatrists were conducting similar clinics. Many of these clinics are little more than 'shifted out-patients' clinics, where the location of the clinic is nearer to the patient's home, and is unstigmatized—so attendance rates are better. Psychiatrists often see community nurses at these clinics who are seeing other patients of the practice, but contact with GPs may be no better than with conventional out-patient clinics. Another problem is that few new patients are seen with this type of clinic—they are mainly those who have been on the psychiatrist's ward. Creed and Marks (1989) described a consultation relationship, in which the psychiatrist sees new patients with the GP, and advises the GP on the patient's future care. This has the advantage that both GP and patient may benefit from the psychiatrist's visit, yet the psychiatrist does not take over the patient's care.

Relationships with community mental health teams

CMHTs are increasingly aligning themselves geographically to PHCTs and may in the future align themselves to primary care groups (PCGs). This improves communication between the two teams particularly if each team has a lead contact. Both teams need to know how best to communicate key information. This may seem fundamental but most inquiries after tragedies, where things have gone wrong, conclude that poor interagency communication had been causative. The teams need to understand each other's roles and responsibilities (aided by multi-professional learning) and develop joint protocols for care.

'Link-workers' between the two services

A problem with psychiatrists providing the relationship with primary care is that they cannot be generalized to the whole set of GPs looking after the psychiatrist's patients—there are simply too many GPs to provide a service to all of them. An alternative relationship between the two services is for keyworkers in the CMHTs to arrange their caseloads so that they are looking after patients cared for by, say, only two GPs. The link-worker acts as a 'culture carrier' between the two services, and makes sure that patients needing services from other members of the CMHT obtain them. The relationship with the GPs is much closer than

with the more usual arrangements (Goldberg and Gournay, 1998). It is possible for these workers—who are usually nurses—either to see patients in their homes, or to have their own clinics in primary care.

Shared care registers and shared care plans

A shared care register is usually a computerized record of all patients jointly cared for by the two services. It might consist of all those who have been discharged from hospital in the past 2 years, all those who have been on a psychotropic drug for longer than a year, and all psychotic patients known to the GP, who have not had an admission to hospital. The record gives information about the keyworker, out-patient clinics are held in the surgeries, and 'good practice protocols' may be developed so that the case register can be audited against what other teams agree is good clinical practice (Strathdee, 1993).

'Shared care plans' follow on from this development. Such a plan gives the primary care staff information about symptoms which they may expect while the patient is well, likely symptoms in relapse, the name of the keyworker and full details of who to contact in an emergency, both during the day and at night. The plan makes clear who is responsible for medication, and gives an acceptable alternative should the GP find it necessary to vary the medication. It is essential that these plans are mutually agreed between the two teams, rather than being imposed by one team on the other.

A recent multi-professional working group published consensus views about the shared care of schizophrenia (Burns and Kendrick, 1997) whether in a crisis or in planning shared care. Another expectation is of shared training and transmission of skills (e.g. in training and supervising PHCT staff in administering depot medication and assessing mental state concurrently). One way of highlighting skills deficits can be by using critical incident analysis (e.g. discussing suicides or suicide attempts). Mental Health Trusts are also increasingly appointing GPs onto their boards to ensure better communication.

Counselling in primary care

In primary care, the entire spectrum of mental health problems is seen and at the mildest end this includes worry, grief, emotional reactions to physical illness or threat of it, or events such as the loss of a job. GPs have reported a noticeable increase in patient demand for counselling and psychological treatment that could not be met by secondary services (Department of Health, 1996). Many GPs have responded to the difficulties of obtaining psychological services for these patients by employing counsellors, counselling psychologists, clinical psychologists, psychotherapists and CPNs within their practices, and in the early 1990s around a third of practices declared someone who provided counselling in the practice (Sibbald *et al.*, 1993). The number of personnel who provide counselling in primary care has grown rapidly mainly because such patients would not be a priority in the psychiatric services, yet they have needs which cannot be met within a 10-minute GP consultation either through a real or perceived lack of GP skills, or insufficient time available. Generalists need to use listening skills and within the confines of everyday consultations help their patients formulate problem lists and apply problem solving as well as help their patients come to terms with insoluble problems. Such patient needs are ubiquitous, and the public prefers to be listened to rather than to receive pills, as a majority consider these to be addictive (Paykel *et al.*, 1998). Public satisfaction with counselling is also found in primary care randomized controlled trials of counselling which have been unable so far to demonstrate any benefit over 'treatment as usual' by GPs (Friedli *et al.*, 1997; Harvey *et al.*, 1998). Such studies also demonstrate satisfaction amongst GPs, possibly because they gain respite from that patient for a while. However, resources are finite, and the mental health needs of those with moderate and severe mental illness are often not being met. It is essential that primary care counselling services adopt more clearly defined protocols and are properly managed, organized, supervised, monitored and evaluated.

Needs for more formal psychological therapy, such as cognitive therapy, should be recognized and met, which will entail a close working relationship with psychological services and shared training. Many attenders in primary care have moderate mental health problems that could become disabling and chronic if undertreated. Well proven psychological treatments for this large group can be provided by clinical psychologists, nurse therapists and CPNs. Such services, however, because of high prevalence of disorder and low manpower, vary in availability to primary care yet need to be essentially primary care led, perhaps by finding an enhanced role for primary care nurses with referral as appropriate to secondary care services (Goldberg and Gournay, 1997).

Patients with severe and enduring mental illness such as schizophrenia, bipolar disorder, dementia and 'treatment-resistant' depression are best managed by the community mental health services with assistance from primary care. Examples of such assistance would be the provision of generalist medical services such as cervical cytology, helping with patient review, providing medication, watching for signs of deterioration and relapse and notifying CMHTs of any changes (Burns and Kendrick, 1997; Bebbington and Tylee, 1998).

The role of the primary care nurse

Practice nurses are involved increasingly in sharing the care of mental illness in primary care, mainly in the chronic disease management of the common mental disorders such as depression and anxiety, but increasingly with the severely mentally ill. Such collaboration often follows a similar pattern to the chronic disease management of conditions such as asthma and diabetes, although unlike for these other two conditions, in the UK there is as yet no financial reward for doing so. Practice nurses undertaking such work need proper training and supervision yet are still often required to administer depot medication without such training and support. Expecting an untrained practice nurse to administer depot without support and training is unacceptable—

training is needed in how to: give the injection, review the suitability of this form of medication, monitor for side effects, assess mental state for signs of deterioration, when to involve colleagues or refer to the CMHT, and crisis management. The mental health training needs of primary care nurses are therefore being recognized increasingly. Practice nurses potentially have a key role in the management of the common mental disorders in primary care (Goldberg and Gournay, 1997) unless there is a dramatic increase in the numbers of CPNs, psychologists and nurse therapists.

Practice nurses increasingly collaborate with other primary care nurses (community nurses, health visitors, nurse practitioners, midwives, CPNs, etc.) in integrated nursing teams. In such teams, they can tailor individual skills to patient need but also attempt to avoid duplication so that a patient is not being seen concurrently by two or three nurses when one would do. Health visitors trained in counselling have been shown to benefit women with postnatal depression (Holden *et al.*, 1989), and Appleby and colleagues (1997) have targeted the same group of patients with a nurse-led intervention.

Future patterns of service

In the past, psychiatry was practised in asylums; more recently in departments of the general hospital. In the future, we must look to a situation in which specialized mental health teams are working closely with primary care teams. Psychiatry in general practice is here to stay. Seen from the vantage point of the CMHT, the PHCT team should and could be an extension of their services, and close collaboration between the two is highly desirable. In the UK, purchasing of health care will progressively be done by PCGs, which is likely to have major implications for mental health care. GPs are likely to cause more resource to be directed towards staff who can help them in primary care settings, so that we can confidently expect an enlarged mental health role for practice nurses, community nurses and counsellors. The emphasis on evidence-based medicine ought to influence the kinds of psychotherapies made available by coun-

sellors—with a progressive emphasis on structured treatments such as cognitive behaviour therapy, interpersonal therapy and problem solving—and away from non-directive counselling.

At present, there are insufficient trained staff to take this burden, and there is a major training task which is likely to involve both psychologists and psychiatrists. The work of the CMHT with more severely ill patients needs to be co-ordinated more closely with primary care, who do and can take some responsibility for monitoring them. The scale of the training task is formidable but, if successful, a working partnership between the two teams will be the reward. In this way, psychiatry will remain in touch with a wide range of psychological problems, rather than being marginalized and confined to the care of the dangerous and the disruptive—which would represent a return to the alienism with which the 20th century began.

References

Appleby, L., Warner, R., Whitton, A. and Faragher, B. (1997) A controlled study of fluoxetine and cognitive-behavioural counselling in the treatment of postnatal depression. *British Medical Journal*, 134, 932–936.

Bebbington, P. and Tylee, A. (1998) The management of schizophrenia in the community: primary and secondary care. *Primary Care Psychiatry*, 4, 51–62.

Bennett, D.H. (1973) Community mental health services in Britain. *American Journal of Psychiatry*, 130, 1065–1070.

Burns, T., Kendrick, T. (1997) The primary care of patients with schizophrenia: a search for good practice. *British Journal of General Practice*, 144, 593–620

Creed, F. and Marks, B. (1989) Liaison psychiatry in general practice: a comparison of the liaison attachment scheme and the shifted out-patients models. *Journal of the Royal College of General Practitioners*, 39, 514–517

Department of Health (1996) *NHS Psychotherapy Services in England: Review of Strategic Policy*. London: Department of Health.

Friedli, K., King, M.B., Lloyd, M. and Horder, J. (1997) Randomised controlled assessment of non-directive psychotherapy versus routine general practitioner care. *Lancet*, 350, 1662–1665.

Garralda, M.E. and Bailey, D. (1986) Children with psychiatric disorders in primary care. *Journal of Child Psychology and Psychiatry*, 27, 611–624.

Garralda, E. (1994) *Primary Care Psychiatry*. In *Child and Adolescent Psychiatry* (ed. Rutter, M., Hersor, L., Taylor, E.). Oxford: Blackwell Science

Goldberg, D.P. (1995) Epidemiology of mental disorder in primary care. *Epidemiologic Reviews*, 17, 182–190

Goldberg, D. and Gournay, K. (1997) *The General Practitioner, the Psychiatrist and the Burden of Mental Health Care*. Maudsley Discussion Document. London: Maudsley.

Goldberg, D. and Huxley, P. (1992) *Common Mental Disorders. A Biosocial Model*. London: Routledge.

Goldberg, D.P., Privett, M., Ustun, B., Simon, G. and Linden, M. (1998) The effects of detection and treatment on the outcome of major depression in primary care: a naturalistic study in 15 cities. *British Journal of General Practice*, in press.

Harvey, C.A., Pantelis, C., Taylor, J. *et al.* (1998) The Camden schizophrenia surveys. II: high prevalence of schizophrenia in an inner London borough and its relationship to socio-demographic factors. *British Journal of Psychiatry*, 168, 418–426.

Holden, J.M., Sagovsky, R. and Cox, J.L. (1989) Counselling in a general practice setting: controlled study of health visitor intervention in treatment of postnatal depression. *British Medical Journal*, 298, 223–226.

Mann, A.H., Jenkins, R. and Belsey, E. (1981) The twelve-month outcome of patients with neurotic illness in general practice. *Psychological Medicine*, 11, 535–550.

Marks, I. (1999) Computer aids to mental health care. *Canadian Journal of Psychiatry*, 44, 548–555.

OPCS (Office of Population Censuses and Surveys) (1995) *The Prevalence of Psychiatric Morbidity Among Adults Living in Private Households*. Report 1. HMSO: London.

Ormel, J., Von Korff, M., Van den Brink, W., Katon, W., Brilman, E. and Oldehinkel, T. (1993) Depression, anxiety and social disability show synchrony of change. *American Journal of Public Health*, 83, 385–390

Paykel, E.S., Hart, D. and Priest R.G. (1998) Changes in public attitudes to depression during the Defeat Depression Campaign. *British Journal of Psychiatry*, 173, 519–522.

Sibbald, B., Addington-Hall, J., Brenneman, D. and Freeling, P. (1993) Counsellors in English and Welsh general practices; their nature and distribution. *British Medical Journal*, 306, 29–33.

Strathdee, G. (1993) *The Nunhead Service: A Community Mental Health Service with a Focus on Primary Care*. PRiSM Occasional Paper 13. London: Institute of Psychiatry

Strathdee, G. and Williams, P. (1984) A survey of psychiatrists in primary care: the silent growth of a new service. *Journal of the Royal College of General Practitioners*, 34, 615–618

Upton, M.W., Evans, M., Goldberg, D.P. and Sharp, D.J. (1999) Evaluation of ICD10-PHC mental health guidelines in detecting and managing depression in primary care. *British Journal of Psychiatry*, 175, 476–482.

Ustun, T.B. and Sartorius, N. (eds) (1995) *Mental Illness in General Health Care. An International Study*. Chichester: John Wiley and Sons.

Ustun, B., Goldberg, D.P., Cooper, J., Simon, G. and Sartorius, N. (1995) A new classification of mental disorders based upon management for use in primary care. *British Journal of General Practice*, 45, 211–215

World Health Organization (1975) *Organizations of Mental Health Services in Developing Countries*. Sixteenth Report of the WHO Expert Committee. WHO Technical Report Series, 564. Geneva: WHO.

World Health Organization (1996) *Diagnostic and Management Guidelines for Mental Disorders in Primary Care ICD-10*. Chapter V Primary Care Version. Bern: Hogrefe and Huber.

35 | *Developing integrated health and social welfare services*

John Carpenter and Diana Barnes

Introduction

Deinstitutionalization, observed Bachrach (1997), involves not just the decanting of the long-stay hospitals and preventing or diverting potential new admissions, but also the development of community programmes which combine psychiatric services with those providing social support. People living with severe mental illness have multiple and complex needs. They typically require long-term help in coping with the disabling aspects of their illnesses on themselves and their families and with the stigmatizing responses of the societies in which they live. Further, people with mental illness are likely to experience disadvantage on the grounds of social class, unemployment, poverty and homelessness. Many will also experience racial and sexual discrimination within mental health services as well as in the communities where they live. Effective mental health services must address all these issues.

As discussed elsewhere in this volume, community mental health care typically is made up of a patchwork of services, including primary care clinics, community mental health centres, day- and out-patient services, community support and outreach teams, residential and group homes, supported employment, education and training. These services are provided, in different measure and in different proportions in countries of the economically developed world, by a variety of health, social welfare and housing agencies operated by national and local governments, voluntary, not-for-profit, and church organizations, and private companies. This pattern commonly is referred to as the 'welfare mix', or the 'mixed economy of care', and at the end of the 1990s could be observed in all western countries.

This chapter will focus on the relationships within the welfare mix between health and social welfare services for people with severe and long-term mental health problems. We will describe the various ways in which services are funded, noting the discretionary nature of financial support for non-medical services, the restrictive nature of insurance-based systems and how governments have sought to control social welfare costs. We will identify sources of conflict between health and social care workers, arising from different models of mental illness and different approaches to care and treatment. In a search for possible solutions to organizational and interprofessional problems, we will examine attempts to integrate, or at least 'harmonize' health and social services provision in the UK, particularly in relation to models of case management.

Financing social care for people with mental illness

It is important to recognize the variety of models of financing mental health provision in the developed countries (Goodwin, 1997). These may be understood historically, politically and culturally. Two key dimensions may be identified: the relationship between central and local governments and the extent to which services are funded out of general taxation or through sickness and invalidity insurance.

Social welfare services, including social services, supported housing, and leisure and recreation, are generally the responsibility of local government. Central government may, as in the welfare states of Scandinavia and the UK, contribute to their financing directly, as well as through social assistance for those individuals who are unable to support themselves. The balance of contributions and the devolving of financial responsibility from central to local government frequently is a source of tension, as will be seen in the examples of Spain and the UK described below.

The development of a national framework of integrated health and social care services is facilitated in countries where central government takes responsibility for mental health. In the USA, in addition to the federal legislative framework, each state has its own policy and laws which, as Bachrach (1997) points out, local governments (counties) may modify, extend or abridge. Consequently, the organization and coverage of community services vary greatly both within and between states. Further, there are independent mental health services such as the Veterans' Affairs services, and numerous privately owned and operated agencies (behavioural health care organizations) which determine their own policies and services (Freedman, 1990). The result is that whilst some community-based services in the USA are understandably held up as models of excellence in providing locally integrated mental health care, they are the exception rather than the rule. Bachrach (1997) points out that around 40 million Americans have no health insurance of any kind and that even for those who are insured, mental health services are often very limited or even non-existent.

Australia, like the USA, is a federation but, mindful of the limitations of uneven development across the country, in 1992 the federal (Commonwealth) government agreed with the governments of the states a national mental health strategy. The strategy aims to provide an integrated network of community treatment and social support, and annual reports compare performance between states (e.g. Commonwealth of Australia, Department of Health and Family Services, 1998).

The development of community and social models of mental health care has been inhibited in most countries by the discretionary nature of financial support for 'non-medical services'. For example, in Spain, a ministerial committee on psychiatric reform (1985) recommended the development of community-based support services, including primary and community mental health teams (CMHTs), for discharged hospital patients (Poveda, 1987). Responsibility was devolved from provinces to local authorities but, according to Comelles and Hernaez (1994), this ceding of authority was exploited centrally as an opportunity to reduce budgets. Instead, professional psychiatric power was reinforced in university and general hospitals with little funding for community initiatives. Since Spain has not developed a welfare state, social security benefits are low and there are few social services, social care services remain sparse and patients are discharged to the care of their families.

Although the UK has a developed welfare state in which health care services are, at least in theory, available to all, a similar pattern of central and local government relations may be seen in relation to social welfare services. General mental health treatment services, including hospitals, out-patient services and primary care, are funded through general taxation with money disbursed from central government through local health authorities. Local government is responsible for social services and housing, raising money from local taxes and receiving a further amount from central government according to a formula. Long-term community care was funded through a combination of 'dowry' payments from health authorities with respect to people resettled from hospitals and, until 1993, social security payments to individuals provided by central government. Social security payments for residential care had been rising at a rate which alarmed central government and, it was argued, services were not being allocated on the basis of an adequate assessment of need. This was one of the factors which led to changes in the financing of community care (Beecham *et al.*, 1996), with the assessment of individual needs and the responsibility for purchasing of services being transferred to local authority social services departments. The additional money which was made available to local government soon proved inadequate to the task, and social services were forced to introduce tight 'eligibility criteria' (i.e. restricting services to those with severe disabilities) in addition to means testing in order to contain costs (Lewis *et al.*, 1997). Further, central government proceeded to impose general spending limits on local authorities, declined to safeguard (ring-fence) community care budgets and penalized any attempts to raise additional funds through local taxes. Consequently, annual social services per capita expenditure on mental health services in the UK varies by a factor of 10, between £3 and £30 per head. However, the majority of local authorities spend less than £9 per head of population per year (Barnes, 1998).

In Sweden, which is another much quoted example of a welfare state, hospitals have been the responsibility of local government county councils since 1967. Social welfare services, including financial support for people with mental illness and housing, are the responsibility of local communities (Brink, 1994). These district level authorities are required to pay the costs of institutional care for voluntary patients who have stayed in hospital for over 6 months in the previous 3 years. This provides an incentive to assess needs and develop support systems. In a move with similarities to the community care legislation in the UK (Department of Health, 1989), a 1994 law gave people with a 'lowered level of functioning', including those with mental illness, the right to an assessment of need for treatment and support. Social services were required to engage in case finding and to provide outreach services, group homes or supported accommodation, and activities for those who cannot take up employment. It is not yet clear whether these initiatives will encounter the financial problems experienced in the UK. A Swedish government commission in 1992 found that neither a lack of resources nor ignorance of the health and welfare system caused the failure to provide a good service. Rather, they concluded that the causes lay in poor co-ordination and co-operation, and they blamed the various agencies for looking first to the needs of their own organization (Brink, 1994).

In insurance-based systems, such as Germany and the USA, only medical treatments may be reimbursed. In the USA, this has led to conflict between psychiatrists and other mental health professionals over the definition of treatment. The American Psychiatric Association has resisted the designation of psychologists, clinical social workers and marital and family therapists as treatment providers. Thus insurance policies may provide perverse incentives for in-patient care. Brady *et al.* (1986) reported that many policies in the USA provided a month's full coverage for in-patient treatment, but only 50% of costs for a limited number of out-patient sessions.

Similarly, although all Dutch citizens are required by law to have insurance cover for mental health treatment, this does not cover social care, which is the responsibility of municipal and provincial authorities. These, according to Giel (1987), have not provided sufficient money to fund community support services. Giel reports clashes between hospitals and agencies providing residential care in the community over who should provide for service users.

In Germany, patients in hospital are graded as either 'active treatment' or 'care' cases on the basis of prognosis and length of in-patient stay (Brink, 1994). The former receive sickness insurance, but care cases, including people with severe and enduring mental illness, receive only means-tested social assistance. This lays a long-term financial burden on the family (Hollingsworth, 1992). Community services cannot provide 'treatment'. Local authorities are responsible for 'complementary' care, including counselling and social welfare, and supervised accommodation but, according to Brink (1994), they have hesitated to take on this responsibility in the tighter financial climate which followed reunification.

In Spain, the highest rate of financial return from insurance companies to the hospitals is in the first 10 days of admission. The consequence, according to Comelles and Hernaez (1994), has been brief and multiple admissions to hospital. Spanish psychiatrists are apparently strongly wedded to a biomedical model and receive little or no education in social sciences so that psychiatric intervention takes no account of social needs.

In general, it would appear that because of perverse economic incentives and illogical distinctions between treatment and care, people with enduring mental illness fare less well in insurance-based systems. However, even in taxation-based systems such as the UK, social care services usually carry a means-tested charge. Thus, whilst attendance at a day hospital will be free, service users participating in a very similar programme of activities at a centre run by social services may have to contribute to the cost.

In conclusion, the development of comprehensive services which provide for the social as well as health care needs of people with severe and long-term mental health problems has undoubtedly been hindered by the discretionary nature of financing for social care (and, in some countries, health care) and the reluctance of central and local governments in most countries to assume full responsibility, particularly financial responsibility. However, there are further difficulties in the development of integrated services. These include the different orientations of health and social care professionals involved, difficulties in working in partnership between agencies with different cultures, and practical obstacles to the harmonization of organizational systems.

Interprofessional relations

Difficulties in collaboration between health and social care professionals may arise from different models of mental health and illness, conflicting value systems, divergent approaches to care and treatment, and distinct organizational cultures.

Social workers are trained in a humanistic as distinct from a scientific paradigm, with a knowledge base drawn broadly from the social sciences and typically comprising sociology, social policy, psychology and law as applied to social work practice. There is no requirement to study human biology or health, indeed social workers in the UK, at least, are taught to be wary of the 'medical model'. The medical model is characterized (some would say caricatured) as focusing solely on individual pathology and ignoring the social factors which impact on people's lives. In failing to recognize and counter the 'structural oppressions' of sexism, racism, ageism and disabilism, it is argued, medicine and psychiatry contribute further to oppression (e.g. Thompson, 1993). While many would suggest that this is an extreme view, redolent of the anti-psychiatry movement of the 1960s, it is undoubtedly the case that social workers favour a social model for understanding

the impact of disability in which society's response to an individual is seen as disabling. From this perspective, psychiatry's concern to formulate a diagnosis on the basis of observed signs and symptoms of disease, and thence to prescribe a treatment, is restrictive, to say the least. It curtails enquiry into the social and environmental causes of mental ill health, such as physical, emotional and sexual abuse within families, racial harassment and homelessness. Without an understanding of these factors, the patient becomes identified with the diagnosis, and psychiatric treatment is limited to the suppression of symptoms. A social model, on the other hand, is concerned with the individual service user in the context of his or her family and social relationships and the communities in which they live, and aims to alleviate the socio-economic causes of mental ill health.

In theory at least, social workers are trained to identify strengths and skills rather than focus on pathology and deficits. In the context of case management carried out by social workers in community mental health services in the USA, this has been termed the 'strengths model' (Rapp and Wintersteen, 1989). Social workers in the UK have embraced this approach on the grounds that a focus on an individual's strengths and resources, and how they can be used and developed, is potentially a more participatory and empowering approach (Stevenson and Parsloe, 1993). Further, a strengths model should not ignore the very real handicaps which people with mental illness experience, but should challenge the negative assumptions and discriminatory attitudes and behaviour of health and social service workers (e.g. Broverman *et al.*, 1970). This is not to say that some other mental health professionals would not subscribe to a similar approach, but clearly this is a potential source of conflict. Such conflict is particularly likely over compulsory admissions to hospital, where a social worker's value of 'respect for persons', expressed as a concern for civil liberties and for care in 'the least restrictive environment', may clash with a doctor's value of 'respect for life', expressed in the belief that the need for treatment of the illness predominates (Sheppard, 1991).

Similar interprofessional rivalries have been reported in other European countries (Freeman *et al.*, 1985), Canada (Williams and Luterbach, 1976) and the USA (Thompson, 1994). For example, the American Psychiatric Association reported concerns that the integration of community mental health services would erode the role of psychiatrists, with the medical model being replaced by a social one, and social workers taking the top administrative jobs and 'calling the shots' (APA, 1998).

Huntingdon (1981) has drawn attention to the different occupational cultures of social work and health professionals. Social workers employed by local government agencies may not share the same assumptions about teamworking and medical leadership. They are accountable to senior staff within their own hierarchical and bureaucratic organization rather than to senior health service colleagues. Social class and gender differences between psychiatrists and social workers (predominately a relatively poorly paid, female group) are also likely to play a part in constraining discourse between these professions (Rogers and Pilgrim, 1996, p. 101).

Partnerships between health and social services

The different occupational cultures found in health and social welfare services are, along with the problems of financing discussed, a significant impediment to the development of interagency working. Only when effective partnerships have been established at a local level can structural and organizational issues be tackled.

There have been, over the last 15 years, repeated efforts by the Department of Health in the UK to encourage joint working between health and social services. These have ranged from financial incentives for joint initiatives to legal requirements to produce joint plans for community care services. Major structural change has, however, been ruled out. Successive governments have, except in the case of Northern Ireland, rejected the option of creating a new joint authority for health and social care.

There is, however, some evidence of successful joint working between health and social services. Barnes (1996) reported a study of mental health partnerships in eight localities in the UK. She noted that there were no consistent areas of success; what was achieved in one area was often

Table 35.1 *Requirements for effective partnerships between health and social services*

A shared vision of what community mental health services should try to achieve

An emphasis on action, seeking out and securing early success

Leadership, and commitment at all levels of the respective organizations, including a willingness to take risks

Enabling structures, such as agencies being responsible for planning and operating in the same geographical areas, formal mechanisms for getting together people with the power to make decisions, and information sharing

Interagency understanding of cultures, roles and values

An appreciation of political and financial constraints

A willingness to listen and to communicate clearly and unambiguously

Sharing responsibility, especially when the inevitable problems occur causing difficulties in another. She identified common stimuli for effective partnerships (Table 35.1). Joint training was perceived as an important means of facilitating interprofessional and interagency collaboration. It was required not only on specific issues such as the operation of the care programme approach (see below), but also on issues which would increase basic understanding of agency roles, values, systems and protocols. Training should be planned jointly, jointly attended and be part of an integrated strategy.

Partnerships were easier, Barnes (1996) observed, and significantly more progress had been made in authorities where a clear focus on mental health services had been maintained. Effective partnerships required staff with time and commitment and, in many cases, the appointment or secondment of staff with specific expertise. An important factor was the willingness to prioritize joint work. It is not an optional extra and relationships take time and effort to build up. Nor can partnerships be taken for granted once they are established; they need regular review and regeneration, and a continual commitment must be made to improving communication and co-operation. As Barnes commented, reasons not to co-operate can always be found.

Integrating health and social welfare services

As we have already indicated, a number of countries including Australia, Sweden, the UK and the USA are attempting to improve the co-ordination of community mental health services. At a strategic level, common features of these efforts are the use of financial incentives and the encouragement to form new structures to deliver comprehensive services. At an organizational level, we can see the development of multi-disciplinary and interagency CMHTs. In addition, at the level of service to the individual user, case management systems are being developed for the co-ordination of health and social welfare services.

Financial changes

In the USA, the impetus for integration has emerged as part of 'managed care'. Managed care strategies, according to Mechanic and colleagues (1995), involve financial and organizational arrangements and regulation which have the primary intention of containing costs while ostensibly maintaining quality of service. As Salzer (1999) points out, managed care has gone through a number of transformations with a current emphasis on managed outcomes, where cost savings are emphasized along with the demonstration of service effectiveness. Federal funding of state programmes is to be based on Performance Partnership Grants, where objectives will be assessed through measures of capacity, process and outcomes. States, in turn, are contracting with behavioural health organizations to provide comprehensive, co-ordinated health and welfare services with a stress on alternatives to expensive hospitalization, such as assertive community treatment and home-based services.

In the UK, the government has announced an intention to legislate to remove financial impediments to joint working (Department of Health, 1998). Proposals include pooled budgets, where both agencies put a proportion of their funds into a joint budget; lead commissioning, where one party transfers funds to the other which will then take responsibility for commissioning both health and social care; and integrated provision. Integrated provision, where one organization provides both health and social care, would allow health services to provide social care, or social services to provide community health services. The effectiveness of these arrangements remains to be seen, but it is already clear that they will do nothing to enhance the coherence of interagency relationships nationally, since the government clearly expects local authorities and health services to decide between themselves which, if any, of the arrangements should be applied.

Community mental health teams

CMHTs are discussed in detail in Chapter 39. They are a feature of community mental health services in the USA, Italy, Spain, France, Belgium and The Netherlands as well as the UK (Goodwin, 1997, Chapter 1). They have been promoted by the Department of Health as the 'most effective' way of delivering multi-disciplinary services for people with severe mental illness (Department of Health, 1995, p. 35), although no evidence is offered to support this assertion. Onyett *et al.* (1997) described CMHTs as the main vehicle for co-ordinating health and social care services in the UK. However, the evidence suggests that their development is patchy. Barnes (1999) found that only just over half of social services departments were able to report having one or more CMHTs which were integrated with a health trust. On the other hand, most of the social services teams described as offering community mental health services were separate from health services. There is clearly some way to go in establishing this service model. Setting up integrated teams requires agreeing financial and management arrangements and paying careful attention to goals and operational policies, including clarification of the roles of team members.

The role of the social worker within a multi-disciplinary team may be particularly difficult to establish if there are philosophical differences with psychiatric staff of the kind noted above, together with tensions over professional autonomy. Studies in the UK of multi-disciplinary team functioning and interprofessional attitudes, currently being directed by the authors, show that even in integrated mental health teams, social workers score comparatively poorly in terms of both team and professional identification; they are also less clear about team objectives (Carpenter *et al.*, 1999). Further, social workers consider their status in society to be significantly lower than that of other mental health professionals. They are also inclined to believe that other professionals have a poor opinion of their knowledge and professional competence, significantly lower than is actually the case (Carpenter and Barnes, 1999).

Case management

In the USA, case management has, according to Salzer (1999), received renewed emphasis. In a case management system, service users are assigned a nurse or social worker with responsibility for ensuring access to and co-ordination of the range of care and treatment (see Chapter 21). The assumption is that enhanced co-ordination will improve outcomes and reduce relapse rates, thereby lessening the need for intensive, expensive hospital treatment. The empirical evidence from the USA to support this assumption is not strong however (Rubin, 1992). Nevertheless, early follow-up in the community of patients discharged from hospital has emerged as an important quality indicator.

Similarly in the UK, concern about the poor follow up and co-ordination of care for former patients led to the introduction of the care programme approach (CPA) (Department of Health 1990). The implementation of the CPA, for which health services have the primary responsibility, and its relationship with care management provided by local authorities, provides an interesting case study of the integration of health and social welfare services for people with severe mental health problems. We will draw on data from two complementary surveys of local authorities (Barnes, 1998) and health trusts (Schneider *et al.*, 1999), to explore the extent to which harmonization has been achieved. First, however, we will outline the two approaches and indicate how care management has been implemented in local authorities.

The detailed operation of the CPA was left to local agreement between health authorities and local government social services departments, but central government defined the key elements. These included an integrated approach to assessment and care planning:

- systematic arrangements for assessing the health *and social care needs* of people accepted by specialist psychiatric services [emphasis added.]

- the formulation of a care plan which addresses the identified health *and social care needs*

- the appointment of a keyworker (usually a community mental health nurse or a social worker) to stay in close touch with the patient and monitor care

- regular review (UK Department of Health, 1990),

The underlying principles of the CPA include the involvement of users (patients) and carers, and multi-disciplinary and interagency working. At around the same time, the government resolved that from 1993, local government should be the 'lead agency' responsible for the community care of people with disabilities, including those with mental illness (Department of Health, 1989). This responsibility was to be exercized through the operation of a brokerage model of case management, in which assessment of social care needs and the planning and purchasing of care are separated from the provision of care. The intention was that care managers (as they are called) should not provide the care themselves and thus potential conflicts of interest would be avoided. This model was clearly at variance with the clinical model of case management which underlies the CPA, and there has, understandably, been confusion between the two approaches (Burns, 1997). Further, Onyett (1992, Chapter 4) argued for the importance of case managers developing a close and consistent working relationship with mental health service users who are frequently difficult to engage, and Marshall (1996) pointed out that there was no evidence to support the efficacy for the brokerage model (and some against).

In practice, many local authorities have been reluctant to adopt the brokerage model wholesale, especially the devolving of budgets to front line care managers. Across all service user groups, 64% of departments retained responsibility with managers rather than practitioners (Challis *et al.*, 1998). According to Lewis *et al.* (1997), who studied implementation in five local authorities, reasons for this included a concern to minimize transaction costs and the difficulty of arriving at a formula by which to distribute money to a large number of care managers. As noted above, spending limits on local government have resulted in the introduction of eligibility criteria.

A national survey of local authorities found that 84% had established specific eligibility criteria for mental health services, the majority of which prioritized people with severe and enduring mental illness (Barnes, 1998). As Barnes observes, these are the people who receive priority attention from health services through the CPA (Department of Health, 1995). Costs of care packages are controlled further in 56% of local authorities by means of a weekly 'ceiling' with, in 1997, a mean value across authorities of £229 per week (Challis *et al.*, 1998). The bulk of this expenditure is made up of the costs of residential care, followed by home support and day care.

With the collaboration of a national multi-disciplinary reference group of community mental health service co-ordinators ($n = 135$), Schneider *et al.* (1999) developed a set of criteria for assessing the degree of integration. These include organizational arrangements, mental health teams policies and procedures concerning case management, information systems and joint training (Table 35.2). These criteria were employed to assess the extent of integration between health services trusts and their partner local authorities. Of particular importance are the acceptability of assessments and flexibility of roles.

Barnes (1998) found that assessments made under the CPA were acceptable for the purposes of care management in 59% of 118 local authorities (90% response rate), thus enabling access to social services monies to provide services such as residential care. In a further 24% of local authorities, systems were being developed. This provides a good indicator of interagency working. However, although social workers acted as keyworkers under the CPA in 57% of local authorities, health workers were able to take the role of care manager in less than one-third (31%). Reasons given for nurses not carrying out care management included the lack of appropriate training for community psychiatric nurses (CPNs) on the management of complex care packages and CPNs' reluctance to take on the task, given their high caseloads. The legality of health professionals acting as care managers has also been questioned. However, Parker and Gordon (1998, p. 28) advise that health service employees may, under Section 113 of the Local Government Act 1972, be designated to act for the local authority and to commit the authority's resources.

Table 35.2 *Frequency of positive responses to criteria of integration of interagency approach to care programme approach and care management in England* (Schneider *et al.*, 1999)

Criteria applying to health and social services agencies (some are mutually exclusive)	Percentage yes
Organization arrangements and policy	
Interagency management arrangements for monitoring integration of CPA and care management	66%
Operational co-ordinator for CPA and care management systems	55%
Joint health and social services community mental health team	63%
Separate community teams with a shared base[a]	30%
Shared definition of severe mental illness	64%
Agreed confidentiality policy for exchange of information on patients	60%
Common complaints procedure	22%
Case management processes	
Joint communications strategy to inform public and service users	44%
Consistent initial screening process/forms	55%
Common assessment protocol for CPA and care management	55%
Single care plan agreed between all agencies	75%
Single keyworker able to co-ordinate the work of other professionals	80%
Social services staff can be keyworkers	57%
Social services staff can access health resources	64%
Health staff can access social services resources	46%
Proportion of users with SMI on CPA also on SSD caseloads 60–79%[a]	13%
Proportion of users with SMI on CPA also on SSD caseloads 80%+	17%
Information systems	
Shared information systems on service provision and use, population needs and service commissioning	28%
Shared database for CPA	27%
Shared supervision register of 'at-risk' patients	31%
Joint training of health and social services staff in past 12 months	71%

n = 145 (79% response rate); maximum score 38.

[a]Scores 1, all other indicators score 2.

Using Schneider *et al.*'s (1999) criteria, harmonization scores were calculated for 145 trusts (75% response rate). Overall, the mean score for harmonization was 19.8 (standard deviation 7.5, range 1–35) out of a possible 38. A large variation was found: 13% of trusts and social services departments fulfilled 79% of the harmonization criteria, scoring at least 30 points, but 10% scored less than 10, indicating very little harmonization, and 32% scored less than 20 points. According to this measure, significant progress has been made in some areas but there is some way to go before harmonization can be said to have been achieved nationally in England.

Conclusion

The development of integrated health and social welfare services for people living in the community with severe mental illness has been hindered by a variety of factors. These include the discretionary nature of financial support for social care, interprofessional conflicts over models of mental illness and mental health care, and difficulties in working in partnership between organizations with different cultures. Integration can be fostered through financial change, commitment to interagency working, joint training and organizational developments including CMHTs and case management.

Acknowledgement

We would like to thank Dr Justine Schneider for comments on a draft of this chapter.

References

American Psychiatric Association (1998) Psychiatrists should take leadership roles as public agencies integrate services for mentally ill. *Psychiatric News*, 18 September 1998.

Bachrach, L. (1997) Lessons from the American experience in providing community-based services. In: Leff, J. (ed.), *Care in the Community. Illusion or Reality?* Chichester: Wiley, pp. 21–36.

Barnes, D. (1996) *Effective Partnerships in Mental Health*. University of Durham: Centre for Applied Social Studies.

Barnes, D. (1998) *Local Authority Health and Social Care Joint Working and Interface Issues Survey 1998*. London: Social Services Inspectorate, Department of Health.

Barnes, D., Carpenter, J. and Dickinson C. (2000) Interprofessional Education for Community Mental Health: attitudes to community care and professional stereotypes. *Social Works Education*, 19(6).

Beecham, J., Knapp, M.R.J. and Schneider, J. (1996) Policy and finance for community care: the new mixed economy. In: Watkins, M., Hervey, N., Carson, J. and Ritter, S. (eds), *Collaborative Community Mental Health Care*. London: Arnold, pp. 41–57.

Brink, U. (1994) Psychiatric care and social support for people with long-term mental illness in Germany. *International Journal of Social Psychiatry*, 40, 258–268.

Brady, J., Sharfstein, S. and Muszynski, I. (1986) Trends in private insurance coverage for mental illness. *Psychiatric Services*, 48, 1276–1279.

Broverman, I., Broverman, D., Clarkson, F., Rosenkrantz, P. and Vogal, S. (1970) Sex role stereotypes and clinical judgements in mental health. *Journal of Consulting and Clinical Psychology*, 34, 1–7.

Burns, T. (1997) Case management, care management and care programming. *British Journal of Psychiatry*, 170, 393–395.

Carpenter, J., Schneider, J., Brandon, T. and McNiven, F. (2000) *The Care Programme Approach and Care Management in Mental Health. A Comparative Study of Models of Integration, Their Outcomes and Costs*. Report to the Department of Health. University of Durham: Centre for Applied Social Studies.

Challis, D., Darton, R., Hughes, J., Stewart, K. and Weiner, K. (1998) *Mapping and Evaluation of Care Management Arrangements for Older People and Those with Mental Health Problems*. London: Social Services Inspectorate, Department of Health.

Comelles, J. and Hernaez, M. (1994) The dilemmas of chronicity: the transition of care policies from the authoritarian state to the welfare state in Spain. *International Journal of Social Psychiatry*, 40, 283–295.

Commonwealth of Australia, Department of Health and Family Services (1998) *Fourth Annual Report. Changes in Australia's Mental Health Services Under the National Mental Health Strategy 1995–6*. Canberra, Australia: Department of Health and Family Services.

Department of Health (1989) *Caring for People in the Next Decade and Beyond*. London: HMSO.

Department of Health (1990) *The Care Programme Approach for People with a Mental Illness Referred to the Specialist Psychiatric Services.* London: Department of Health.

Department of Health (1995) *Building Bridges. A Guide to Inter-agency Working for the Care and Protection of Severely Mentally Ill People.* London: Department of Health.

Department of Health (1998) *Partnership in Action.* London: Department of Health.

Freedman, A.M. (1990) Mental health programs in the United States: idiosyncratic roots. *International Journal of Mental Health*, 18, 81–98.

Freeman, H., Fryers, T. and Henderson, J. (1985) *Mental Health Services in Europe: 10 Years On.* WHO: Copenhagen.

Giel, R. (1987) The jig-saw puzzle of Dutch mental health care. *International Journal of Mental Health*, 16, 152–163.

Goodwin, S. (1997) *Comparative Mental Health Policy. From Institutional to Community Care.* London: Sage.

Hollingsworth, J. (1992) Falling through the cracks: care of the chronically mentally ill in the United States, Germany, and the United Kingdom. *Journal of Health, Politics, Policy and Law*, 17, 899–928.

Huntingdon, J. (1981) *Social Work and General Medical Practice. Collaboration or Conflict?* London: Allen and Unwin.

Lewis, J., Bernstock, P., Bovell, V. and Wookey, F. (1997) Implementing care management: issues in relation to the new community care. *British Journal of Social Work*, 27, 5–24.

Marshall, M. (1996) Care management: a dubious practice. *British Medical Journal*, 312, 523–524.

Mechanic, D., Schlesinger, M. and McAlpine, D. (1995) Management of mental health and substance abuse services: state of the art and early results. *Milbank Quarterly*, 73, 19–55.

Onyett, S. (1992) *Case Management in Mental Health.* London: Chapman and Hall.

Onyett, S. (1997) The challenge of managing community mental health teams. *Health and Social Care in the Community*, 5, 40–47.

Parker, C and Gordon, R. (1998) *Pathways to Partnership. Legal Aspects of Joint Working in Mental Health.* London: Sainsbury Centre for Mental Health.

Poveda, J. (1987) Mental health care in Spain. *International Journal of Mental Health*, 16, 182–197.

Rapp, C.A. and Wintersteen, R. (1989) The strengths model of case management: results from twelve demonstrations. *Psychosocial Rehabilitation Journal*, 13, 23–32.

Rogers, A. and Pilgrim, D. (1996) Mental health workers and the state. In: Rogers, A. and Pilgrim, D. (eds), *Mental Health Policy in Britain.* Basingstoke: Macmillan, pp. 96–120.

Rubin, A. (1992) Is case management effective for people with severe mental illness? *Health and Social Work*, 17, 138–150.

Salzer, M. (1999) United States mental health policy in the 1990s: an era of cost-effectiveness, research and consumerism. *Policy and Politics*, 27, 75–84.

Schneider, J., Carpenter, J. and Brandon, T. (1999) Operation and organisation of services for people with severe mental illness in the UK: a survey of the care programme approach. *British Journal of Psychiatry*, 175, 422–425.

Sheppard, M. (1991) General practice, social work and mental health sections: the social control of women. *British Journal of Social Work*, 21, 663–683.

Stevenson, O. and Parsloe, P. (1993) *Community Care and Empowerment.* York: Joseph Rowntree Foundation.

Thompson, J. (1994) Trends in the development of psychiatric services. *Hospital and Community Psychiatry*, 45, 987–992.

Thompson, P. (1993) *Antidiscriminatory Practice.* Basingstoke: Macmillan.

Williams, J. and Luterbach, E. (1976) The changing boundaries of psychiatry in Canada. *Social Science and Medicine*, 10, 15–22.

36 | *Community alliances*

Susan J. Grey

Who provides mental health care ?

Traditionally, the statutory psychiatric services are seen as central to the mental health care system, with the voluntary sector and the community playing a peripheral part. However, it has been argued that, in practice, more mental health care is provided by the voluntary sector, non-mental health agencies and the families of psychiatric patients than by the psychiatric services (Hatfield and Lefley, 1987) and that much more emphasis should be placed on responding to the whole spectrum of suffering brought about by mental ill-health. Hodgson (1996) recommends an active policy of mental health promotion, which should have a place alongside crime prevention, physical health promotion and pollution control in the way we organize our communities. Such a policy would include enhancing the well-being of the general population and those at risk of developing a mental illness as well as those with a recognized disorder. In a similar vein, Kuipers and Westall (1993) argue that mental health issues warrant public education campaigns on the same scale as those mounted in relation to AIDS. Hodgson and Abbasi (1995) and Mrazek and Haggerty (1994) describe a growing body of evidence that psychological and social interventions can be effective in a range of situations, such as bereavement, divorce, unemployment and physical illness, in which people are at risk of developing mental health problems. These interventions can involve a number of organizations, including schools, the workplace, social services, the church, trade unions and the media.

Obstacles to strengthening the role of the community

Despite the arguments in favour of a broader-based response to mental illness, the focus remains on the statutory agencies. One reason for this lies with public attitudes towards mental illness. Lewis (1991) argues that, amongst the public in general, mild disabilities are often found acceptable, but severe disabilities, particularly those involving antisocial behaviour, are more likely to result in stigma and rejection. In a review of the early research into stigma, Hayward and Bright (1997) report that the public are generally quite slow to label unusual or abnormal behaviour as mental illness, often defining it in terms of being in hospital or receiving treatment (Cummings and Cummings, 1957; Star, 1957). However, once the label is applied, it can be accompanied by extremely negative attitudes (Nunnally, 1961). Scheff's (1966) labelling theory suggests that once a person has acquired the label of mental illness they are treated differently by others, leading to further abnormalities in their behaviour.

In the past, the adoption of the asylum system for the treatment of mental illness effectively circumvented the issue of community rejection. However, there has always been a tension between the function of the mental hospital as a treatment facility and as a residence for socially troublesome people (Goffman, 1968), and recent attempts to move away from a custodial function have brought the issue of rejection to the fore. Recent research into public attitudes towards people with mental illness shows very varied results and, although some of this can be attributed to differences in methodology, it is clear that there is much to be done to dispel fears about mental illness, change expectations about treatment and promote wider acceptance (Bhugra, 1993). In the USA, Aubrey *et al.* (1995) examined public attitudes to tenants of neighbouring community mental health hostels and found high levels of receptiveness on the part of community members. Smith (1981), on the other hand, found that acceptance of individuals with severe mental illness was greater in a neighbourhood adjacent to a mental hospital than in a more distant neighbourhood, but was less among those residents immediately next to the hospital. The likelihood of rejection of psychiatric patients living in the neighbourhood is influenced by a combination of factors including both severity of the disorder and the size, proximity and intrusiveness of the hostel.

Particular groups within the community can have a special contribution to mental health care. For example, the clergy have always had a role in the care of people with mental health problems (Gordon, 1946; Barbery and Kew, 1949; Hall, 1955, 1992; Sutherland, 1996). In the USA, Gurin *et al.* (1960) reported that 42% of their subjects would turn to a clergyman first to seek help, and Dohrenwend (1961) found that clergymen scored higher than other community representatives in recognizing the seriousness of mental illness. Churches with trained counsellors among their members can run a range of services including drop-in centres, befriending services and professional counselling and support. The hospital chaplain may also assist by providing emotional and spiritual care alongside that provided by the hospital team. How-ever, Sutherland (1996) describes some of the tensions between statutory services and the clergy. He notes the historical hierarchical relationship between institutional centres of professional excellence and community-based generalists. This is characterized in the mental health field by a wide acceptance of the superiority of the medical model, as adopted by psychiatrists, and the perception of community-based workers as more lowly than their institutional counterparts. The resulting resentments and power inequalities across the hospital and community divide can lead to relationships in which barriers are reinforced rather than overcome, as a means of reducing conflict.

Liaison between mental health services and people from ethnic minorities can also be problematic. Extensive networks usually exist informally between local voluntary agencies, police and local clergy, but mental health professionals do not always have access to them. Furthermore, the attitudes of members of ethnic minorities towards the statutory services may be soured by experiences of discriminatory treatment practices (Moodley, 1993).

So, despite the fact that much mental health care is already carried out by non-professionals and there are compelling arguments for bringing mental health issues into the mainstream of social policy, there are obstacles in the form of negative public attitudes, interprofessional tensions and cross-cultural barriers. Furthermore, in recent years, the entire mental health care system has been operating against a backdrop of continuous political and organizational change.

Changes in the role of the voluntary sector

Voluntary organizations have a historic role in stimulating new services by identifying unmet need and campaigning on behalf of marginalized sectors of society (Ramon, 1992; Brown and Dixon, 1996). Their members include patients, carers and other interested individuals. Brown and Dixon argue that changes in social policy and legislation threaten the campaigning function of some of these organizations by increasing their reliance on state funding. Up to the 1980s, grants from local authorities and other government or health agencies constituted the most common method of funding for voluntary organizations. These were awarded in response to applications initiated by the voluntary organization and were reviewed periodically. This arrangement allowed innovative projects to develop and provided a degree of autonomy and independence for the voluntary organization. It also allowed the organization to continue its campaigning function.

In Community Care: Agenda for Action (Griffiths, 1988), Griffiths recognized the value of the voluntary sector in fulfilling the following functions: self-help support groups; sources of information and expertise; befriending agencies; advocacy; constructive critics of services; public educators; and campaigners. The White Paper, Caring for People (Department of Health, 1989), recommended that health and local authorities should work towards funding in partnership with the voluntary sector and should involve voluntary organizations at an early stage in the negotiation of contracts. Mental health professionals have also recognized that a comprehensive service should include the work of service users and other community groups (Strathdee and Thornicroft, 1995). However, despite these endorsements of the important role of the voluntary sector, some concerns have been expressed about the consequences of bringing voluntary organizations into the mainstream of service provision. For example, it has been claimed that development of the contract culture in the USA has merely led to an increase in bureaucracy (Gutch, 1992). Brown and Dixon (1996) warn that in Britain the voluntary sector is becoming increasingly managerially and financially dependent on the statutory sector which now takes the lead in deciding which services to commission. There is a danger that this could lead to a stifling of innovation and a weakening of the autonomous campaigning function of the voluntary organizations.

Lewis (1993) is more optimistic about the position in Britain, but recommends that the redefined relationship requires the voluntary organizations to become equal partners in the planning process and make a real contribution to decisions about which services are commissioned. The creation of genuine partnerships has always been difficult, since community representatives enter the relationship as unequal partners lacking the apparent technical knowledge and sophistication of the professionals. One way to redress the balance is described by Landsberg and Hammer (1978) who improved the expertise of community volunteers by involving them in research and evaluation projects carried out by a community mental health service.

Involvement of the wider community in service planning

Links are needed between the statutory services and the voluntary sector which allow local people to contribute to service planning, allow innovative projects to flourish and do not compromise the campaigning function of voluntary organizations. The mechanisms of public participation in the USA identified by Arnstein and described by Lewis (1991) range from public education exercises in which the bureaucrats and professionals pass on information to passive recipients, through consultation and partnership models in which the public have some opportunity to voice preferences, to full delegation, where citizens have full control over management and decision making. Public consultation is used increasingly in the British NHS, but often serves merely as a placatory gesture, prior to the implementation of policies which have already been decided.

Another method of participation involves direct contact between special interest groups and representatives of the statutory services or of government. Government ministers, members of parliament, civil servants and professionals can be invited by voluntary organizations to conferences about specific topics, allowing the flow of information between professional organizations such as the Royal Colleges, the Department of Health and representatives of the interest groups. Lewis (1991) criticizes some of these initiatives on the grounds that they are technocratic, involve mainly the elite of the interest groups, exclude user groups and reach only a select group of politicians. Despite these criticisms, there have been occasions when campaigning coalitions between interest groups, professionals and government representatives have succeeded in influencing policy and legislation. One example of this is the UK 1983 Mental Health Act which came about as a result of campaigning by MIND (National Association for Mental Health), together with a number of professionals and Members of Parliament (MPs), to enhance the civil liberties of detained patients. More recently, the campaigns of two voluntary organizations, the NSF (National

Schizophrenia Fellowship) and (SANE) Schizophrenia: A National Emergency, have succeeded in slowing down the closure of psychiatric hospital beds and highlighting the need for improved alternative facilities in the community. It is unfortunate, however, that elements of the SANE campaign, which highlighted violent incidents as examples of inadequate resource provision, involved a down-grading of the social image of people with schizophrenia and the inflaming of public fears and prejudices, counter to the aims of normalization (Ramon, 1991). The challenge is for those individuals participating in such campaigns to ensure that they genuinely represent the broader interests of service users rather than of minority groups of public or professionals.

In the British NHS, prior to the reforms of 1991, the District Health Authority comprised lay members, appointed by the Secretary of State on the basis of their expertise and interest in health, and members nominated by the local authority. The latter could claim to have a local mandate and were, to a limited degree, accountable to the local area. Meetings were held regularly in public, giving members of staff, trade unions, voluntary organizations and other interested people an opportunity to hear what was being discussed. Access to agendas and minutes of meetings allowed campaigning groups or individuals to organize more effectively and lobby their representatives. Since the NHS reforms, Health Authorities have become commissioning bodies with just five appointed non-executive members. These arrangements were criticized because the new bodies were less accountable to the local community and appeared to be conducting their business in a less open manner than before (Colenutt and Ellis, 1993; Grey, 1993). The Department of Health has since produced a Code of Practice on Openness in the NHS which sets out the obligations of Health Authorities to give members of the local community access to meetings and related documents and to consult on major policy decisions (Department of Health, 1995).

Community Health Councils (CHCs) were set up in 1973 with a monitoring, complaints and planning remit. Through their statutory responsibility to represent the public and help express patients' views, they provide an alternative forum for public participation. They consist of lay members who provide a link between the public and the statutory services. Although CHCs tend to comprise mainly middle class, middle aged, white members, they are able to co-opt additional members with special knowledge to deal with specific issues. They have often been successful in campaigning for better services for disadvantaged groups, particularly those in residential care, and they also give priority to their service planning function.

Examples of good practice in developing alliances with the wider community

The All-Wales Strategy for mental handicap

In the UK, public participation may be easier in Wales and Scotland than in England. The populations are smaller and the Welsh Office and Scottish Office are multi-purpose territorial departments, unlike the Department of Health in England. The All-Wales Strategy for mental handicap provides an exceptional model for high level public participation in the planning process (Hunter and Wistow, 1987; Welsh Office, 1983; McGrath, 1988). The Secretary of State for Wales took a leading role and there was wide consumer participation throughout the planning process, including the involvement of carers. The Central Planning Group consisted of six professionals from social services, education and health authorities, with six lay members co-ordinating local district representation plus a member from a non-mental handicap voluntary body to promote broader community links. At the local level, carers and front line workers met to make decisions which were forwarded to the Central Planning Group. The formal participation continued in the All-Wales Advisory Panel which included members from Mencap and SCOVO (campaigning organizations which seek to remove discrimination and provide support for people with a learning disability). This method of planning came about because Mencap was already a credible and effective campaigning group in Wales and because members of the public and a sympathetic MP wanted to ensure that decisions were taken only with consultation. The process was not without its difficulties. Many of the participants lacked knowledge and experience of the planning process. Some active carers dropped out after finding the procedures too time-consuming and the committee process slow and frustrating, leaving an experienced but potentially unrepresentative minority. Finally, all participants found it difficult to reconcile conflicting views on service priorities (Lewis, 1991). These difficulties notwithstanding, the process provides a model which could be used more widely in health service development.

Inequalities, health and the new Scotland

The Health Education Board for Scotland provides another example of constructive dialogue between the community, professionals and politicians in the development of a positive health strategy (HEBS, 1988). A programme of discussion and consultation took place early in 1998 to build an alliance of representatives from six key sectors, namely, government, business, health boards, community services, the voluntary sector and local authorities. The delegates identified through this process then attended a major conference to develop a shared response to the Green Paper, 'Working Together for a Healthier Scotland'. Participants tackled problems occurring in a fictional Scottish community (Easthill). Data were provided on the socio-economic, health, poverty, transport, housing and work characteristics of the area, plus the findings of a community survey and needs assessment. Representatives of the key sectors then presented their perspectives on health inequalities, their priorities and their potential contribution. Groups of participants then worked on specific tasks, such as developing mechanisms for ensuring that health service provision reaches stigmatized and socially excluded

groups; deciding how to divide a community chest award between different areas; and making recommendations to the health board on local projects to reduce the stress caused by poverty, insecurity and isolation. A further objective of the conference was to examine (in the real world) the Green Paper proposal to set up an 'Expert Group' to address issues of health inequality. Participants had criticisms of this recommendation, saying that it represented a 'top-down' approach which did not make use of existing community networks and did not make clear how the group would be selected or in what way it would be accountable. The Minister for Health and Arts in Scotland responded there and then by agreeing to reconsider the name and composition of the group.

Participation at a local level

The examples described above did not focus primarily on services for people with mental health problems, yet neither was free of difficulties and controversy. When local projects are targeted specifically at people with mental illness, the planning process can be even trickier. As already noted, the support of the local community cannot be taken for granted, particularly where the prospective users of the project appear to have the potential for aggressive or sexually inappropriate behaviour. This presents a dilemma for service developers who have to decide when, how and with what to inform the local community. These difficulties are likely to occur whenever facilities for people with mental health problems are to be provided in mainstream settings, but are especially acute where housing projects are involved.

Zippay (1997) notes that, in the USA, federal anti-discrimination legislation supports the setting up of mental health housing projects without advance notification of the neighbours. Examining this issue further, Zippay interviewed representatives from 72 mental health agencies in Massachusetts, asking questions about their siting strategies for group housing projects and the communities' responses to them. A significant association was found between advance notification and greater community opposition. In contrast, a telephone survey of New Jersey group home providers (Hogan 1986) suggested that an active programme of community preparation at an early stage resulted in greater community support. This preparation included meetings with municipal officials, involvement with the immediate neighbours, use of local personal contacts and invitations to open days. In Hong Kong, a retrospective examination of a community campaign opposing the establishment of a psychiatric halfway house highlighted some of the lessons to be learned (Cheung, 1990). Cheung recommends the involvement of community leaders at the planning stage and the use of broad-based community education strategies, including the mass media, to raise general levels of public understanding of mental health issues. Wolff *et al.* (1996) found that a public education campaign focused on the neighbours of a sheltered home resulted in reduction in anxieties about mental illness and an increased willingness to socialize with the project residents. Leff (1997) argues that attempts to open community homes unobtrusively may be counterproductive and lead to more opposition than if well-constructed educational campaigns are undertaken, with the continued involvement of the neighbours after the project is established.

Examples of good practice in developing local alliances

Housing projects

As already stated, a significant contribution to mental health care is provided by non-mental health agencies and by non-professional individuals. Craig and Timms (1992) investigated psychiatric morbidity among people using facilities for the homeless. They found that whilst rates of severe mental illness were higher than would be expected given population norms, these people did not necessarily have a long history of psychiatric hospitalization. It seems that many people with diagnosable psychiatric illness have found a refuge of sorts in these institutions where the symptoms of their illness are tolerated and few

social demands are placed upon them (Timms and Fry, 1989), but where they remain out of touch with specialist services (Scott, 1993). Craig and Timms conclude that current levels of homelessness amongst the mentally ill cannot be attributed entirely to psychiatric hospital closure, but point out that community care is failing to reach significant numbers of homeless people with psychiatric disorders.

A later study by Commander *et al.* (1998) found that psychiatric service utilization was reasonably good among people living in residential homes for the mentally ill and among residents of small hostels for the mentally ill. However, this was less true for people with diagnosable psychiatric disorders housed in larger hostels not specifically designated for the mentally ill. Interestingly, many of the residents of these larger hostels were highly mobile, having only been at the current address for a matter of days or weeks and had no registered GP (family doctor), making it harder for psychiatric services to reach them.

Phelan and Strathdee (1994) report an innovative project designed to increase awareness of mental health issues amongst housing officers employed by the local authority to allocate public housing. Although many people with mental illnesses are dependent on local authority housing for their accommodation, communication between housing and health agencies tends to be limited to dealing with the patient's initial placement or with subsequent crises. Each party often feels disappointed in the failures of the other to meet expectations, and there may be limited mutual understanding or respect. The training project was undertaken by a sectorized community mental health team in inner London and grew from an earlier training course developed for residential hostel workers (Conning *et al.*, 1992).

Housing officers from each neighbourhood office were consulted about areas of training need. The initial data revealed that most housing officers had had recent experiences with people with mental health problems. These included dealing with violence and intoxication, experiencing abuse, feeling overwhelmed by clients' problems, being given inadequate or incorrect information by the referring agencies, having to complete rapid assessments of people who were incomprehensible, and being unsure of the appropriate referral route to mental health services. The training course was based on these identified needs and was completed by 90 housing officers in six neighbourhood offices over a 6-month period. The content of the course consisted of a lecture on the nature of mental illness, its prevalence in the community and the changes following deinstitutionalization; a group exercise designed to develop insight into the experiences of the mentally ill and the need for good communication, empathy and respect for individual rights; a role-playing task to improve interviewing skills; and group discussion of recent violent incidents and ways of modifying the work environment or procedures to prevent further incidents. Although not evaluated formally, the course was well received and would appear to serve the dual purpose of raising the levels of expertise in this staff group and forging links between the two agencies which would go some way to reducing the tensions between them.

Work schemes

Many studies have demonstrated an association between unemployment and mental illness (Warr, 1982; Furnham, 1985; Fryer and Payne, 1986; Warr *et al.*, 1988). Job loss may be followed by lower self-esteem and minor psychiatric problems which in turn lead to difficulties in finding new employment. However, for people with severe mental illness, work can also be stressful (Watts, 1983; Floyd, 1984), involve too much or too little stimulation (Wing and Freudenberg, 1961) or be located in environments which may have a damaging effect on self-esteem (Lipsedge and Summerfield, 1987).

Dick and Shepherd (1994) examined the relationship between mental health and perception of the working environment among employees at four sheltered workshops run by the Richmond Fellowship (a charitable organization providing therapeutic environments for people with mental health problems). Perceptions of the working environment were assessed using the Work Environment Survey (WES), a scale incorporating

the nine dimensions identified by Warr (1987) as relevant to psychological well-being. These dimensions include the content of the job and the physical environment, as well as certain aspects of the social environment, the money earned and the work's perceived social value. The study revealed that the WES has acceptable reliability and validity for the most part, but, interestingly, that the only significant relationship between perceived features of the work environment and mental health was that between 'valued social position' and self-esteem. This suggests that individuals who believe that the public do not value their work are likely to have lower self-esteem. As Dick and Shepherd acknowledge, this does not necessarily indicate a causal relationship between patients' perceptions of the social value of their work and their self-esteem, but it does suggest that the social value attached to work is of importance and is consistent with the philosophy of normalization described by Wolfensberger (1972).

Mental health staff in mid-Wales set up an Employment Initiative Group to assist mental health service users in gaining access to mainstream employment (Hutchings and Gower, 1993). They initially surveyed the caseloads of the local community mental health team (CMHT) and found that although 33% were unemployed, the majority had had no specialist help in finding employment. A panel was set up consisting of a local Disablement Resettlement Officer, an adult guidance officer, an occupational therapist and a Training Agency Manager. In the first 6 months, this multi-agency panel interviewed 12 clients and helped four into employment and six into some form of training. Following these promising beginnings, funds were sought for a Mental Health Employment Co-ordinator to develop the service for clients who needed more help than could be provided by a single interview. The proposal, which had the support of the local MP, was subsequently funded by the Employment Services Agency and the local Training and Enterprise Council, with additional support from the Adult Guidance Service and the Health Authority. The scheme is strengthened by its origins in the identification of local clients' needs and by its use of expertise from several agencies including those not solely involved with mental health problems.

Another multi-agency attempt to overcome barriers to employment for people with psychiatric disorders is described by McCrum *et al.* (1997). In Northern Ireland, several bodies have been involved in the promotion of training and employment opportunities for people with mental illness, namely the Department of Economic Development, voluntary sector organizations such as the Industrial Therapy Organization and the Department of Health and Social Services (NI). The Antrim Job Clinic was set up by a Disablement Employment Adviser (DEA), a placement officer from the Industrial Therapy Organization and an Occupational Therapist from the local CMHT. The local area had had a rise in unemployment following the closure of a large manufacturing plant, and pockets of public housing were vacant with an increase in petty crime and vandalism.

The formation of the Job Clinic was publicised among local GPs, CMHTs, local employment agencies and employers. Referrals were accepted for any client who had mental health problems and was experiencing difficulties with employment. Clients were assessed by the team and encouraged to discuss their work strengths and weaknesses, and related issues such as concentration, punctuality and independence. Interpersonal skills were also assessed in terms of the types of interaction tolerated by the client, ability to give or accept criticism or instructions, etc. An individual plan was produced recommending suitable work or training opportunities and, in some cases, followed up by a staff member who gave additional help with job applications, rehearsal for job interviews and other training in other job-related skills. Of 77 clients referred in the first 15 months, the majority (88%) had been in employment at some time in their lives, but all except two also had a history of unemployment, particularly just prior to attending the Job Clinic. Of 71 clients who attended for assessment, 46 entered some form of training and a further 19 went into either sheltered or full-time employment. Others pursued either further education or voluntary work. Unfortunately, no data were reported on the effect of contact with the clinic or

subsequent work experience on clients' work-related skills or mental health. However, several positive outcomes were identified on an anecdotal basis. Because the scheme co-ordinates the work of staff from different agencies who would previously have seen many of the same clients separately, it seems likely that duplication of effort is avoided both for staff and clients. There is an additional spin-off in raising awareness of mental health issues in the non-mental health agencies such as government bodies, NGOs (non-governmental organizations) and the business community. The scheme also provides local employers with an opportunity to inform the mental health and employment agencies about their expectations of prospective employees.

A shift in perspective for the professionals?

As psychiatric services move away from institutions and into the community, greater links are needed between statutory services and the wider public, for both service planning and delivery. This change implies a more explicit recognition of the responsibilities of the community for providing mental health care and a greater requirement for people to accept the presence of the mentally ill in their midst. The potential benefits of greater community involvement include a reduction in suspicion and fear of mental illness, more influence in determining local health policies and better prospects of an appropriate and acceptable response in the event of personal mental health problems. The process of deinstitutionalization also affects the professionals. A shift towards the more egalitarian dynamics of the community may help the professionals to understand the positions of the public in general and service users in particular. Professional practice and interagency relations may be enriched by tapping into the expertise already demonstrated in many local projects and campaigns, and by accommodating alternative ways of understanding mental illness.

References

Aubrey, T.D., Tefft, B. and Currie, R.F. (1995) Public attitudes and intentions regarding tenants of community mental health residences who are neighbours. *Community Mental Health Journal*, 31, 39–52.

Barbery, H.L. and Kew, C.E. (1949) The nature and function of a church clinic. *Journal of Pastoral Care*, 3, 17–25.

Bhugra, D. (1993) Attitudes towards mental illness. In: Bhugra, D. and Leff, J. (eds), *Principles of Social Psychiatry*. Oxford: Blackwell Scientific Publications, pp. 385–399.

Brown, R. and Dixon, R. (1996) The role of the voluntary sector. In: Watkins, M., Hervey, N., Carson, J. and Ritter, S. (eds), *Collaborative Community Mental Health Care*. London: Arnold, pp. 197–213.

Commander, M.J., Odell, S., Sashidaram, S.P. and Surtees, P. (1998) An epidemiological survey of communal establishment residents: implications for mental health purchasers. *Journal of Mental Health*, 7, 385–392.

Cheung, F.M. (1990) People against the mentally ill: community opposition to residential treatment facilities. *Community Mental Health Journal*, 26, 205–215.

Colenutt, B. and Ellis, G. (1993) The next quangos in London. *New Statesman and Society*, March 1993.

Conning, A.M., Phelan, M. and Strathdee, G. (1992) *What Mental Health Training Do Hostel Workers Want?* Unpublished research report.

Craig, T. and Timms, P. (1992) Out of the wards and onto the streets? Deinstitutionalisation and homelessness in Britain. *Journal of Mental Health*, 1, 265–275.

Cumming, E. and Cumming, J. (1957) *Closed Ranks: An Experiment in Mental Health Education*. Cambridge, MA: Harvard University Press.

Department of Health (1989) *Caring for People*, London: HMSO.

Department of Health (1995) *Code of Practice on Openness in the NHS; Annex B. Purchasers of Healthcare: District Health Authorities and Family Health Service Authorities*. London: NHS Executive.

Dick, N. and Shepherd, G. (1994) Work and mental health: a preliminary test of Warr's model in sheltered workshops for the mentally ill. *Journal of Mental Health*, 3, 387–400.

Dohrenwend, B., Bernard, V. and Kolb, L. (1961) The orientations of leaders in an urban area toward problems of mental illness. *American Journal of Psychiatry*, 118, 683–691.

Floyd, M. (1984) The employment problems of people disabled by schizophrenia. *Journal of Social and Occupational Medicine*, 34, 93–95.

Fryer, D.M. and Payne, R.L. (1986) Being unemployed: a review of the literature on the psychological experience of unemployment. In: Cooper, C.L. and Robertson, I. (eds), *International Review of Industrial and Organizational Psychology*. London: Wiley.

Furnham, A. (1985) Youth unemployment: a review of the literature. *Journal of Adolescence*, 8, 109–124.

Goffman, E. (1968) *Asylums*. Harmondsworth: Penguin Books.

Gordon, J.B. (1946) The relation of the church to mental hospitals. *Psychiatric Quarterly*, 20 (Suppl.), 23–29.

Grey, S.J. (1993) What has happened to accountability? *Journal of Mental Health*, 2, 189.

Griffiths, R. (1988) *Community Care: agenda for action*. Section 4.3, London: HMSO.

Gurin, G., Verof, J. and Field, S. (1960) *Americans View Their Mental Health*. New York: Basic Books.

Gutch, R. (1992) Contracting lessons from the US. *Local Economy*, 7, 188.

Hall, C. (1955) The function of the psychiatric chaplain *Journal of Pastoral Care*, 9, 145–152.

Hall, C. (1992) *Head and Heart: The Story of the Clinical Pastoral Education Movement*. Dectur, GA: Journal of Pastoral Care Publications.

Hatfield, A. and Lefley, H. (eds) (1987) *Families of the Mentally Ill*. London: Cassell.

Hayward, P. and Bright, J. (1997) Stigma and mental illness: a review and critique. *Journal of Mental Health*, 6, 345–354.

HEBS (Health Education Board for Scotland) (1998) *Inequalities, Health and the New Scotland*. Edinburgh: HEBS.

Hodgson, R.J. (1996) Mental health promotion. *Journal of Mental Health*, 5, 1–2.

Hodgson, R.J. and Abbasi, T. (1995) *Effective Mental Health Promotion, Literature Review*. Cardiff: Health Promotion Wales (Technical Report 13).

Hogan, R. (1986) Gaining support for group homes. *Community Mental Health Journal*, 22, 117–126.

Hunter, D.J. and Wistow, G. (1987) *Community Care in Britain: Variations on a Theme*. London: King Edward's Hospital Fund for London.

Hutchings, J. and Gower, K. (1993) Unemployment and mental health. *Journal of Mental Health*, 2, 355–358.

Kuipers, L. and Westhall, J. (1993) The role of facilitated relative's groups and voluntary self-help groups. In: Bhugra, D. and Leff, J. (eds), *Principles of Social Psychiatry*. Oxford: Blackwell Scientific Publications, pp. 562–572.

Landsberg, G. and Hammer, R. (1978) Involving community representatives in CMHC evaluation and research. *Hospital and Community Psychiatry*, 29, 245–247.

Leff, J. (1997) Aiding resocialisation of the chronic psychotic patient. *International Clinical Psychopharmacology*, 12 (Suppl. 4), S19–S24.

Lewis, A. (1991) Public participation in decision-making. In: Ramon S. (ed.), *Beyond Community Care: Normalisation and Integration Work*. Basingstoke, UK: Macmillan, pp. 137–161.

Lewis, J. (1993) Developing the mixed economy of care: emerging issues for voluntary organizations. *Journal of Social Policy*, 22, 173–192.

Lipsedge, M. and Summerfield, A. (1987) *The Employment Rehabilitation Needs of The Mentally Ill. Final Report to the Manpower Services Commission*. London: MSC.

McCrum, B.W., Burnside, L.K. and Duffy, T.L. (1997) Organizing for work: a job clinic for people with mental health needs. *Journal of Mental Health*, 6, 503–513.

McGrath, M. (1988) Inter-agency collaboration in the all-Wales strategy – initial comments on a vanguard area. *Social Policy and Administration*, 22, 53-67.

Moodley, P. (1993) Setting up services for ethnic minorities. In: D. Bhugra and J. Leff (eds), *Principles of Social Psychiatry*. Oxford: Blackwell Scientific Publications, pp. 490–501.

Mrazek, P.J. and Haggerty, R.J. (eds) (1994) *Reducing Risks for Mental Disorder*. Washington, DC: National Academy Press.

Nunnally, J.C. (1961) *Popular Conceptions of Mental Health: Their Development and Change*. New York: Holt, Rinehart and Winston.

Phelan, M. and Strathdee, G. (1994) Living in the community: training housing officers in mental health. *Journal of Mental Health*, 3, 229–233.

Ramon, S. (1991) Policy issues. In: Ramon S. (ed.), *Beyond Community Care: Normalisation and Integration Work*. Basingstoke, UK: Macmillan, pp. 167–194.

Ramon, S. (ed.) (1992) *Psychiatric Hospital Closure*. London: Chapman and Hall.

Scott, J. (1993) Homelessness and mental illness. *British Journal of Psychiatry*, 162, 314–324.

Scheff, T.J. (1966) *Being Mentally Ill: A Sociological Theory*. Aldine: Chicago.

Smith, C.J. (1981) Hospital proximity and public acceptance of the mentally ill. *Hospital and Comunity Psychiatry*, 32, 178–180.

Star, S.A. (1957) *The Public's Ideas about Mental Illness*. University of Chicago (unpublished): National Opinion Research Centre.

Strathdee, G. and Thornicroft, G. (1995) The principles of setting up mental health services in the community. In: Bhugra, D. and Leff, J. (eds), *Principles of Social Psychiatry*. Oxford: Blackwell Scientific Publications, pp. 473–489.

Sutherland, M.R. (1996) Shifting into community focus: a pastoral perspective. In: Watkins, M., Hervey, N., Carson, J. and Ritter, S. (eds), *Collaborative Community Mental Health Care*. London: Arnold, pp. 197–213.

Timms P.W. and Fry, A.H. (1989) Homelessness and mental illness. *Health Trends*, 21, 70–71.

Warr, P. (1982) Psychological aspects of employment and unemployment. *Psychological Medicine*, 12, 7–11.

Warr, P. (1987) *Work, Unemployment and Mental Health*. Oxford: Oxford University Press.

Warr, P., Jackson, P. and Banks, M. (1988) Unemployment and mental health: some British studies. *Journal of Social Issues*, 44, 47–68.

Watts, F. (1983) Employment. In: Watts, F.N. and Bennett, D.H. (eds), *Theory and Practice of Psychiatric Rehabilitation*. Chichester: Wiley and Sons, pp. 214–240.

Welsh Office (1983) *The All Wales Strategy fo rthe Services for Mentally Handicapped People*. Cardiff: Welsh Office.

Wing, J.K. and Freudenberg, R.K. (1961) The response of severely ill chronic schizophrenic patients to social stimulation. *American Journal of Psychiatry*, 118, 311–322.

Wolfensberger, W. (1972) *The Principles of Normalisation in Human Services*. Toronto: National Institute on Mental Retardation.

Wolff, G., Pathare, S., Craig, T. and Leff, J. (1996) Public education for community care: a new approach. *British Journal of Psychiatry*, 168, 441–447.

Zippay, A. (1997) Trends in siting strategies. *Community Mental Health Journal*, 33, 301–310.

37 | *Responding to migration and upheaval*
Richard F. Mollica

Introduction

The 21st century will probably continue as a century of migration. International migration has grown so dramatically in volume since 1945, especially accelerating in the 1980s, that the absolute number of people living outside of their countries of birth is the highest in history (Hirschman *et al.*, 1999). Associated with the revival of immigration after the Second World War and the large number of migrants are major changes in their countries of origin and receiving nations. Before 1985, 85% of all international migrants originated in Europe. Since 1960, Europe has contributed only a small fraction of emigrants to world migration flows; the new migrant-producing nations now include those in Africa, Asia and Latin America. In addition to traditional immigrant-receiving nations such as Canada, the USA, Australia, New Zealand and Argentina, countries throughout western Europe now attract significant numbers of immigrants. Even long-time sending countries such as Italy, Spain and Portugal have begun to receive immigrants.

By the late 1990s, international migration had become a global phenomenon. This fact is readily apparent in the developed nations of today where ethnic diversity of local communities, not only in large urban areas, is becoming the norm. For example, in the USA, the proportion of foreign-born persons is approximately 10% of the total population; more than 50 million Americans are immigrants or children of immigrants. Similar population trends exist in Europe, especially in northern European countries such as Germany. Douglas S. Masey, a leading contributor to international migration studies, has stated:

"International migration will surely continue. Barring all international catastrophes of unprecedented proportions, immigration will likely expand and grow for none of the causal forces for immigration show any signs of moderating. The market economy is expanding to ever farther reaches of the globe, labor markets in developed countries are growing more rather than less segmented, national immigration and trade networks are expanding, large stocks of migration-related human and social capital are forming in sending countries everywhere, and the power of the nation-state is faltering in the face of transnational onslaught. The twenty-first century will be one of globalism and international migration will no doubt figure prominently within it." (Masey, 1999, p. 52)

The general mental health community has been slow to acknowledge the impact of the new diversity of cultures and languages on mainstream psychiatric services that serve native populations. Over the past two decades, interest in migrant mental health has been mixed. On the other hand, modern psychiatry has pioneered the psychiatric care of a special subcategory of migrant, the refugee patient who has been exposed to mass violence and torture (Masey, 1999). This work has been greatly enriched by the clinical and scientific interests of medical anthropologists who have dramatically expanded psychiatry's interest and appreciation of the mental health world view and healing traditions of non-western countries (Kleinman, 1978). Unfortunately, the mental health field's significant scientific attention on migration before the Second World War seems to have vanished. These historic trends in psychiatric interest in migration may be partially due to not only the changing cultural background of migrants but also the withering attacks of a new generation of sociologists of migration on the previously accepted canons of assimilation and acculturation (Alba *et al.*, 1999). The older mental health theories of migration that were wedded to these canons held that all migrants eventually acculturated to the dominant society and that this process of assimilation was inherently stressful, resulting in the migrants' greater vulnerability to mental illness than native-born or non-migrants of similar background. The fact that this mental health 'belief' is no longer considered valid and has never been demonstrated scientifically does not negate the reality that a wide range of clinical phenomena exist and are associated with the migrant experience.

A comprehensive model of mental health and migration has not been forthcoming. This chapter will not attempt to formulate one. This chapter instead will present a scientifically validated approach to the identification and treatment of serious mental illness in resettled migrant populations. Clearly, the modern psychiatric practitioner must learn to practise a new global method of psychiatry since he/she is now called upon to care for the mental health needs of local citizens who have come to their communities from around the world. The psychiatric practitioner no longer exists in a mainstream homogeneous society in which the mental health care of those 'different' from the native population can be relegated to the margins of conventional diagnosis and treatment. Instead, globalization has brought the migrant into the mainstream of psychiatric practice.

Terms and definitions

Within all scientific facts are embedded scientific theories. The same claim can be made for medical and sociological definitions of terms fundamental to the mental health care of migrant populations. There are a bewildering number of terms used to describe those individuals who were not born within their new host society and the psychosocial processes associated with their adjustment to their new environment.

Transnational migrants

Contemporary observers of late 19th century migration were well aware of the fact that immigrants maintained close ties to family and friends in their countries of origin. Many returned home on a regular basis; others routinely sent money to relatives in their native land. Yet, in the 1950s, Oscar Adlin in a classic history of US immigration, *The Uprooted* (Handlin, 1973), described a static situation in which American immigrants were almost totally cut-off from contact with their countries of origin. This perceived reality, of course, was believed to allow the immigrant to move along fully with the process of assimilation. This view of immigration was most probably as far from the truth then as it is today. Extensive research on modern immigration reveals that immigrants maintain an extensive transnational network of social communication and related activity. As N.G. Schiller has stated (Schiller, 1999), "To adopt transnational migration as the research paradigm is to change the unit of analysis; persons in sending and receiving societies become participants in a single social unit" (p. 99). The term, transnational migrant, therefore, increases the social domain in which the traditional migrant lives and operates psychosocially. Migrants no longer are perceived as individuals and families cut-off from their cultural roots within their host countries. In this chapter, the transnational character of migration will be implied whenever the term migrant is used.

Migrants are divided further into two main categories: immigrants and refugees. Although these terms primarily describe legal distinctions made by international and national covenants and laws, respectively, immigrants and refugees have been treated very differently by mental health researchers and clinicians. *Immigrants* are defined as legal migrants who have entered a country voluntarily, often to seek out new economic opportunities within the host society. "From the point of view of the receiving state, persons are immigrants when they become incorporated into their country; from the point of view of the sending state, persons are emigrants when they leave home and settle abroad" (Schiller, 1999).

Many countries are faced with illegal immigrants who attempt to enter a country without knowledge or permission of that country.

Refugees, in contrast to immigrants, are migrants who have been forced out of their homes by violence within their country of origin. Although the US government and those of western Europe have specific legal definitions of refugee status, these definitions usually conform to UN definitions defined by the 1951 UN Convention relating to the status of refugees and later modified by the 1967 Protocol (United Nations High Commissioner for Refugees, 1993, 1988). The latter states:

"Any person is a refugee who owing to well-founded fear of being persecuted for reasons of race, religion, nationality, membership of a particular social group or political opinion, is outside the country of his nationality and is unable, or owing to such fear, is unwilling to avail himself of the protection of that country; or who, not having nationality and being outside the country of his former habitual residence is unable, or owing to such fear, is unwilling to return to it."

Refugees are considered by migration specialists to have similar patterns of transnational networking as immigrants— but ones that have been severely restricted by the violent destruction of their local communities that resulted in their refugee status. Refugees may also be forced to resettle in host countries that do not have established communities of similar cultural background to the refugee. Unlike many immigrants, refugees may be resettled in local environments with little access to fellow countrymen, friends or relatives.

Displaced persons are refugees who have not been able to relocate themselves across an international border, remaining homeless within their native land. Displaced persons, because they are not protected by international conventions, have little hope of resettlement and extreme difficulty in obtaining international protection and humanitarian assistance. *Exiles* are a subclass of refugees who are individuals forcibly expelled from their countries by their governments, usually through legal measures. The exile fears return because he/she will be captured, imprisoned and possibly killed or tortured by the police, military or paramilitary groups. *Asylum seekers* are refugees who are awaiting a refugee determination in the host country where they are seeking asylum.

Since the Second World War, an exponential increase in the number of refugees and displaced persons has occurred worldwide (United Nations High Commissioner for Refugees, 1998). For example, in 1930, there were only 2.5 million refugees receiving international protection through the UN; by 1999 there were 23 million refugees and at least an additional 50 million displaced persons. In 1998, the majority of refugees came from over 40 developing nations; the overwhelming majority were also being hosted within the developing world. In spite of this trend, the resettlement of refugees in developed nations over the last quarter of a century has been very large. In addition, the number of asylum seekers filing claims in Europe and the USA during the period of 1989–1998 has amounted to approximately one-half million persons per year, with the most claims going to Germany, The Netherlands, Switzerland, the UK and the USA (US Committee for Refugees, 1999).

Psychosocial processes related to migration

Assimilation and acculturation are the two major terms relevant to the psychosocial adaptation of migrants to their new host countries. In 1921, the American sociologists Park and Burgess gave the central concept of assimilation its classic formulation: a process of interpretation and fusion in which persons and groups acquire the memories, sentiments and attitudes of other persons and groups; and, by sharing their experience and history, are incorporated with them in a common cultural life (Park and Burgess, 1921, p. 735).

The early concepts of assimilation were associated with a 'straight-line assimilation' process through which all traces of a migrant's prior ethnic identity is totally erased. The ultimate end point, a totally assimilated person completely similar to his/her native counterpart, was believed to be accomplished by the increasing adaptation of each new generation of immigrant children within the host society.

Acculturation, in contrast to assimilation, has a much more limited meaning. Acculturation refers mainly to the newcomer's ability to adopt the cultural practices of the new host society, such as food and drink. While migrants appear to have considerable control over their use of native culture and behaviours, they usually cannot assimilate into mainstream social structures such as the educational system unless these opportunities are provided to them.

Unfortunately, these two concepts rarely have been distinguished from each other by the mental health field. They have been used interchangeably without full appreciation of the inherent theoretical problems caused by this confusion. In addition, many mental health practitioners may still believe in the straight-line process of assimilation that will lead to a well-adjusted citizen. A corollary to this belief is that the psychological distress of this transformation in some migrants may lead to serious mental illness (Shural, 1982). In spite of this negative outcome, the alternative to assimilation, the development of a marginated citizen alienated from the benefits of the mainstream society, may have dire mental health consequences. These attitudes toward migrant patients by mental health practitioners have not been clearly articulated but remain an unspoken social bias.

Recent studies by migration sociologists reveal three new possible scenarios on assimilation that may be of some theoretical and clinical value to mental health practitioners (Runbaut, 1999). The new scenarios, called segmented assimilation theory, offer a different framework for understanding the observed changes in adaptation of migrants to the host society. Three possible pathways associated with assimilation have been empirically identified. First, the complete assimilation of second- and third-generation immigrant children remains a possibility as outlined by Park and his predecessors. Secondly, the assimilation process leads the next generation of immigrant children into socially deviant behaviour and poverty as they become a permanent underclass within the host society. Thirdly, rapid acculturation and penetration into the social structures of

mainstream society occur simultaneously with the maintenance of traditional values and community solidarity. Clearly, many factors such as economic opportunity, family cohesion and host–migrant relations such as racism will affect the assimilation process and mental health outcomes.

Race, ethnicity and nationality

The terms race, ethnicity and nationality, although often applied interchangeably in mental health practices when describing migrants, have radically different meanings (Bahr *et al.*, 1979). The concept of race and racial categories, although often used in psychiatry and medicine to identify a patient, probably has very limited clinical utility. Racial classifications have their origins in Linnaeus' 18th century attempts to classify all living organisms, including human beings. Unfortunately, this and later attempts at racial classification have led to many social abuses in which pseudoscientific evidence has been presented publicly to prove that one race is biologically superior or inferior to another. The radicalization of immigration policy in the history of US immigration highlights how the concept of race has been applied negatively to social values given to so-called 'black' migrants, including immigrants from southern and eastern Europe and most recently developing nations. Southern and eastern Europeans initially were characterized as members of the black race by American society at the turn of the 19th century and considered to be socially inferior to northern European immigrants. These groups were eventually able to 'pass' as whites, which is not the case for many persons who are migrants today.

Because of the negative social history associated with race, many social scientists have suggested that this concept be abandoned completely in favour of the concept of ethnicity. As Barr *et al.* (1979, p.4) state:

"The term ethnicity refers to shared culture and background. Shared background includes common ancestry, and the shared culture embraces language, religion, customs and national or political identification. The essential determinant of ethnic group membership is social identification. If the group defines a person as similar enough to belong to it, and if that person identifies with that group, then he or she belongs to that group, whatever his or her real ancestry may be."

These authors furthermore embedded the concept of ethnicity in Max Weber's sophisticated notion of social interactions that lead to a shared concept of social affinity and ethnic identity. Weber's sociological description of the origins of ethnicity is definitely worthy of a review by mental health practitioners caring for culturally diverse migrant populations (Weber, 1968).

Nationality is a very common term used by ethnic groups, particularly in the USA, to describe ethnic background and country of origin. Some social theorists such as W. Newman (1973) actually agree with this narrower view of ethnicity that describes people by the nations from which they have originated. Montagu (1972) and Shermenhorn (1970), however, recommend the broader use of the original Greek term, *ethnos* which referred not to nationality but to a number of people living together, such as a tribe, group, nation or people—bringing us back again to the modern concept of ethnicity.

Mental health practitioners must take note of the terms migrants use to describe themselves as well as the clinical implications of the terms used to describe their migrant patients.

Identification and diagnosis of serious mental illness

Community diagnosis

New terminologies such as 'transnational migrants' give rise to appreciation in clinical medicine and psychiatry of new approaches to the identification and treatment of mental illness in members of culturally diverse communities. The old but commonly used convention of identifying a patient by racial features, "Mr. X is a 23-year-old black single male ..." now seems almost meaningless. The mental health practitioner must begin the psychiatric evaluation with a comprehensive overview of the migration history and ethnic background of the patient. Not all foreign-born migrants or their children are alike in social class background, educational history and relative degree of assimilation into the host country. The Chilean exile living in Europe who is a famous professor in his home country has little in common with other Spanish-speaking immigrants from Central and Latin America. The distinction between refugee and immigrant needs to be made by the mental health practitioner at the onset since refugees are most likely to have experienced much more trauma and violence than non-refugee members of their own local ethnic communities (e.g. Vietnamese boat people resettled in the USA in the 1980s were considerably more traumatized then the Vietnamese population air-lifted out of South Vietnam in 1975 at the end of the Vietnam War).

Psychiatric evaluation of culturally diverse migrant patients must begin with a culturally valid assessment approach to the identification of psychiatric symptoms and diagnosis. In order to achieve the latter, the commonalities and differences in psychiatric concepts of illness must first be acknowledged. Every society has a unique way of classifying emotional distress associated with human suffering (Hahn, 1995). In western countries, this distress is called mental illness. A person is considered to have a mental illness when emotional suffering is associated with problems in thinking, behaviour and deterioration in functioning. It is generally considered that the more severe the emotional suffering becomes, the more functionally impaired the patient becomes. As the patient recovers, functioning usually returns to normal. Western patients usually express their emotional distress through physical and emotional symptoms. Some may also feel spiritually disturbed. Many patients will show signs of abnormal thinking and actions at work, at home and in the community. These signs and symptoms of mental illness are labelled and treated in western medicine as 'mental disorders' and 'psychiatric diseases'.

In contrast, in many immigrant and refugee cultures and societies, the western terms for mental illnesses are not known. In fact, developing nations have different local terms for describing and classifying states of emotional suffering. The term 'categories of emotional distress' (CED) has been coined recently to describe these local taxonomies of human suffering (Mollica *et al.*, 1999). For example, over the past 20 years, the Harvard research group has been able to describe over 20 CEDs in Cambodian culture (Lavelle *et al.*, 1996). These Cambodian CEDs are a system of classifying states of emotional distress commonly used by Cambodian society. Specific CEDs are popular diagnoses given by the community. Each CED has its own signs and symptoms which can be observed and identified by the ill person, family and friends, or the traditional healer. A person who is ill from a CED is expected by the community to seek help from a traditional or religious healer and/or a family elder. Rarely does the community or the ill person believe that their emotional distress should be treated by a medical doctor. However, the patient will bring his/her CED to the medical doctor seeking a cure, especially if traditional treatments have failed. CEDs are rarely written down; they are usually informally passed along from generation to generation. Within every ethnically diverse refugee and immigrant community, there will be different degrees of knowledge of CEDs based upon the relative assimilation and westernization of the migrant patient. For example, even within Cambodia, western-educated Cambodian professionals rarely subscribe to CED concepts; they adhere almost exclusively to western explanations of physical and mental illness. Mental health practitioners who care for refugee and migrant patients must seek to learn the most common CEDs used by their patient's communities in order fully to appreciate their mental health world view.

General symptoms of emotional distress

All patients express their emotional distress through physical and emotional idioms that are usually not associated with any specific CED or western psychiatric diagnosis (Kleinman, 1977). For example, the most common symptoms of emotional distress for Cambodian refugee patients are demonstrated in Table 37.1 (Mollica *et al.*, 1998). If these culture-specific symptoms are

Table 37.1 *General symptoms of emotional distress*

Dizziness
Weakness
Breathing problems
Vision problems
Headaches
Sadness
Fainting
Ringing in the ears
Warm inside the body
Cold hands/cold feet
Sweating
Joint pain
Difficulty falling asleep
Poor appetite
Loss of memory
Forgetfulness
Loss of ambition
Shortness of breath

presented as a chief complaint by the patient to their medical doctor or mental health practitioner, the latter must check to see if the signs and symptoms of a specific CED or a western psychiatric diagnosis are also present. Only by making a proper diagnosis can the mental health practitioner offer effective treatment.

Assessment of traumatized refugee patients

Highly traumatized refugee patients have been shown to exhibit special problems in revealing their symptoms during conventional psychiatric interviews (Bosnian HTQ and Manual, Allden *et al.*, 1998). The psychiatric interview should consist of guided open-ended questions since it has been demonstrated widely that most refugee patients are easily overwhelmed by their emotional response to the examiner's questions. Over the past 20 years, simple screening instruments have been culturally validated which can help refugee patients 'put words' around their feelings of emotional distress as well as help them describe their traumatic history without having to relive their traumatic experiences within the psychiatric interview. These screening instruments (Hopkins-Symptom Checklist-25, Mollica *et al.*, 1987b; Harvard Trauma Questionnaire, Mollica *et al.*, 1992) are now widely used for evaluating symptoms of depression, anxiety and post-traumatic stress disorder (PTSD) in highly traumatized refugee patients.

Psychiatric diagnosis

An extensive amount of literature has developed investigating the cultural validity and clinical relevance of western psychiatric diagnoses such as those described by ICD-10 and DSM-IV (Jablensky *et al.*, 1991). One approach previously mentioned has avoided these controversies in migrant and refugee patients by using both local CEDs and DSM-IV (ICD-10) diagnostic criteria. What emerges for the clinician from this mixture of culture-specific and western diagnosis is the relative strengths of each diagnostic approach in designing effective treatment. For example, clinical work with Cambodian patients has revealed that there is considerable overlap in the criteria for Cambodian CEDs and DSM-IV criteria for major depression and psychosis. In contrast, the DSM-IV has no diagnosis comparable with the CED 'spirit possession' and the Cambodian CED has no diagnosis comparable with the DSM-IV category of 'organic brain syndromes'. The DSM-IV criteria for PTSD, interestingly, are being used by many refugee cultures since so many members of refugee communities today suffer from the symptoms of PTSD. Family problems common to

Cambodian patients are largely ignored by the DSM-IV; other social problems such as domestic violence and dependence on alcohol would not be considered by the Cambodian refugee community as a mental health problem except in the most extreme situation. Finally, any suffering related to sexual violence is considered a 'taboo' topic by the majority of Southeast Asian refugee women (Mollica *et al.*, 1989). The diagnosis of sexual violence has to be approached by the western therapist in a slow, patient and extremely confidential manner, and it sometimes may take years before the issue is even mentioned by the refugee patient.

As Englehardt (1976) and other philosophers of medicine have expertly articulated, all disease entities are a combination of disease phenomena and disease explanations. Many CEDs and DSM-IV diagnoses may recognize similar symptoms of human suffering, but offer the sufferer different disease explanations, resulting in radically different treatment expectations, therapeutic approaches and possible outcomes. Western practitioners will be most effective if they are aware of these differences in medical and psychiatric world views within the refugee and migrant communities they serve.

Risk and resiliency factors

This chapter will not be able to review the hundreds of innovative treatment approaches that are being practised worldwide in the mental health care of refugee and migrant patients. A major review of the mental health care of torture survivors by the US National Institute of Mental Health (Keane *et al.*, 1998) has revealed the core therapeutic features of these treatment approaches as applied to refugee and torture survivors. In spite of this plethora of treatment methods, little empirical research has been forthcoming to validate as well as compare the efficacy of different techniques and methods.

Our understanding of the social processes that affect transnational migrants such as different assimilation scenarios and the nature of the mental health effects of mass violence and torture on refugee populations has, in fact, led to a revolution in the analysis of the causes and consequences of negative mental health outcomes associated with the migration and refugee experience. Susser (1981) originally suggested an approach that can be modified to help modern day treatment of the refugee and migrant patient. The classic epidemiologic triad of agent–host–environment relationship has rarely been used to understand the mental health sequelae associated with migration. Unfortunately, in prior studies of migrants, there was an underlying pre-supposition that migration itself was a 'toxic' agent producing serious mental health problems. Mental health investigators whether conscious of it or not, subscribed to the straight-line assimilation canon, that is complete assimilation reduced conflict and stress leading to normal levels of mental illness within the host society (Odegaarde, 1932). These early migration researchers did not have the conceptual tools and empirical data now available to us indicating that migrants are sometimes physically healthier, more economically productive and educationally successful, and better socially adapted (including less suicide and involvement in crime) than comparable native members of the host society (Rumbaut, 1999). If 'migration' has temporarily lost its scientific sanctity as a negative mental health agent, then what can replace it?

Over the past two decades, investigators have repeatedly demonstrated that the violence experienced by refugees has serious mental health consequences (Mollica *et al.*, 1993). Refugees in countries of resettlement and in refugee camps have levels of major depression and PTSD many orders of magnitude higher than comparable non-traumatized populations (Kinzie and Jaranson, 1998). Violence is also associated with many physical symptoms and chronic medical conditions affecting all organ systems (Goldfeld *et al.*, 1988). Furthermore, recent studies of Bosnian refugees have revealed the serious physical disability associated with psychiatric co-morbidity in these individuals (Mollica *et al.*, 1999).

Figure 37.1 reveals a schematic model for assessing these risk and resiliency factors that contribute to medical and psychiatric illnesses and disability in refugee and migrant patients and communities. The clinician as well as the public health official can use this model to investigate the agent, individual and environmental factors affecting negative mental health outcomes. Knowledge of the real-life social and economic situation of refugee and migrant patients can now be seen to be absolutely essential in making psychiatric assessments and in planning interventions.

Stereotypical characterizations of the refugee and migrant pre-migration, resettlement and

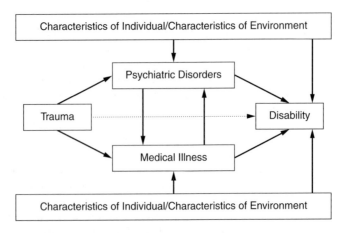

Figure 37.1 *A schematic model for assessing risk and resiliency factors that contribute to medical and psychiatric illnesses and disability in refugee and migrant patients and communities.*

assimilation/acculturation experiences will not provide useful treatment data and might impede a successful treatment outcome. For example, in considering trauma, the mental health practitioner must know the full range of violence experienced by the patient and the community during all time periods (Mollica *et al.*, 1987a). The mass violence experienced by the Cambodian patient under the Pol Pot regime may be replaced by further violence in an American ghetto. Many refugees and migrants experience the racial abuse they receive in their new host countries as extremely disturbing with many negative health consequences.

Personality characteristics in these communities include traditional coping styles, cultural concepts of ethnic identity, gender-related behaviours and strong religious, political and cultural belief systems (Basoglu *et al.*, 1997). Environmental characteristics include the positive and negative features of family life, marriage and kinship ties. As transnational migration research has revealed, family ties and support are not just local but may extend to the migrant's community of origin. The surrounding local community, in addition, may show the strength of cultural solidarity or the negative pressure to participate in antisocial behaviours. Conflict between different generations may also prove to be extremely destructive to parents and children or may be enriching to family unity; similar possibilities exist for the different educational and work experiences of spouses and children (Beiser, 1988). The mental health practitioner must know the patient's family and community well enough to attempt to reduce those risk factors contributing to the patient's illness while supporting those resiliency factors contributing to the patient's recovery.

Organization of refugee and immigrant mental health services

Mental health services for refugees and immigrants have been organized very differently in different countries depending upon that nation's

tradition of dealing with the medical and psychiatric problems of culturally diverse populations (Magruder *et al.*, 1998). However, two major service organizations seem to have emerged over the past two decades correlating with the upswing of human rights interest in the care of torture survivors, who generally come from asylum seekers and resettled refugee groups.

These two major treatment approaches to the psychiatric care of migrants can be described as (i) human rights treatment centres and (ii) community-based mental health care. A noble example of the former is the model developed by the Danish group (Ortmann *et al.*, 1987) and others which focuses specifically on the medical and psychiatric rehabilitation of torture survivors. These specialized torture treatment centres generally care for torture survivors from many diverse geopolitical backgrounds. In contrast to the human rights clinics, community-based psychiatric programmes (Mollica and Lavelle, 1988) primarily focus on the general mental health needs of a specific ethnic community or the resident members of a specific neighbourhood or catchment area. All community residents are encouraged to seek mental health care regardless of the specific nature of their diagnosis or trauma history. The focus of these neighbourhood health centres is on care by members of the ethnic community they serve. It would, therefore, not be uncommon for foreign-born immigrants, traumatized refugees and their children's generation from the same cultural background to seek mental health care at the same facility. In contrast to torture rehabilitation centres, these community-based mental health clinics often are able to employ many paraprofessional and professional mental health practitioners with similar cultural background to that of the local community residents.

In spite of these differences in orientation, psychiatric services to diverse populations are remarkably similar to those services provided to native populations. Modern emphasis on the linkage of clinical out-patient psychiatric care to general hospital in-patient care where brief hospitalization can occur has also been remarkably effective in the total delivery of psychiatric care to refugees and migrants. The traditional mental hospital (or asylum) can almost always be totally by-passed, especially if a designated general hospital in-patient unit has staff trained in the care of refugee and migrant patients. Avoidance of the mental hospital is especially critical in the in-patient care of migrants because historically these facilities were often used in countries of resettlement to incarcerate immigrant populations without adequate treatment. For example, in America and western Europe, the role of the mental hospital in the radicalization of immigrant mental health care, leading to extraordinary abuses, is well documented and remembered by local migrant communities (Malzberg, 1964). In many developing countries that are the source of today's migrants and refugees, the mental hospital was feared by local residents for its oppression and prison-like environment. Mental hospitals were also used to incarcerate political prisoners and may have also served as places where torture occurred. This fear of the mental hospital combined with cultural resistance to psychiatric in-patient hospitalization of any kind by migrant and refugee patients demands that out-patient strategies, including day programmes and home visits, be maximized even for the most seriously ill patients.

The clinical work of dedicated mental health practitioners in resource-poor environments with culturally diverse migrant patients has led to many service innovations. These innovations in providing culturally effective mental health care are too numerous to describe in this section. However, there are two service delivery elements which appear to be fundamental to the care of refugees and migrants (Mollica, 1988). These include (i) the role of the primary health care facility and (ii) utilization of the bi-cultural paraprofessional.

Role of the primary health care facility

Refugees and migrants will seek out health care consistent with their cultural expectations and traditional health-seeking behaviours. Many members of culturally diverse populations are unfamiliar with western psychiatrists and mental health practitioners. In general, as the previous discussion of CEDs revealed, common physical symptoms of emotional suffering are considered by these patients to be the appropriate domain of medical practitioners; in contrast, emotional stress and related social problems are believed to be brought most appropriately to family, friends, elders and religious leaders. Furthermore, many refugees and immigrants associate shame and humiliation with their perceived need to seek help for a 'broken mind or spirit'. These negative attitudes of refugees and immigrants toward mental health commonly is reinforced by the immigration policies of host countries, which prevent migrants from resettlement if they are discovered to have a medical history of psychiatric illness. In effect, these barriers to mental health care result in the general medical clinic or primary health care setting being the major portal of entry for most psychiatric illnesses within ethnic communities. Consequently, the location of refugee and migrant mental health services within primary health care settings with close ties between mental health practitioners and primary care physicians has been shown to maximize the identification and treatment of mental illness in refugee and migrant communities.

The bicultural paraprofessional

Two realities in psychiatric services to ethnic communities reinforce each other, resulting in limited and sometimes harmful mental health care (Putsch, 1985). First, it has been well documented that western mental health practitioners with limited knowledge of the ethnic patient's culture consistently misdiagnose serious mental illness; in fact they have a tendency to recommend organic treatments such as ECT and high doses of medication without the use of supportive psychotherapies or counselling. In addition, 'black' migrant patients, in particular, are over-rated as being dangerous, paranoid and violent when compared with native-born white patients revealing similar symptoms. This may be due again not only to the lack of knowledge of patterns of human suffering in ethnic populations but also to racial prejudices inherent in the host society.

Secondly, combined with these racial biases may be a lack of mental health professionals from the refugee or immigrant's culture who are capable of countering these tendencies. In spite of the obvious need for skilled communication between patients and psychiatric professionals, a bizarre range of inappropriate interpreting procedures occurs, including the use of untrained hospital staff such as kitchen workers, children interpreting for their parents, males reviewing sexual history with female patients, torturers interpreting for patients they have tortured, and husbands interviewing suicidal wives about possible marital infidelity. Confidential and culturally skilled medical and psychiatric interpreting is essential in the mental health diagnosis and treatment of refugee and migrant patients. Fortunately, the scientific literature on the importance of competent cross-cultural communication in clinical medicine and psychiatry is expanding rapidly. No longer are medically untrained interpreters sufficient or acceptable in medical practice. (Putsch, 1985; Westermeyer, 1990; Lavelle *et al.*, 1993). Yet in many refugee and immigrant communities, clinically trained medical professionals are not available. This lack of available professional staff has led to the training of bicultural paraprofessionals from the local communities. These paraprofessionals are not just 'interpreters' or 'translators'; they are highly specialized mental health clinicians who can move conceptually between western models of disease and treatment and the unique medical and psychiatric world of their own culture. Many continue their education to eventually receive degrees in the health care professions, eventually creating a cadre of mental health professionals from the migrant communities themselves.

Acknowledgements

This manuscript is dedicated to the late Professor Douglas Bennett.

References

Alba, R. and Nee, Y. (1999) Rethinking assimilation theory for a new era of immigration. In: Hirschman, C., Kasinitz, P. and DeWind, J. (eds), *The Handbook of International Migration*. New York: Russell Sage Foundation, pp. 137–160.

Allden, K., Frani_kovi, T., Lavelle, J., Mathias, M., McInnes, K., Mollica, R.F. and Moro, L. (1998) *Harvard Trauma Questionnaire: Bosnia-Herzegovina Version*. Cambridge: Harvard Program in Refugee Trauma (Available in English and Bosnian).

Bahr, H.M., Chadwick, B.A. and Strauss, J.H. (eds) (1979) *American Ethnicity*. Lexington, MA: DC Heath and Co.

Basoglu, M., Mineka, S., Paker, M., Aker, T., Liuanoa, M. and Gok, S. (1997) Psychological preparedness for trauma as a projective factor in survivors of torture. *Psychological Medicine*, 27, 1421–1433.

Beiser, M. (1988) Influence of time, ethnicity, and attachment on depression in Southeast Asian refugees. *American Journal of Psychiatry*, 145, 46–51.

Berry, J.W., Kim, U., Minde, T. and Mok, D. (1987) Comparative studies of acculturation stress. *International Migration Review*, 21, 491–511.

Englehardt, T. (1976) Deology and ethiology. *Journal of Medicine and Philosophy*, 1, 256–268.

Goldfeld, A., Mollica, R.F., Pesavento, B. and Faraone, S. (1988) The physical and psychological sequelae of torture: symptomatology and diagnosis. *Journal of the American Medical Association*, 259, 2725–2729.

Hahn, R.A. (1995) *Sickness and Healing: An Anthropological Perspective*. New Haven, CT: Yale University Press.

Handlin, O. (1973) *The Uprooted: The Epic Story of the Great Migrations That Made the American People*, 2nd edn. Boston: Little Brown.

Hirschman, C., Kasinitz, P. and DeWind, J. (eds) (1999) *The Handbook of International Migration*. New York: Russell Sage Foundation.

Jablensky, A., Sartorius, N., Gulbinat, W. and Ernberg, G. (1991) Characteristics of depressive patients contacting psychiatric services in four cultures. *Acta Psychiatrica Scandinavica*, 63, 367–383.

Keane, T., Gerrity, E. and Tuma, F. (1998) *Mental Health Consequences of Torture and Related Violence*. Washington, DC: NIMH.

Kinzie, J.D. and Jaranson, J. (1998) Refugees and asylum seekers. In: Keane,T., Gerrity, E. and Tuma, F. (eds), *Mental Health Consequences of Torture and Related Violence*. Washington, DC: NIMH.

Kleinman, A. (1977) Depression, somatization and the 'new' cross-cultural psychiatry. *Social Science and Medicine*, 11, 3–10.

Kleinman, A., Eisenberg, L. and Good, B. (1978) Culture illness and care: clinical lessons from an theopologic and cross-cultural research. *Annals of Internal Medicine*, 88, 251–258.

Lavelle, J., Tor, S., Stedman, W., Mollica, R.F. and Sath, S. (1993) *Curriculum for Khmer Mental Health Training and Certification Program on the Thai–Cambodian Border*. Boston: Harvard Program in Refugee Trauma.

Magruder, K.M., Mollica, R. and Friedman, M. (1998) Mental health services research: implications for survivors of torture. In: Keane, T., Gerrity, E. and Tuma, F. (eds), *Mental Health Consequences of Torture and Related Violence and Trauma*. Rockville MD: National Institute of Mental Health.

Malzberg, B. (1964) Mental disease among native and foreign born whites in New York State. 1949–1951. *Mental Hygiene*, 48, 478–499.

Masey, D.S. (1999) Why does immigration occur? a theoretical synthesis. In: Hirschman, C., Kasinitz, P. and DeWind, J. (eds), *The Handbook of International Migration*. New York: Russell Sage Foundation, pp. 34–52.

Mollica, R.F. (1988) The trauma story: the psychiatric care of refugee survivors of violence and torture. In: Ochberg, F.M. (ed.), *Post-traumatic Therapy and Victims of Violence*. New York: Brunner/Mazel.

Mollica, R.F. (1999) The mental health and psychosocial effects of mass violence. In: Leaning, J., Briggs, S.M. and Chen, L. (eds), *Humanitarian Emergencies: The Medical and Public Health Response*. Cambridge, MA: Harvard University Press, pp. 125–142.

Mollica, R. and Chan, S. (1996) Causes and treatment of depression. In: *Harvard Guide to Khmer Mental Health*. Lavelle, J., Tor, S., Mollica, R.F., Allden, K. and Potts, L. (eds), Boston: Harvard Program in Refugee Trauma.

Mollica, R.F. and Lavelle, J. (1988) Southeast Asian refugees. In: Comas-Diaz, L. and Griffith, E.E.H. (eds), *Clinical Guidelines in Cross-Cultural Mental Health*. New York: Wiley & Sons.

Mollica, R.F. and Son, L. (1989) Cultural dimensions in the evaluation and treatment of sexual trauma: an overview. *Psychiatric Clinics of North America*, 12, 363–379.

Mollica, R.F., Wyshak, G. and Lavelle, J. (1987a) The psychosocial impact of war trauma and torture on Southeast Asian refugees. *American Journal of Psychiatry*, 144, 1567–1572.

Mollica, R.F., Wyshak, G., de Marneffe, D., Tu, B., Yang, T., Khuon, F. and Lavelle, J. (1987b) Hopkins Symptom Checklist-25: a screening instrument for the psychiatric care of refugees. *American Journal of Psychiatry*, 144.

Mollica, R.F., Caspi-Yavin, Y., Bollini, P., Truong, T., Tor, S. and Lavelle, J. (1992) Harvard Trauma Questionnaire: validating a cross-cultural instrument for measuring torture, trauma, and posttraumatic stress disorder in Indochinese refugees. *Journal of Nervous and Mental Disease*, 180, 111–116.

Mollica, R.F., Donelan, K., Tor, S., Lavelle, J., Elias, C., Frankel, M., Bennett, D., Blendon, R.J. and Bass, R. (1993) The effect of trauma and confinement on functional health and mental health status of Cambodians living in Thai–Cambodia border camps. *Journal of the Americn Medical Association*, 270, 581–586.

Mollica, R.F., Tor, S. and Lavelle, J. (1998) *Pathways to Healing: Viewmaster Guide to Khmer Mental Health*. Boston: Harvard Program in Refugee Trauma.

Mollica, R.F., McInnes, K., Sarajlic, N., Lavelle, J., Sarajlic, I. and Massagli, M. (1999) Disability associated with psychiatric comorbidity and health status in Bosnian refugees living in Croatia. *Journal of the American Medical Association*, 282,

Montagu, A. (1972) *Statement on Race*. New York: Oxford University Press.

Newman, W.M. (1973) *American Pluralism*. New York: Harper and Row.

Odegaarde (1932) Emigration and Insanity. *Acta Psychiatrica et Neurologica*, 4, 1–206.

Ortmann, J., Genefke, I.K., Jakobsen, L. and Lunde, I. (1987) Rehabilitation of torture victims: an interdisciplinary treatment model. *American Journal of Social Psychiatry*, 7, 161–167.

Park, R.E. and Burgess, E.W. (1921) *Introduction to the Science of Sociology*. Chicago: University of Chicago Press.

Putsch, R.W. (1985) Cross-cultural communication. the social case of interpreters in health care. *Journal of the American Medical Association*, 254, 3344–3348.

Rumbaut, R.G. (1999)Assismiliation and its discontents: ironies and paradoxes. In: Hirschman, C., Kasinitz, P. and DeWind, J. (eds), *The Handbook of International Migration*. New York: Russell Sage Foundation, pp. 172–195.

Schermerhorn, R.A. (1970) *Comparative Ethnic Relations: A Framework for Theory and Research*. New York: Random House.

Schiller, N.G. (1999) Transmigrations and nation-states: something old and something new in the US immigrant experience. In: Hirschman, C., Kasinitz, P. and DeWind, J. (eds), *The Handbook of International Migration*. New York: Russell Sage Foundation, pp. 94–119.

Shural, J. (1982) Migration and Stress. In: Goldberger, L. and Breznitz, S. (eds), *Handbook of Stress*. New York: Colliers, Macmillan.

Susser, M. (1981) The epidemiology of life stress. *Psychological Medicine*, 11, 1–8.

United Nations High Commissioner for Refugees (1993) *The State of the World's Refugees: The Challenge of Protection*. Penguin: New York.

United Nations High Commissioner for Refugees (1988) *Handbook on Procedures and Criteria for Determining Refugee Status*. Geneva: UNHCR.

United Nations High Commissioner for Refugees (1998) *The State of the World's Refugees 1997–1998: A Humanitarian Agenda*. New York: Oxford University Press.

US Committee for Refugees (1999) *World Refugee Statistics, World Refugee Survey*. Washington, DC: USCR.

Weber, M. (1968) Economy and society. In: Roth, G. and Wittich, C. (eds), New York: Bedminister Press, pp. 387–398.

Westermyer, J, (1990) Working with an interpreter in psychiatric assessment and treatment. *Journal of Nervous and Mental Disease*, 178, 745–749.

38 | *Community attitudes towards mental disorder*

Richard Warner

"I have often been fraught with a profound guilt over my diagnosis of schizophrenia . . . .I had little idea how dehumanising and humiliating the hospital would be for me . . . .I felt that I had partly lost my right to stand among humanity . . . and that for some people I would be forevermore something of a subhuman creature . . . . Mental health professionals often treated me . . . as if I were a stranger or alien of sorts, set apart from others by reason of my label" (Anonymous, 1977, p. 4).

Public attitudes

With the growth of interest in community psychiatry in the 1950s and 1960s, attention in the industrial world was focused on the question of the stigma of mental illness. Star (1955), using vignettes depicting people with psychotic symptoms, conducted a nationwide survey of members of the American public in 1950 and found the general reaction to the mentally ill to be negative and poorly informed. Cumming and Cumming (1957), using the same techniques in 1951, uncovered similar attitudes among residents of a rural town (which they called Blackfoot) in Saskatchewan, Canada, and found that the negative attitudes were untouched after a 6-month educational campaign. Following a survey of residents of the Champaign-Urbana area of Illinois in the 1950s, Nunally (1961) concluded that the mentally ill were viewed by the general public with "fear, distrust, and dislike." "Old people and young people" reported Nunally, "highly educated people and people with little formal training—all tend to regard the mentally ill as relatively dangerous, dirty, unpredictable and worthless" They were considered, in short, "all things bad" (p. 46).

In the following years, a dispute has arisen over whether the initial impressions of high levels of stigma attached to mental illness continue to hold true. A number of researchers in the 1960s concluded that the public tolerance of the mentally ill had improved (Lemkau and Crocetti, 1962; Meyer, 1964; Bentz *et al.*, 1969; Crocetti *et al.*, 1971). In the late 1970s, 20 years after Nunally's original survey, Cockerham (1981) again analysed public attitudes towards the mentally ill in Champaign-Urbana and found them to be somewhat more tolerant. Rabkin (1980) argued in 1980 that attitudes had improved but had subsequently reached a plateau. Other researchers found no improvement in popular mental health attitudes between the 1960s and 1970s (Olmsted and Durham, 1976); a second survey of public tolerance of the mentally ill in Blackfoot, Saskatchewan, 23 years after Cummings' original study, revealed that virtually no change had occurred (D'Arcy and Brockman, 1976).

As recently as 1993, public surveys conducted in two English communities revealed a similar failure to identify mental illness as in Star's 1950 US study; the authors argued that there was a reluctance to label someone as mentally ill because of the negative associations of the term (Hall *et al.*, 1993). The same study revealed that public tolerance of the mentally ill was scarcely better in a district which had been served for 10 years by a model community psychiatry programme than in the area which had no such service (Brockington, 1993; Hall *et al.*, 1993).

Positive attitudes towards treatment and community integration, however, were noted in a 1997 survey conducted in England, Scotland

and Wales (Market and Opinion Research International, 1997). Most respondents felt that schizophrenia was treatable, that treatment should be in the community and that they willingly would work alongside someone with the disorder. Only 13%, however, would have been happy for a son or daughter to marry someone with the illness.

Misconceptions continue to abound. In Britain, 50% of survey respondents believed that setting fire to public buildings was a 'very likely' consequence of mental illness (O'Grady, 1996) and, in an American survey, 58% blamed 'lack of discipline' as a cause while 93 blamed drug and alcohol abuse (Borenstein, 1992). The World Psychiatric Association Programme Against Stigma and Discrimination Because of Schizophrenia (described below) lists a number of widespread misconceptions about schizophrenia including the following:

- Nobody recovers from schizophrenia.
- Schizophrenia is an untreatable disease.
- People with schizophrenia are usually violent or dangerous.
- People with schizophrenia are likely to infect others with their madness.
- People with schizophrenia are lazy and unreliable.
- Schizophrenia is the result of a deliberate weakness of will.
- Everything people with schizophrenia say is nonsense.
- People with schizophrenia are completely unable to make rational decisions about their own lives.
- People with schizophrenia are unpredictable.
- People with schizophrenia cannot work.
- Schizophrenia is the parents' fault.

Media images

Media representations of the mentally ill have shown little change since the Second World War. In the late 1970s and early 1980s, US media were still projecting a sensational image of people with mental illness (Steadman and Cocozza, 1978); TV dramas represented the mentally ill much of the time as violent or homicidal (Gerbner *et al.*, 1981). A US media survey in 1983 (Shain and Phillips, 1991) found the same misconceptions of mental illness reflected as Nunally had found in 1961. In the following years, the US lobbying group, the National Alliance for the Mentally Ill, grew in influence and confronted the issue of media coverage, and by 1988 press reporting had improved somewhat; there was less focus on crime, and more on causes of illness and treatment, but dangerousness was still a dominant focus (Shain and Phillips, 1991). A 1993 review of British news coverage revealed that the mentally ill were almost always portrayed in a negative light—as violent criminals, murderers or rapists, at best figures of fun (Barnes, 1993). A 1994 study of British media coverage of mental illness found that accounts of violence outweighed sympathetic reports by four to one (Philo, 1994). Fear-mongering by tabloids continues to be common; a recent British headline trumpeted, "Hospital Bungle Released Beast for Sex Spree" (Wolff, 1997) and another vilified health services which were ". . . Setting Patients Free to Kill and Rape" (Wolff, 1997).

Prejudice, discrimination and stigma

People with mental illness are subject to prejudice, discrimination and stigma. Branded as 'psychos' in popular parlance, they encounter discrimination in housing and employment (Miller and Dawson, 1965; Wolff, 1997) and generate fear as to their dangerousness (Monahan and Arnold, 1996). In a recent American study, it was found that 40% of landlords immediately rejected applicants with a known psychiatric disorder (Alisky and Iczkowski, 1990). Citizens fight to exclude treatment facilities and living quarters for the mentally ill from residential neighbourhoods, even though group homes for the mentally ill have not been shown to have adverse effects on communities (Boydall *et al.*, 1989). According to a recent survey of the American public (Robert Wood Johnson Foundation, 1990), the 'not in my backyard' phenomenon is a widespread obstacle to the community integration of people with mental illness. The status afforded the mentally ill has been shown to be the very lowest—lower than that of ex-convicts or the developmentally disabled (Tringo, 1970). Even after 5 years of normal living and hard work, according to one early US survey, an ex-mental patient was rated as less acceptable than an ex-convict (Lamy, 1966).

The agencies serving the mentally ill are tainted by association, and mental health professionals themselves sometimes hold attitudes towards mental patients which are similar to those of the general public; they may even be *more* rejecting. In one study, mental hospital staff were considerably less likely than members of the public to take the trouble to mail a sealed, addressed letter which they believed to have been accidentally lost by a mental hospital patient (Page, 1980).

The mentally ill themselves often accept the stereotype of their own condition. Young patients in rural Ireland viewed their "spending time in the 'madhouse' . . . as a permanent 'fall from grace' similar to a loss of virginity" (Scheper-Hughes, 1979, p. 89). A number of studies have shown that psychiatric patients can be as negative in their opinions of mental illness as the general public (Giovannoni and Ullman, 1963; Manis *et al.*, 1963; Crumpton *et al.*, 1967). Some reports, indeed, indicate that patients are *more* rejecting of the mentally ill than are family members or hospital staff (Bentinck, 1967; Swanson and Spitzer, 1970).

Moderating factors

Some individual factors are known to moderate stigma and improve public tolerance of the mentally ill. Younger and better-educated people are usually more tolerant (Rabkin, 1980; Brockington *et al.*, 1993; Wolff, 1997). Prior contact with someone who suffers from mental illness decreases stigma and fear of dangerousness, as does knowledge of the person's living situation (Penn *et al.*, 1994). Those who do not perceive the mentally ill as violent are relatively tolerant (Link *et al.*, 1987; Penn *et al.*, 1994). Residential facilities for the mentally ill are better accepted in downtown, transient districts with low social cohesion and less well accepted in single-family neighbourhoods (Trute and Segal, 1976).

Stigma in the developing world

People with psychotic disorders in the developing world are often viewed differently by their community. In the past, psychiatrists working in developing countries often noted the low level of stigma which attaches to mental disorder. Among Formosan tribesmen studied by Rin and Lin (1962), mental illness was free of stigma. Sinhalese families freely refer to psychotic family members as *pissu* (crazy) and show no shame about it; tuberculosis in Sri Lanka is more stigmatizing than mental illness (Waxler, 1977).

The World Psychiatric Association Programme Against Stigma and Discrimination Because of Schizophrenia has identified a number of factors in the developing world which promote greater tolerance and community support for people with serious mental illness. These include:

- the absence of large-scale institutional care from the traditional mental health care system;
- the rural agrarian nature of the society;
- the strength of the extended family system;
- explanatory models which place the cause of the illness external to the patient;
- the fact that symptoms of psychosis are more readily reversible and outcome from schizophrenia better in the developing world.

The authors of a WHO follow-up study of schizophrenia suggest that one of the factors contributing to the good outcome from schizophrenia in Cali, Colombia, is the high level of tolerance of relatives and friends for symptoms of mental disorder—a factor which can help the readjustment to family life and work after discharge (World Health Organization, 1979). An Indian 5-year follow-up study of people with schizophrenia found that 80% of families preferred that a disturbed family member continue to stay with the family (Indian Council of Medical Research, 1988). Another Indian study found home-based treatment of schizophrenia to be better accepted and less disruptive for families than hospital care (Pai and Kapur, 1983).

The lower degree of stigma in parts of the developing world may be partly a result of different folk-diagnostic practices. Throughout the non-industrial world, the features of psychosis are likely to be given a supernatural explanation; people with these symptoms may be considered to be victims of witchcraft or, conversely, shamans or spiritualists (Warner, 1984). When urban and rural Yoruba with no formal education in Nigeria were shown Star profiles of mentally ill people, only 40% thought that the person with paranoid schizophrenia was mentally ill (Erinosho and Ayonrinde, 1981) [nearly all Americans label the subject of this vignette as mentally ill (D'Arcy and Brockman, 1976)]. Only a fifth of Yoruba respondents considered the person with simple schizophrenia to be mentally ill (three-quarters of American respondents call this case mentally ill). A third of the Yoruba, moreover, would have been willing to marry the person with paranoid schizophrenia and more than a half would have married the person with simple schizophrenia (Erinosho and Ayonrinde, 1981).

When such people are labelled as being 'mad', however, the situation changes. When skilled workers from the area of Benin in mid-western Nigeria were asked their opinions about someone specifically labelled a 'nervous or mad person', 16% thought that all such people should be shot and 31% believed that they should be expelled from the country. These educated Nigerians conceived of mad people as 'senseless, unkempt, aggressive and irresponsible' (Binitie, 1970).

There is evidence that the stigma of mental illness is increasing in parts of the developing world with advancing industrialization and urbanization. Early studies in India found high levels of tolerance and sympathy, willingness to interact with the mentally ill, optimism about treatment, and

absence of concealment (Sathyavathi *et al.*, 1971: Verghese and Beig, 1974). More recent Indian studies point to decreasing tolerance. A recent survey of public attitudes in New Delhi (Prabhu *et al.*, 1984) concluded that "the mentally ill are perceived as aggressive, violent and dangerous" by city dwellers. "A pervasive defeatism exists about the possible outcome after therapy. There is a tendency to maintain social distance from the mentally ill and to reject them" (p. 12).

In other industrializing parts of the developing world, reaction against people labelled as mentally ill can be extreme. Since the 1980s, there has been a vigorous movement in Hong Kong which opposes the placement of psychiatric halfway houses in residential districts. The movement, supported by a political party, is based on a fear of violence by the mentally ill. One halfway house was opposed on the basis that it was too near a butcher's shop where, it was believed, the sight of a meat cleaver would drive patients to homicide. Angry residents even threatened to demolish psychiatric facilities and used video cameras to track the movements of outpatients (K.S. Yip, personal communication, 1998). It is clear that attitudes to the mentally ill vary from culture to culture and are influenced by the label which is applied to the person with psychosis.

Labelling theory

In the early post-war period, research on the stigma of mental illness was fuelled by interest in labelling theory. Once a deviant person has been labelled 'mentally ill', argued Scheff (1966), society responds in accordance with a predetermined stereotype and the individual is launched on a career of chronic mental illness from which there is little opportunity for escape. There is evidence to support Scheff's position. Phillips' (1966) study of the attitudes of residents of a small New England town showed that a normal person of an 'ideal type' who was described as having been in a mental hospital was socially rejected to a much greater degree than was a person with schizophrenia who sought no help or who instead consulted a clergyman.

In Rosenhan's (1973) study, normal volunteers presented themselves for voluntary admission to a dozen different psychiatric hospitals with complaints of auditory hallucinations. Every pseudopatient was admitted and, although they reverted to normal behaviour and denied psychotic symptoms immediately upon admission, each one was labelled schizophrenic at the time of discharge. Staff described the normal behaviour of the pseudopatients as if they were pathological. None was discharged in less than a week—one was detained for almost 2 months. Such studies suggest that patients with schizophrenia may be subject to pressure to conform to stereotypic expectations which could influence their hope of recovery and their behaviour.

Critics of labelling theory argue that the approach understates the importance of the initial deviance and of the inherent pathology of mental illness in causing a label to be attached, and that it minimizes the capacity of mental patients to shake off the harmful effects of stigma (Gove, 1975). Of a dozen studies conducted after 1963 assessing the relative importance of the mental illness label versus the person's behaviour in determining public attitudes, most found the effect of labelling to be significant but nearly all found the person's behaviour to be more potent (Link *et al.*, 1987). Similarly, in a more recent study, knowledge of the symptoms of a person's acute schizophrenic episode created more stigma than the label 'schizophrenia' (Penn *et al.*, 1994).

Regardless of the relative potency of the illness label, patients and families continue to report that stigma is a significant obstacle to community integration (Penn *et al.*, 1994), and it seems likely that labelling has a significant effect in shaping the self-concept, behaviour and symptoms of the mentally ill person. Strauss and Carpenter (1981) conclude that

"Labelling is an important variable affecting the course . . . of schizophrenia . . . .Who can doubt the devastating impact on a fragile person of perceiving that the entire social milieu regards him (wittingly or not) as subhuman, incurable, unmotivated, or incompetent to pursue ordinary expectations . . . ? Can we doubt that a deteriorating course of disorder is fostered when fundamental roles are changed by social stigma and employment opportunities become limited?" (p. 128)

How stigma influences the course of illness

How does the stigma of mental illness affect symptoms of schizophrenia and shape the course of the illness? The author has suggested (Warner, 1984) that patients who accept the diagnosis of mental illness feel internal pressure to conform to the stereotype of incapacity and worthlessness, becoming more socially withdrawn and adopt a disabled role. As a result, their symptoms persist and they become dependent on treatment and others in their lives. Thus, insight into one's illness may be rewarded with poor outcome.

The author's view is confirmed by Doherty's (1975) study of self-labelling by psychiatric inpatients. Hospitalized patients who accepted that they were mentally ill were rated as showing the least improvement and those who denied that they were mentally ill did better. A study by the author and his colleagues (Warner *et al.*, 1989) supported this finding. Patients who accepted that they were mentally ill had lower self-esteem and lacked a sense of control over their lives. Those who found mental illness most stigmatizing had the worst self-esteem and the weakest sense of mastery. The study suggested that patients could only benefit from accepting that they were ill if they also had a sense of control over their lives. Such patients were few and far between, however, since a consequence of accepting the illness label was loss of a sense of mastery. Thus, stigma creates a Catch 22 for people with schizophrenia—accepting the illness can mean losing the capacity to cope with it.

Social isolation

Partly as a consequence of their pariah status, people with schizophrenia in the developed world lead lives of social isolation. Many studies have shown that such patients have networks of social contacts which are much more restricted than is usual in our society. People with schizophrenia are found to have close contacts with a third to a fifth of the number of people which is average for other members of the community. A third of the chronically mentally ill have no friends at all. In the USA, the relationships of people with schizophrenia tend to be one-sided, dependent and lacking in complexity and diversity. Although family relationships deteriorate less than contact with friends, a considerable disintegration of family ties does occur (Pattison *et al.*, 1975; Cohen and Sokolovsky, 1978; Lipton *et al.*, 1981; Pattison and Pattison, 1981).

The social isolation of the person with schizophrenia in the west stands in contrast to the more effective social reintegration of people with psychosis in the developing world. Although disruptive and violent individuals living in villages who have been designated 'mad' do have restricted social networks (Westermeyer and Pattison, 1981), the problem does not apply, to the same extent, to less chronic and severely disturbed people with psychosis in the developing world (Warner, 1984). In both the developed and developing world, however, social isolation has been shown repeatedly to be associated with poor outcome (World Health Organization, 1979; Strauss and Carpenter, 1981; Brugha *et al.*, 1993). For example, regardless of symptom severity, people with schizophrenia who have broader and more complex social networks are less likely to be readmitted to hospital (Cohen and Sokolovsky, 1978).

Families of people with schizophrenia

The stigma which attaches to mental illness also taints the relatives. Some react by talking to no one about the illness for years, not even to close friends. Those who do discuss the matter openly may find themselves snubbed by acquaintances. Other families respond by withdrawing socially. One-third of the wives in an early US study followed a course of aggressive concealment including dropping and avoiding friends or even moving to a new residence (Yarrow *et al.*, 1955).

Although there is a tendency for family members to deny the stigma, their concealment and withdrawal point to an underlying sense of shame and lead them into social isolation (Kreisman and Joy, 1974).

In a survey of relatives of people with schizophrenia in Washington, DC, Hatfield (1978) observed "a picture of unremittingly disturbed family life marked by almost constant stress" (p. 358) as a consequence of caring for a patient at home. Marital disruption, blame, grief and helplessness were common results. In a study of British families in which someone with schizophrenia was living at home, half of the family members reported severe or very severe impairment of their own health as a consequence of their relative's psychiatric condition (Creer, 1975).

What can be done to reduce stigma?

Neighbourhood campaigns

Surveys of public attitudes reveal negative attitudes but also a substantial amount of goodwill toward the mentally ill. When neighbours of a new group home for people with mental illness in south London were surveyed, two-thirds expressed a willingness to help the new facility and showed interest in learning more about mental illness (Reda, 1995). Organizers found that this goodwill could be mobilized by a focused education campaign which encouraged neighbours to initiate social contact with mentally ill residents (Wolff, 1997). During the campaign, informational packets (video tapes and written materials) were distributed, and social events and informal discussion sessions were organized. The campaign decreased fearful and rejecting attitudes and increased contacts between group-home residents and their new neighbours. Thirteen percent of the neighbours made friends with patients or invited them into their homes, whereas no neighbours did so in an area which was not exposed to the educational program (Wolff, 1997). Campaigns which increase contact with patients can be expected to improve attitudes, since personal knowledge of someone with mental illness is associated with greater tolerance (Penn *et al.*, 1994). Such projects suggest that neighbourhood action campaigns are feasible and effective. Can broader societal campaigns achieve a similar impact? To answer this question, we can look at some of the advances in modern communication technology.

Social marketing

Since the unsuccessful anti-stigma campaigns of the post-war period, public education methods and techniques for health promotion have improved dramatically. Such 'social marketing' campaigns, as they are known in the communication field, have been used successfully around the world in reducing infant mortality, AIDS prevention, family planning, improving nutrition, smoking cessation and a variety of other causes (Rogers, 1995). Carefully designed campaigns can have substantial effects on behaviour (Rogers *et al.*, 1995). Effectiveness is increased by 'audience segmentation'—partitioning a mass audience into subaudiences that are relatively homogeneous and devising promotional strategies and messages that are more relevant and acceptable to those target groups (Rogers *et al.*, 1995; Rogers, 1996).

In developing such campaigns, it is important to conduct a needs assessment which gathers information about cultural beliefs, myths and misapprehensions, and the media through which people would want to learn about the topic. The needs assessment method may incorporate focus groups, telephone surveys and information from opinion leaders. A pre-testing mechanism is then established which allows the promotional strategy to be refined continuously (Rogers, 1995). Initially, specific objectives, audiences, messages and media are selected, and an action plan is drawn up. These messages and materials are pre-tested with specific audiences and revised. The plan is implemented and, with continuous monitoring of impact, a new campaign plan is developed and constantly refined.

Health promotion campaigns aim to heighten awareness and to provide information; the former is possible without the latter, but not the reverse.

Awareness campaigns need to be supported by an infrastructure which can link people to sources of information and support—for example, a telephone number to call and trained people to respond to the caller. Ideally, the infrastructure should be a central organization with a local network.

Entertainment media, such as popular songs and soap operas, can heighten awareness and provide information, and are especially useful for socially taboo topics such as mental illness. Soap operas have been successful in advancing social messages in several countries. For example, a TV soap opera in China called 'Ordinary People', which promotes smaller family size and AIDS education, began broadcasting in 1995 and will, in due course, reach 16% of the world's population (Rogers *et al.*, 1995). A radio soap opera encouraging AIDS awareness and family planning gained a wide audience in Tanzania and was effective in changing attitudes and sexual behaviour. Similarly, a TV programme centred on a character named Maria and aired in Mexico for 40 years has promoted, among other things, adult education (Rogers *et al.*, 1995).

Focus groups of local experts and representatives of interest groups help generate the 'moral messages' for such serial dramas, and scriptwriters develop positive, negative and transitional characters. Transitional characters switch from positive to negative behaviour, or vice versa, to illustrate the rewards and consequences of their decisions. Characters are devised to reflect a variety of age ranges of both genders so that listeners can find someone with whom to identify. The approach embraces social learning theory and the concept that people model their behaviour on others.

Pure entertainment soap operas can also be adapted to incorporate characters with a social message. In the USA, a group calling itself the 'Soap Summit' analyses the content of soap operas (looking at such topics as teenage sexual behaviour), lobbies scriptwriters to change the content of their programmes to create positive social messages, and measures the impact of their lobbying on soap opera content. A character with schizophrenia recently was introduced into one of the most widely watched programmes in Britain,

'EastEnders'. The National Schizophrenia Fellowship reports that this storyline has attracted unprecedented attention and done more to reduce stigma than any number of worthy media appeals. The programme has humanized the illness and exploded the myths that schizophrenia means someone has a split personality and/or that it is likely to make someone violent (Frean, 1997).

The Australian film 'Shine' is an example of the successful use of a mainstream entertainment medium to heighten awareness and to communicate information about serious mental illness. This Oscar-winning movie conveyed several stigma-busting messages:

- People recover from schizophrenia;
- Most people with schizophrenia can work even if they have symptoms;
- Work helps people recover from schizophrenia;
- People's responses and attitudes towards someone with schizophrenia can influence the course of the illness;
- People with schizophrenia can and should be included in the community.

'Shine' can be criticized, however, for failing to communicate the important message:

- Poor parenting does not cause schizophrenia.

Nevertheless, the subsequent public appearances of David Helfgott as a concert pianist around the world have reinforced the positive messages in the movie.

A national anti-stigma campaign

Building on advances in communication technology, the Defeat Depression Campaign was conducted in Britain between 1991 and 1996 with the goals of reducing the stigma associated with depression, educating the public about the disorder and its treatment, encouraging people to seek treatment early and improving professional treatment expertise. Campaign media directed at the general public included newspaper and magazine articles, television and radio interviews, acknowledgement by celebrities of their own episodes of depression, press conferences, books, leaflets in multiple languages, audio cassettes and a self-help video. A programme to educate GPs, which included conferences, consensus statements, practice guidelines and training video tapes, was also launched (Paykel *et al.*, 1997).

The results of the campaign were clearly positive. Knowledge about and attitudes towards depression and its treatment were tested before, during and after the campaign, and showed progressive improvement of around 5–10%. At all stages of testing, counselling was regarded positively. Antidepressants were viewed with suspicion, as being addictive and ineffective, but attitudes towards them improved substantially during the campaign. By the end, members of the general public regarded people suffering from depression as being more worthy of understanding and support, and were more likely to acknowledge the experience of depression in themselves and in close friends. They saw depression as more like other medical disorders and were increasingly positive about GPs' capacity to treat the disorder (Paykel *et al.*, 1998).

A global anti-stigma campaign

The World Psychiatric Association recently has initiated an educational programme on schizophrenia focusing on social aspects of the illness, effective and humane treatment, and rehabilitation. The project aims to reduce stigma and increase awareness of the public health importance of schizophrenia. The programme, which is being distributed throughout the world, will be sensitive to differences between cultures by combining internationally and locally produced materials. The 3-year programme is field-testing materials, such as teachers' guides, brochures, posters and an Internet web page, in different settings, and is preparing them in multiple translations (Sartorius, 1997).

The first pilot project of this global campaign was launched in Calgary, Alberta, in 1997. The local action committee, made up of representatives of consumer organizations, mental health professionals, health policy makers, researchers and representatives of the press and the clergy, selected the following target groups:

- health care professionals, including emergency room personnel, medical students and senior health care policy makers;
- teenagers aged 15 and 17;
- community change agents such as the clergy, business leaders and journalists; and
- the general public.

For each target group, messages and appropriate media were selected. In the case of the teenage target group, the messages were:

- No-one is to blame for schizophrenia (a message about causes)
- People recover from schizophrenia (a message of hope)
- People with schizophrenia are *people* with schizophrenia (a message of humanity and caring).

The media used were:

- Speakers' bureaux of consumers, family members and professionals, organized by the local chapter of the Schizophrenia Society (the Canadian national advocacy group), addressed senior and junior high school classes across the region.
- Health teachers in high schools were provided with a well-researched, attractively designed teaching guide on schizophrenia.
- An Internet web page (www.openthedoors.com) was created with information on schizophrenia (developed by a World Psychiatric Association panel) with access doors for different types of users: teenagers, health professionals and consumers and family members.
- A competition for high school students to produce anti-stigma materials was launched. The winners received $500 prizes and public recognition.
- Posters promoting the campaign and advertising the competition were posted in the high schools.

- Radio advertising was conducted for a month over five stations, including a teen-oriented station.

The following is an example of one of the 30-second radio spots:

Dr. Dickson: "My name is Dr Ruth Dickson and this is voice of someone who has recovered from schizophrenia."

Michelle: "I saw visions of angels on the walls. I heard two voices, a male and a female voice, arguing back and forth about me, making derogatory remarks towards me, like 'She's stupid, she's dumb. Why doesn't she just kill herself and get out of this world?'"

Dr. Dickson: "This is just one of the people who have received treatment and the support of friends and family. But because of society's fears and prejudices, others may go for years without treatment. Without treatment they become isolated, homeless, or turn to drugs—even suicide." "Schizophrenia is a treatable brain illness. Find out how we can begin to treat the people who suffer from it like human beings.

Call 1-800-685-4004. Or visit our website at: www.openthedoors.com"

Outcome results for the teenage campaign were positive. The proportion of students achieving a perfect score in a knowledge test about schizophrenia increased from 11 to 24%. Attitude scores also improved substantially. The proportion of students expressing the least possible social distance improved from 15 to 25%, and the proportion expressing a high degree of social distance decreased from 13 to 7%. Results for other target groups are not yet available at the time of writing.

A stigma-reducing campaign need not be expensive. Many of the interventions used in Calgary were low cost, and more expensive media, such as radio and bus advertising, were only used to the extent that funding was available. The 2-year budget for the Calgary project, including a limited media campaign directed at the general public, was under US$150,000 (plus a good deal of volunteer time). Even if funds had been more limited, it would still have been possible to introduce education about schizophrenia into the high school curriculum, thus reducing the massive ignorance about this condition throughout an entire generation.

Summary

Around the world, the stigma associated with schizophrenia is high, though it is less severe in parts of the developing world, where symptoms of psychosis are at times regarded in a more positive light. Post-war attempts to reduce stigma in industrial countries were largely unsuccessful. Media hyperbole, biased reporting and negative attitudes among the general public continue to be major problems. Modern communication technology offers the possibility of more successful assaults on stigma in schizophrenia, and the World Psychiatric Association is harnessing these approaches in a new worldwide educational campaign.

References

Alisky, J.M. and Iczkowski, K.A. (1990) Barriers to housing for deinstitutionalized psychiatric patients. *Hospital and Community Psychiatry*, 41, 93–95.

Anonymous (1977) On being diagnosed schizophrenic. *Schizophrenia Bulletin*, 3, 4.

Barnes, R.C. (1993) Mental illness in British newspapers (or my girlfriend is a Rover Metro). *Psychiatric Bulletin*, 17, 673–674.

Bentinck, C. (1967) Opinions about mental illness held by patients and relatives. *Family Process*, 6, 193–207.

Bentz, W.K., Edgerton, J.W. and Kherlopian, M. (1969) Perceptions of mental illness among people in a rural area. *Mental Hygiene*, 53, 459–465.

Binitie, A.O. (1971) Attitude of educated Nigerians to psychiatric illness. *Acta Psychiatrica Scandinavica*, 46, 391–398.

Borenstein, A.B. (1992) Public attitudes towards persons with mental illness. *Health Affairs*, Fall issue, 186–196.

Boydall, K.M., Trainor, J.M. and Pierri, A.M. (1989) The effect of group homes for the mentally il on residential property values. *Hospital and Community Psychiatry*, 40. 957–958.

Brockington, I.F., Hall, P., Levings, J. and Murphy, C. (1993) The community's tolerance of the mentally ill. *British Journal of Psychiatry*, 162, 93–99.

Brugha, T.S., Wing, J.K., Brewin, C.R. *et al.* (1993) The relationship of social network deficits with deficits in social functioning in long-term psychiatric disorders. *Social Psychiatry and Psychiatric Epidemiology*, 28, 218–224.

Cockerham, W.C. (1981) *Sociology of Mental Disorder*. Englewood Cliffs, NJ: Prentice-Hall.

Cohen, C.I. and Sokolovsky, J. (1978) Schizophrenia and social networks: ex-patients in the inner city. *Schizophrenia Bulletin*, 4, 546–560.

Creer, C. (1975) Living with schizophrenia. *Social Work Today*, 6, 2–7.

Crocetti, G., Spiro, J.R. and Siassi, I. (1971) Are the ranks closed? Attitudinal social distance and mental illness. *American Journal of Psychiatry*, 127, 1121–1127.

Crumpton, E., Weinstein, A.D., Acker, C.W. and Annis, A.P. (1967) How patients and normals see the mental patient. *Journal of Clinical Psychology*, 23, 46–49.

Cumming, E. and Cumming, J. (1957) *Closed Ranks: An Experiment in Mental Health Education*. Cambridge, MA: Harvard University Press.

D'Arcy, C. and Brockman, J. (1976) Changing public recognition of psychiatric symptoms? Blackfoot revisited. *Journal of Health and Social Behavior*, 17, 302–310.

Doherty, E.G. (1975) Labeling effects in psychiatric hospitalization: a study of diverging patterns of inpatient self-labeling processes. *Archives of General Psychiatry*, 32. 562–568.

Erinosho, O.A. and Ayonrinde, A. (1981) Educational background and attitude to mental illness among the Yoruba in Nigeria. *Human Relations*, 34, 1–12.

Frean, A. (1997) EastEnders praised for breaking taboo on schizophrenia. *The Times*, May 10, 1997.

Gerbner, G., Gross, L., Morgan, M. and Signorielli, N. (1981) Health and medicine on television. *New England Journal of Medicine*, 305, 901–904.

Giovannoni, J.M. and Ullman, L.P. (1963) Conceptions of mental health held by psychiatric patients. *Journal of Clinical Psychology*, 19, 398–400.

Gove, W.R. (1975) Labelling and mental illness. In: Gove, W.R. (ed.), *The Labelling of Deviance: Evaluating a Perspective*. New York: Halsted, pp. 35–81.

Hall, P., Brockington, I.F., Levings, J. and Murphy, C. (1993) A comparison of responses to the mentally ill in two communities. *British Journal of Psychiatry*, 162, 99–108.

Hatfield, A. (1978) Psychosocial costs of schizophrenia to the family. *Social Work*, 23, 355–359.

Indian Council of Medical Research (1988) *Multicentred Collaborative Study of Factors Associated with Cause and Outcome of Schizophrenia*. New Delhi, India: Indian Council of Medical Research.

Kreisman, D.E. and Joy, V.D. (1974) Family response to the mental illness of a relative: a review of the literature. *Schizophrenia Bulletin*, 10, 34–57.

Lamy, R.E. (1966) Social consequences of mental illness. *Journal of Consulting Psychology*, 30, 450–455.

Lemkau, P.V. and Crocetti, G.M. (1962) An urban population's opinions and knowledge about mental illness. *American Journal of Psychiatry*, 118, 692–700.

Link, B.G., Cullen, F.T., Frank, J. and Wozniak, J.F. (1987) The social rejection of former mental patients: understanding why labels matter. *American Journal of Sociology*, 92, 1461–1500.

Lipton, F.R., Cohen, C.I., Fischer, E. and Katz, S.E. (1981) Schizophrenia: a network crisis. *Schizophrenia Bulletin*, 7, 144–151.

Manis, M., Houts, P.S. and Blake, J.B. (1963) Beliefs about mental illness as a function of psychiatric status and psychiatric hospitalization. *Journal of Abnormal and Social Psychology*, 67, 226–233.

Market and Opinion Research International (1997) *Attitudes Towards Schizophrenia: A Survey of Public Opinions*. Study conducted for Fleishman Hillard Eli Lilly, September.

Meyer, J.K. (1964) Attitudes toward mental illness in a Maryland community. *Public Health Reports*, 79, 769–772.

Miller, D. and Dawson, W.H. (1965) Effects of stigma on re-employment of ex-mental patients. *Mental Hygiene*, 49, 281–287.

Monahan, J. and Arnold, J. (1996) Violence by people with mental illness: a consensus statement by advocates and researchers. *Psychiatric Rehabilitation Journal*, 19, 67–70.

Nunally, J.C. (1961) *Popular Conceptions of Mental Health: Their Development and Change*. New York: Holt, Rinehart and Winston.

O'Grady, T.J. (1996) Public attitudes to mental illness. *British Journal of Psychiatry*, 168, 652.

Olmsted, D.W. and Durham, K. (1976) Stability of mental health attitudes: a semantic differential study. *Journal of Health and Social Behavior*, 17, 35–44.

Page, S. (1980) Social responsiveness toward mental patients: the general public and others. *Canadian Journal of Psychiatry*, 25, 242–246.

Pai, S. and Kapur, R.L. (1983) Evaluation of home care treatment for schizophrenic patients. *Acta Psychiatrica Scandinavica*, 67, 80–88.

Pattison, E.M. and Pattison, M.L. (1981) Analysis of a schizophrenic psychosocial network. *Schizophrenia Bulletin*, 7, 135–143.

Pattison, E.M., DeFrancisco, D., Wood, P. et al. (1975) A psychosocial kinship model for family therapy. *American Journal of Psychiatry*, 132, 1246–1251.

Paykel, E.S., Tylee, A. Wright, A. et al. (1997) The Defeat Depression Campaign: psychiatry in the public arena. *American Journal of Psychiatry*, 154 (Suppl. 6), 59–65.

Paykel, E.S., Hart, D. and Priest, R.G. (1998) Changes in public attitudes to depression during the Defeat Depression Campaign. *British Journal of Psychiatry*, 173, 519–522.

Penn, D.L., Guynan, K., Daily, T. et al. (1994) Dispelling the stigma of schizophrenia: what sort of information is best? *Schizophrenia Bulletin*, 20, 567–578.

Phillips, D.L. (1966) Public identification and acceptance of the mentally ill. *American Journal of Public Health*, 56, 755–763.

Philo, G. (1994) Media images and popular beliefs. *Psychiatric Bulletin*, 18, 173–174.

Prabhu, G.C., Raghuram, A., Verma, N. et al. (1984) Public attitudes towards mental illness: a review. *NIMHANS Journal*, 2, 1–14.

Rabkin, J.G. (1980) Determinants of public attitudes about mental illness: summary of the research literature. Presented at the *National Institute of Mental Health Conference on Stigma Toward the Mentally Ill*, Rockville, MD, January 24–25.

Reda, S. (1995) Attitudes towards community mental health care of residents in north London. *Psychiatric Bulletin*, 19, 731–733.

Rin, H. and Lin, T. (1962) Mental illness among Formosan aborigines as compared with the Chinese in Taiwan. *Journal of Mental Science*, 108, 134–146.

Robert Wood Johnson Foundation (1990) *Public Attitudes Toward People with Chronic Mental Illness*. New Jersey: The Robert Wood Johnson Foundation Program on Chronic Mental Illness, April.

Rogers, E.M. (1995) *Diffusion of Innovations*, 4th edn, New York: The Free Press.

Rogers, E.M. (1996) The field of health communication today: an up-to-date report. *Journal of Health Communication*, 1, 15–23.

Rogers, E.M., Dearing, J.H., Rao, N. et al. (1995) Communication and community in a city under siege: the AIDS epidemic in San Francisco. *Communication Research*, 22. 664–677.

Rosenhan, D.L. (1973) On being sane in insane places. *Science*, 179, 250–258.

Sartorius, N. (1997) Fighting schizophrenia and its stigma: a new World Psychiatric Association educational programme. *British Journal of Psychiatry*, 170, 297.

Sathyavathi, K., Dwarki, B.R. and Murthy, H.N. (1971) Conceptions of mental health. *Transactions of All India Institute of Mental Health*, 11, 37–49.

Scheff, T.J. (1966) *Being Mentally Ill: A Sociological Theory*. Chicago: Aldine.

Scheper-Hughes, N. (1979) *Saints, Scholars and Schizophrenics: Mental Illness in Rural Ireland*. Berkeley: University of California Press.

Shain, R.E. and Phillips, J. (1991) The stigma of mental illness: labeling and stereotyping in the news. In: Wilkins, L. and Patterson, P. (eds), *Risky Business: Communicating Issues of Science, Risk and Public Policy*. Westport, CT: Greenwood Press, pp. 61–74.

Star, S. (1955) The public's idea about mental illness. Presented at the *National Association for Mental Health Meeting*, Chicago, IL, November.

Steadman, H. and Cocozza, J. (1978) Selective reporting and the public's misconceptions of the criminally insane. *Public Opinion Quarterly*, 41, 523–533.

Strauss, J.S. and Carpenter, W.T. (1981) *Schizophrenia*. New York: Plenum.

Swanson, R.M. and Spitzer, S.P. (1970) Stigma and the psychiatric patient career. *Journal of Health and Social Behavior*, 11, 44–51.

Tringo, J.L. (1970) The hierarchy of preference towards disability groups. *Journal of Special Education*, 4, 295–306.

Trute, B. and Segal, S.P. (1976) Census tract predictors and the social integration of sheltered care residents. *Social Psychiatry*, 11, 153–161.

Verghese, A. and Beig, A. (1974) Public attitude towards mental illness: the Vellore study. *Indian Journal of Psychiatry*, 16, 8–18.

Warner, R. (1984) *Recovery from Schizophrenia: Psychiatry and Political Economy*, 2nd edn. London: Routledge.

Warner, R., Taylor, D., Powers, M. and Hyman, J. (1989) Acceptance of the mental illness label by psychotic patients: effects on functioning. *American Journal of Orthopsychiatry*, 59, 398–409.

Waxler, N.E. (1977) Is mental illness cured in traditional societies? A theoretical analysis. *Culture, Medicine and Psychiatry*, 1, 233–253.

Westermeyer, J. and Pattison, E.M. (1981) Social networks and mental illness in a peasant society. *Schizophrenia Bulletin*, 7, 125–134.

Wolff, G. (1997) Attitudes of the media and the public. In Leff, J. (ed.) *Care in the Community: Illusion or Reality?* New York: Wiley, pp. 144–163.

World Health Organization (1979) *Schizophrenia: An International Follow-up Study*. Chichester: Wiley.

Yarrow, M., Clausen, J., Robbins, P. (1955) The social meaning of mental Illness. *Journal of Social Issues*, 11, 33–48.

| *Users and their advocates*

David Pilgrim and Anne Rogers

Introduction

Most community mental health workers are probably familiar with the notion of 'user involvement in mental health services'. In this chapter, we will introduce some wider considerations from social science about the role of psychiatric patients. We will explore the various ways in which psychiatric patients have traditionally been portrayed and conceptualized and examine how moves from institutional to community services have impacted on this portrayal.

In the British context, the term 'user' of mental health services has generally been common in recent years. Potentially the concept refers to a wide range of people, not just designated patients, who have contact with mental health services. Mental health services interface with, or are accessed by, a range of statutory and civil groups in wider society: the criminal justice system, social services, the immigration service, primary health care and relatives of people entering the psychiatric patient role. We will not examine this wider notion of service utilization (cf. Pilgrim and Rogers, 1999, Chapter 10), but focus only on four ways of viewing those who are designated patients: the user-as-patient; the user-as-consumer; the user-as-survivor; and the-user-as-provider.

The user-as-patient

The traditional way in which users of psychiatric services have been portrayed is as objects of the 'clinical gaze' of mental health professionals (Armstrong, 1980). This is clearly seen in the academic literature that forms the basis of most psychiatric and psychological knowledge. Clinical research in the area of mental health has tended to either exclude the views of patients or portray them as passive objects of study. Their individual characteristics and feelings are mostly variables to be 'controlled out' as it is assumed that their mental illness prevents them from holding valid views. Explicitly or implicitly, 'mental patients' are portrayed in a way that emphasizes their pathology. There are four forms in which patients are denied a valid viewpoint. (A fuller exploration of the points is given in Rogers *et al.*, 1993.)

- The disregarding by researchers of those users' views that do not coincide with the views of mental health professionals. For example, findings that some users of services prefer contact with non-professionals to contact with health service personnel have not always been viewed as a convincing expression of ways of meeting users' needs.

- The notion that psychiatric patients are continually irrational and so incapable of giving a valid view. Therapists often suggest that the consumer cannot adequately judge the treatments they are given (Lebow, 1982; Davidhazar and Wehlage, 1984).

- Patients and relatives are assumed to share the same perspective, and where they do not, the views of the former may be down-played or disregarded.

- Framing patient views in terms which are more akin to professional ways of working (Furnham, 1984; Teasdale, 1987; McIntyre *et al.*, 1989), for example giving greater salience to the value of therapeutic interventions than is evident from the responses provided by patients.

Thus the user-as-patient construction has two main implications for community mental health work. The agency and competence of people with mental health problems are considered to be flawed by their illness; this necessitates a paternalistic role for professionals (which may be expressed in a benign or coercive way). For those only socialized in a clinical role, it may be difficult to transcend this user-as-patient discourse and its practical consequences.

The user-as-consumer

An alternative way of conceptualizing psychiatric patients is not as the objects of clinical interventions but as consumers of services. The term 'consumerism' implies the existence of choice between products and an active insistence on value for money. Consumerism characterized health policy making in Britain between the mid-1980s and the 1997 General Election. It was linked to the introduction of general management principles in the National Health Service, which tended to modify the clinical view of services noted above. The administration of the health services by consensus decision making amongst different clinical groups was replaced by the concentration of responsibility for services and management in the general manager. Part of this trend towards general management involved what Offe (1984) referred to as the 'commodification' of welfare services. This introduced the logic of the wider economic system into the health service. Whilst the significance attributed to consumerism oscillates according to changes in government, the 'marketization' of the NHS and the emphasis on consumerism has left a trace in that 'quality assurance' remains an important building block of the new NHS agenda of 'clinical governance' (Department of Health, 1998a). Quality assurance programmes place an emphasis on user outcomes—are consumers satisfied with the service they receive?

There are a number of difficulties associated with viewing patients as consumers. Although during the 1980s general management encouraged a market-influenced system permitting consumer choice, the extent to which the health service actually achieved this was restricted by the 'clinical autonomy' exercized by the medical profession. A study (Britten, 1991) showed that consultants who adhered to a biomedical rather than psychosocial model of illness were less likely to agree with a proposed policy of patient access to their own records. Thus, the paternalism noted earlier of the user-as-patient can undermine a health policy based upon consumerism.

There are also doubts about whether users of health services can make fully informed choices. Consumers of health care do not have the same access to clinical knowledge as professionals, who have many years of training and experience on which to base their decisions. Informed consent, in which the benefits and negative effects of treatment are made available to patients, has only recently been acknowledged as an area that needs attention. Patients do not have access to information about their treatment, whereas professionals do. In particular, there is the bias set up by professionals selectively withholding information that might alarm or demoralize the patient.

There are also objections to the notion of 'consumer' being used specifically in relation to psychiatric patients. 'Consumer' tends to denote a positive choice from a range of alternatives. As one user representative put it:

"Consumer tends to be rejected because of its connotations with Tory consumerism but also because consumer implies you are getting something of value. The majority of people in the users' movement do not feel that they have consumed anything of value and many say quite clearly that the real consumers of mental health services are relatives, the police and the state." (cited in Rogers and Pilgrim, 1991, p. 136)

Psychiatric patients can be forced into the sick role by means of compulsory admission. Being excluded from employment, in the main, psychiatric patients are also a group with very little 'buying power' so their access to private care is restricted. In measuring satisfaction in the area of mental health, we need to consider a number of differences between patients who use services for acute physical problems and those who receive psychiatric services:

(i)   Contact with services for those with mental health problems is far more extensive than for most others who use the health and social services. (Although they have this in common with some groups of physically disabled people.) Those who enter hospital for acute physical problems, such as appendicitis, are patients for a short time only, whether or not they experience their hospitalization as positive or negative. Thus, the quality of service and treatment does not have as many long-term consequences as for those who are psychiatric patients. The latter often spend many years of their lives in contact with the services and professionals.

(ii) The consequences of being labelled 'ill' are often greater for a person who is given a psychiatric diagnosis. For the majority of those with physical problems, the diagnosis itself is often only a temporary one and is usually not stigmatizing. The diagnosis of a person as 'mentally ill' risks invalidating their whole identity or sense of self. Mental illness brings with it a common stigmatizing assumption of a permanent susceptibility to irrationality. To have been deemed to have lost one's reason indicates a permanent vulnerability rather just than a temporary deficit. Again certain physical disabilities (such as epilepsy) may carry with them stigma, and so the mental patient is not unique.

(iii) There are social and economic consequences of contact with psychiatric services that apply much less often when acute medical services are used. Those labelled as mentally ill are discriminated against by present and prospective employers and, as a result, are often subjected to a life of poverty (Sayce, 2000). Educational opportunities are curtailed, family and intimate relationships affected and making social contact with people is fraught with difficulties. Again some of these impediments to citizenship often apply to people with long-term physical disabilities (Pilgrim *et al.*, 1997).

Thus the consumerist depiction of psychiatric patients is problematic. Firstly, professionals under the sway of biomedical paternalism may not accept the role. Secondly, in Britain since 1997, government support for consumerism has diminished. Thirdly, the socio-economic position of chronic dependency by many psychiatric patients on the State for basic material provision is incompatible with a consumer role. Fourthly, the coercive powers of psychiatry negate the notion of voluntary choice, which is at the heart of the concept of consumerism.

The user-as-survivor

There have been analyses of users' views of services by those who do not work directly with people in service settings, either as clinicians or as managers. The position of psychiatric users in a wider social context is their object. Two perspectives can be identified. The first has adopted a phenomenological approach to understanding the social position of the mental patient. The second has tried to analyse the structural position of users as a social group within wider society. In particular, there is an interest in users campaigning collectively, thus constituting a version of a 'new social movement'.

An example of the phenomenological approach is provided by the work of Barham and Hayward (1991) who used personal accounts by mental patients to explore their experiences of living outside of hospital. In adopting this approach, their work takes us beyond the measuring of consumer satisfaction. Rather, the concern is with identity and social position in everyday life. The themes identified from the subjects themselves were:

- Exclusion from participation in social life.
- Burden, which refers to the stigma and disability resulting from having a mental health problem.
- Reorientation, which refers to 'coping' with vulnerabilities.

Everyday encounters reported by subjects suggested the continuing marginalization of people labelled as 'schizophrenic'. Participants in the study were reluctant to enter or re-enter patient-hood. Most wanted to establish their credibility as ordinary people with rights of citizenship, such as adequate employment and housing. The participants were only marginally more willing to be incorporated into community services than the old institutional ones. This suggests a fundamental questioning of the utility of services from the perspective of users themselves. Such questioning is not acknowledged by the other two views (patient or consumer) discussed above. Phenomenological analysis gives primacy to the individual experience of the patient in relation to the mental hospital or community.

Turning now to the second strand of work on the 'user-as-survivor', other literature situates users within a wider set of new social movements which have arisen in civil society to challenge marginalization or oppression (e.g. feminism and the black movement).

The growing collective activities of mental health users over the last two decades have been noted by a number of commentators (Haafkens *et al.*, 1986; Burstow and Weitz, 1988; Chamberlin, 1988; Rogers and Pilgrim, 1991). There have been a number of examples from the British survivors' movement of activism in the area of user participation and mental health services. These have included campaigns against the changes being advocated by the Royal College of Psychiatrists to the 1983 Mental Health Act which proposed Community Treatment Orders to treat patients in the community on a compulsory basis; opposition to a poster campaign, run by SANE (Schizophrenia a National Emergency) in the early 1990s; and a lobby of the opposition spokespeople in Parliament by a national network of 56 user groups during the same period. More recently, there have been protests at the celebration of the 750th anniversary of the Bethlem Hospital and against the commonly accepted view of psychiatry as a form of enlightened and benign humanism.

User political action has now reached such a point that, in terms of numbers and organizations (globally as well as nationally), it constitutes a 'new social movement'. Social movements can be defined as groups engaged in informal efforts to promote their interests in opposition to dominant forms of power and organization preferred by the State (Toch, 1965). 'New' social movements can

be distinguished conceptually from 'old' social movements in that they are further removed from the arena of production than the latter. Additionally, rather than seeking to defend existing social and property rights from erosion by the State, they are a source of innovation, generating new ideals for living, questioning the existence of the status quo and seeking to establish new agendas and conquer new territory (Habermas, 1981).

Scott (1990) contrasts new social movements with the labour, or workers', movement (the focus of the Marxian tradition in sociology). The latter movement has become a part of the political process through organized industrial action and negotiation. Its organization has become formalized or bureaucratized and its aims have been economic and political. In contrast, the new social movements (feminism, ecology, black and gay liberation, etc.) have mainly had social and cultural aims and have emphasized direct action and non-hierarchical forms of organization. Some social scientists have gone as far as arguing that the absorption of the labour movement into the established political process in capitalist society leaves the new social movements as the only remaining radical challenge to the status quo (Marcuse, 1964; Scott, 1990). The mental health service survivors' movement seems to fit conceptually into this new political pattern of radicalism (Crossley, 1999).

Whilst the rise of survivors' groups suggests that there is a groundswell of dissatisfaction, which health and social services overall have failed to contain, this new social movement is not homogenous. Disparities in ideology between British users' groups over attitudes to conceptualizing mental health problems, professionals and treatment are clearly evident. Some groups uncritically accept the paradigm of mental illness, whilst others are wholly rejecting of the medical model and its treatments (Rogers and Pilgrim, 1991).

In the USA, where the movement is more developed, user groups have been classified according to two models—'structural' and 'clinical'. The first is concerned with offering self-help services and is oriented towards social change through legal advocacy, public education and providing information. The second model (which conceptually shades into our point below about user-providers) is concerned with individual change though group support meetings, drop-in centres and alternative therapies. The analysis of the relationship between these groups and professionals shows that the former are more likely to develop partnerships than the latter. However, both types of group tend to reject alliances with mental health professionals having a narrow clinical conception of mental illness (Emerick, 1990).

Sang (1989) has pointed out that the term 'advocacy' has been co-opted by professionals and is used loosely by them to include 'meeting clinical needs'. Sang notes that information giving and a patient-centred approach to care by responding to expressed client need can be framed by professionals as acting as an advocate for clients. He distinguishes this professional discourse from two separate notions from service users themselves: citizen advocacy and self-advocacy. In the first, ordinary citizens (i.e. not professionals) form a relationship with a psychiatric patient to represent their interests as if they were their own. In the second, psychiatric patients work together to represent their individual and collective interests independently of non-patients.

A final point about survivors' groups is that they have shared several concerns first highlighted by critical professionals during the 1960s (the so-called 'anti-psychiatry' movement) (Pilgrim, 1997a). Whereas that critique was highly theoretical, the more recent critique has come from service users directly and is less conceptually orientated. Practical direct action characterizes its form. However, the 'clinical' group described in the USA clearly draws upon the therapeutic alternatives which the 'anti-psychiatrists' developed and advocated earlier. An example was the use of therapeutic communities for psychotic patients (Cooper, 1967).

The user-as-provider

A further trend is the development of user-led service innovations. This represents a departure from viewing people with mental health problems as the passive recipients of therapeutic interventions or as protesters about a mental health system that is failing to meet expressed need or is seen as oppressive. User-led services can be found in the voluntary sector in Britain, and occasionally they are supported by statutory authorities. The reasons for voluntary organizations spawning user-led initiatives are twofold. First, the voluntary sector has a history of providing alternatives services not available within the mainstream NHS (e.g. crisis lines, tranquilliser withdrawal groups). In this regard, voluntary organizations have arguably been more responsive to expressed need than mainstream services. Secondly, whilst professional boundaries prevent the participation by users in the delivery of services, these barriers are less evident in the voluntary sector. Active engagement in collectively providing and promoting services is something that users highly value as a part of being able to participate in local community life (Rogers *et al.*, 1993).

The large range of user-controlled facilities available in the USA is reviewed by Mowbray *et al.* (1997). Activity varies from patients being self-caring and mutually supportive within professionally led services and self-help groups, through to independent funded projects managed and staffed by users themselves (Chamberlin, 1988; Lindow, 1994). The type of services the latter provide (such as safe houses and drop-in day centres) reflect the users' movement's priorities of voluntary relationships, alternatives to hospital admission, crisis intervention and personal support.

In recent years, service providers have, to various degrees in different localities, sought the collaboration of users to support service developments. This has included: the formal acceptance by professional providers of innovations, such as patients councils; users being trained to train mental health staff (Crepaz-Keay *et al.*, 1998); and users' and carers' groups being called upon to improve services in collaborative experiments in service development (Carpenter and Sbaraini, 1997).

User-led services have also introduced an alternative philosophical base to the management and treatment of mental health problems. At times, this has an impact on traditional services. The Hearing Voices Network, informed by the work of Romme, works positively with people's experiences of hearing voices. Rather than attempting to eradicate or suppress the voices, as a traditional symptom-based approach might do, this user-led initiative attributes meaning to voice-hearing. This offers alternative means of coping with voices that may at times be distressing. The limits of the user-as-provider role are essentially set by the willingness (or lack of it) to encroach upon the social control role which professionals traditionally have taken in community, as well as hospital, settings (e.g. powers compulsorily to detain or treat people). It is unlikely that user-led projects would want such a role, given that user initiatives have on the whole been opposed to coercion. The advantage of such services is that they are more likely to develop voluntaristic ways of dealing with 'difficult to manage' patients who have proved harder to engage in mainstream service provision (Lindow, 1994).

User participation and community settings

The possibility of increased user participation discussed in the section above has been facilitated by changes in wider society. The way in which we view users has changed as a result of a number of social and political processes:

(i)   *Deinstitutionalization.* When people were confined in the old asylums, the citizenship of patients was simply repressed. Once a policy of hospital closure began, the 'asylum' began to symbolize a form of repression and the 'community' a site which held out the hope of demarginalization and restoration of civil and political rights. The issue of citizens' rights was immediately opened up and became an arena for struggle by patients.

(ii) *The crisis of biomedical legitimacy.* Since the Second World War, the legitimacy of institutional biomedical psychiatry has been under recurring pressure. Hospital scandals

exposed its failings (Martin, 1985) by demonstrating that the large-scale separation of people with mental health problems from wider society led to a 'corruption of care'. The latter term was used by Martin to describe the recurring evidence that institutionally based staff neglected and abused those in their charge. Internal dissenters or 'anti-psychiatrists' exposed the epistemological problems of applying a medical model to social and existential dimensions of madness, which only utilized symptoms (i.e. communication) not 'hard' biological signs (Szasz, 1961; Laing, 1968). These weaknesses undermined patient confidence in orthodox psychiatric practice and encouraged a user interest in defining good quality care and criticizing psychiatric diagnosis. This crisis of psychiatry was amplified by critiques from other professionals, such as clinical psychologists, making a bid for legitimacy in the clinical and research arenas of mental health work (e.g. Bentall *et al.*, 1988; Boyle, 1991). Moreover, dissent in the 1960s and 1970s from internal critics such as Laing, Cooper and Szasz did not disappear permanently. It re-surfaced during the 1990s, with further critiques of psychiatry from a minority within its ranks (e.g. Fernando, 1992; Bracken and Thomas, 1998).

(iii) *The relevance of a philosophy of community, public health and legalism.* Deinstitutionalization for those with mental health problems has been accompanied by a wider movement towards the demarginalization of excluded groups. This 'normalization' movement began first with the closure of the large mental handicap hospitals and then mental illness hospitals (Ramon, 1991). Normalization emphasizes people with mental health problems having a right of access to ordinary resources and a right to be treated as equally as others in society. Also there has been a growth in primary care services that have an ethos of treating people in the localities where they live. A 'new public health' paradigm has drawn attention not only to the social conditions which are implicated in the genesis and recovery from mental health problems, but also to social exclusion and vulnerability of disadvantaged groups on the one hand and the capacity for community action that such groups have on the other. The community development movement during the 1980s resonated with the emergence of non-traditional political movements around specific issues (e.g. eco-politics). The mental health arena was also influenced by the legalism underlying many of the changes represented in the 1983 Mental Health Act in the UK and similar legislation elsewhere. This drew attention to the issue of patients' rights, informed consent and compulsory detention, even though the changes introduced by the Act in the UK were modest (Bean 1986).

(iv) *Patient-centred professional care.* Professionals operating in community and primary care settings have tended to embrace a holistic and patient-centred philosophy more than hospital-based specialists.

Despite these factors, and the consumerism discussed above, creating a facilitative context for user involvement, there have also been constraints. There remains the possibility that a halt or break to user-led initiatives might occur as a result of a set of countervailing processes (Pilgrim and Waldron, 1998). These include:

(i) *Reinstitutionalization.* Although the large old hospitals have now mainly closed, hospital-based facilities and nursing homes still absorb the bulk of mental health investment by the state. Moreover, there are signs that when new money is being made available, this may be prioritized for hospital beds (Department of Health, 1998b). Thus a question arises of whether we are now in a phase of reinstitutionalization (Pilgrim and Rogers, 1994).

(ii) *The failure to gain public and political legitimation for the social inclusion of users.* In the UK, the 'demonisation' of psychiatric patients through an amplification of untoward events involving psychiatric patients and the exaggeration of the link between mental illness and dangerousness (especially homicide) has brought with it demands for greater control over psychiatric patients. This has been reinforced by central government. Such 'concerns' have been placed centrally in a review of mental health legislation, which pre-figures a new mental health act (Department of Health, 1999).

(iii) *The patchy impact of the users' movement.* Despite points made earlier about the rise of a new social movement of disaffected patients, this has not been sufficiently strong across all localities to ensure consistent support for user involvement. Moreover, the demand for greater involvement and participation in the delivery of services and the rights afforded to other citizens has had a variable impact. There have been variations in the receptiveness of statutory agencies to user involvement (Barnes, 1999). The demand for greater involvement and participation in the delivery of services and for rights afforded to other citizens (e.g. in employment and discrimination) has had a variable impact. There is some ambivalence too from parts of the users' movement about getting involved with the details of training and service delivery in a locality at the expense of wider campaigning.

(iv) *The retention of psychiatry's social control role.* The ethos of voluntary and democratic negotiations implied by user participation in mental health service planning and evaluation is contradicted by the continuing scope for psychiatric social control. As long as psychiatric services exist in part in order to regulate the daily disruptions surrounding madness, both the principle and practice of user involvement will be undermined. The expectation of a continuing coercive role has been formalized in the British government's mental health policy which brings to the foreground the issue of public safety (Department of Health, 1998b, 1999).

Conclusions

This chapter has not been able to address all parties utilizing mental health services (the courts, the police, relatives, etc.). Instead it has focused on the ways in which psychiatric patients have been conceptualized in relation to services. We have drawn attention to social processes that require attention when understanding these conceptualizations. If users are understood solely as patients then their views will be ignored or the validity of those views will be cast in doubt because of their 'loss of reason'. Professional paternalism is a natural corollary. If users are understood as consumers, then we have to clarify in what sense they 'consume' services. In particular, their use of services in competition with the groups we have not had the space to address in this chapter needs to be borne in mind. This raises the question of services acting in the interest of parties other than patients. The latent function of psychiatric treatment can be understood as social control in two senses. First, the coercive imposition of treatment is linked to the removal of people with mental health problems from civil society without trial. Secondly, admission and delayed discharge from psychiatric in-patient facilities may be linked to the absence of appropriate accommodation in open society in every locality. Psychiatric admission and detention, *inter alia*, reflect the containment of one group of difficult to place people in society.

If we shift our attention from social control, a question arises of whether in-patient wards can create mental health gain for those who temporarily inhabit them. A recent national audit of British in-patient facilities described them as 'non-therapeutic' (Sainsbury Centre, 1998). An earlier study found that what psychiatric patients liked most about hospital was 'their ability to leave' (McIntyre *et al.*, 1989). Whilst reviews of interventions in in-patient settings suggest that

around half have an evidence base (Pilgrim, 1997b), there is no clear evidence (i) that the *siting* of these interventions positively influences their degree of efficacy and (ii) that patient-reported outcomes endorse the positive benefit of having an in-patient stay. In-patient stays have also been shown to remove rights of tenancy and access to welfare benefits, thus creating or amplifying social disadvantage—an iatrogenic effect of service contact (Bean and Mounser, 1993).

Brugha and Lindsay (1996) suggest that mental health gain should be operationalized as improved quality of life in the community. If this definition is accepted, and the debatable therapeutic impact of in-patient care taken into account, then the notion of 'user-as-survivor' makes some sense. In this context, users 'survive' their 'non-therapeutic' experience as in-patients and then confront the extent to which their quality of life can be sustained and improved in community settings when discharged from hospital. In such open settings, it is not so much the iatrogenic impact of professional attention which is the main challenge, but a whole range of other threats to citizenship and personhood: labour market disadvantage; stigma and prejudice; poverty; and the lack of choice over affordable accommodation—in short, 'social exclusion' (Sayce, 2000). In these circumstances, it is not surprising that the survivors' movement has campaigned about citizenship and that researchers in the phenomenological tradition have been concerned to understand the subjective experience of social exclusion endured by patients.

Finally, it is significant that user-controlled service provision eschews actions that traditionally have reflected the interests of others. The emphasis upon a unique appreciation of the person's distress contrasts with a traditional psychiatric approach which engages with problem formulation by emphasizing diagnosis. The emphasis upon voluntary relationships is an alternative to the coercive imperative that can be deployed by psychiatry *in loco parentis* and demanded by relatives. The more we shift our understanding of users from being patients to being consumers, survivors and providers, the more the interests of professionals and the identified patient's significant others are thrown into relief. Accordingly, focusing on identified patients also allows us to elucidate the sociological features of other stakeholders in the mental health system.

References

Armstrong, D. (1980) Madness and coping. *Sociology of Health and Illness*, 2, 393–413.

Barham, P. and Hayward, R. (1991) *From the Mental Patient to the Person*. London: Routledge.

Barnes, M. (1999) Users as citizens: collective action and the local governance of welfare. *Social Policy and Administration*, 33, 73–90

Bean, P. (1986) *Mental Disorder and Legal Control*. Cambridge: Cambridge University Press.

Bean, P. and Mounser, P. (1993) *Discharged from Mental Hospitals*. London: Macmillan.

Bentall, R.P., Jackson, H. and Pilgrim, D. (1988) Abandoning the concept of schizophrenia: some implications of validity arguments for psychological research into psychotic phenomena. *British Journal of Clinical Psychology*, 27, 303–324.

Boyle, M. (1991) Schizophrenia: a scientific delusion. London: Routledge.

Bracken, P. and Thomas, P. (1998) A new debate in mental health. *Open Mind*, 89, February, 17.

Britten, N. (1991) Hospital consultants' views of their patients. *Sociology of Health and Illness*, 13, 83–97.

Brugha, T.S. and Lindsay, F. (1996) Quality of mental health service: the forgotten pathway from process to outcome. *Social Psychiatry and Psychiatric Epidemiology*, 31, 89–98.

Burstow, B. and Weitz, D. (eds) (1988) *Shrink Resistant: The Struggle Against Psychiatry in Canada*. Vancouver: New Star.

Carpenter, J. and Sbaraini, S. (1997) *Choice, Information and Dignity: Involving Users and Carers in Care Management in Mental Health*. London: Policy Press.

Chamberlin, J. (1988) *On Our Own*. London: MIND Publications.

Cooper, D. (1967) *Psychiatry and Anti-Psychiatry*. London: Tavistock.

Crepaz-Keay, D., Binns, C. and Wilson, E. (1998) *Dancing with Angels: Involving Survivors in Mental Health Training*. London: CCETSW.

Crossley, N. (1999) Working utopias: an investigation using case study materials from radical mental health movements in Britain. *Sociology*. 33, 4, 809–830.

Davidhazar, D. and Wehlage, D. (1984) Can the client with chronic schizophrenia consent to nursing research? *Journal of Advanced Nursing*, 9, 381–390.

Department of Health (1998a) *A First Class Service*. London: HMSO.

Department of Health (1998b) *Modernising Mental Health Services: Safe, Sound and Supportive*. London: HMSO.

Department of Health (1999) *Reform of the Mental Health Act 1983: Proposals for Consultation*. London: HMSO.

Emerick, R.E. (1990) Self help groups for former patients: relations with mental health professionals. *Hospital and Community Psychiatry*, 41, 401–407.

Fernando, S. (1992) 'Psychiatry'. *Open Mind*, 58 (Aug/Sept).

Furnham, A. (1984) Lay conceptions of neuroticism. *Personality and Individual Difference*, 5, 95–103.

Haafkens, J., Nijhof, G. and van der Poel, E. (1986) Mental health care and the opposition movement in the Netherlands. *Social Science and Medicine*, 22, 185–192.

Habermas, J. (1981) New social movements. *Telos*, 48, 33–37.

Laing, R.D. (1967) *The Politics of Experience and the Bird of Paradise*. Harmondsworth: Penguin.

Lebow, J. (1982) Consumer satisfaction with mental health treatment. *Psychological Bulletin*, 91, 244–259.

Lindow, V. (1994) *Self-help Alternatives to Mental Health Services*. London: MIND Publications.

Marcuse, H. (1964) *One Dimensional Man*. London: Routledge and Kegan Paul.

Martin, J.P. (1985) *Hospitals in Trouble*. Oxford: Blackwell

McIntyre, K., Farrell, M. and David, A. (1989) What do psychiatric inpatients really want? *British Medical Journal*, 298, 159–160.

Mowbray, C.T., Moxley, D.P., Jasper, C.A. and Howell, I.L. (eds) (1997) *Consumers as Providers in Psychiatric Rehabilitation*. Columbia: International Association of Psychosocial Rehabilitation Services.

Offe, C. (1984) *Contradictions of the Welfare State*. London: Hutchinson.

Pilgrim, D. (1997a) *Psychotherapy and Society*. London: Sage.

Pilgrim, D. (1997b) Some reflections on 'quality' and 'mental health'. *Journal of Mental Health*, 6, 567–576.

Pilgrim, D. and Rogers, A. (1994) Something old, something new: sociology and the organisation of psychiatry. *Sociology*, 28, 2, 531–38.

Pilgrim, D. and Rogers, A. (1999) *A Sociology of Mental Health and Illness*, 2nd edn. Miton Keynes: Open University Press.

Pilgrim, D. and Waldron, L. (1998) User involvement in mental health service development: how far can it go? *Journal of Mental Health*, 7, 95–104.

Pilgrim, D., Todhunter, C. and Pearson, M. (1997) Accounting for disability: customer feedback or citizen complaints? *Disability and* Society, 1, 3–15.

Ramon, S. (1991) *Beyond Community Care.* Basingstoke: Macmillan.

Rogers, A. and Pilgrim, D. (1991) 'Pulling down churches': accounting for the rise of the British mental health users' movement. *Sociology of Health and Illness*, 13, 129–148.

Rogers, A., Pilgrim, D. and Lacey, R. (1993) *Experiencing Psychiatry: Users' Views of Services.* London: Macmillan.

Sainsbury Centre (1998) *Acute Problems: A Survey of Quality of Care in Acute Psychiatric Wards.* London: Sainsbury Centre for Mental Health.

Sang, B. (1989) The independent voice of advocacy. In: Brackx, A. and Grimshaw, C. (eds), *Mental Health Care in Crisis.* London: Pluto Press.

Sayce, L. (2000) *From Psychiatric Patient to Citizen: Overcoming Discrimination and Social Exclusion.* London: Macmillan.

Scott, A. (1990) *Ideology and The New Social Movements.* London: Unwin Hyman.

Szasz, T.S. (1961) The uses of naming and the origin of the myth of mental illness. *American Psychologist*, 16, 59–65.

Teasdale, K. (1987) Stigma and psychiatric day care. *Journal of Advanced Nursing*, 12, 339–346.

Toch, H. (1965) *The Social Psychology of Social Movements.* New York: Bobbs Merrill.

Introduction

In this chapter, carers are family members—parents, partners, children, siblings, other extended family and close friends who carry out an informal care-giving role for a relative with a major mental illness. Carer organizations refer to mental health support groups that were started predominantly for and by family members. The most developed of these organizations are involved in a wide range of activities that have moved beyond support groups for family members into community services for people with mental illness, advocacy for better mental health services and anti-stigma campaigns. Given the growing awareness of the need for collaboration between major stakeholders, many of these activities are being carried out in conjunction with professional workers and consumers.

International overview of carer organizations

National and regional organizations of families of people with mental illness have been formed in many countries, in spite of major economic and social obstacles. Johnson (1994a) surveyed organizations worldwide that were focused on families of people with serious mental illnesses. These organizations were commenced mainly by family carers, but recent developments have seen the inclusion of primary consumers as members of some executive boards, reflecting the growing understanding that improvements in mental health services delivery will not happen unless greater collaboration is developed between all major stakeholders.

Family organizations rely heavily on a volunteer workforce, though most of the national bodies have some paid staff. Johnson reported that while the emphasis is on voluntary activity—"a concept new to the citizens of the former Soviet Union and many Europeans who are accustomed to extensive state-run social programs" (p. 29)—the groups have made efforts to work with mental health professionals while endeavouring to keep administrative and policy control in the hands of relatives and consumers. Professionals in many nations have had a key role in supporting and fostering the organizations. All the organizations reported having mutual support functions primarily led by members, but sometimes started and led by interested mental health professionals.

Information was obtained from Australia, Bermuda, Belgium, Canada, Germany, Holland, India, Ireland, Israel, Japan, New Zealand, Russia, South Africa, Spain, Sweden, Switzerland, Ukraine, the UK, the USA and Uruguay. Several countries known to have carer organizations did not respond, for example France, Austria, Denmark, Norway, Portugal, Romania and several organizations in Italy. Some organizations are newly formed. Others such as Zenkaren in Japan, and the National Alliance for the Mentally Ill in the USA, have been in existence for over 20 years. In December 1992, the European organizations developed the European Federation of Family Associations of Mentally Ill People (EUFAMI).

In 1982, what is now called the World Fellowship for Schizophrenia and Allied Disorders (WFS), was founded in Toronto by representatives of an eight-nation coalition of family charities. The WFS comprises dedicated volunteer professionals, most of whom care for a family member with mental illness. Since its inception, approximately 50 new family organizations have commenced operation. Mutual exchange visits have been made to Russia, India, Chile, China,

Mexico, Kenya, Uganda, Turkey and Bermuda. Mutual exchange educational packages and correspondence initiatives have resulted in groups in Iran, Slovakia, Uzbekistan, Argentina and Columbia, with several other locations in the process of starting family groups. WFS works in partnership with a worldwide spectrum of user, carer and professional groups.

The aim of the WFS mutual exchange programme is to build more international relationships with families, professionals and existing organizations who have a specific interest in mental illness. Such individuals and groups would be supported to begin and sustain their own self-help community-based groups to further the objectives and goals of their Fellowship. The WFS spearheads many of their initiatives by suggesting what can be done to help families and their mentally ill relatives directly. For example, APEF (the Spanish initials for the Argentine Association of Help for Persons with Schizophrenia and Their Families) reports that "the commencement of our organization was pushed by our belief in the importance of self-help groups, but when we got to know of the existence of similar organisations in other countries and we got in touch with the WFS, our strength grew enormously. The same happens with the small groups we start in different towns of Argentina. Being part of a net empowers families and family organizations" (Piatigorsky, 1997, p. 3). The WFS in turn learns a great deal from its involvement in these countries and helps with efforts to promote their work to governments and others in authority.

In his survey, Johnson reported that the goals and objectives of the various national organizations were similar, although the organizations differed in size, membership requirements, advocacy orientations, funding and other sources of support. Families in many nations have organized to advocate for better services, to counter stigma and to support research. In recent years, organizations have been funded for the delivery of mental health services such as rehabilitation and employment programmes, supported housing, and 'drop-in' centres.

Financial support was reported by Johnson to be inadequate, with many difficulties occurring when national bodies were seen to be in competition with local and regional groups for the same government monies. All organizations reported serious dissatisfaction with mental health services. Nowadays, in developed countries where reform has been implemented, the response is more likely to indicate 'patchy' improvement.

Historical development of carer organizations

Why did carer organizations develop?

In 1960, in England, John Pringle's son developed schizophrenia. For the next 9 years, in the face of evasion by physicians and without intelligible professional guidance, his parents tried to cope with the moods, the fits of aggression and the extreme social regression that developed as a result of their son's mental illness. John Pringle felt that they were on their own; he realized that this tragic problem was one that the community and public authorities in Britain were not confronting. He sent an article to *The Times* which was published on May 9th, 1970. Health officials took no notice, but relatives of people with schizophrenia with problems like those of the Pringles wrote mailbags of letters. In 1971, the National Schizophrenia Fellowship was founded to meet the needs of relatives caring for people with schizophrenia. A decade later, NSF had more than 100 groups in Britain. The NSF has been the model for many organizations, most notably Australia, Canada and New Zealand.

In response to a questionnaire, Hatfield (1979) found that friends, relatives and support group members were of far greater help to families than the various forms of professional therapy; half the sample reported no benefit at all. Families gave as their highest priorities an understanding of the illness, practical guidance in patient management and community resources such as housing. Self-help groups served these needs better than family therapy provided by professional workers.

Families as primary carers

Accompanying deinstitutionalization was the failure to provide families with appropriate and sufficient education, training and emotional support for their care-giving role. Added to this omission was the attribution of blame:

"Relatives become used to being targets for hostile criticism, either for allegedly being implicated in the causation of the condition in the first place, or for their clumsy handling of it afterwards . . .. but relatives have things to teach as well as to learn . . .. (Mental health workers) must be prepared to accept information derived from the untutored fumblings of people so lowly regarded in most professional circles as relatives." (Wing, 1977, p. 1)

In eastern societies, the relationship between families and mental health professionals has been different:

"In contrast to those in the west, mental health professionals in India generally have not dealt with families on the basis of any aetiological presupposition regarding their role in causation of illness. Because of this, professional–family interactions have been on a relatively even keel and the ideological see-saw from viewing families as schizophrenogenic in the 1950's to viewing families as equal treatment partners in the 1980's, has not taken place in India." (Shankar and Menon, 1991)

Apart from a difficult care-giving role, problems for family carers relate to stigma and the dearth of resources. These problems are extreme in developing countries where caring is aggravated by poverty. The presence of populations facing life-threatening diseases makes it more difficult to advocate for the needs of the mentally ill.

How did carer organizations develop?

Self-help groups were started by family members for family members. Some included consumers/users from the beginning, but the drive and initiative came from families. Katz and Bender (1976) defined self-help groups as voluntary, small group structures formed by peers who have come together for mutual assistance in satisfying a common need and bringing about social and/or personal change, such as improvement in confidence and the development of problem-solving skills. They develop values through which members may attain an enhanced sense of personal identity. Members of such groups perceive that their needs are not being met by existing social institutions.

Self-help implies that those who help others also receive help themselves. This principle has an added dimension for helpers who have the same problem as the person they are helping. They are able to see themselves as an example of someone who has come to terms with, and learned the best ways of coping with, the same set of problems. This, in turn, instils a sense of hope in the recipients of help. Recipients of help are often then able to become helpers themselves. 'Experiential knowledge' is accumulated by family carers through their care-giving experiences. This is able to be shared with other families in an atmosphere that is informal, accepting, understanding and non-judgemental. Self-help/mutual support groups fill gaps by providing for unmet needs.

Subsequent economic, social and political changes have been responsible for some of the developments that have taken place in carer organizations in more recent years. Two are especially noteworthy:

The employment in self-help groups of professional workers, who, in the main, were not family carers

Self-help groups applied for government funding to help them set up offices because the workload for volunteers working from 'kitchen tables' became too great. Accountability for government monies led to the need for suitably qualified professional people to be employed. Governments then began to 'purchase' services from community 'providers.' Many self-help organizations became the developers of community mental health services such as rehabilitation programmes, accommodation support services and drop-in centres.

Community-based services developed by professional workers employed in the self-help organizations dominated their development, and the family carer voice seemed to lose impetus. The burden of care-giving for families was still not widely understood or appreciated. In spite of the growing evidence of neurobiological causation of mental illness lessening the attribution of family blame, the needs of families were still largely ignored.

The consumer voice started to gain ground

The consumer voice frequently was hostile to families. Families, either through guilt, their own low self-esteem, loss of confidence or exhaustion as a result of their care-giving responsibilities, were silenced by this hostility. Mental health systems supported consumers, but rarely supported their family carers. Although many family support organizations have become substantial service providers, the family support groups within these organizations have continued—a testament to their importance in spite of the many obstacles they encountered.

Established methods to begin and sustain carers' groups

Groups commence when a family carer feels they want to start a support group and there has been some indication that a support group is needed. Alternatively, an empathic mental health professional can initiate the development of a group and then stand back when a suitable carer feels ready and able to take on a group leadership role. Techniques for the beginning and sustaining of support groups are described in handbooks developed by self-help organizations. Guiding principles include the following:

(i) Group convenors may need some training in the management and administration of groups. Convenors need to be able to:

(a) delegate tasks to other group members

(b) develop clear administrative procedures for organizing, running and publicizing the meetings, arranging the venue and running the meeting

(c) set realistic goals, particularly for the convenor. He/she should not have to bear total responsibility. The essence of groups should be the sharing of all aspects of support group functions, particularly the sharing of phone calls that become the 'life-blood' for many family carers in between group meetings.

(ii) Convenors need a back-up resource person, usually from the organizations' central administration. Where there is no formal organization, the support person could be found from a mental health service that is sympathetic to the function of self-help support groups.

(iii) Each group needs to determine clear eligibility for membership. Is the group to be for family carers, or a mixture of family carers and mental health consumers? Separate meetings of consumers and carers can be organized if necessary.

(iv) There should be a clear rationale underlying the functions of a support group. Groups might have as their goal to help family carers change from 'passive minding' to 'assertive caring.' Passive minding has been described by Alexander (1991) as not setting limits on inappropriate behaviour, fostering dependency, paying attention only to the sick person and dedicating one's whole life to caring. Assertive carers become aware that unlimited, unconditional self-sacrifice on behalf of someone with a serious mental illness is fatal to caring. They learn to set goals for appropriate independence, to pay attention to the needs of other members of the family and to take care of themselves.

(v) There needs to be recognition of the changing needs of group members. Over time the needs of group members change from unresolved problems that brought them to the group, to problem resolution and the development of effective coping. When energy, confidence and self-esteem return, some family members are ready to become advocates or to work voluntarily in the non-government organizations.

(vi) Protocols for managing difficult group situations. Difficult situations include:

(a) Competing interests of group members. Some carers just want support; others might want to fundraise, or to be advocates. If there are competing interests, groups can form sub-committees who carry out specific tasks.

(b) Overly critical and negative influences. 'Sad, hopeless stories' and the 'getting nowhere' feeling can at times pervade a group that is not properly managed. Convenors need to be trained in the management of negativism, with an approach that stresses that there is always something that can change for the better.

(c) Dominant talkers, immovable beliefs. Protocols for group management can build-in the idea that everyone must have an opportunity to talk, and time is limited for each participant. People are entitled to their beliefs, but must not force them upon others, particularly controversial issues such as unscientifically proven theories about treatment.

(d) Declining membership. Strategies to gain new membership include approaching local mental health services to explain the work of the group and suggest new referrals; placing notices in local papers, churches, libraries, and any other forms of relevant publicity.

If problems seem insurmountable, there is always the option of closing the group, and starting again at a later date. Some groups may serve a purpose for a time, but that purpose can be fulfilled and there may be no good reason to continue. This does not mean that the group is a failure. Some people may prefer a time-limited group.

The role of carer groups within the framework of statutory services

For family members to become effective carers, they need:

Information:
- to understand early warning signs of mental illness in order to take measures to prevent relapse.
- to learn about medications and other treatments
- to appreciate the nature of symptoms in order to create an optimal social and emotional environment for the mentally ill person.

Training in the management of mental illness:
- to cope with the unusual nature of the symptoms of mental illness
- to learn problem-solving approaches to behavioural difficulties created by mental illness.

Understanding of mental health services:
- to become aware of what mental health services can and should provide, and how to access these services
- to help plan for the future when they are no longer able to provide care.

Emotional support:
- to resolve feelings of grief, loss, anxiety, fear and other distressing feelings which family members experience. The resolution of emotional problems enhances their capacity to cope.
- to appreciate that instinctive responses to caring for someone with a mental illness, may not be helpful.
- through referral to family support organizations.

Respite care services:
- to provide 'breaks' from care-giving.

The ongoing relationship with mental health service providers is enhanced when professionals meet these needs through initial positive family contacts. It allows the development of collaborative care which strongly endorses the role of carers as equal partners. Consumers' and carers' 'lived experience' of mental illness must be listened to, heard and acted upon effectively. This knowledge is as important to planned treatment, care and rehabilitation as is the professional knowledge of clinicians. Information from families that is vital to mental health workers concerns differing cultural customs about the role of families, particularly the role of women as care-givers. Family traditions need to be understood and respected if treatment and care plans are not to founder through lack of appreciation of socially and culturally different methods of family interaction (Bloch *et al.*, 1994).

Members of carer groups can become:

- **Educators and trainers of mental health professionals.** Traditional mental health education and training has emphasized the clinician–patient relationship This does not change easily to a triad of clinician, consumer and carer within mental health. Nevertheless, the education and training of the professional mental health workforce must involve learning how to work with family carers. This is best achieved by working together with family members in a reflective learning process at undergraduate and post-graduate levels as well as in-service workplace training.

- **Advisors in policy development for mental health services.** Family and consumer perspectives must inform mental health policies through advisory groups alerting governments to mental health issues.

- **Advocates for community acceptance of mental illness.** Carer organizations have an important role in mental health advocacy, particularly through community awareness campaigns.

- **Educators and trainers of other families.** Programmes are being developed by carer organizations where family members educate and train other families. Trained family members have the advantage of personal experience in care-giving. These programmes are cost-effective in that families support other families without payment.

Conflicts of interest between carers, users and professionals

Potential conflicts of interest occur when consumers blame their families for their problems, often when symptoms of mental illness (paranoia for example) are directed at family members; when involvement of the family raises concern over breaching confidentiality; and when consumers and carers do not have the same goals. Mental health workers can experience divided loyalties in situations of family conflict. Good clinical care should aim to resolve these issues.

In Australia, federal and state governments have formed 'Consumer Advisory Groups,' made up of consumers and family carers. These groups are invited to comment on policies that the government develops in mental health. They can take problems to government authorities. Consumers and carers had great difficulty at first in meeting together, but have gradually developed greater respect for each other's viewpoints.

Doctor–patient confidentiality and the need of family carers for information

Confidentiality has become a 'shibboleth' masking a wide range of other issues where good practice methods need to be developed.' (Furlong and Leggatt, 1996, p. 620). One of the reasons that family carers have been ignored in western cultures comes from the belief in the right of the individual to privacy in relation to his or her psychiatric condition. Doctors and other health professionals are trained to maintain confidentiality. Nowadays, the legal system and the threat of being sued are powerful forces working towards the preservation of patient privacy.

In western cultures, the enforcement of confidentiality often assumes precedence over other treatment and care issues which may be of greater benefit to the consumer. Eastern cultures are different, exhibiting a high regard for an open sharing of knowledge, particularly among the members of the immediate family. If confidentiality is a reflection of learned, cultural behaviours, then it is not a theoretically necessary component in the therapeutic process. Indeed, the opposite may be true; therapy may be best achieved where open dispersal and discussion of information is encouraged.

Ignoring family carers leads to exacerbations of family tensions through insensitive responses from clinical services. Without the information that people in close contact with a mentally ill person can give professionals, inadequate and inappropriate plans for treatment and care can occur. Failure to take into account the information from immediate carers on the 'early warning signs' of relapse, for example, has led to difficult and sometimes tragic consequences.

Confidentiality is not absolute. There are situations where it is legal and ethical to breach confidentiality (Zipple *et al.*, 1990; Bloch *et al.*, 1994; Furlong and Leggatt, 1996). Confidentiality is the right of the patient, not the professional. Professionals often fail to ask patients whether or not they would like family members to be involved. Problems with maintaining confidentiality can be largely overcome if professionals develop a commitment to ongoing involvement with family carers by establishing an equal partnership with them. This will encourage a process that becomes sensitive to the needs of families as well as to the needs of consumers.

Clinicians require training in how to give families the information they need and to accept that helping families in their own right should be standard practice. This commitment is necessary if 'best practice' is to be achieved, given the substantial evidence we now have that family involvement produces positive results for consumers.

In the process of engaging with family carers, clarification is needed on what information can be divulged, and what information a consumer has the right to know can remain private. It is legally, ethically and morally possible to help family members without breaching confidentiality through divulging personal and private information that is unique to particular individuals. For example, immediate decisions that need to be made should take into account the future

outcomes for patients. The patient may lack the capacity for consent, or may have the capacity but will not give it for reasons to do with their illness/disability, yet carers need information as they are involved with the person's care. Helping families here is in the patient's longer term best interest, even if the patient cannot agree at this stage. In many of the research projects where families, consumers and clinicians are working together in an equal partnership, the problems associated with confidentiality do not occur.

Research evidence of the effects of supporting carers in terms of their own well-being and that of their affected relatives

In recent years, research programmes have studied ways of educating and training families in effective coping. These studies were influenced by findings that showed that 30–40% of patients with schizophrenia relapsed even while on medication (Leff and Wing, 1971). There was a gradual realization by some mental health professionals that the primary burden of care had become the responsibility of the family of the patient (Katschnig and Konieczna, 1989). 'Expressed emotion' (Brown *et al.*, 1972)—a research tool developed to measure aspects of the home environment that were thought to precipitate relapse, namely hostility, critical comments and marked emotional overinvolvement—was researched further by Leff *et al.* (1982, 1985) and became the basis for the development of many family psychoeducational interventions.

Programmes for families can be described in various ways:

Family education

Family education 'packages' have provided knowledge about mental illness, but any long-term effect on the reduction of family burden is dubious or unknown. The evidence to date tends to caution against the organization of short education packages without other intervention components (Lam, 1991).

Family psychoeducation, family intervention

Goldstein (1995) states that family intervention programmes have been termed 'psychoeducational' because they involve a "combination of didactic material about schizophrenia for patients and relatives, and therapeutic strategies designed to improve stress management by all family members through enhanced communication and problem-solving skills." Other elements of psychoeducation are 'family support and crisis management.' (Dixon and Lehman, 1995, p. 631).

Service delivery methods of family intervention have ranged from relatives-only groups, individual family plus relatives' groups, individual family units, multiple family groups (with consumers), and parallel patient and relatives' groups (Goldstein, 1996). The most rigorous assessment of family interventions in schizophrenia that met the criteria for randomized controlled trials was carried out by the Cochrane Collaboration (Mari *et al.*, 1997). This assessment concluded that family interventions resulted in a decrease in the number of relapses, fewer admissions to hospital over a period of 2 years, better compliance with medication and greater stability in employment. Dixon and Lehman's review (1995) of the existing evidence and effectiveness of psychoeducational family interventions reports some suggestive though not conclusive evidence for improvements in patient functioning and family well-being. They conclude that more research is needed to try and understand "the critical ingredients of family interventions, to expand the groups of patients included in these studies, and to evaluate a broader range of outcomes."

Studies that do not meet the 'gold standard' for randomized controlled trials nevertheless suggest positive results for the family members themselves. SANE—Australia's review (1999, p. 4) cites research outcomes such as greater optimism (Smith and Birchwood, 1987); reduced feelings of blame (Tarrier and Barraclough, 1986); less negative emotion, greater adaptability and better

intrafamily communication (Berkowitz, 1986); a better understanding of mental illness and a consequent rise in confidence and skill in working with professionals and negotiating the mental health system (Smith and Birchwood, 1987); the development of working alliances between family carers, professionals and consumers (Greenberg *et al.*, 1988); and a greater capacity for advocacy (Lundwall, 1996). Reduced isolation and stronger support networks result when families are part of group education and training (McFarlane *et al.*, 1995b).

Families helping families

The reaction of families to the lack of recognition of their problems and the failure of mental health services to provide appropriate assistance has resulted in carer organizations developing their own education and support programmes such as 'Understanding and coping with schizophrenia: 14 principles for the relatives' (Alexander, 1991), and the 'Family-to-family education programme' (Burland, 1998). The family carers who developed these programmes claim that their experiences have given them the knowledge which mental health professionals do not have—the personal 'lived experience' of day to day coping with mental illness in a close relative. These programmes have not been subjected to rigorous evaluation. Nevertheless, thousands of family carers attest to their importance claiming that the only substantial help they have ever received has been through attending these 'peer support' educational courses (SANE—Australia, 1999).

An extension of 'peer support' is the 'Learning to cope together' project (Shore, 1998). Mental health professionals and family carers combined to develop and implement pilot programmes of education and training for carers. Evaluation of the programmes comparing pre- and post-training scores for each individual showed significant improvement for the 'Understanding schizophrenia' scores and 'General health questionnaire' scores, and a non-significant improvement in the 'Family distress' score. A training programme to enhance partnerships between mental health professionals and family care-givers (Farhall *et al.*,

1998) was the impetus for the development of the 'Family-sensitive training' programme where trained family care-givers and mental health professionals jointly developed a programme to facilitate the "crucial but complex relationship between mental health workers and family members and other carers of people living with mental illness." (Bouverie Centre, FAST video series kit, 1997).

A review of family burden studies by Johnson (1994b) concludes that the greater emphasis in family interventions has been on outcomes for the consumer. It is assumed that positive outcomes for consumers necessarily imply better outcomes for carers. There is some evidence that family interventions have been successful in reducing burden on families, but there are still problems with what constitutes burden. Szmukler (1996) criticizes the simplistic division of burden into objective and subjective. What may be more appropriate for understanding 'care-giving' is the implementation of a 'stress–appraisal–coping' paradigm since it deals directly with the responses of normal people, such as carers, to stressful circumstances. Johnson suggests that family burden should be conceptualized as 'stress and the need for stress reduction.' In effect, this means regarding subjective burden (distressing emotional reactions to mental illness) as the result of stress, and a primary objective for preventive efforts. Behaviours and events considered as objective burden would be viewed as stressors, with interventions being aimed at optimal management and reduction of stressful events.

Further research should develop and refine outcome measures such as patients' social role performance and reduction of carer distress. Subjective reports of the impact of psychoeducational interventions should be studied from families', patients' and clinicians' perspectives. (Lam, 1991).

Implications for future service development

Roles for carers and carer organizations in collaborative care with consumers and mental health professionals still face many problems.

Educational and social 'treatments' are not seen as important

Many mental health professionals see medical treatment as the main treatment modality for schizophrenia, and are sceptical about the benefits of psychoeducational (social) treatments. It is also common to find families who believe that all the answers lie in finding the right medications.

Research findings that have shown the efficacy of education, training and support for families have not been disseminated widely. Family interventions are still viewed as an 'optional extra' and not as 'core business'. There is a lack of clarity about the goals of family interventions. For families, being 'trained' can mean that the responsibility of caring will be on their shoulders. Training for families should emphasize 'shared care' between themselves and professional carers. Resistance from families often relates to previous poor interactions with mental health professionals. They are not prepared to try something new for fear of again being 'put down', 'blamed' or 'not listened to'. Problems also arise over definitions and responsibilities. Should these be treatment programmes, and funded by health departments? Or should they be social programmes, and funded from welfare or rehabilitation budgets?

Problems with models of care

A number of models of family psychoeducation have been developed. This has led to controversies about which is the better, more productive method for the implementation of family education, training and support. Programmes developed by family members in family support organizations could become a substitute for, and therefore prevent or delay the implementation of, comprehensive psychoeducational family interventions involving collaboration between carers, consumers/patients and clinicians.

Some authors are critical of programmes that have targeted high expressed emotion families as those most likely to benefit from 'psychoeducational interventions' (Hatfield *et al.*, 1987; Kanter *et al.*, 1987; Lefley, 1992). While criticizing the validity of the expressed emotion construct, they argue that 'expressed emotion' has become another way of blaming families. These programmes ignore the needs of 'low expressed emotion' families (Hatfield *et al.*, 1987). While professionals may believe working with families is useful if intrafamily communication can be improved, many families have become wary about involvement with professionally led family programmes.

Consensus on the basic principles which need to be in place in mental health services regardless of any particular method of family work has been developed by the WFS (1998). Different circumstances in different countries, particularly different levels of resources, will dictate which particular style of family work is implemented.

Structural problems in mental health services

In western countries, there is a growing acceptance of the need to involve families, but the necessary structural changes in mental health services have yet to be made. In eastern countries such as India, the problem is more the complete lack of resources for mental health in many areas.

Problems with services encountered so far, include:

- Lack of support from managers and professional colleagues who are not yet prepared to work with families. Mental health services are not accustomed to families becoming involved and have anxieties about how families will fit into a system that has worked predominantly within the 'doctor–patient' relationship.

- The results of family work take time to become evident. Failure to see improvements in the short term may deter staff from continuing.

- Overloaded staff feel they have no time to involve families. Around the world the mental health workforce is coping with huge caseloads. This works against implementing better methods of treatment and care, especially when this means extra work to implement the new techniques—at least in the short term. 'Current crises' interfere with the development of longer term projects.

- There is often poor continuity of care between clinical and social needs of consumers, let alone the needs of the family carers. Allied staff in community agencies often have no contact with the medical/clinical teams of their patients/consumers. This leads to fragmentation of care, misinterpretations and sometimes conflicting treatment goals.

Costs

Family psychoeducational research studies give an indication of cost reductions (McFarlane, 1995b). In countries where governments purchase both medication and psychosocial programmes, it is still likely that new medications will take priority over other forms of treatment.

Inadequate education and training of the mental health workforce

Psychoeducation requires training in collaborative partnerships based on sharing knowledge and skills. Clinicians educated and trained to work in hierarchical systems find this change in status and power threatening and difficult to manage. Goldstein (1995, p. 68.) believes that "family psychoeducational techniques can be easily disseminated to community practitioners ... However, we have also observed a resistance to applying these techniques among community practitioners who are used to individual therapy or case management models ... many practitioners have never worked with families and understandably find the prospect quite intimidating. Thus the training of practitioners in psychoeducational family models should not be separated from training in traditional family therapy, including techniques for joining and alliance building, maintaining neutrality, reframing and relabelling, and thinking in terms of family system dynamics."

In England (Duggan, 1997) and Australia (Deakin Human Services, 1999), workshops and consultations have been carried out between the major mental health professional groupings—psychiatrists, clinical psychologists, psychiatric nurses, occupational therapists and social workers, with substantial input from family carers and consumers. There were positive statements about the roles of consumers and carers in the education and training of the workforce. In the British report, recommendation 6 stated . . ."that options for encouraging user and carer involvement in curriculum planning, training and delivery and setting service standards relating to continued fitness for purpose and assessment of competence should be developed and implemented. This should be done following consultation with user and carer organisations."

The Australian report, a 'Statement of Principle', developed by consumers and carers, confirms the need to involve them in all levels of mental health education and training. They are to be remunerated adequately for this work, and encouraged to develop their 'bodies of knowledge' to form the basis for education and training of the mental health workforce.

Carer organizations started out as small groups of family members meeting to give each other support. From these small beginnings, the growth of the family movement in mental health has been impressive. The diversity of functions now undertaken by carer organizations has spearheaded many reforms, making them a substantial political and social asset in the modern treatment, care and rehabilitation of the mentally ill.

References

Alexander, K. (1991) *Understanding and Coping with Schizophrenia: 14 Principles for the Relatives.* Australia: Schwartz and Wilkinson.

Berkowitz, R. (1984) Educating relatives about schizophrenia. *Schizophrenia Bulletin*, 10, 418–429.

Bloch, S., Hafner, J., Harari, E. and Szmukler, G. (1994) *The Family in Clinical Psychiatry.* Oxford: Oxford University Press.

Bouverie Centre (1997) *Family Sensitive Training Video Series Kit.* Flemington, Australia: The Bouverie Centre.

Brown, G.W., Birley, J.L.T. and Wing, J.K. (1972) Influence of family life on the course of schizophrenia: a replication. *British Journal of Psychiatry*, 121, 241–258.

Burland, J. (1998) Family-to-family: a trauma and recovery model of family education. *New Directions for Mental Health Services*, 77, 33–41.

Deakin Human Services (1999) *Learning Together: Education and Training Partnerships in Mental Health Service.* Australia: Commonwealth Department of Health and Aged Care.

Dixon, L.B. and Lehman, A.F. (1995) Family interventions for schizophrenia. *Schizophrenia Bulletin*, 21, 4.

Duggan, M. (1997) *Pulling Together—The Future Roles and Training of Mental Health Staff.* London: Sainsbury Centre for Mental Health.

Farhall, J., Webster, B., Hocking, B., Leggatt, M., Reiss, C. and Young, J. (1998) Training to enhance partnerships between mental health professionals and family caregivers: a comparative study. *Psychiatric Services*, 49, 11.

Furlong, M. and Leggatt, M. (1996) Reconciling the patient's right to confidentiality and the family's need to know. *Australian and New Zealand Journal of Psychiatry*, 30, 5.

Goldstein, M.J. (1995) Psychoeducation and relapse prevention. *International Clinical Psychopharmacology*, 9 (Suppl. 5), 59–69.

Goldstein, M.J. (1996) Psycho-education and family treatment related to the phase of psychotic disorder. *International Clinical Psychopharmacology*, 11 (Suppl. 2), 77–83.

Greenberg, L., Fine, S., Cohen, C., Langton, K., Michaelson-Baily, A., Rubington, P. and Glick, I. (1988) An interdisciplinary psychoeducation program for schizophrenic patients and their families in an acute care setting. *Hospital and Community Psychiatry*, 39, 277–282.

Hatfield, A. (1979) Taking issue. *Hospital and Community Psychiatry*, 38, 341.

Hatfield, A. (1997) Help-seeking behaviour in families of schizophrenics. *American Journal of Community Psychiatry*, 17, 5.

Hatfield, A., Spaniol, L. and Zipple, A. (1987) Expressed emotion: a family perspective. *Schizophrenia Bulletin*, 13, 221–226.

Johnson, D.L. (1994a) Families around the world form organisations for the mentally ill. *Innovations and Research*, 3, 25–30.

Johnson, D.L. (1994b) Current issues in family research: can the burden of mental illness be relieved? In: Lefley, H.P. and Wasow, M. (eds), *Helping Families Cope with Mental Illness.* Newark, NJ: Harwood Academic, pp. 309–328.

Kanter, H., Lamb, R. and Loeper, C. (1987) Expressed emotion in families: a critical review. *Hospital and Community Psychiatry*, 43, 591–598.

Katschnig, H. and Konieczna, T. (1989) What works in work with relatives? An hypothesis. *British Journal of Psychiatry*, 155 (Suppl. 5), 144–150.

Katz, A. and Bender, E. (eds) (1979) *The Strength in Us:*

Self-help Groups in the Modern World. New York: Franklin Watts.

Lam, D.H. (1991) Psychosocial family intervention in schizophrenia: a review of empirical studies. *Psychological Medicine*, 21, 423–441.

Leff, J.P. and Wing, J.K. (1971) Trial of maintenance therapy in schizophrenia. *British Medical Journal*, 141, 594–600.

Leff, J.P., Kuipers, L., Berkowitz, R., Eberlein-Fries, R. and Sturgeon, D. (1982) A controlled trial of social intervention in schizophrenia. *British Journal of Psychiatry*, 141, 121–134.

Leff, J.P., Kuipers, L., Berkowitz, R. and Sturgeon, D. (1985) A controlled trial of social intervention in the families of schizophrenia patients. *British Journal of Psychiatry*, 146, 594–600.

Lefley, H. (1992) Expressed emotion: conceptual, clinical and social policy issues. *Hospital and Community Psychiatry*, 43, 591–598.

Lundwall, R. (1996) How psychoeducational support groups can provide multidiscipline services to families of people with mental illness. *Psychiatric Rehabilitation Journal*, 20, 64–71.

Mari, J.J., Adams, C.E. and Streiner, D. (1997) Family intervention for those with schizophrenia. In: Adams, C.E., Anderson, M. and Mari, J. (eds), *Schizophrenia Module of the Cochrane Database Systematic Reviews.* London: British Medical Journal Publishing Group. The Cochrane Library 2. Update Software (1998).

McFarlane, W.R., Link, B., Dushay, R., Marchal, J. and Crilly, J. (1995a) Psychoeducational multiple family groups: four-year relapse outcome in schizophrenia. *Family Process*, 324, 127–144.

McFarlane, W.R., Lukens, E., Link, B., Dushay, R., Deakins, S., Newmark, M., Dunne, E., Horan, B. and Toran, J. (1995b) Multiple family groups and psychoeducation in the treatment of schizophrenia. *Archives of General Psychiatry*, 52, 679–687.

Piatigorsky, M. (1997) *Psychologist and Social Worker Pioneer Family Support. Living With Schizophrenia.* Mundelein IL: Eli Lilly.

SANE—Australia (1999) *Blueprint Guide to Carer Education and Training.* Australia: SANE.

Shankar, R. and Menon, M.S. (1991) Interventions with families of people with schizophrenia: the issues facing a community rehabilitation center in India. *Psychosocial Rehabilitation Journal*, 15, 85–90.

Shore, L. (1998) *Learning to Cope Together.* Implementation and evaluation of the NSF/Sainsbury Centre for Mental Health Carers' Education Support Project (CESP).

Smith, J. and Birchwood, M. (1987) Specific and non-specific effects of educational intervention with families living with a schizophrenic relative. *British Journal of Psychiatry*, 150, 645–652.

Szmukler, G. (1996) From family 'burden' to caregiving. *Psychiatric Bulletin*, 20, 449–451.

Tarrier, N. and Barrowclough, C. (1986) Providing information to relatives about schizophrenia: some comments. *British Journal of Psychiatry*, 149. 401–405

Wing, J.K. (1997) *Schizophrenia and its Management in the Community.* Kingston upon Thames: National Schizophrenia Fellowship.

World Fellowship for Schizophrenia (1998) Families as partners in care. e- mail:wsf@inforamp.net

Zipple, A., Langle, S., Spaniol, L. and Fisher, H. (1990) Client confidentiality and the family's need to know: strategies for resolving the conflict. *Community Mental Health Journal*, 26, 374–380.

41 | *Primary prevention of mental disorders*

Norman Sartorius

Introduction

The term primary prevention has its origin in the concept of linear progression of conditions from a state without disease to a disease, from there to impairment, then to disability (an incapacity to perform in social roles) and finally to handicap (describing the social disadvantage that a person has because of his disability) (see Figure 41.1).

These terms and the scheme shown in Figure 41.1 express the views that the World Health Organization has adopted as a basis for its International Classification of Impairments, Disabilities and Handicaps (WHO, 1980). Since then, this way of viewing the progression of conditions has been losing popularity because of the recognition of multiple and complex relationships between diseases, impairments, disabilities and handicaps. Diseases can handicap persons, and impairments and disabilities are risk factors that can lead to relapses of the disease that has produced them, and to other illnesses. The scheme therefore today has to be amended (see Figure 41.2).

As a consequence of these conceptual changes, it is more appropriate to speak of the prevention of diseases, the prevention of impairments, the prevention of disability and the prevention of handicaps than to speak about primary, secondary, tertiary and quartenary prevention: but for a while it is likely that the latter terms will be used, by force of habit, parallel to the more precise terms that are being proposed now.

The specific features of prevention in the field of mental health

Most mental disorders are the result of the action of a number of biological, social and (personal) psychological factors. These risk factors also contribute to the occurrence of non-psychiatric disorders: poor perinatal care, for example, is likely to act as a risk factor for a variety of illnesses. The ways in which these risk factors interact with each other and the manner in which they lead to the appearance of diseases often is not clear. As a general rule, the more risk factors are present the more likely it is that a mental disorder will appear: it is important to recognize that the number of factors present seems to be more important than their type.

Several important guidelines for preventive action stem from these facts. First, it is useful and necessary to join efforts to prevent mental disorders with efforts to prevent other illness. Secondly, the fact that it is the number of factors that is more important than their type means that diseases often can be prevented by choosing factors which can be neutralized so that mental disorders do not manifest themselves, although a number of risk factors cannot be changed and remain present. Thirdly, taking into account the complex pathogenesis of mental disorder, research into the causes of mental disorders is less likely to make a contribution to their prevention (at least in the near future) than concerted action of different social sectors to control risk factors. Fourthly, the effects of interventions undertaken

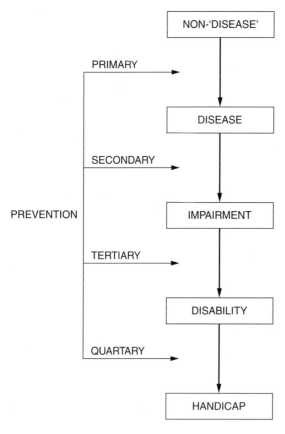

Figure 41.1 *Concept of relationships between disease, impairment, disability and handicap in the 1980s.*

reached the threshold. Research, however, shows that treatments of mental disorders have very low specificity and that 'subthreshold disorders' produce severe suffering and disability (Judd *et al.*, 1997). Yet, 'subthreshold' disorders do not appear in results of surveys of prevalence of mental disorders and it is therefore possible that a preventive intervention can be shown to have reduced the severity of clinical symptoms (and thus also the incidence of mental disorders which now do not reach the threshold) without reducing the suffering and disability that these disorders will produce in their 'subthreshold' form. Conversely, it is imaginable that a preventive intervention will reduce suffering and disability due to mental disorders without this being visible in changes of prevalence or incidence of the disorder. Mental disorders are not only defined vaguely; their definition also changes with time and by the country in which they are used. Consequently, it is possible to reduce the numbers of mental disorders by changing their definition, a fact that has had its effects, for example, in reviews of changes of effectiveness of psychiatric treatment over time.

Possibilities for the prevention of mental disorders

The possibilities for the prevention of mental disorders can be examined from different points of view. First, it is possible to assess which

to prevent physical disorders may show effects in the diminution of incidence of mental disorders *and vice versa*, which adds to the difficulty of evaluating preventive interventions in psychiatry.

A particular problem that has to be kept in mind in designing interventions aimed at preventing mental illness and in measuring their effects is that the borders of mental disorders are vague and consensual. The thresholds of mental disorders have been set by psychiatrists who used the best of their experience and available knowledge: the validity of these thresholds was supposed to be confirmed by a positive reaction to specific treatments and by similar consequences which were more severe than those of disorders that have not

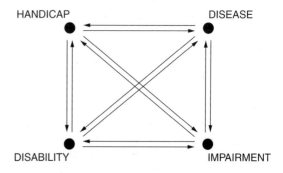

Figure 41.2 *Current concepts of relationships between disease, impairment, disability and handicap.*

measures can prevent a particular disorder: thus, we can list mental disorders and indicate which measures can reduce their incidence. This list of measures soon becomes repetitive and sometimes looks like an election programme of a political party—better nutrition, adequate housing, more tolerance, less war and violence will all appear on these lists several times while specific measures will be in a minority.

Alternatively, the preventive measures could be examined by the social service sector which should undertake them. The health sector and particularly the primary health care services can make a major contribution to the prevention of mental disorders; but equally, other Ministries, for example of education, labour and social security, could through their agents in the field and by promulgating appropriate legislation significantly diminish risk factors contributing to the occurrence of mental disorders.

Another possibility for examining possibilities of preventive action is to examine measures by reference to the level at which they have to be implemented. Thus, at the governmental level, we could list legislation and allocation of (earmarked) funding for preventive activities; at the district level some other measures, for example water sanitation control; and at the community level support to a mutual help association that could alleviate the burden of mothers looking after severely impaired children at home.

There are advantages and disadvantages of each of these presentations: in presentations to medically qualified people, it is probably better to present measures grouping them by group of disorders; for decision makers responsible for a particular sector (e.g. Education) it will be better to describe specifically the various health, mental health and other (e.g. political) benefits that will accrue if a particular intervention is introduced in schools. For health care planners, the presentation by level of responsibility will be the most convenient, particularly if proposals for preventive interventions are accompanied by specific suggestions about indicators of effectiveness of the measures proposed.

These considerations are listed here because psychiatrists cannot do much preventive work themselves: most of the interventions that can be recommended today are best done by agencies or sectors outside of the health sector; when the health sector has the responsibility it will be health services other than psychiatry (e.g. maternal and child health units) that will have to undertake the measures; and when the mental health services have the opportunity to do something it will be mainly mental health staff other than psychiatrists who will have to act (Sartorius and Henderson, 1992). For psychiatrists, the main task will lie in advocacy of the implementation of measures by others; and, to be successful advocates, psychiatrists will have to think of the best ways to present their proposals to the executive agencies that have the opportunity—and the moral duty—to intervene.

Synoptic review of interventions that can prevent the occurrence of mental disorders

Mental retardation is one of the most frequent among disorders classified in Chapter F (Mental and Behavioural Disorders) of the 10th Revision of the International Classification of Diseases (ICD-10) While its most severe forms reach the prevalence of 0.3–0.5% of the population, less severe forms are much more frequent and can strike as many as 4% of the population. The incidence of the condition (both in its severe and in its less severe forms) is approximately 30% higher in the developing than in developed countries: the difference is due largely to poor health care and poor conditions of life. In absolute numbers, the difference amounts to some 40 million people, in whom mental retardation would not have occurred had the conditions of their life been similar to those in industrialized countries. The total gain that could be expected if the current knowledge about the condition was to be applied fully is, however, much higher: in developed countries also, mental retardation occurs where it could have been prevented by relatively simple interventions. Appropriate prenatal and perinatal care, immunization, child spacing, control of epilepsy and other convulsive conditions in childhood, better day care, prevention of accidents, support to families at risk, teaching of parenting skills, early recognition and correction of minor sensory deficits (e.g. myopia), prevention of alcohol, nicotine and other drug abuse in pregnancy, and an improvement of psychosocial care in longterm care institutions for children are among the most obvious measures that could be taken.

The gains of the application of these measures would be considerable. By way of an example, an improvement of nutrition by the addition of iodine in the form of iodinized salt and water or the administration of iodinized oil could have prevented the occurrence of cretinism and related disorders in at least 6 million people. Among fairly well documented areas of interventions are the prevention of the foetal alcohol syndrome, of phenylketonuria and of Down's syndrome (WHO, 1998b): obtaining precise estimates of the benefits that would accrue if health care and conditions of life were to improve is difficult, but the gain could not be less than that of the current difference of the developed and developing countries' prevalence rates of mental retardation.

While listing the above possible interventions that are likely to reduce the incidence of mental retardation, two points have to be recalled: first, that most of the measures listed would not only reduce the incidence of mental retardation but also diminish the incidence of other diseases and contribute to the quality of life of the populations concerned; and secondly, that many of the above measures have to be undertaken by sectors other than health.

Acquired lesions of the central nervous system

Damage to brain tissue is a major cause of mental (and neurological) disorders. Its causes are many—including trauma, bacterial, viral and parasitic infections, malnutrition, extended or intensive exposure to pollutants (e.g. carbon monoxide, heavy metals, fertilizers and insecticides), arterial hypertension, alcohol and other drug abuse, as well as congenital damage due to untoward events during pregnancy. The above list of causes of brain damage is also a list of targets for preventive interventions. Some of them are easy, others require a major investment or changes in society. Countries will differ in the choice of intervention that they might use: here again, it is likely that measures that prevent more than one negative consequence will have priority, as will measures that will be seen as being politically advantageous to the government in power.

Several of the causes listed above will produce the clinical picture of dementia: a point worth stressing to dispel the gloom resulting from our inability to prevent certain forms of dementia, for example Alzheimer's disease.

An issue arising in the instance of Huntingdon's chorea and likely to arise in the period between the discovery of genetic markers for Alzheimer's disease (and for psychotic disorders) and the development of specific preventive or treatment measures for these conditions is the necessity to develop clear ethical guidelines covering the handling of information about diseases that will appear at a later point in life.

Problems related to the abuse of alcohol and other drugs

The area of substance abuse is characterized by uncertainty about epidemiological facts and by political, moral and religious overtones. These factors play a role in the aetiology of alcohol and drug abuse and in shaping preventive, curative and rehabilitative action. Preventive action is clearly dependent on the categorization of alcohol-related problems: these were first seen as a vice, than as a disease and more recently as a set of behavioural syndromes, of which some are profoundly imbedded in cultural and social traditions defining a population group (e.g. ritual drinking and ingestion of hallucinogenic drugs), some are primarily medical (e.g. delirium tremens and Korsakov's syndrome) and some are partial causes of problems determined by the behaviour of the persons ingesting alcohol and by the circumstances in which they find themselves (e.g. traffic accidents due to drunken driving). Preventive action has therefore also taken several routes including: (i) the reduction of alcohol intake and nutritional supplementation to prevent the even more sinister consequences of alcohol abuse and dependence (e.g. delirium tremens); (ii) the prevention of alcohol-related problems through the reduction of availability of alcohol (e.g. by pricing policies and control of alcohol outlets); (iii) campaigns of information of the general public and of groups at particularly high risk (e.g. adolescents) to prevent the ingestion of alcohol altogether; and (iv) reducing the incidence of alcohol-related problems by making it difficult that persons under the influence of alcohol find themselves in situations in which their state might result in an accident or other problem (e.g. by regular control of alcohol blood levels in pilots or long-haul truck drivers).

The prevention of alcohol- and drug-related problems (as well as the prevention of some other problems related to psychiatric disorders) also raises an important ethical question: just how much restriction can a society impose on its citizens in the name of preserving their health ? Also, connected to this, who should decide on the application of these measures—the medical profession, a referendum, the Ministry of the Interior or the health authorities?

The effects of prevention of alcohol-related problems are sometimes measured in terms of reduction of per capita alcohol intake after comprehensive campaigns to reduce drinking (e.g. in Australia) and sometimes expressed in terms of life expectancy of people with alcohol problems. Unfortunately, it is often difficult to interpret the numbers that are reported and to be certain of their validity. The numerous confounding factors as well as the political and economic considerations (e.g. income from alcohol trade and customs taxes) that affect the conduct of studies also play their role in the analysis of data, in the reporting of information and in its public use. The situation is even worse in the instance of abuse of illicit drugs in which international as well as national interests are involved in addition to problems arising from the complexity of the phenomena, from the influence of criminal forces and from the lack of agreement about basic concepts still prevailing among the health professionals.

Neurotic psychotic and personality disorders

Knowledge about factors which contribute to the risk of occurrence of neurotic, psychotic and personality disorders indicates that preventive action will probably have to be directed at the reduction of exposure of individuals and groups to putative risk factors. Data on which such a statement can be based are results of studies showing that groups exposed to certain factors have a higher probability of having the disease than others who were not exposed: at present there is no absolute certainty that these associations are causal nor has it yet been proven—for a variety of reasons—that the removal of one or another risk factor reduced the incidence of the diseases in question.

While specific examples of preventing a particular neurotic, personality or psychotic disorders are still lacking, there is considerable literature about the improvement of competence and reduction of certain behavioural symptoms in children and adolescents. Most of these studies have been carried out in affluent countries and dealt with severely deprived families or children who were both shown to benefit from material and educational support, better conditions of life and better health care. Some studies have shown that appropriate interventions can reduce behavioural problems There has been a fair amount of work aimed at improving marital relationships, to learn how to deal with separation and divorce, to enhance personal development and to cope with a variety of life stresses ranging from losing a job to caring for a sick relative. The success of these programmes has varied: details of the contribution that such improved coping skills might have made to the prevention of mental disorders have, however, not been provided (Mrazek and Haggerty, 1994).

With admirable pragmatism, Paykel and Jenkins (1994) summarized the available evidence about social causative factors of neurotic and psychotic—but probably also of other psychiatric conditions—as a possible target for primary prevention saying:

"... social causative factors have implications for primary prevention. Here an important general conclusion emerges: it is better to think small than to think big. In psychiatry targeted preventive medicines are likely to be more profitable than universal measures. It is easier to modify the social micro environment of the family than the macro environment of society as a whole. Similarly, it is easier to tackle precipitating factors where the link with onset of disorders is closer rather than predisposing factors. Coping responses are more amenable to intervention than is removal of social stresses themselves many of which are bound up with the inevitable consequences of the life cycle. What is not at present feasible in primary prevention is to change dramatically cultures or societal structures except for the most deprived. Nor is it possible to avoid interpersonal life events or, as yet, to prevent functional disorders by tackling fundamental biological causes and mechanisms" (Paykel and Jenkins, 1994).

Suicide and attempted suicide

Suicide is among the most important causes of death in many industrialized and some non-industrialized countries. It is often under-reported for a variety of reasons ranging from the stigma that will mark the family in which a suicide has taken place to administrative and religious reasons. Attempted suicide is usually estimated at rates that are several times higher than those of suicide. Although both suicide and attempted suicide can have a variety of reasons, mental disorders are often involved: usually it is estimated that two-thirds to four-fifths of all suicides are related to mental disorders including substance abuse problems. Among the preventive measures are the treatment of mental disorders, particularly depression and substance misuse, and support to individuals at elevated risk for suicide because of long-lasting and painful physical illness, unemployment and poverty, family problems and marital breakdown, and control of methods used

for suicide. An example of a possible intervention in this respect would be the replacement, by a less deadly variety, of the currently widely used phosphor-based insecticides serving as the main method in the current epidemic of suicide of young women in China. These insecticides are particularly lethal and there is no effective treatment for those who have ingested them.

Prevention of suicide in institutions has received more urgency because of its growing frequency in prisons, long-term care institutions and mental hospitals. Reductions of numbers of staff for economic reasons and the increased emphasis on providing in-mates of such institutions with some freedom of movement and action may be among the main reasons for this trend of increase which is particularly difficult to tolerate since those who attempt suicide are supposed to be well looked after in a health care system of controled quality.

Excessive risk-taking behaviours

Certain forms of behaviour expose individuals to an unnecessary risk of physical or mental illness. In young people, such behaviour often takes the form of experimenting with drugs, sexual activity without appropriate precautions against (teenage) unwanted pregnancy or sexually transmitted diseases, and driving at excessive speed. Similar behaviours can also be observed in people at other ages, but somewhat less frequently; in their case there are also others, e.g. those related to work style. Most of such behaviours could be changed—thus reducing risks to health—but changes often require modifications of the immediate and broader physical and social environment which are out of reach of the individuals concerned and of health services.

These behaviours are mentioned here because they illustrate the difficulty of defining reasonable limits of primary prevention in psychiatry. Changes of behaviour that expose the individuals to risk of damaging their health are not directed specifically to the prevention of a mental disorder but could prevent their occurrence as well; the techniques used to change the behaviour are only in part stemming from psychiatry and psychology, the rest coming from the domain of other sciences and social sectors; the change of behaviour that is to be expected at a certain age (e.g. that of seeking opportunities to face challenges in adolescence) and might be contributory to the development of an individual raises the issue of ethically permissible limits of health system interventions; and finally, the yield of the interventions that could be proposed is probably greater in terms of physical health than in terms of mental health.

Summary and conclusions

Primary prevention of a number of psychiatric disorders is possible. The role of psychiatrists in the field of prevention will usually be restricted to that of an advocate of measures that others have to undertake—those in the mental health team, those in other parts of the health system or those in other parts of the social sectors that can contribute to the reduction of incidence of mental and neurological disorders. The prevention of mental disorders has important secondary impacts: it eliminates prolonged stress that mental disorders exert on carers and brings psychiatry closer to the other medical disciplines since so many of the preventive measures have to be taken in concert with other medical disciplines.

There are legal instruments that could be used to invigorate preventive programmes in the field of psychiatry. The World Health Assembly, the supreme international body composed of Ministers of Health or other representatives of the 170 Member States of the World Health Organization, has for example adopted a special resolution (WHA, 39.25) requesting Member states to undertake preventive programmes and national health programmes in many countries which make references to the need to introduce preventive programmes in psychiatry (WHO, 1988a). The gains of introducing appropriate programmes of primary prevention of mental disorders could be enormous: a significant proportion of mental disorders that are one of the main contributors to the burden of disease (Murray and Lopez, 1996)

could have been prevented by primary prevention, and numerous others could be reduced in duration and consequences by appropriate treatment (which would have also reduced the risks for mental disorders in carers).

Despite the fact that effective prevention interventions exist and that there is a legal framework that would facilitate their application, primary prevention of mental disorders has few advocates and there is no country in which there is a coherent policy of a comprehensive implementation of measures preventing the occurrence of mental disorders. In part, this is probably due to the difficulties of evaluating the effects of primary prevention of mental disorders which would require long-term prospective studies and a resolution of the terminological chaos that still characterizes mental health action. In part also, this is due to the fact that mental disorders are due to the action of a number of risk factors that are by and large non-specific, and that preventive measures depend on the simultaneous action of a number of social sectors often not accustomed to collaboration.

Interventions enhancing coping and other capacities are, strictly speaking, not measures of primary prevention of mental disorders. They are useful because in our time of evidence-based action they confirm the obvious, for example that appropriate stimulation, good health care, adequate nutrition and harmonious family life are likely to be useful in the development of a child's capacity and mental set-up. They are, however, also carrying a risk that providing adequate nutrition and other conditions of life or the elimination of racial discrimination will be seen as a medically useful interventions rather than as the fulfilment of basic ethical imperatives of societies towards its citizens—regardless of whether they will increase the intelligence quotient or not.

References

Judd, L.L., Akiskal, H.S. and Paulus M.P. (1997) The role and clinical significance of subsyndromal depressive symptoms in unipolar major depressive disorders. *Journal of Affective Disorders*, 45, 5–18.

Murray, C.J.L. and Lopez, A.D. (1996) *The Global Burden of Disease.* Cambridge, MA: Harvard University Press

Mrazek, P.J. and Haggerty, R.J. (1994) *Reducing Risks for Mental Disorders.* Washington, DC: National Academy Press.

Paykel, E.S. and Jenkins, R. (eds) (1994) *Prevention in Psychiatry.* London: Gaskell.

Sartorius, N. and Henderson, A.S. (1992) The neglect of prevention in psychiatry. *Australian and New Zealand Journal of Psychiatry,* 26, 550–553.

World Health Organization (1980) *International Classification of Impairments, Disabilities, and Handicaps.* Geneva: WHO.

World Health Organization (1998a) *Prevention of Mental, Neurological and Psychosocial Disorders.* Document WHO/MINH/EVAI88. 1. Geneva: WHO.

World Health Organization (1998b) *Primary Prevention of Mental Neurological and Psychosocial Disorders.* Geneva: WHO.

42 | *Secondary prevention of mental disorders*

Patrick McGorry

From secondary prevention to early intervention

Conceptual issues

"Is 'an ounce of prevention worth a pound of cure'? . . . sometimes perhaps 15 ounces of prevention are worth a pound of cure." Eaton and Harrison (1996, p. 142).

What exactly is prevention in psychiatry? What is cure? What lies in between? What emphasis is most cost-effective for a particular disorder? A key obstacle to developing effective preventive interventions in psychiatry has been the lack of an agreed conceptual framework. The lack of clarity regarding the scope of prevention and of related concepts such as early intervention and mental health promotion has been addressed only recently. If we were less confused about such issues, then perhaps we could deploy our finite resources in a more cost-effective manner across the spectrum of mental disorder.

Traditional definitions

The most familiar framework consists of primary, secondary and tertiary prevention (Commission on Chronic Illness, 1957; Caplan, 1964). Primary prevention, the reduction of incidence, is an ideal but elusive goal. This is because, while it is the most cost-effective form of prevention at least for high incidence disorders, it requires a good knowledge of the causal risk factors, especially those with large population attributable risk, and of the causal sequence in the onset of disorder, so that the most efficient intervention point can be selected. Such knowledge is still lacking for many

mental disorders. Even when the knowledge base for primary prevention is present, other obstacles, such as policy failure, cost factors and logistic deficits, interfere with its implementation. This is obvious in many developing countries for a range of physical diseases, and has been described as a failure of *knowledge utilization*. In the developed world, there is an ambivalence concerning primary prevention for a variety of reasons, especially in the mental health field, because of earlier false dawns (Jenkins, 1994), and primary responsibility for its implementation falls outside the usual role of clinicians and clinical services. In contrast, secondary prevention, aimed at the reduction of prevalence, falls clearly within the mandate of clinical services and health professionals. Even so, it too has been slow to emerge in real world settings.

Recent conceptual advances

Building on the ideas of Gordon (1983), Mrazek and Haggerty (1994) developed a more sophisticated framework for conceptualizing, implementing and evaluating preventive interventions for mental disorders within the full spectrum of interventions for mental disorders. They classified preventive interventions as universal, selective and indicated.

- *Universal* preventive interventions are targeted to the general public or a whole population group that has not been identified on the basis of individual risk, e.g. use of seat belts, immunization and prevention of smoking.
- *Selective* preventive measures are appropriate for subgroups of the population whose risk of

becoming ill is above average. Examples include special immunizations such as for people travelling to areas where yellow fever is endemic and annual mammograms for women with a positive family history of breast cancer. The subjects are clearly asymptomatic.

- *Indicated* preventive measures apply to those individuals who on examination are found to manifest a risk factor that identifies them, individually, as being at high risk for the future development of a disease, and as such could be the focus of screening. Gordon's view was that such individuals should be asymptomatic and 'not motivated by current suffering', yet have a clinically demonstrable abnormality. An example would be asymptomatic individuals with hypertension. Mrazek and Haggerty (1994) adapted Gordon's concept as follows:

"Indicated preventive interventions for mental disorders are targeted to high-risk individuals who are identified as having minimal but detectable signs or symptoms foreshadowing mental disorder, or biological markers indicating predisposition for mental disorder, but who do not meet DSM-111-R diagnostic levels at the current time."

This major definitional shift allows individuals with early and/or subthreshold features (and hence a degree of suffering and disability) to be included within the focus of indicated prevention. Some clinicians would regard this as early intervention or an early form of treatment; however, the situation with these individuals is not so clear cut. While some of these cases will clearly have an early form of the disorder in question, others will not. They might, however, have other less serious disorders, and many individuals' subthreshold for a potentially serious disorder nevertheless may have crossed a clinical threshold where they either require or request treatment. This will either be because they have reached a diagnostic threshold for other co-morbid syndromes, or because the subthreshold symptoms of the putatively core disorder have become disabling or distressing. As any clinician knows, help-seeking and treatment need in psychiatry are not perfectly correlated with diagnostic threshold; not surprisingly, patients do not always conform to the DSM or

ICD categories and thresholds (Frances, 1998; Regier *et al.*, 1998; Spitzer, 1998).

In community settings, co-morbidity is common, with patients manifesting admixtures of symptoms, mainly anxiety and depression, with some syndromes more prominent than others. Strictly speaking they could be seen as receiving treatment for one syndrome and an indicated preventive intervention for another. This way of looking at it makes particular sense if the disorder that has already reached diagnostic threshold, say depression, is known regularly to form part of the prodromal phase of another serious syndrome, such as acute psychosis or schizophrenia, for which some subthreshold features have emerged. So treating the depression would be worthwhile in its own right and possibly reduce the risk of emergence of frank psychosis. It would also be feasible to intervene specifically with subthreshold features of psychosis. This could be seen as indicated prevention, which also clearly involves providing treatment to a proportion of the group who would not have developed psychosis anyway. This aspect is analogous to uniform maintenance therapy following recovery from psychosis or depression, where a proportion will not have required this.

Indicated prevention, therefore, sits within an ambiguous zone between primary and secondary prevention. These problems are really an artefact of a categorical model of diagnosis. In a field with high levels of co-morbidity, a syndrome-based system of classification and the definite possibility that one syndrome may act as a risk factor or precursor for another, the primary–secondary distinction has limited utility.

Beyond the subthreshold or prodromal phase, two additional secondary prevention foci can be discerned. First, early case detection aimed at shortening delays in accessing treatment will reduce prevalence provided there is an effective form of treatment available. The related task of increasing the treated incidence, particularly for high incidence disorders, also aims to reduce prevalence, and can be achieved through similar strategies (see below). Secondly, the notion that optimal treatment of the early phase of a disorder could shorten the duration of illness and thus

Table 42.1 *Roles of clinical service in prevention and treatment*

Prevention level	Role
Universal	Partnership with other agencies
Selective	High risk groups, e.g. unemployed—risk factor is common and potent Intervention = mental health promotion (MHP) (asymptomatic)
Indicated	High risk groups, e.g. unemployed with symptoms Intervention = early treatment and MHP, e.g. pre-psychotic phase
Early case detection	High risk groups, e.g. unemployed Intervention = ECD General population Full range of primary agencies Interventions = Education; improve access; improve engagement
Optimal intervention early treatment	First-episode psychosis—e.g. EPPIC model Other disorders
Treatment	Optimal treatment
Rehabilitation	Mental health promotion (MHP)

reduce the prevalence of the disorder, and further have a positive medium- to long-term effect on the course and outcome, is an attractive idea. Although the idea of a 'critical period' during which the disorder is more responsive to intervention has been developed principally for psychotic disorders (Falloon, 1992; Loebel, 1992; Birchwood and Macmillan, 1993; McGorry and Singh, 1995; Birchwood *et al.*, 1998; McGorry and Jackson, 1999), it could also apply to relapsing and persistent mood and anxiety disorders as well. Optimizing and intensifying early phase treatment is a third subtype of secondary prevention which could be implemented and evaluated within mental health services at the present state of knowledge. Mental health professionals and services could also explore indicated prevention and early case detection as secondary preventive strategies. These three foci can be termed collectively '*early intervention*'. A fourth subtype of secondary prevention, relapse prevention in the context of full remission between episodes of disorder, genuinely falls within the scope and definition of secondary

prevention. While there is substantial evidence supporting its widespread use, space considerations preclude its further consideration here. The remainder of the chapter will confine itself to early intervention as defined above. The potential role of mental health services across this spectrum of prevention and treatment is presented in Table 42.1.

The Global Burden of Disease report (Murray and Lopez, 1996) makes reference to the cost-effectiveness of interventions and the concept of 'best buys'. Even when good knowledge of risk factors for a disorder is available, and primary prevention possible, if the disorder is of low incidence, secondary prevention (indicated prevention and early detection) may be more cost-effective, as suggested by Eaton and Harrison (1996). This may be especially so if a knowledge of the clinical epidemiology of onset is interwoven with an understanding of developmental psychiatry and implementation of consumer-friendly models of service provision, as described in the next section. If not yet a "best buy", this is probably a "best bet".

Developmental psychopathology and the clinical epidemiology of onset: a preventive opportunity

Epidemiological surveys have demonstrated that vulnerability to most psychiatric disorders of adults is expressed for the first time in adolescence or early adult life. The Epidemiologic Catchment Area (ECA) study (Regier *et al.*, 1984) showed that the median age for first expression of symptoms of mental disorder was approximately 16 years. Indeed, the median value for onset of nearly all disorders individually (including depression which has actually fallen from 40 to 25 years) was 25 years or below. Clearly there are some exceptions to this pattern, yet one could argue that these are exceptions which emphasize a striking pattern, one which is of great potential utility for early intervention. A key element of this pattern is the extent of *discontinuity* between childhood and adult psychiatric disorder, which is substantial, and the consequent clustering of onsets in the adolescent–young adult period. This is not to say that many key risk factors for adult onset disorders do not operate during the pre-pubertal period, but their effects are delayed and may require other risk factors in order to come into play. The complementary perspectives of epidemiology and developmental psychopathology, a set of research approaches that capitalize on developmental variations and psychopathological variations to ask questions about mechanisms and processes (Rutter, 1988; Lechman, 1999), can be harnessed to guide early intervention efforts for adult-type disorders.

Rutter and colleagues (Rutter and Smith, 1995) have concluded that there has been a substantial rise in the incidence of psychosocial disorders in adolescents and young adults aged between 12 and 26 years in recent decades. This rise is paradoxical in view of the improvements in physical health during this period and, despite much indirect evidence and much theorizing, it remains an obscure phenomenon. The recent Australian National Survey of Mental Health and Well-being (1998) provides further evidence of this phenomenon, demonstrating that the 18–24 age group manifests the highest rate of psychiatric 'caseness' (27%) of any age group. Indeed, the level of morbidity and mortality may still be rising in this age group, given the continuing rapid increase in substance abuse and a range of profound socioeconomic changes (Rutter and Smith, 1995; Booth *et al.*, 1999; Davis, 1999). The deterioration in the mental health of young people, which pertains particularly to high incidence disorders and co-morbid mixtures of these, is especially concerning because we know that people at this phase of life are especially sensitive to the damaging psychosocial consequences of developing a psychiatric or psychosocial disorder. Kessler *et al.* (1995) showed that the vocational trajectory of adolescents is seriously affected, and a whole range of other adverse consequences, including increased risk of other psychiatric syndromes or substance abuse, suicide, unemployment, trauma, physical ill-health and homelessness, have been described (McGorry, 1992, 1996; Herman *et al.*, 1998).

Thus if the onset of psychiatric disorder could be delayed and its initial effects cushioned, this might result in significant reductions in morbidity and a consequent fall in both the human and economic costs of the disorder. Similarly, Lee Robins (in Rutter and Smith, 1995) has suggested that for other potentially self-limited disorders such as substance abuse and crime, a 'damage control' strategy might be effective. Creating a 'holding pattern' and minimizing secondary damage, such as reducing the risks of secondary forms of morbidity, e.g. substance abuse or post-psychotic depression, is a related idea (McGorry, 1992). There are powerful social and economic arguments to support preventive efforts focused on this age group. *The Global Burden of Disease* report (Murray and Lopez, 1996) asks the question "are years of healthy life worth more in young adulthood than in early or late life?" If people are forced to choose between saving a year of life for a 2-year-old and saving it for a 22-year-old, most choose to save the 22-year-old. Many studies confirm this social preference to 'weight' the value of a year lived by a young adult more heavily in contrast to that of a very young child and of an older adult.

There is strong nexus therefore between the premium placed on this phase of life and the fact that it is the peak age of onset for most adult forms of psychiatric morbidity, that such morbidity may be uniquely damaging during this developmental period. The evidence that the level of this morbidity appears to be increasing enhances the salience of this nexus. This alarming scenario presents a major challenge to current service systems that typically have been seriously inaccessible and unresponsive to this age group. The fact that the 12–26 age range has evolved an increasingly well defined cultural identity for itself has led the commercial world as well as a number of more responsive government agencies, e.g. employment services, to focus on them as a specific subculture. Health services and psychiatry in particular have lagged behind. Psychiatry is particularly important here because most health problems in this physically healthy period of life, as Rutter has emphasized, tend to be predominantly psychosocial or psychiatric in nature. There is an urgent imperative rapidly to develop and disseminate effective mental health care models for this subcultural group, a process which would automatically create an opportunity to deliver effective secondary prevention under an early intervention banner.

Real world models for early intervention in community psychiatry

In discussing an approach to secondary prevention and early intervention in psychiatric disorder, I will make a somewhat artificial distinction between *high incidence disorders* (HIDs) and *low incidence disorders* (LIDs). I have used the term *incidence* (even though we are considering secondary prevention here, which is concerned with *prevalence*) because it makes the distinction between these types of disorder more clear cut, and also because we are focusing upon onset and detection issues. Some of the LIDs are quite prevalent because they have a long duration, and some of the HIDs tend to be of brief duration, so if we used the terms low and high *prevalence* disorders there would be less diagnostic separation and consequently less clarity.

The term 'serious mental illness' warrants discussion here. This term is based around a core of chronic schizophrenia with associated co-morbidities, and neuropsychiatric diagnoses with similar or more severe levels of disability. It is a disability-based concept and emphasizes care over treatment. The disorders involved are low in incidence but proportionately much higher in prevalence because of their persistence and tendency to recurrence; hence people with these conditions accumulate in service systems and dominate in every respect. Onset cases with ambiguous features, less disability and a different range of needs will appear atypical, and perhaps 'not appropriate' for or deserving of access to specialist mental health services. Despite deinstitutionalization, many traditional services have merely evolved into a restructured ('mainstreamed') community-based asylum and have continued to focus on the same subset of patients and the same phases of illness, specifically 'chronic schizophrenia'. 'Serious mental illness' has been important as a strategic way of focusing the work of specialist mental health services in a resource-poor environment, but in its concrete and inflexible form it can be inhibitory to efforts to prevent or reduce the prevalence of even 'serious mental illness' itself. The evidence for this is the degree of difficulty experienced by patients and relatives in gaining access to mental health services for the first time (Lincoln *et al.*, 1998).

For both the LIDs and the HIDs, since effective treatment is available, the twin goals of increasing the treated incidence and reducing delays in accessing treatment, if achieved, should result in a reduction in prevalence. Early intervention strategies, logically targeted preferentially at young people, the age group with peak rates of onset, who currently have the poorest access to mental health services, should increase treated incidence and reduce delays. In practice, there will be much overlap in the preventive strategies required for the LID and HID groups and the distinction is merely intended to highlight the different emphasis required for the two categories. For the HIDs, the emphasis will be on the treated incidence, for the LIDs, this is assumed, perhaps incorrectly (van Os *et al.*, 2000), to be high as a proportion of the total incidence, and hence greater emphasis may need to be placed on the reduction of delays.

Finally, there is an important distinction between the epidemiological and developmental psychopathology perspectives. The former is categorical and seeks to define exactly what constitutes a *case*, a task which is supported by the operationalized systems of psychiatric diagnosis. This is notoriously difficult and arbitrary in the real world, especially in relation to the preventive psychiatry of onset. Most disorders, especially the HIDs such as anxiety and depression, but also many LIDs such as psychosis and obsessive–compulsive disorder, are diagnosed on the basis of the dimensional severity of the experiences plus their social impact, rather than the *form* of the disorder. Even to diagnose accurately may be insufficient: "to confuse making a mental disorder diagnosis with demonstrating treatment need, however, would be a serious mistake" (Spitzer, 1998, p. 120). Developmental psychopathology takes the opposite stance and treats the arbitrariness of the threshold for case definition and the consequent grey areas as a matter of interest, rather than as a problem to be overcome (Rutter, 1988). This makes sense from an aetiological perspective; however, from an intervention point of view, we seem to have little choice other than to adopt definitions of caseness, though this is still a complex and contentious endeavour (Regier *et al.*, 1998, Spitzer, 1998). If a more complete and seamless community–primary care–specialist care matrix could be established, this problem might become less salient in a practical sense.

Low incidence disorders

Psychosis, including, but not solely, schizophrenia, which covers the key group of conditions managed in most integrated systems of commu-nity-based care will be used as the paradigmatic disorder group for the purposes of this discussion. The three phases of early intervention will be considered briefly in turn.

Indicated prevention

The notion of pre-psychotic or prodromal intervention in schizophrenia and related psychoses has a long pedigree (Sullivan, 1927; Meares, 1959), and finally research is providing increasing support for the logic of subthreshold intervention (McGorry *et al.*, 2000b,c). The careful work of Häfner and colleagues (Häfner *et al.*, 1995, 1999) has shown that deficits in social functioning are established primarily during the pre-psychotic or prodromal phase. The level of social development achieved by the end of the prodromal phase, when the first psychotic symptom appears, determines the further social course of the disorder by setting a 'ceiling' for recovery (Häfner *et al.*, 1995). This is congruent with earlier work which showed that, during childhood, most people with subsequent schizophrenia are only very subtly, if at all, different from their peers, and even less so from those who later develop an affective illness (Jones *et al.*, 1994; van Os *et al.*, 1997). This means that in children it is far too early to make any accurate predictions regarding subsequent psychosis in adolescence or adulthood. While an early vulnerability may exist in a proportion of cases, other environmental risk factors (Mahy *et al.*, 1999) and putative problems with adolescent brain development processes (a second stage process, termed neurodegenerative or neurotoxic by some) (Rapoport *et al.*, 1999) clearly come into play during adolescence or later, though months or years prior to the emergence of the diagnostically defining features of psychotic disorder (Häfner *et al.*, 1995).

Until recently, it has not been possible systematically to identify those at incipient risk of transition to psychosis, that is people in the late prodromal phase of illness. However, within the rubric of indicated prevention, a new research model, the 'close-in' strategy (Bell, 1992), has shown that it is possible to provide clinical access to the subgroup of young people who are at ultra

Table 42.2 *Intake criteria for the PACE clinic*

Group 1 Attenuated/low grade psychotic symptoms	Group 2 Transient psychotic symptoms	Group 3 Trait and state risk factors
Ideas of reference, magical thinking, perceptual disturbance, paranoid ideation, odd thinking and speech, not at intensity or duration of acute psychosis	Ideas of reference, magical thinking, perceptual disturbance, paranoid ideation, odd thinking and speech, above an operationally defined threshold	First-degree relative with a psychotic disorder or client has schizotypal personality disorder
Symptoms deviate significantly from normal	Duration of episode of <1 week	Significant decrease in mental state or functioning, maintained for at least 1 month
Symptoms occur several times per week	Symptoms resolve spontaneously	
Change in mental state has been present for at least 1 week in the past year and for not more than 5 years	The change in mental state occurred in the past year	The decrease in functioning occurred within the past year

high risk (UHR) of a first episode of psychosis, are already distressed and functioning poorly and who are willing to accept professional help (Yung *et al.*, 1996, 1998; McGorry *et al.*, 1999a, 2000b,c). These studies have shown that even with excellent psychosocial care, 41% of operationally defined UHR patients make the transition to first-episode psychosis within a 12-month follow-up period (Table 42.2). Several clinical features, such as depression and various negative and positive symptoms, enhance the capacity to predict transition to psychosis even though a very diverse range of clinical features are present (Yung *et al.*, 1998; McGorry *et al.*, 1999b; Schultze-Lütter and Klosterkötter, 1999). Prediction is better for those in the late prodromal phase, but there is clearly a less specific early prodromal phase where prediction will be much less feasible. Non-specific interventions helpful in the reduction of risk from a range of disorders may find a place during this less differentiated phase.

A recent randomized controlled trial in this clinical population has shown a significant reduction in transition rate to psychosis for patients receiving specific treatment—very low dose risperidone (1–2 mg/day) and cognitive therapy—in comparison with non-specific treatment—supportive psychotherapy and symptomatic treatment (Phillips *et al.*, 1999a; McGorry *et al.*, 2000a). A range of ethical and conceptual issues need to be considered in relation to this emerging field; however, it is clear that these young people are a help-seeking clinical population and are both distressed and disabled by their symptoms, whatever their ultimate diagnosis. As defined in Table 42.2, they also have a very substantial risk of developing a frank psychotic illness, usually schizophrenia. While research is urgently required to clarify the range of treatments which will alleviate their distress and disability and reduce their risk of subsequent psychosis, in the interim there is a need for a clinical response from community mental health services and primary care. The offer, at least, of initial psychosocial treatment, including the emerging range of cognitive therapies, with or without syndrome-based drug treatments, aimed at the relief of such distress and disability in young people seems eminently justifiable as a component of youth-oriented mental health care (Häfner *et al.*, 1999; McGorry *et al.*, 2000b). If this offer is refused initially, as it may well be in this age group, this decision can be accepted, although some kind of assertive follow-up is also justifiable, combined with family contact because, in addition to the risk of psychosis, there is also a higher than expected rate of substance abuse, deliberate self-harm and suicide in this subset of the pre-psychotic population (Phillips *et al.*, 1999b).

Enhanced early case detection

The currently accepted threshold for treatment with antipsychotic medication is at the first clear and sustained emergence of psychotic features. Despite this, for a substantial proportion of people, such treatment is delayed, often for very prolonged periods (Padmavathi *et al.*, 1998; Carbone *et al.*, 1999). For others, especially in the developing world (Padmavathi *et al.*, 1998), treatment is never accessed. The duration of untreated psychosis (DUP), as a marker of delay in delivering effective specific treatment, is a potentially important variable in improving outcome in first-episode schizophrenia, and more widely in first-episode psychosis (Harrigan *et al.*, 2000). Indeed, psychosis may be an easier and less conflicted target to detect than schizophrenia (McGorry, 1995; Driessen *et al.*, 1998). DUP is important because, unlike other prognostic variables such as genetic vulnerability, gender and age of onset, it is a potentially malleable variable which can become the focus of intervention strategies.

There is a strong literature supporting a correlational link between DUP and both short- and long-term outcome (McGlashan, 1999). This raises one obvious and central question. Is the association causal, i.e. is delay (prolonged DUP) in treatment a risk factor for worse outcome? Or is the link due to a common underlying factor, namely a more severe form of illness which has a more insidious onset with more negative symptoms, more paranoid ideation, less salience and awareness of change and less willingness to seek and accept treatment? Even if so, DUP may still be a key intervening variable through which these clinical features influence outcome.

The classic study of May *et al.* (1976) reanalysed by Wyatt (1991) is the most compelling evidence in favour of a causal link. Essentially, DUP, or, more accurately, time to commencement of antipsychotic medication, was varied randomly in this comparison of psychological versus biological therapies. Delay in receiving antipsychotics led to significantly poorer short- and medium-term outcomes. More recently, an alternative, quasi-experimental design has been proposed and implemented by McGlashan and colleagues (McGlashan, 1996, 1998). This involves a two-step process, first aiming to reduce the duration of DUP, and secondly estimating whether the outcome is correspondingly improved. The early results appear promising in having substantially reduced DUP in the experimental sector (Johannessen *et al.*, 1999). However, a number of unforeseen methodological problems have surfaced which make interpretation complex.

In summary, even though it is not yet clearly proven that reducing DUP improves outcome, as clinicians we might agree with McGlashan (1999) that delayed treatment is already a major public health problem and that: "DUP, by itself, is reason enough for early intervention on a large and intensive scale" (p. 901).

What justifies such a statement is an appreciation of the destructive effects of delay and the range of negative psychosocial outcomes which accumulate during the period of untreated psychosis (McGorry *et al.*, 1996; Lincoln *et al.*, 1998). These include vocational failure, self-harm, offending behaviour, family distress and dysfunction, aggression, substance abuse and victimization by others. The effect of early intervention strategies in community psychiatry settings will probably be twofold. First, if intensive efforts are made to improve mental health literacy, and access to and engagement with services, then the duration of untreated psychosis for the average case should be substantially reduced. Secondly, there will be an increase in treated incidence, which should reduce the prevalence of hidden psychiatric morbidity in the community. These effects will be complex to measure and monitor.

To achieve them, an initial change in the culture of clinical practice will be required with reciprocal effects upon the complexion of the service.

Intensive phase-specific intervention in first-episode psychosis and the 'critical period'

Although it may not be as challenging as the previous two preventive foci, more intensive phase-specific treatment in first-episode psychosis and beyond into the critical period may be even more potent, and is still the most feasible proposition for most clinicians and researchers interested in secondary prevention, since access to patients during this period is at least assured. Several monographs have appeared on this subject recently (McGorry and Edwards, 1997; McGorry, 1998; Aitchinson *et al.*, 1999; McGorry and Jackson, 1999). In addition, a number of recent research studies have focused on the treated course of early psychosis. These have shown that the early course of illness for both schizophrenia and affective psychosis is turbulent and relapse prone, with up to 80% of patients relapsing within a 5-year period (Strakowski *et al.*, 1998; Wiersma *et al.*, 1998; Robinson *et al.*, 1999a,b; Vazquez-Barquero *et al.*, 1999). These findings suggest that drug therapy should be continued for most if not all patients for longer than 12 months after recovery from a first psychotic episode. However, it should be remembered that a subsample, at least 20%, never relapse, that some will not relapse for a prolonged period, and that relapse prevention is not the sole consideration in treatment but rather a means to an end. Adaptation to illness is a challenging, often overwhelming task for these young people and they usually need to be given time and special help to come to an acceptance of the need for maintenance treatment (McGorry, 1995). An important earlier study (Mason *et al.*, 1995) has also shown that outcome at 13 years was much more positive than expected, supporting the notion of an early critical period, which may be turbulent but seems to abate after 2–5 years.

In general, the intensive treatment of young people at this phase of illness appears effective (McGorry *et al.*, 1996; McGorry and Edwards,

1998; Power *et al.*, 1998; McGorry and Jackson, 1999) and cost-effective (Mihalopoulos *et al.*, 1999) in real-world settings, at least in the short term, though more research is certainly required to examine the longer term impact and to determine the most appropriate service models. Whether it is possible to reduce the intensity of treatment over a longer time frame or not (Birchwood *et al.*, 1998) is an important secondary research question.

High incidence disorders

HIDs, such as depression, manifest in the community as co-morbid admixtures of syndromes. From the categorical perspective of clinical epidemiology, a particular individual may be above threshold for caseness for one syndrome and subthreshold for one or more other syndromes. The fact that these clinical pictures are generally not different in form from normal subjective emotional experiences, except in terms of their severity, persistence and disabling effects, has to be taken into account in the design of early intervention models.

First, in the context of HIDs, given the sheer volume of morbidity, the prospect of primary prevention becomes more attractive. The spontaneous remission and placebo response rates may be relatively high, yet the problem of untreated incidence and prevalence is serious and more salient than the secondary issue of treatment delay. Currently, only a minority of cases receive treatment and the majority of these receive it in primary care or non-psychiatric settings. Yet while epidemiological surveys consistently demonstrate high levels of point and period prevalence for a range of non-psychotic disorders, it remains unclear how to determine which people among this multitude genuinely need treatment (Ferdinand *et al.*, 1995; Regier *et al.*, 1998; Spitzer, 1998). Criteria could be developed which might include severity, distress, co-morbidity, persistence and disability. If this issue were to be clarified, then it would make sense to blend the primary goal of increasing the treated incidence with the secondary goal of shortening delay in

identifying and treating the first episode of disorder, under the banner of early intervention. Given the epidemiology of onset, this would lead to a predominant (but not exclusive) focus on young people, as discussed earlier.

In summary, a 'high incidence' strategy for secondary prevention would be to increase the treated incidence of first episodes of HIDs, because of their disproportionate impact on the life trajectory of the person and a still hypothetical enhanced responsivity to treatment in a biopsychosocial sense. On the other hand, increasing treated incidence of relapsing cases and of first episodes in older people would still fall within the scope of secondary prevention.

Early intervention for disorders of high incidence could be considered, as with the LIDs, under the three headings of indicated prevention; reduction of delays in case detection; and intensive phase-specific treatment of the initial episode and a critical period beyond. Unfortunately, there is little evidence to date to review in relation to these three strategies. We do know (Eaton *et al.*, 1995) that subthreshold depressive symptoms are a potent risk factor for subsequent major depression and that many people presenting to GPs have subthreshold symptoms which confer significant levels of disability (Olfson *et al.*, 1996). Family history of depression confers an increased risk (Weissman *et al.*, 1987), and this could be integrated into an indicated prevention model. Indicated prevention would certainly be worth considering, though the intervention itself would probably have to be inexpensive and highly effective in order to be cost-effective.

Early detection and increased treated incidence of first episodes of depression to my knowledge has never been attempted, but it would be most appropriate and might prove to be a key weapon in the reduction of rates of suicide, since many cases are in retrospect a consequence of unrecognized clinical depression. The same case as developed for phase-specific intensive treatment of first episodes of psychosis could be made for disorders such as depression. Like psychosis, depression can be conceptualized as a complex biopsychosocial vulnerability that fluctuates. Its propensity to recur can be influenced by a range of factors:

medication, psychological interventions and social influences. If these are addressed more fundamentally in the initial onset phase and a more secure form of *remission*, which could be termed *recovery*, achieved, then future relapses might be less likely and the prevalence of the disorder thereby reduced. This might be less likely with brief, symptomatic and more superficial forms of therapy, which is generally all that is available. This issue could be examined using research methodology and, ultimately, cost-effectiveness criteria as well as consumer input should help to determine what model is implemented.

The elements involved in early intervention models for HIDs inevitably depend even more heavily on partnerships between community, primary care and specialist care. We know that the mental health literacy of the general community is not conducive to early treatment by mental health professionals (Jorm *et al.*, 1997). Primary care professionals have a major role in recognition and treatment of the HIDs, a role for which they currently are poorly equipped. Resources need to be found so that they can be supported in this role by mental health specialists linked to, or part of, mental health services.

Conclusion

This chapter has sought to present progress in thinking about secondary prevention, a way of working which is highly compatible with the core objectives and activities of integrated community mental health services. The synergy between the perspectives of developmental psychopathology and clinical epidemiology have been utilized to highlight the potential for enhanced secondary prevention in targeting young people in the early phases of a range of psychiatric and psychosocial disorders. In this way, early intervention may be used as a proxy for secondary prevention since it captures most of its key elements as defined in this chapter. Progress in implementing some of these ideas in real-world settings is beginning to occur, particularly, and somewhat surprisingly so, in schizophrenia and psychotic disorders. The distinction is made between high and low inci-dence disorders in order to highlight the different emphasis and approach that is required in implementing early intervention strategies. In an ideal world of skilled, well-resourced and well-integrated systems of primary and specialist care, such a distinction might be of lesser importance.

References

Aitchinson, K., Meehan, K. and Murrary, R. (1999) *First Episode Psychosis*. London: Martin Dunitz Ltd.

Australian Bureau of Statistics (1998) *Mental Health and Wellbeing: Profile of Adults, Australia*. Canberra: Commonwealth of Australia.

Bell, R.Q. (1992) Multiple-risk cohorts and segmenting risk as solutions to the problem of false positives in risk for the major psychoses. *Psychiatry*, 55, 370–381.

Birchwood, M. and MacMillian, F. (1993) Early intervention in schizophrenia. *Australian and New Zealand Journal of Psychiatry*, 27, 374–378.

Birchwood, M., Todd, P. and Jackson, C. (1998) Early intervention in psychosis: the critical period hypothesis. *British Journal of Psychiatry*, 172 (Suppl. 33), 53–59.

Booth, A., Crouter, A.C. and Shanahan, M.J. (1999) *Transitions to Adulthood in a Changing Economy. No Work, No Family, No Future?* Westport, CT: Praeger.

Caplan, G. (1964) *Principles of Preventive Psychiatry*. New York: Basic Books.

Carbone, S., Harrigan, S., McGorry, P., Curry, C. and Elkins, K. (1999) Duration of untreated psychosis and 12-month outcome in first-episode psychosis: the impact of treatment approach. *Acta Psychiatrica Scandinavica*, 100, 96–104.

Commission on Chronic Illness (1957) *Chronic Illness in the United States*, Vol. 1. Cambridge, MA: Harvard University Press.

Davis, N.J. (1999) *Youth Crisis. Growing Up in the High-risk Society*. Westport, CT: Praeger.

Driessen, G., Gunther, N., Bak, M., van Sambeek, M. and van Os, J. (1998) Characteristics of early- and late-diagnosed schizophrenia: implications for first-episode studies. *Schizophrenia Research*, 33, 27–34.

Eaton, W.W. and Harrison, G. (1996) Prevention priorities. *Current Opinion in Psychiatry*, 9, 141–143.

Eaton, W.W., Badawi, M. and Melton, B. (1995) Prodromes and precursors: epidemiologic data for primary prevention of disorders with slow onset. *American Journal of Psychiatry*, 152, 967–972.

Falloon, I.R.H. (1992) Early intervention for first episode of schizophrenia: a preliminary exploration. *Psychiatry*, 55, 4–15.

Ferdinand, R.F., van der Reijden, M., Verhulst, F.C., Nienhuis, F.J. and Giel, R. (1995) Assessment of the prevalence of psychiatric disorder in young adults. *British Journal of Psychiatry*, 166, 480–488.

Frances, A. (1998) Problems in defining clinical significance in epidemiological studies. *Archives of General Psychiatry*, 55, 119.

Gordon, R. (1983) An operational classification of disease prevention. *Public Health Reports*, 98, 107–109.

Häfner, H., Nowotny, B., Löffler, W., an der Heiden, W. and Maurer, K. (1995) When and how does schizophrenia produce social deficits? *European Archives of Psychiatry Clinical Neurosciences*, 246, 17–28.

Häfner, H., Löffler, W., Maurer, K., Hambrecht, M. and an der Heiden, W. (1999) Depression, negative symptoms, social stagnation and social decline in the early course of schizophrenia. *Acta Psychiatrica Scandinavica*, 100, 105–118.

Harrigan, S.M., McGorry, P.D. and Krstev, H. (2000) Does treatment delay in first-episode psychosis really mater? *Schizophrenia Research*, 41, 177.

Herman, D., Susser, E., Jandorf, L., Lavelle, J. and Bromet, E. (1998) Homelessness among individuals with psychotic disorders hospitalized for the first time: findings from the Suffolk County Mental Health Project. *American Journal of Psychiatry*, 155, 109–113.

Jenkins, R. (1994) Principles of prevention. In: Paykel, E.S. and Jenkins, R. (eds), *Prevention in Psychiatry*. Dorchester: Gaskell, pp. 11–24.

Johannessen, J., Larsen, T., Horneland, M., Mardal, S., Bloch Thorsen, G., Vaglum, P. and McGlashan, T. (1999) Strategies for reducing duration of untreated psychosis. *Schizophrenia Research*, 36, 342–343.

Jones, P., Rodgers, B., Murray, R. and Marmot, M. (1994) Child developmental risk factors for adult schizophrenia in the British 1946 birth cohort. *Lancet*, 344, 1398–1402.

Jorm, A., Korten, A., Rodgers, B., Pollitt, P., Jacomb, P., Christensen, H. and Jiao, Z. (1997) Belief systems of the general public concerning the appropriate treatments for mental disorders. *Social Psychiatry and Psychiatric Epidemiology*, 23, 1988–1998.

Kessler, R.C., Foster, C.L., Saunders, W.B. and Stang, P.E. (1995) Social consequences of psychiatric disorders: I. Educational attainment. *American Journal of Psychiatry*, 152, 1026–1031.

Lechman, J.F. (1999) Incremental progress in developmental psychopathology simply complex. *American Journal of Psychiatry*, 156, 1495–1498.

Lincoln, C., Harrigan, S. and McGorry, P. (1998) Understanding the topography of the early psychosis pathways. *British Journal of Psychiatry*, 172 (Suppl. 33), 21–25.

Loebel, A., Lieberman, J.A., Alvir, J.M., Mayerhoff, D.I., Geisler, S.H. and Szymanski, S.R. (1992) Duration of psychosis and outcome in first-episode schizophrenia. *American Journal of Psychiatry*, 149, 1183–1188.

Mahy, G., Mallett, R., Leff, J. and Bhugra, D. (1999) First-contact incidence rate of schizophrenia on Barbados. *British Journal of Psychiatry*, 175, 28–33.

Mason, P., Harrison, G., Glazebrook, C., Medley, I., Dalkin, T. and Croudace, T. (1995) Characteristics of outcome in schizophrenia at 13 years. *British Journal of Psychiatry*, 167, 596–603.

May, P., Tuma, A., Yale, C., Potepan, P. and Dixon, W. (1976) Schizophrenia—a follow-up study of results of treatment, II: hospital stay over two to five years. *Archives of General Psychiatry*, 33, 481–486.

McGlashan, T. (1996) Early detection and intervention with schizophrenia: research. *Schizophrenia Bulletin*, 22, 327–345.

McGlashan, T. (1998) Early detection and intervention of schizophrenia: rationale and research. *British Journal of Psychiatry*, 172 (Suppl. 33), 3–6.

McGlashan, T. (1999) Duration of untreated psychosis in first-episode schizophrenia: marker or determinant of course? *Biological Psychiatry*, 46, 899–907.

McGorry, P.D. (1992) The concept of recovery and secondary prevention in psychotic disorder. *Australian and New Zealand Journal of Psychiatry*, 26, 3–17.

McGorry, P. (1995) A treatment-relevant classification of psychotic disorders. *Australian and New Zealand Journal of Psychiatry*, 29, 555–558.

McGorry, P.D. (ed.) (1998) Preventive strategies in early psychosis: verging on reality. *British Journal of Psychiatry*, 172 (Suppl. 33), 1–136.

McGorry, P. and Edwards, J. (eds) (1997) *Early Psychosis Training Pack*. Cheshire, UK: Gardiner-Caldwell Communications Ltd.

McGorry, P. and Edwards, J. (1998) The feasibility and effectiveness of early intervention in psychotic disorders: the Australian experience. *International Journal of Clinical Psychopharmacology*, 13 (Suppl. 1), 47–52.

McGorry, P.D. and Jackson, H.J. (eds) (1999) *The Recognition and Management of Early Psychosis: A Preventive Approach*. Cambridge: Cambridge University Press.

McGorry, P.D. and Singh, B.S. (1995) Schizophrenia: risk and possibility. In: Raphael, B. and Burrows, G.D. (eds), *Handbook of Studies on Preventive Psychiatry*. Amsterdam: Elsevier.

McGorry, P., Edwards, J., Mihalopoulos, C., Harrigan, S. and Jackson, H. (1996) EPPIC: an evolving system of early detection and optimal management. *Schizophrenia Bulletin*, 22, 305–326.

McGorry, P., Jackson, H., Edwards, J., Hulbert, C., Phillips, L., Henry, L., Power, P., Francey, S. and Cocks, J. (1999a) Preventively-oriented psychological interventions in early psychosis, in *Psychological Treatments for Schizophrenia*. Manchester: Institute of Psychiatry, The University of Manchester.

McGorry, P.D., Phillip,s L.J., Yung, A.R., Francey, S., Velakoulis, D., Brewer, W., Yuen, H.P., Hallgren, M., Patton, G., Adlard, S., Hearn, N., Crump, N. and Pantelis, C. (1999b) The identification of predictors of psychosis in a high risk group. *Schizophrenia Research*, 36, 49–50.

McGorry, P.D., Phillip, L.J., Yung, A.R., Francey, S., Germano, D., Bravin, J., MacDonald, N., Hearn, N., Amminger, P. and O'Dwyer, L. (2000a) A randomised controlled trial of interventions in the pre-psychotic phase of psychotic disorders. *Schizophrenia Research*, 41, 9.

McGorry, P., Phillips, L. and Yung, A. (2000b) Recognition and treatment of the pre-psychotic phase of psychotic disorders: frontier or fantasy?. In: Mednick, S., McGlashan, T. Libiger, J. and Johannessen, J. (eds), *Early Intervention in Psychiatric Disorders*. Dordrecht, The Netherlands: Kluwer, in press.

McGorry, P.D., Yung, A.R. and Phillips, L.J. (2000c) 'Closing in': what features predict the onset of first episode psychosis within a high risk group? In: Zipursky, R.B. (ed.), *The Early Stages of Schizophrenia*. Washington, DC: American Psychiatric Press, in press.

Meares, A. (1959) The diagnosis of prepsychotic schizophrenia. *Lancet*, i, 55–59.

Mihalopoulos, C., McGorry, P. and Carter, R. (1999) Is phase-specific, community-oriented treatment of early psychosis an economically viable method of improving outcome. *Acta Psychiatrica Scandinavica*, 100, 47–55.

Mrazek, P.J. and Haggerty, R.J. (eds) (1994) *Reducing Risks for Mental Disorders: Frontiers for Preventive Intervention Research*. Washington, DC: National Academy Press.

Murray, C.J.L. and Lopez, A.D. (eds) (1996) *The Global Burden of Disease*. Geneva: WHO.

Olfson, M., Broadhead, W.E., Weissman, M.M., Leon, A.C., Farber, L., Hoven, C. and Kathol, R. (1996) Subthreshold psychiatric symptoms in a primary care group practice. *Archives of General Psychiatry*, 53, 880–886.

Padmavathi, R., Rajkumar, S. and Srinivasan, T. (1998) Schizophrenic patients who were never treated—a study in an Indian urban community. *Psychological Medicine*, 28, 1113–1117.

Phillips, L., Yung, A., Hearn, N., McFarlane, C., Hallgren, M. and McGorry, P. (1999a) Preventive mental health care: accessing the target population. *Australian and New Zealand Journal of Psychiatry*, 33, 912–917.

Phillips, L., McGorry, P., Yung, A., Francey, S., Cosgrave, L., Germano, D., Bravin, J., MacDonald, A., Hallgren, M., Hearn, N., Adlards, S. and Patton, G. (1999b) The development of preventive interventions for early psychosis: early findings and directions for the future. *Schizophrenia Research*, 36, 331–332

Power, P., Elkins, K., Adlard, S., Curry, C., McGorry, P. and Harrigan, S. (1998) Analysis of the initial treatment phase in first-episode psychosis. *British Journal of Psychiatry*, 172 (Suppl. 33), 71–76.

Rapoport, J., Giedd, J., Blumenthal, J., Hamburger, S., Jeffires, N., Fernandez, T., Nicolson, R., Bedwell, J., Lenane, M., Zijdenbos, A., Paus, T. and Evans, A. (1999) Progressive cortical change during adolescence in childhood-onset schizophrenia. *Archives of General Psychiatry*, 56, 649–654.

Regier D.A., Myers J.K., Kramer M., Robins L.N., Blazer D.G., Hough R.L., Eaton W.W. and Locke B.Z. (1984) The NIMH epidemiologic catchment area program. Historical context, major objectives, and study population characteristics. *Archives of General Psychiatry*, 41, 934–941.

Regier, D.A., Kaelber C.T., Rae, D.S., Farmer, M.E., Knauper, B., Kessler, R.C. and Norquist, G.S. (1998) Limitations of diagnostic criteria and assessment instruments for mental disorders. *Archives of General Psychiatry*, 55, 109–115.

Robinson, D., Woerner, M., Alvir, J., Bilder, R., Goldman, R., Geisler, S., Koreen, A., Sheitman, B., Chakos, M., Mayerhoff, D. and Lieberman, J. (1999a) Predictors of relapse following response from a first-episode of schizophrenia or schizoaffective disorder. *Archives of General Psychiatry*, 56, 241–247.

Robinson, D., Woerner, M., Alvir, J., Geisler, S., Koreen, A., Sheitman, B., Chakos, M., Mayerhoff, D., Bilder, R., Goldman. R. and Lieberman, J. (1999b) Predictors of treatment response from a first-episode of schizophrenia or schizoaffective disorder. *American Journal of Psychiatry*, 156, 544–549.

Rutter, M. (1988) Epidemiological approaches to developmental psychopathology. *Archives of General Psychiatry*, 45, 486–495.

Rutter, M. and Smith, D.J. (eds) (1995) *Psychosocial Disorders in Young People: Time Trends and Their Causes*. Chichester: John Wiley and Sons.

Schultze-Lütter, F. and Klosterkötter, J. (1999) What tool should be used for generating predictive models? *Schizophrenia Research*, 36, 10.

Spitzer, R.L. (1998) Diagnosis and need for treatment are not the same. *Archives of General Psychiatry*, 55, 120.

Strakowski, S., Keck, P., McElroy, S., West, S., Sax, K., Hawkins, J., Kmetz, G., Upadhyaya, V., Tugrul, K. and Bourne, M. (1998) Twelve-month outcome after a first hospitalization for affective psychosis. *Archives of General Psychiatry*, 55, 49–55.

Sullivan, H.S. (1927) (1994: reprinted) The onset of schizophrenia. *American Journal of Psychiatry*, 151, 135–139.

Van Os, J., Jones, P., Lewis, G., Wadsworth, M. and Murray, R. (1997) Developmental precursors of affective illness in a general population birth cohort. *Archives of General Psychiatry*, 54, 625–631.

Van Os, J., Bill, R. and Ravelli, A. (2000). Strauss (1969) revisited: A psychosis continuum in the general population? *Schizophrenia Research*, 41(1), 8.

Vazquez-Barquero, J., Cuest, M., Castanedo, S., Lastra, I., Herran, A. and Dunn, G. (1999) Cantabria first-episode schizophrenia study: three year follow-up. *British Journal of Psychiatry*, 174, 141–149.

Weissman, M.M., Gammon, G.D., John, K., Merikangas, K.R., Warner, V., Prusoff, B.A. and Sholomskas, D. (1987) Child of depressed parents. Increased psychopathology and early onset of major depression. *Archives of General Psychiatry*, 44, 847–853.

Wiersma, D., Nienhuis, F., Slooff, C. and Giel, R. (1998) Natural course of schizophrenic disorders: a 15-year followup of a Dutch incidence cohort. *Schizophrenia Bulletin*, 24, 75–85.

Wyatt, R. (1991) Neuroleptics and the natural course of schizophrenia. *Schizophrenia Bulletin*, 17, 325–351.

Yung, A., McGorry, P., McFarlane, C., Jackson, H., Patton, G. and Rakkar, A. (1996) Monitoring and care of young people at incipient risk of psychosis. *Schizophrenia Bulletin*, 22, 283–303.

Yung, A., Phillips, L., McGorry, P., McFarlane, C., Francey, S., Harrigan, S., Patton, G. and Jackson, H. (1998) Prediction of psychosis. *British Journal of Psychiatry*, 172 (Suppl. 33), 14–20.

43 | *Tertiary prevention of mental disorders*

Martin Gittelman

Introduction

Tertiary prevention can be defined as the minimization of the disabilities and impairments which are consequent upon illnesses or disorders. In this chapter, I will discuss tertiary prevention largely using illustrations in relation to schizophrenia. In this context, tertiary prevention is largely synonymous with psychosocial rehabilitation. Historically, following the introduction of neuroleptic medicine and the associated deinstitutionalization, the need and intent were to establish in the community most of the services previously provided by the mental hospital. Early in the period of transition, there were those (John Wing, Douglas Bennett, Irving Blumberg and Benjamin Pasamanick, among others) who understood that it would be necessary to ensure continuity of care, from acute to tertiary preventive, and make available in the community all of the elements taken for granted in hospital: food, shelter, dental, general health and mental health care, work and recreation. Most importantly, there would have to be a way to monitor patients' adherence to their medication regimen.

Various countries, particularly in the more industrialized world, approached these requirements from different standpoints. For example, the USA instituted the community mental health centre movement, which, unfortunately, was relatively short-lived, largely because of a lack of sustained funding. In the UK, the major problem was seen to be maintenance of contact between the mental hospital staff and the local health authority staff (Goldberg, 1967). In France, continuity between hospital and community care was assured by assigning full responsibility for all treatment, care and rehabilitation to geographically determined sector teams (Gittelman, 1972).

No matter what approach was used, however, it soon became clear that neuroleptic medication and community follow-up were not sufficient in themselves to ensure that the seriously mentally ill could avoid relapses and cope adequately with life in ordinary society. Tertiary prevention, or *psychosocial rehabilitation*, appeared on the scene to help meet these needs. Its *definition and objectives* are to reduce and prevent disability, complications and handicap; to avoid acute relapses; and to enable people with mental illness to live satisfactory lives in the community.

This is accomplished most effectively by a partnership with the prescribing clinician and by:

- monitoring behaviour and medication adjustment;
- assisting the disabled to learn or relearn the skills necessary for their daily living so that they can make the best possible use of their residual capacities in as normalized an environment as possible; and
- teaching people with mental illness and their care-givers (family members or community care staff) to recognize signs of an impending relapse so that medication can be adjusted appropriately and learn health risk reduction measures.

A contingent goal of psychosocial rehabilitation is to improve the quality of life of the mentally disabled and their families and to help reduce both stress and the general stigma associated with mental illness. This involves appropriate education of physicians and other mental health professionals, of the afflicted themselves, and of their families and communities.

Coping with schizophrenia

Though psychosocial rehabilitation can be applied to a broad range of disorders, the relevant research and practice have tended to focus on psychotic conditions, primarily schizophrenia. In fact, psychosocial rehabilitation has become an essential component of the management of serious mental illness (Gittelman and Blumberg, 1975), particularly in public health approaches to such illness.

Schizophrenia is difficult to manage. After the acute episode, which often requires hospitalization, many persons discharged into the community do not follow through with their treatment: they neglect to take their prescribed medication and/or to appear for periodic evaluations. They may not acknowledge the importance of strictly following instructions with regard to medications, or not understand the directions given to them by a busy practitioner; they may cease taking their prescribed medication because of side effects, such as dyskinesia or deficits in attention, memory and cognition (Ayd, 1961); often, they have negative symptoms such as anergia or withdrawal. They may not realize that their illness is likely to take a fluctuating course (Ciompi, 1987) and require changes in medication dosage, hence regular follow-up by a mental health professional.

Whatever its cause, non-compliance with medication is a major problem in dealing with people with schizophrenia. In a meta-analysis of 24 studies, Cramer and Rosenheck (1998) found that compliance in people with mental disorders ranged from 24 to 90%, the combined average being only 54% adherence. Mak (1998) found that over the course of time, non-adherence rates climbed to 74%; and in the absence of adherence, relapse rates have been shown to reach over 70%.

In an effort to cope with this problem, new medications with lesser side effects, especially fewer extrapyramidal effects (at least at lower doses) (Schooler, 1997), have been developed. Despite this possible advantage, they have not yet proved to be more effective in preventing relapses than traditional neuroleptics, except in in-patients who do not respond to the latter (Dixon *et al.*, 1995; Lehman and Steinwachs, 1998; Geddes, 2000).

In any case, there is now substantial research to support the view that for most people with schizophrenia in remission, medication, or secondary prevention, is necessary, but not sufficient alone, to prevent relapses or reduce negative symptoms. It has been shown, however, that tertiary prevention methods, when combined with medication, considerably enhance the effects of medication by 20–40%. Also, in patients who do not respond to the usual medications, the effect of combining psychosocial rehabilitation with newer, atypical drugs is also greater.

If patients take their prescribed medication and are closely monitored (as in clinical drug trials), relapse rates fall to about 20% at 2 years after their initial episode (Davis and Garver, 1978). Also, if their compliance and clinical state are monitored and their medication is effective, it may be possible, eventually, to lower the dose, which means there will be fewer unwanted side effects and better all-round results.

Although low doses enhance compliance, decreases in medication dosage have been found to increase the risk of relapse (Schooler *et al.*, 1997). This risk can be mitigated by ensuring clinical monitoring of the patient by a trained care-giver (Hogarty *et al.*, 1991; Schooler *et al.*, 1997). The system seems to work best when someone, e.g. the trained patient, a family member, a case manager or a rehabilitation worker, really takes responsibility.

In the treatment of mental illness, negative symptoms and handicap (e.g. lowered social functioning) have tended to be neglected—in effect, only half of the illness has been treated (Gittelman and Freedman, 1988). Moreover, serious mental illness, such as schizophrenia, can be associated with increased risk for co-occurring disorders, such as alcohol and/or substance abuse, obesity, diabetes, nicotine addiction, depression and suicide; increased susceptibility to circulatory and respiratory diseases; and a general deterioration in physical health that can lead to a significantly shorter life span than would otherwise be expected. Stroup (2000) has described some of the factors which may cascade and result in 10 years less life expectancy for persons with schizophrenia in developed countries. In fact, even in countries with excellent and abundant health services, suicide rates are 10 times higher among the mentally ill, and overall mortality more than twice as high, than among the general population (Allebeck, 1989). Three or four of every 10 persons with schizophrenia attempt suicide, and completed suicides eventually occur in 10%.

The association between mental illness and other diseases is complex: some may be side effects of medication, e.g. obesity or tardive dyskinesia; some may be associated with diminished awareness of risk, which may be the result of cognitive deficiencies (Andreason *et al.*, 1998) or insufficient access to health risk information, e.g. diseases associated with nicotine addiction; and some are still of unknown aetiology, e.g. depression. The fact remains, however, that mental illness is associated with complications that need to be, and can be, reduced and prevented.

Tertiary prevention techniques

The earliest psychosocial interventions were adapted from physical rehabilitation, including vocational assessment and training. In this context, the plan was to assist in developing a normative milieu for the person in a work context. This model is still being followed in many programmes. In addition, what has been notable has been the gradual acceptance of behavioural and cognitive methods of instruction of the mentally ill and their families or other care-providers.

Among the strategies that psychosocial rehabilitation employs in its efforts to help the mentally ill are health education and promotion, social and occupational skills training, recreation interventions with families, and intensive case management. An appropriate programme should be initiated upon first contact with the patient and his family and continue indefinitely or until such time that it seems not to be needed. Because it is often carried out by ancillary personnel (who have, however, been specially trained in the requisite techniques), tertiary prevention generally is less costly than other types of treatment.

Because tertiarty rehabilitation may be carried out by supervised and trained ancillary personnel it shows promise as an intervention with a large potential impact on mental illness outcome and cost reduction (WHO, 2000). Having shown robust efficacy in enhancing antipsychotic medication compliance and effectiveness in both developed (Hogarty, 1991) and developing countries (Zhang Mingyuan *et al.*, 1993; Chen Yanfang *et al.*, 1996), it mat well prove advantageous in reducing other disease burden measures.

Social skills training

It should be noted that since the early studies of May (1968) and Pasamanick and colleagues (1964, 1967) demonstrated the effectiveness of medication, tertiary prevention has been studied as an add-on to medication; and various psychosocial interventions, such as skills training or family interventions, have been studied in conjunction with the use of psychotropic drugs.

A major influence on increased application of psychosocial rehabilitation was Wolpe's (1958) introduction of learning theory into psychiatry, specifically in the treatment of neuroses. Wolpe's training of clinicians and researchers at the Eastern Pennsylvania Psychiatric Institute emphasized the use of cognitive and behavioural interventions and the combination of medication with behavioural and cognitive therapy for mental disorders (Gittelman, 1965, 1981; Falloon *et al.*, 1982; Tarrier *et al.*, 1988). Nevertheless, before the 1980s, many physicians received little training in the relevant educational methods and depended largely on traditional, authoritative prescribing of drugs in treating their patients. This may have been sufficient for simple, time-limited disorders, but often failed in dealing with complex, chronic disorders with a fluctuating course.

Skills training utilizing a behavioural and cognitive approach was introduced gradually in the 1960s when the efficacy of teaching complex behavioural sequences for behaviour problems was demonstrated and rapidly found use in a broad range of disorders (Wolpe, 1958; Gittelman, 1965). Such training originated in the 1950s with the advent of behavioural and cognitive treatment, and was used initially in the treatment of anxiety and neurotic disorders (Wolpe, 1958) in children and adults (Gittelman, 1965), then gradually with persons with mental illness (Liberman *et al.*, 1989; Tunnell *et al.*, 1987).

The focus has been on using behavioural and cognitive teaching to improve social skills and competence. Most of the interventions utilize behaviour rehearsal (e.g. modelling), role reversal, assertiveness training and reinforcement. Participants are usually started with easily accomplished tasks and then gradually presented with more difficult material (Liberman *et al.*, 1989; Meuser, 1989; Bellack and Meuser, 1993) and given graded assignments in performing increasingly complex skills involving conversation, assertiveness, heterosexual contact and communication, and medication management.

Research support for the additive efficacy of social skills training has come from the work of Hogarty and colleagues (1986, 1991). They found that social skills training alone and combined with family intervention (both interventions being combined with medication) was associated with lower relapse rates in the first year of treatment, but that this effect did not persist in the second year or beyond the duration of the experiment. These findings, Hogarty suggests, may simply indicate that the subjects in the experiment may have received more attention, support and encouragement to continue taking their medication during the experiment and, since they were carefully supervised, may have had medication adjustments when needed. Moreover, it should be noted in trying to interpret this landmark study, that the families involved were not necessarily characteristic of those of most patients with schizophrenia since all of those chosen had high 'Expressed Emotion', which made them arguably somewhat atypical of many families with a member suffering from schizophrenia.

In many areas, social skills are fostered by the patient's participation in activities at day centres, special clubhouses and supervised residences where the mentally disabled care for themselves with the assistance of trained 'house parents' or special social workers.

Vocational rehabilitation

The objective of vocational rehabilitation is to restore or enhance relatively independent social functioning. By normalizing behaviour and improving skills, it helps to reduce stigma. It may be introduced gradually during recovery or, most often, during remission periods in the course of mental illness. Vocational rehabilitation, or industrial therapy, as it is sometimes called, was started in the UK following the First World War (Black, 1970) by the British Ex-Serviceman's Mental Welfare Society at a company termed Thermega, outside London, which provided work for 'shell-shocked' veterans.

Since the introduction of antipsychotic medication, vocational rehabilitation has spread rapidly throughout the industrialized countries that have been experimenting with community psychiatry. Further impetus has been given to the development of vocational rehabilitation, especially in Europe, by national and EU policies that subsidize industrial therapy, sheltered workshops, small enterprises and employers willing to hire the mentally disabled.

The classic programme that has evolved from physical rehabilitation consists of:

- an initial assessment of the person's strengths, including interests and abilities unaffected by the mental disorder, and of the milieu, family and community in which the client lives; some skills training is undertaken on the job to see if the client can meet the job requirements;
- pre-vocational training;
- transitional employment;
- supported employment; and
- vocational counselling and educational services, job clubs and counselling, including that offered during employment.

One of the interesting developments in France has been the creation of the Centres for Work Therapy (Centres d'Ergotherapie), of which there are more than 150 throughout France. These centres are small, non-profit businesses that obtain work from neighbouring towns, villages or enterprises. The people who work at the centres may reside outside or at the particular centre, paying rent out of their salaries and benefits. Psychiatric treatment is provided by the area primary and specialist services. Skills training tends to be on the job, i.e. clients are presented with a variety of tasks to be performed and then assisted in learning the required skills on site. Such programmes have been found to be cost-effective and self-financing.

An analysis of social security expenditures in Germany (Stark, 1999) found that annual costs for subsidized, regular employment cost less (19 000 DM) per participant than unemployment benefit payments plus the usual psychiatric care (60 000 DM). Part of the cost differential is explained by the fact that employed workers, even though their employer is being subsidized for hiring a disabled worker, is required to pay taxes and social security. Of course, these findings are not based on randomized comparisons, and those hired may be less subject to acute relapses and therefore require less costly services than some of the other mentally disabled persons. However, it is interesting to note that in programmes that operate on a part- or full-time basis, the client is observed with great frequency, and a supervisor or employer is often able to note changes in behaviour or appearance that signal a possible relapse and assist in obtaining clinical assistance to prevent it. Moreover, such programmes are of benefit to families both for the needed respite from constant care they offer and for the additional income. Systems research in which randomized controlled studies on the effectiveness of industrial therapy compared with day care activities and family care is required. Certainly, there is no *a priori* reason why such programmes should not be as effective as efforts focusing on trained and supported families.

The initial enthusiasm for vocational rehabilitation was tempered somewhat by Bennett's (1967) observation that some patients require limited and part-time work schedules and also seem to function better when not placed in situations requiring a high degree of social interaction. Moreover, Wing (1978) found that vocational rehabilitation, when utilized excessively, produced high relapse rates. Despite these findings, however, vocational rehabilitation can be an important component of psychosocial rehabilitation programmes.

Family interventions

A number of family interventions have demonstrated validity in research studies, among them education, various types of support and crisis elements, and it is not yet clear which of them are responsible for producing the desired results of compliance with medication, better functioning of the patient and fewer relapses.

In most industrialized countries, the majority of patients return to the families following hospital discharge. Families are a vital part of the natural support system of persons with mental illness, and it has been shown that those who live with families fare better than others (NY State Commission of Quality of Care for the Mentally Disabled, 1996).

Schooler and associates (1997) reviewed family intervention strategies and found that, when combined with medication, they were superior to routine medication and other individual strategies such as social skills training. Dixon *et al.* (1995), in their review of psychosocial interventions such as support, education about the illness and training in problem solving, found that when combined with pharmacotherapy, these interventions reduced 1-year relapse rates from 40–53% to 23% or lower. They recommend that such interventions should be used with all care-givers, not just family members.

Appropriately trained families have been enabled to note the appearance of changes in the patient's condition and head off relapses by arranging for dosage adjustment (Schooler *et al.*, 1997; Chen Yanfang *et al.*, 1996). Effective monitoring also permits clinicians to use lower doses of psychotropic medications, which reduce medication-related side effects, enhance productive capacity and improve adherence to the medication regimen.

In 1988, in an effort to enhance the scope and effectiveness of the Chinese psychiatric hospital system, Dr. N. Shinfuku, then Regional Director for Mental Health of the World Health Organization, in co-operation with the Chinese Ministry of Public Health, instituted a series of training institutes for leading Chinese psychiatrists (Gittelman and Bailly-Salin, 1988; Gittelman and Olly, 1990). This programme was to have important ramifications for both developing and developed countries.

The objective of the programme was to devise a simple method that could be utilized to provide services to large at-risk populations at low cost. Carried out by primary care health workers, often with only high school level education and working under the supervision of a psychiatrist, the programme aimed to 'educate' families about mental illness and how to cope with an afflicted family member and to monitor the patient collaboratively with the family. At a series of training sessions in various cities of China, social skills training and family and patient psychoeducation were undertaken. Initially only families participated; but after a few successful trials, it was found that patients profited from psychoeducation as well.

The results of these training sessions have been evaluated in a carefully controlled, multi-centere study by Zhang Mihgyuan *et al.* (1993). In one of the largest studies evaluating tertiary prevention methods (>3200 subjects participated, 2298 in the experimental group), it was found that the relapse rate for the experimental group was reduced to 20.4%, whereas that of the control group remained about level at 31.1%. The hospitalization admission rate dropped from 22.9 to 11.7%.

These researchers have also studied a similar cohort (Zhang Mingyuan and Yan Heqin, 1993), using similar methods, for a 2-year period and found a similar and significant advantage 'for a combined medication and psychoeducation group'. Moreover, social disability and family burden were significantly reduced.

Subsequent training and research in China (Chen Yanfang *et al.*, 1996) have confirmed the effectiveness of combining psychosocial rehabilitation with medication, including studies using two different drugs, chlorpromazine and a newer, atypical, antipsychotic medication, clozapine. The combined treatment reduced relapse rates regardless of which drug was used. Professor Chen and his colleagues found that while combining medication and psychosocial methods robustly reduced relapse there were no significant differences which resulted from the use of either conventional (chlorpromazine) nor newer atypical antipsychotic (clozapine) medications.

Families have been receiving considerable attention in efforts to help them cope with their mentally disabled members, but it should be noted that not all families are eager to participate and collaborate in such efforts. Many families are either unable to provide adequate care for their disabled member or are reluctant to do so unless needed assistance and respite are assured. Too few countries recognize the economic and emotional cost of providing care for a disabled relative (Eggert *et al.*, 1975). Needed are financial and

homemaker aid plus some respite from the constant care, particularly since, as is usually the case, no end is in sight. This is a problem that requires further research and important consideration by those who determine social policies. Too much is asked and expected of families in caring for their physically or mentally disabled members.

Conclusions

There are three fundamental considerations in planning tertiary prevention for persons with mental illness. The first is how treatment and rehabilitation services are to be organized and funded so as to ensure a comfortable, comprehensive and continuous fit between the characteristics of the illness and its course. Since the 1950s, it has been recognized that unless systems of treatment and rehabilitation are comprehensive, coordinated and continuous, people with mental illness cannot be expected, on their own, to find and obtain the care they must have.

Among the well co-ordinated systems that have evolved is the French system of sectorization, initiated by Paumelle and Lebovici in the 13th arrondissment of Paris (Gittelman, 1972) and subsequently adopted, in various forms, in parts of Europe (Thornicroft and Johnson, 1993), the USA (Test and Stein, 1978) and Asia (Zhang Mingyuan *et al.*, 1993). Sectorization is discussed in more detail by Hansson in this book. More recently, managed care systems have arisen in a number of countries, particularly the USA, and a few managed care organizations are beginning to take advantage of the cost savings and effectiveness of psychosocial rehabilitation (Gittelman, 1998).

A second fundamental concern involves specific interventions that, after appropriate assessment, often involve environmental modification and/or educational interventions. Therapeutic communities, partial hospitalization, clubhouses, farming communities and the French Centres D'Ergotherapie have all been shown to be acceptable to clients in reducing relapse and disability, but few studies concerning them have been undertaken with rigour. Cognitive and behavioural therapies have been studied since they appeared on the scene, as have specific and general interventions with patients and their families, but more research is needed. Further research is also needed to explore how simple or elaborate tertiary prevention programs need to be in order to produce results greater than medication alone. Preliminary data from developing countries suggests that even low cost and rudimentary programs may be useful (Sidandi, 1997; Viet, 1991).

A third fundamental consideration involves advocacy, which is required to reduce handicap. Legislation to provide tax incentives for employers to hire the disabled either part- or full-time, campaigns to educate the public about mental illness and efforts to organize family associations and other self-help organizations all reduce the impact of disabilities and help to eliminate handicap and stigma.

Most important is the first consideration—*organization*. Countries vary in the way in which their mental health systems are organized. Most industrialized countries provide some treatment and rehabilitation of mental illness by professional staff funded by public monies from taxes and/or social security, or other insured funds. The systems may be organized according to their geographic and/or social setting or their funding mechanism—whether they are for, or not for, profit. They may specialize in particular types of treatment or offer only certain treatments, for a limited time.

Tertiary prevention, or psychosocial rehabilitation, is gaining increasing recognition as a useful tool in dealing with mental illness as a public concern. Although there is a need for more precise analysis of what factors account for the effectiveness of various psychosocial interventions, the evidence that they are effective is no longer in doubt. We owe much to those pioneers (Bellack, Bennett, Brown, Falloon, Leff, Liberman, Tarrier and others) who have pointed to the need for psychosocial rehabilitative interventions in conjunction with treatment. For the mentally disabled to live in the community, the community will have to change, in both attitude and services provided. This will require the efforts of not just mental health professionals but of policy makers and the public at large.

References

Allebeck, P. (1989) Schizophrenia: a life-shortening disease. *Schizophrenia Bulletin*, 15, 1.

Andreason, N.C., Paradiso, S. and O'Leary, D.S. (1998) Cognitive dysmetria as an integrative theory of schizophrenia: a dysfunction in cortical–subcortical–cerebellar circuitry? *Schizophrenia Bulletin*, 24, 2.

Ayd, F., Jr (1961) A survey of drug-induced extrapyramidal reactions. *Journal of the American Medical Association*, 175,1054.

Bellack, A.S. and Meuser, K.T. (1993) Psychosocial treatment for schizophrenia. *Schizophrenia Bulletin*, 19, 2.

Bennett, D. (1967) Rehabilitation services for the mentally disabled. In: Freeman, H. and Farndale, J. (eds), *New Aspects of the Mental Health Services*. London: Pergamon.

Black, B. (1970) *Industrial Therapy for the Mentally Ill*. New York: Grune and Stratton.

Chen Yanfang, Zhaoping Wang, Dexiang Yu, Lianzhong Yu, Keshang Jia, Gongzheng Lin, Qintong Wang and Gittelman, Martin (1996) The evaluation of psychological education for 855 schizophrenic patients with clozapine or chlorpromazine maintenance in Chinese rural areas. A two-year follow-up control study. Paper presented at the *World Association for Psychosocial Rehabilitation*, World Congress, Rotterdam, The Netherlands. October.

Ciompi, L. (1987) Toward a coherent multidimensional understanding and psychotherapy of schizophrenia: converging new concepts. In: Strauss, J.S. Boker, W. and Brenner, H.D. (eds), *Treatment of Schizophrenia: Multidimensional Concepts, Psychological, Family and Self-help Perspectives*. Toronto: Hans Huber Publishers, pp. 48–62.

Cramer, J.A. and Rosenheck, R. (1998) Compliance with medication regimes for mental and physical disorders. *Psychiatric Services*, 49, 196.

Davis, J.M. and Garver, D.I. (1978) Neuroleptics: clinical use in psychiatry. In: Iverson, L.L., Iverson, S.D. and Snyder, S.H. (eds), *Handbook of Psychopharmacology*. New York: Plenum Press.

Dixon, L.B., Leham, A.F. and Levine, J. (1995) Conventional antipsychotic medications for schizophrenia. *Schizophrenia Bulletin*, 21, 567.

Eggert. G., Morris, R., Grallger, C. V. and Pendleton, S. (1975) Community-based maintenance care for the long-term, patient. Unpublished paper from the Levinson Policy Institute, Brandeis University. Cited by Morris, R. (1977–78) Integration of therapeutic and community services: cure plus care for the mentally disabled. *International Journal of Mental Health*, 6. 9.

Falloon, I.R.H., Boyd, J.L. and McGill, C.W. (1982) Family management in the prevention of exacerbations of schizophrenia. *New England Journal of Medicine*, 306, 1437.

Geddes, J.R. Atypical antipsychotics in the treatment of schizophrenia: Systematic Review, Meta-Regression and Evidence based treatment recommendations, Royal College of Psychiatrry Guideline Development group, Feb. 2000.

Gittelman, M. (1965) Behavior rehearsal as a technique in child treatment. *British Journal of Child Psychiatry and Psychology*, November, p. 251.

Gittelman, M. (1972) Sectorization: the quiet revolution. *American Journal of Orthopsychiatry*, 42, 159–172.

Gittelman, M. (1981) Refining diagnoses and behavioural interventions: key to preventing overmedication. In Gittelman, M. (ed.), *Strategic Interventions for Hyperactive children*. Armonk, NY: M.E. Sharpe, 1–9.

Gittelman, M. (1994) *Promotion of Community-based Psychosocial Rehabilitation for Individuals with Mental Illness*. Geneva: WHO (CHN/MND/006).

Gittelman, M. (1998) Public and private managed care. *International Journal of Mental Health*, 27, 3–17.

Gittelman, M. and Bailly-Salin, P. (1988) *Promotion of Community-based Rehabilitation for the Mentally Ill in China*. Geneva: WHO (MNH/ICP/NHC/002E)WP).

Gittelman, M. and Blumberg, 1. (1975) Rehabilitation. In: Liberman, J. (ed.), *Mental Health. The Public Health Challenge*. Washington, DC: American Public Health Association, pp. 77–82.

Gittelman, M. and Freedman, A. (1988) Treating half the illness. *Hospital and Community Psychiatry*, 39, 347.

Gittelman, M. and Orley, J. (1990) *Promotion of Community-based Rehabilitation for the Mentally Ill*. Geneva: WHO (WP)MNH/CHN/MND/001-E).

Gittelman, M. and Semba, T. (1992) *National Workshop on Comprehensive Programmes on Rehabilitation of Mental Patients*. Geneva: WHO (ICP MND 002) August.

Goldberg, E.M. (1967) The families of schizophrenic patients. In: Freeman H. and Farndale, J. (eds), *New Aspects of the Mental Health Services*. London: Pergamon.

Hogarty, G.E., Anderson, C.M. Reiss, D.J., Kornblith, S.J., Greenwald, D.P. Javna, C.D. and Madonia, M.J. (1986) Family psychoeducation, social skills training, and maintenance chemotherapy in the aftercare treatment of schizophrenia, I. One-year effects of a controlled trial on relapse and expressed emotion. *Archives of General Psychiatry*, 43, 633.

Hogarty, C.E., Anderson, C.M., Reiss, D.J. Kornblith, S.J., Greenwald, D.P., Ulrich, R.F. and Carter, M. (1991) Family psycheducation, social skills training, and maintenance chemotherapy in the aftercare treatment of schizophrenia, 2. Two-year effects of a controlled trial on relapse and adjustment. *Archives of General Psychiatry*, 48, 340.

Lehman, A., Steinwachs, D.M. and the co-investigators of the PORT Project (1998) At issue: translating research into practice: The Schizophrenia Patient Outcomes Research Team (PORT) treatment recommendations. *Schizophrenia Bulletin*, 24, 1.

Liberman R.P., De Risi, W.D. and Meuser, K.T. (1989) *Social Skills Training for Psychiatric Patients*. Boston: Allen and Bacon.

Mak, K.Y. (1998) Compliance in psychiatric treatment. *Canadian Journal of Psychiatry*, 43, 706–713.

May, P. (1968) *Treatment of Schizophrenia*. New York: Science House.

New York Commission on Quality Care for the Mentally Disabled (1996) May.

Pasamanick, B., Scarpitti, F.R., Lefton, M., Dinitz, S., Wernert, J.J. and McPheeters, H. (1964) Home versus hospital care for schizophrenics. *Journal of the American Medical Association*, 187, 117.

Pasamanick, B., Scarpitti, F.E. and Dinitz, S. (1967) *Schizophrenia in the Community*. New York; Appleton Century Crofts.

Schoder, N. (1997) New antipsychotic medication: strategies for evaluation and selected findings. *Schizophrenia Bulletin*, 27, 249.

Schooler, N., Keith, S.J., Severe, J., Mathews, S.M., Bellack, A.S., Glick, I., Hargraves, W.A., Kane, J.M., Ninan, P., Frances, A., Jacobs, M., Liberman, J.A., Mance, R., Simpson, G. and Woerner, M. (1997) Relapse and rehospitalization during maintenance medication. *Archives of General Psychiatry*, 54, 453.

Sidandi, P. (1997) Report from Botsrrana, personal communication.

Stark, M. (1999) *Rehabilitation for the Mentally Ill in Germany*. Paper presented at the annual meeting of the American Psychiatric Association. 20 May.

Stroup, T.S., Gilmore, J.H., Janakog, L.F (2000) Management of medical illness in persons with schizophrenia, *Psychiatric annals*: 30:1.

Test, M.A. and Stein, L.I. (1978) Alternatives to mental hospital treatment. III. Social cost. *Archives of General Psychiatry*, 37, 1243.

Tarrier, N., Barrowclough, C., Vaughn, C., Bamrah, J.S., Porceddu, K., Watts, D. and Freeman, H. (1988) Community management of schizophrenia: a controlled trial of a behavioural intervention with families to reduce relapse. *British Journal of Psychiatry*, 153, 532–542.

Thornicroft, G. and Johnson, S. (1993) The sectorisation of psychiatric services in England and Wales. *Social Psychiatry and Psychiatric Epidemiology*, 28, 45–47.

Tunnell, G., Alpert, M., Gittelman, M. (1987) Preventing disability and relapse in schizophrenia, *International Journal of Mental Health*, 16, 17, 4.

Viet, N. (1991) Report from Vietnam, personal communication.

WHO, The World Health Report 2000, Geneva.

Wing, J.K. (1978) *Schizophrenia: Towards A New Synthesis*. London: Academic Press.

Wolpe, J. (1958) *Psychotherapy by Reciprocal Inhibition*. Stanford, CA: Stanford University Press.

Yan Heqin, Yao Chengde, Ye Jianlin, Zhang Mingyuan, Yu Qingfang, Chou Peijin, Guo Lianfung, Wong Zhen, Cai Jia hua, Shen Minghua, Orley, J. and Gittelman, M. (1993) Effectiveness of psychoeducation of relatives of schizophrenic patients. *International Journal of Mental Health*, 22, 24–47.

Zhang Mingyuan and Yan Heqin (1993) Effectiveness of psychoeducation of relatives of schizophrenic patients: a prospective cohort study in five cities of China. *International Journal of Mental Health*, 22, 47–59.

44 | *Rationing, priorities and targeting*

David J. Hunter

Introduction

The rationing of health care is one of those 'wicked issues' to which there is no easy solution and possibly none at all. In the UK NHS, the term only entered common currency in the early 1990s when the Conservative government introduced its internal market changes. At this point, the process of allocating resources, which up until then had been shrouded in mystery and notions of clinical judgement, became more explicit as a result of the purchaser–provider separation and the emergence of a contract culture.

However, rationing as a phenomenon has always existed and not only in health care. It is the terminology which has changed. Until the 1991 NHS reforms, terms such as 'priority-setting' and 'making choices' were in common usage. As one commentator has put it: 'priority-setting' is viewed as a term which makes rationing "sound a little less grim, and a little more scientific, than in fact it is" (Loughlin, 1996, p. 146).

This chapter reviews the rationing debate in the UK, drawing on the experience of other countries where appropriate, and examines the arguments in favour of explicit and implicit rationing, respectively. It concludes by arguing that rationing is an unwinnable dilemma of public policy. There are no solutions to some problems and we should not allow the rational scientific bias which infuses much public policy to suggest otherwise. Hence the attractions of an approach based on 'muddling through elegantly' (Hunter, 1993, 1998). While we can improve the muddling, it is politically naive to think that there is a formula waiting to be discovered which will serve as a way of handling the rationing dilemma.

The rationing dilemma

The problem of allocating scarce resources in health care has always existed and not just in the UK. It is a truism to assert that setting priorities and choosing where and how to invest resources are unavoidable political and management tasks. However, not all commentators accept that rationing is inevitable or that we should embrace it, however reluctantly. A former US health secretary of state has said: "rationing is not a solution to the problems we face, it is a capitulation of despair" (Califano, 1992). Loughlin (1996, p. 147) takes to task health economists and others who profess to have solutions to problems such as establishing priorities and whose 'toxic effect' is to obscure 'the monstrous irrationality and barbarity' of modern society. He continues: "the assumption that there must be a defensible, determinate answer to questions about who should be allowed to suffer and die, is false" (p. 155).

More fundamentally, Loughlin is critical of the very nature of the narrow parameters within which the rationing debate is being conducted. By definition, these are not givens or objective phenomena, but are politically determined.

"Unwillingness to think about radical changes in the organisation of social reality when trying to determine what is right or best, reflects not realism but the unwillingness to admit any major differences between the way the world is and how it ought to be. It suggests the disposition to believe that the world is just about right as it is, that the social background to health service policy is morally uncontroversial" (Loughlin, 1996, p. 155).

There is also the matter of how rational rationing can be when society as a whole may not in fact be rational. After all, one person's rationality may be another's irrationality. If this view is accepted, then what grounds are there for believing that any explicit rationing system either can or should succeed? Were a robust social consensus possible, then such an approach might just be conceivable, although even then attempts would probably be made to by-pass any rules for rationing and to make covert what is ostensibly presented as being overt.

The dilemma faced by the rational rationers or those who insist upon the purification qualities of making hard choices (at least at a rhetorical level if not in reality) is that their position is simplistic and politically naive. At a normative level, they may be right. It would be intrinsically desirable to have a system of resource allocation bounded by clear rules and procedures. However, no such system can be sensitive to the myriad complexities surrounding the care of people with multiple needs and varying social circumstances. Moreover, we tend to overstate the miracle of modern medicine. As the US Surgeon-General has said, the best estimates are that health services affect about 10% of the usual indices for measuring health: infant mortality, absences through sickness and adult mortality. The remaining 90% are determined by factors over which doctors have little or no control: individual lifestyle, social conditions and the physical environment. In the words of one policy analyst: "no one is saying that medicine is good for nothing, only that it is not good for everything" (Wildavsky, 1979).

Whatever other arguments may be mobilized concerning the defeatism to which a focus on rationing can give rise, the prevailing orthodoxy is that rationing is both inevitable and should be made more explicit so that the public both understands the issue and actively participates in decisions about where resources should go.

Defining terms

The terms 'priority-setting' and 'rationing' are invariably used interchangeably and it seems pointless getting into a narrow, and probably ultimately futile, debate about semantics. Suffice to say, that those favouring the term 'priority-setting' consider it to be a more positive process in contrast to the negative or pejorative overtones associated with the term 'rationing'. To put it bluntly, priority-setting is about deciding what the NHS should provide while rationing is about deciding what the NHS should not provide, or to whom treatment should be denied (British Medical Association, 1995). However, in practice, this distinction does not survive close scrutiny as it is implicit when setting priorities within tight budgets that some services of lower priority will not be available. Denial, if not scarcity, is therefore a feature of both priority-setting and rationing.

Rationing and priority-setting can be defined in a variety of ways. In its evidence to the House of Commons Health Committee (1995), the Association of Community Health Councils for England and Wales identified three distinct forms of rationing:

- withdrawal of the NHS from a particular type of service or treatment (e.g. 'cosmetic' operations, treatment of infertility, tattoo removal, long-term care of the elderly)
- explicit and regular attempts to define how much of which services should be provided and moving resources between services
- restricting access to a service by reference to the characteristics of prospective patients, e.g. their age, personal lifestyle (whether they smoke, take drugs, are heavy drinkers and so on).

Briefly examining each of these in turn, rationing in the NHS can and does occur commonly through a range of devices such as deterrence, delay, deflection, dilution and denial (Harrison and Hunter, 1994, pp. 25–30). As Aaron and Schwartz found in their comparative study of rationing in the USA and Britain, "few of the criteria for rejection are explicitly stated. Age, for example, is not officially identified as an obstacle to treatment" (Aaron and Schwartz, 1984, p. 37). Yet there is very clear evidence that age is a major factor in determining whether treatment is sanctioned or denied (Grimley Evans, 1993). However, it is not clear whether rationing is itself a cause of elderly people being denied treatment from which they could benefit or whether it is a symptomatic reflection of deep-seated ageist attitudes within society which are in turn reflected in the treatment decisions made by professionals. In a society plagued by images of 'a rising tide' of elderly people and by the 'burden of ageing', it is hardly surprising that negative stereotypes prevail. Positive views of ageing would be unlikely to be reflected in rationing decisions currently based on age.

Given the inevitability of exercizing professional judgement in decisions about who to treat and how, it is almost impossible to trace the motivation underlying the decision. What may be denied a patient on the grounds that they would not benefit from the treatment may in fact be inextricably bound up with moral factors whereby a patient is seen as less deserving and as getting their 'just deserts'. While doctors may be forbidden to allow moral judgements to enter into their decision making, it may in practice be difficult to disentangle these from clinical judgements. In sum, the content of medical work is a complex mix of clinical factors, effectiveness of resource use and policing lifestyle (Hughes and Griffiths, 1996).

While those concerned about the value-laden nature of much professional decision making advocate explicit rationing as a way of exposing and holding to account the making of moral judgements, there is no *a priori* reason to believe that explicit rationing would in fact be any more rational. As Hughes and Griffiths state: "It is perfectly possible for doctors to act according to their perceptions of deservingness, while accounting for their actions in terms of medical benefit". In situations of tight resource constraints, making treatment decisions on clinical grounds alone may not be sufficient. Inevitably, therefore, moral factors come into play.

In the NHS, priority-setting has largely been left to health authorities and, in future, to Primary Care Groups and Trusts (in England). Many health authorities have therefore drawn up lists of procedures they will either not fund at all or only in exceptional circumstances. Most of the exclusions relate to lifestyle treatments that cannot be said to result in major discomfort of a life or death nature. For the most part, too, these exclusions do not release significant savings although the resources made available in this way might be deployed more effectively elsewhere.

Most recent discussion of rationing in the NHS has been about whether or not it should become more explicit. This is linked to the issue of the level at which rationing should be conducted—national, local or at the doctor–patient level. In a national health system, should it be central government which takes responsibility for what are essentially political decisions about the areas of care and treatment the NHS should cover and exclude? Or is it reasonable to leave such decisions to the local level where there is more knowledge about needs and about the population's characteristics?

A national or local approach to rationing?

For many years, the British Medical Association and various other health service organizations have been calling on central government to take the lead on rationing and to make explicit decisions instead of looking to health authorities and doctors to make them. Indeed, Richard Smith, editor of the *British Medical Journal*, went so far as to accuse government of a 'failure of leadership' with the result that "Britain has not had the broad, deep, informed, and prolonged debate on rationing that is needed" (Smith, 1995, p. 686). Britain is accused of lagging behind countries such as The Netherlands, Sweden and New Zealand which have all grasped the nettle of explicit rationing, albeit with varying degrees of success (Hunter, 1998).

What international experience demonstrates is that there exist several approaches to tackling rationing, ranging from prescribed lists of treatments to be included in a publicly funded system of health care, through wide-ranging ethical discussions to establish criteria governing resource use, to agreeing broad principles as the basis of a coherent policy framework (Coulter and Ham, 2000). There is no consensus on the best way forward, and all British governments over the years have resisted attempts either to define a set of core services, to rank treatments or to lead a public debate on the issue other than to reassert the founding principles of the NHS as a universal facility accessible to all in need of care and to reaffirm its view that it is for local health authorities not to ration care or deny effective treatments but to establish priorities informed by public opinion.

An exception to this position has been the introduction into the NHS of the drug Viagra manufactured by Pfizer. For the first time, this involved an intervention by the Secretary of State for Health with a view to restricting the circumstances under which it could be prescribed on the NHS. However, the case illustrates all the pitfalls of Ministers taking a lead and is unlikely to be repeated. Moreover, Viagra is not concerned with a life-threatening condition and for a Minister to take a stand on a life and death matter would be extremely unlikely. As Klein has put it, governments seek to diffuse blame and centralize credit (Klein, 1995). Nevertheless, the Viagra example does demonstrate what can happen when governments seek to determine nationally what treatment options should be available and to whom. Having been urged to develop a national policy by clinicians, various NHS organizations and assorted academics, the Secretary of State did so in respect of Viagra, publishing a list of criteria governing its use on the NHS.

The pronouncement triggered an immediate backlash on the grounds that the list excluded all kinds of deserving medical conditions and that doctors on the front-line were best placed to make such decisions since they knew their patients best. That, after all, is the whole point of professional judgement. As a result of the furore, the government extended its list of inclusions and inserted an escape clause which allowed doctors a certain degree of latitude to prescribe the drug in exceptional circumstances. However, there remains criticism of the process and the outcome. Supporters of the government's stance claim that the Minister was absolutely right to react in the way he did even if the resulting decision was defective; but is this not precisely the point? From *somebody's* perspective, the outcome will probably always be

defective. If the political fallout becomes damaging, then it is unlikely that governments will wish to be so explicit in future in quite such a 'hands on' way.

The next best option is to set up a national body to take rationing decisions on behalf of the government but to present them as evidence-based decisions underpinned by robust science and research evidence. The NHS Research & Development strategy, introduced in 1991, and the ensuing evidence-based medicine (EBM) movement have been attempts to do precisely this and they have not been without some success, although there is a risk of raising unrealistic expectations concerning the existence and robustness of an evidence base with respect to all treatments. The effort has also been criticized for being fragmented and not clearly connected to government health policy.

These problems are being addressed with the establishment in April 1999 of the National Institute for Clinical Excellence (NICE) in England and Wales (Scotland is pursuing a similar approach with its own machinery) which will produce a steady stream of clinical guidelines and protocols on what works and what does not work. Clinicians will not be compelled to act on the evidence but they will be held accountable for their decisions and be required to give good reasons for not following the appraisals and guidelines produced by NICE. To ensure that good progress is being made and to assist health authorities, trusts and primary care organizations in changing their practice and behaviour, another new national agency for England and Wales, the Commission for Health Improvement (CHI), was set up towards the end of 1999. It provides support and ultimately sanctions if change in management and/or clinical practice is not forthcoming. It is the closest the NHS has come to having its own independent inspectorate, although the term produces a negative reaction among clinicians. However, the government is impatient to see evidence of real change in clinical practice and, as the NHS Plan published in July 2000 clearly states, will not hesitate to introduce tougher measures if required. The dilemma, is that in order to secure change it needs the support and compliance of clinicians.

It is too soon to judge how successful NICE and CHI will be, but the government regards them as being of critical importance with respect to the rationing issue. Ministers stress that the NHS cannot be expected to provide interventions that are known to be ineffective or where evidence of their efficacy is lacking. However, even where relevant studies exist, their application locally may remain problematic. So while NICE may improve the availability, accessibility and dissemination of data, it will be up to the CHI to work with health service organizations to encourage their uptake where there is a persistent failure to do so. Through these means, Ministers hope that the lottery of so-called 'post-code rationing' will cease and that a uniform level of provision will exist across the country regardless of where a patient happens to live. The price to pay for this degree of standardization is greater centralized decision making and less scope for local variation, clinical discretion and priority-setting. However, it is hard to see how NICE and CHI will altogether end such practices since it is in the nature of health care and medicine that decisions must reflect individual circumstances which are far from uniform.

NICE will appraise both new and existing technologies covering pharmaceuticals, medical devices, diagnostic technologies, procedures and health promotion, and will develop and publish clinical guidelines on the basis of its cost-effectiveness analyses. The guidelines will also be available to the public in the hope that patients can establish reasonable expectations and temper unreasonable demands. The evidence base with respect to drug therapies is better than that in the other categories, especially health promotion, although it is unlikely that NICE will invest a great deal of its scarce resources on this topic leaving this task to the Health Development Agency established in April 2000. NICE's recommendations will fall into one of three categories: that a treatment or procedure be recommended for routine use in the NHS; that it be recommended for use only in clinical trials; that it not be recommended for routine use. A clinical audit system will accompany each guideline to monitor adherence to NICE's recommendations. How much management clout it will have remains unclear.

Rather less is known about the CHI and how it will operate, although its director insists that it will adopt a developmental approach in preference to a punitive one. It is charged with the task of offering an independent guarantee that local systems to monitor, assure and improve clinical quality are in place. It intends visiting all NHS organizations within 4 years through a system of rolling reviews. Its work programme is dependent upon a number of successful secondments from the NHS in order to undertake an extensive visiting programme. The work of the CHI will complement arrangements for clinical governance. It will offer targeted support and be able to intervene by invitation/request and make recommendations to the Secretary of State for Health.

Both NICE and CHI allow Ministers to be kept at arm's length from making decisions about what treatments work and do not work. The Viagra case illustrates how difficult it is for Ministers to win in such cases even with the weight of public opinion on their side. It also illustrates how different it is for minorities not to interfere.

The government regards EBM, and a focus on cost-effectiveness with respect to new and existing treatments and interventions, as representing the best way forward. It amounts to a technocratic solution, or fix, to what is essentially a political and social problem or public policy puzzle. Estimates about the amount of resources squandered on ineffective interventions vary. The first NHS R&D Director, Sir Michael Peckham, estimated that at least £1 billion could be released by terminating ineffective procedures. Commentators, such as David Eddy, maintain however that even eliminating waste, itself very difficult to do, will not obviate the need to ration care (Eddy, 1994). At most, it will buy time, but that assumes that the evidence base is sufficiently robust and that clinicians will act on the evidence and modify their practice. All the available evidence suggests that even if there is progress, it will take a long time to secure. In the meantime, and notwithstanding a generous budget settlement, pressures on NHS resources intensify.

Responding to these, the Rationing Agenda Group, led by the BMJ and King's Fund, have proposed an approach which seeks to be more open and explicit about the principles governing rationing decisions (New and Le Grand, 1996). They suggest three basic characteristics that make some kinds of health care special: unpredictability of the need for that care; information imbalance between doctors and patients; and what might be termed the fundamental importance of the care concerned in allowing people to realize their life goals. The application of these principles (none of which would be sufficient on its own) might help in deciding what should be in the NHS and what should lie outside it.

Some interventions are rather obvious and are already the subject of exclusions in some health authorities (as noted above). Within their schema, New and Le Grand argue that cosmetic surgery to enhance physical attractiveness is not of fundamental importance and should not therefore be provided under the NHS. Other treatments and services are less obvious, such as residential care, which can be predicted. It should not therefore be available free under the NHS. However, adult dental care and *in vitro* fertilization (IVF) should be available because both are unpredictable. Where New and Le Grand draw the line over being explicit and laying down fairly strict rules is over who should receive treatment and how much they should get. Pragmatism, they believe, should prevail here, which means leaving such decisions to clinicians. What a national framework would achieve is an end to the present lottery whereby our place of residence can determine whether or not we have a chance of fertility treatments, continuing care, dentistry or whatever.

A difficulty with New and Le Grand's approach, beguiling though it is in its apparent simplicity and reasonableness, is how the characteristic of 'fundamental importance' is to be defined (Klein, 1997). An illustration of the dilemma is provided by IVF. Whereas New and Le Grand assert its fundamental importance—"is not the inability to have a child of fundamental importance?"—the Dunning Committee in The Netherlands which examined the whole issue of making choices in health care excluded IVF from the basic package on the grounds that "from a community-oriented approach, the answer to the question of necessity would most probably be no" (Ministry of Welfare, Health and Cultural Affairs, 1992, p. 87).

This sharp divergence of view is the nub of the issue. When there exist multiple interpretations of what constitutes necessity or care of fundamental importance then it renders the whole selection criterion 'vacuous' since it "provides no guidance on how conflicting interpretations can be resolved" (Klein, 1997, p. 507). Moreover, for all their efforts to confront 'hard choices' in a hard-nosed fashion, New and Le Grand resort to an 'escape clause' and acknowledge the need for judgement since the three criteria of unpredictability, information imbalance and fundamental importance are not able "to specify action so precisely that the need for further thought and judgement is unnecessary" (New and Le Grand, 1996, p. 52). Individual cases will then need to be assessed so there can be no blanket exclusions. At the end of the day, it would seem that there is no effective substitute for clinical judgement and local discretion, albeit within a broad set of principles governing action. Do these not already exist in terms of the NHS's founding principles and core values as laid down in legislation and endorsed by successive governments in white papers and numerous policy statements?

Engaging the public voice

To resolve the rationing conundrum from another standpoint, which would also have the virtue of tackling what amounts to a significant 'democratic deficit' in the way in which the NHS is run, policy makers have resorted to asserting the rights of the public to be actively involved in decisions about who to treat and about what the NHS should cover. Such a participative approach is now common across the public policy landscape, notably in education and in local government.

A dilemma is that members of the public occupy different roles at different times throughout their lives. They can be patients, carers, users of services, tax-payers and citizens. Their views are likely to differ, and certainly be influenced, by the particular role, or roles, they are playing at a particular point in time. Advocates of explicit rationing vary in the extent to which they believe users of services as opposed to citizens should be involved in decisions about resources and who should receive them. So far, efforts to involve the public in making choices about health care have had only limited success. As Moore (1996, p.15) explains:

"Nationally, 'public debate' ends up as media debate, when issues are inevitably treated in a simplistic way. Locally, purchasers have sometimes met with apathy when attempting to debate general principles, while moves to restrict or close services typically prompt vocal opposition."

There are other problems, too. For example, Moore again:

"Asking the general public to weigh up the merits of different demands can produce results which conflict with public health principles. People frequently rank glamorous, high technology services, such as liver transplants, above far more effective and cost effective interventions, like child immunisation and family planning."

Rather than seeking to involve the public at a strategic macro or meso (i.e. local) level in making trade-offs about which sectors or care groups should receive a higher priority, when information and understanding are absent, a better way of involving the public may be at a micro level, i.e. on a one-to-one basis through a more equal partnership with doctors in making decisions about individual treatment (Hunter, 1993; Moore, 1996). Such an approach is central to effective implicit rationing as articulated through the notion of 'muddling through elegantly'.

This is not to suggest that all attempts at public involvement at a higher level are fatally flawed. To tackle the 'democratic deficit' perceived to exist, there have been numerous experiments with, *inter alia*, health panels, focus groups and citizens' juries (Cooper *et al.*, 1995; Lenaghan, 1997; Richardson, 1997). Citizens' juries have received a great deal of attention in the UK and build on earlier models developed in Germany and the USA. The concept draws on the jury system in the courts, arguably the most participative institution in the British state.

The principle uniting all models of citizens' juries is that ordinary citizens, without vested interests or expertise, are able to make sound polit-ical decisions if they have enough information and time to consider the issue at stake. Citizens' juries attempt to overcome the passivity which representative government generally assumes and to encourage active citizenship through creative participation. They are not intended to make binding decisions but to consider proposals and make comments and recommendations. It has been suggested that citizens' juries should not be seen in isolation but as one of several innovations, such as deliberative opinion polls, mediation groups, referenda and electronic town meetings, designed to strengthen democracy (Stewart *et al.*, 1994). A number of pilot juries have met and been evaluated in the UK. Many valuable lessons can be learned from these pilot schemes. A key one, apart from the high cost of each jury (in the region of £25 000), is that public enthusiasm for juries is tempered by deep cynicism about the possibility of them making a difference. After all, health authorities are not required to take their views into account or even to offer feedback on how the jury's views have been treated.

Richardson, in her evaluation of the Somerset health panels, concluded that, contrary to the doubts of some analysts, ordinary people are not only willing to take part in rationing discussions but are also capable of exploring complex issues and funding priorities with some sensitivity (Richardson, 1997). She asserts that the public can overcome the information asymmetry problem and learn about NHS budget limitations and weigh issues on their merits as well as reflect on the wider implications of their arguments. Richardson believes the results of the Somerset initiative to be sufficiently encouraging to warrant their testing through further similar consultation exercises.

From implicit to explicit rationing and back again?

It appears from reviewing the debate and the reality in the UK, and taking account of developments elsewhere in Europe and beyond, that when all the various initiatives and commission reports on rationing are studied, devising acceptable and agreed criteria for rationing is "a peculiarly intractable endeavour, where practice lags behind rhetoric" (Klein *et al.*, 1996, p. 118). Even in New Zealand, often held up as an example of a country which has done more than any other to involve the public at a macro level in rationing decisions, there is a lack of hard evidence as distinct from speculation as to how effective these efforts have been (Ham and Coulter, 2000). There is no generally acceptable technical fix, such as quality adjusted life years (QALYs), for resolving the dilemma posed by finite resources. Nor is there a universal prescription which can be applied. It is not surprising, therefore, for the World Health Organization (WHO) to conclude its review of health care reform issues in Europe by stating that despite various initiatives to examine priority-setting on a more systematic and explicit basis, "overall, there has not been any substantial reductions in the coverage or package of benefits offered by [countries'] statutory systems" (WHO, 1996, p. 106).

If, in keeping with the spirit of the times, rationing is to be explicit and underpinned by a set of publicly agreed principles, then there are a number of variations on this particular theme. At one end of the spectrum there is the option of specifying very tight criteria governing services to be included (and conversely excluded). This is the core service, or restricted menu or limited list approach. It is sometimes known as the guaranteed entitlement to health care and has, in most countries, been found wanting. New Zealand, where a core service approach was attempted, quickly came to the view that such an approach could not be made to work or be made politically acceptable.

At the other extreme is what may be termed the ethically sound approach. This approach does not seek to exclude any particular service or treatment but rather to establish an agreed public framework of ethics or principles to guide, and not prescribe, decision making over who should and should not receive treatment. Sweden is perhaps the best example of this approach but it is dismissed by the hard men (for it is men) of rationing who favour hard choices and regard the Swedish 'ethical platform' as vague, insufficiently

precise to operationalize and ducking the difficult choices that must be made.

In between these extremes are various approaches, notably the Dutch one, which seeks to combine elements of both approaches: the soft approach to defining and gaining public acceptance for a set of principles to assist in the making of choices, and the hard approach involving the making of specific decisions about who should get treatment (and, by definition, if resources are limited, who should be denied it).

Another middle way, and one adopted by the UK, is to firm-up on the evidence base and to refuse to talk of rationing but, instead, use the term priority-setting. Recalling the point made earlier, whereas rationing may entail the denial of a treatment regardless of its effectiveness simply because there is not enough to go round, priority-setting is much more concerned with choosing on the basis of what is effective and works. As long as ineffective procedures are being provided, it is wrong, or at least premature, to talk of rationing. As the Anti-rationing Group asserts, there is an *a priori* need to terminate ineffective medical interventions (Roberts *et al.*, 1995).

Explicit rationing sounds find in theory—who in an ideal world could possibly be against an open transparent system of arriving at decisions? However, the world is not ideal. It is messy, turbulent, ambivalent and full of paradox. We should not seek to deny or eliminate such aspects but to manage them better. Explicit rationing is not without pitfalls. Five merit brief comment.

Whose voice?

Whose voice is being articulated when public opinion is sought on establishing priorities in health care? Is it the articulate middle class? The 'worried well'? Attempts to engage the public carry the danger of a low priority being attached to the needs of people with a mental illness, a mental handicap, a physical disability, those who are old and those who are poor and inarticulate. Who will act as advocates on their behalf? Participation is inherently inegalitarian. How far it can and should be relied on in rationing decisions are crucial questions. Even those who favour greater public participation warn that "it can advantage the already privileged through their ability to manipulate the information process and can sacrifice the common good to sectional interpretations of it" (Doyal and Gough, 1991). Of course, it is not impossible to access all sections of a community, but the expense and time involved in doing so may act as effective deterrents allowing the more assertive elements of public opinion to hold sway. Implicit rationing is often criticized for sanctioning an inequitable system where 'knowledgeable, sophisticated and aggressive patients are more able to have their needs satisfied than docile patients' (Mechanic, 1995, p. 1657). However, explicit rationing is also susceptible to a similar bias.

Quality of decision making

Could explicit decision making lead to more incremental and conservative decisions at the risk of preventing the development of innovative or different patterns of delivery? Is it possible that reallocating resources from, say, acute to community and primary care or long-term care, difficult though this has been to achieve in the past, could become even more difficult when processes which have been largely implicit become explicit? Merely by increasing the visibility of a decision process, and allowing many more individuals and groups access to it, the potential for conflict among key groups of decision makers is likely to increase (Mechanic, 1995). As Klein (1992, p. 5) argues:

"the greater the visibility of rationing in the sense of prioritisation, the more difficult it may become to steer resources towards the most vulnerable . . . groups. Lack of visibility may be a necessary condition for the political paternalism required to overcome both consumer and producer lobbies."

Power of numbers

As the debate over QALYs and other such techniques has revealed, numbers can have a curiously mesmerizing effect on managers and others required to produce and rely on them. Often, unfounded assumptions of certainty and precision seem to underpin the very hardness of numbers.

Such numbers are, however, an abstraction. They are not an observation of real life: they are generated and produced by a specific set of technical procedures which may be more or less comprehensible to the average manager or non-executive director. It becomes all too easy to forget the value base of numbers and to attach a degree of certainty and precision to them that may be quite unfounded or unwarranted (Carr-Hill, 1989). Whatever their value, such techniques should not supplant other, softer qualitative measures or indicators of quality.

Underfunding is the issue

Explicit rationing carries the danger that attention is diverted from the cause of the problem—lack of resources—to its symptoms. A restricted list or core service approach to health care services could lead policy makers to believe that there is some finite level of health care and level of resources that are appropriate.

When does covert become overt and vice versa?

The assumption that by being explicit and transparent there is no scope for manipulation and inequitable behaviour is simply naive. Explicit rules are by no means inviolable. As Mechanic concludes, "the rich and powerful if sufficiently motivated will always find ways to circumvent explicit criteria" (Mechanic, 1995, p. 1658).

These observations are not intended to imply an uncritical defence of the status quo which suffers from an excess of medical paternalism that is far from satisfactory. However, if advocates of an explicit approach believe human behaviour under an implicit approach to be flawed, then where is the evidence for believing that it should somehow be different under an explicit system? Zimmern (1996), for example, cautions against being too uncritical about the advantages of transparent and explicit decision making. Strengthening the rights and autonomy of the individual might be at the expense of the welfare of the collective. Whether or not this is an acceptable price to pay should at least be debated.

'Muddling through elegantly'

If overt rationing is a minefield strewn with major problems which could well prove to be as, if not more, intractable than those it seeks to address—a 'wicked issue' as it was described at the outset—then why not consider a rather more subtle and incremental approach which acknowledges the complexities of actual priority-setting? Such an approach has been termed 'muddling through elegantly' (Hunter, 1993, p. 1998).

Muddling through elegantly does not entail a conservative defence of the status quo. Rather, it acknowledges that improvements are necessary in how decisions about priorities are made, especially at a micro level where doctors and patients interact, but that these adjustments can be made within current arrangements backed by a system of procedural rights designed to ensure that the exercise of discretion in decision making is undertaken fairly, thereby ensuring that the principles of equity and equal treatment are upheld (Bynoe, 1996; Coote and Hunter, 1996).

Procedural rights are based on the principle of fair treatment (in the non-clinical sense). A set of procedural rights in health care might include: a right to be heard, a right to consistency in decision making, a right to relevance in decision making, a right to unbiased decisions, a right to reasons and a right to review. Procedural rights are different from substantive rights in that they are not about entitlement to substantive services but about entitlement to fair procedures in the way decisions are reached.

There is no mileage in a wholesale switch to a nationally determined and led system of explicit rationing that is itself unproven. Nobody denies that rationing gives rise to complex moral dilemmas. However, to face them explicitly in the manner proposed by the rational rationers may just be too difficult for society to contemplate. In support of this position, Gillon (1994, p. xxvii) writes:

"Until there is far greater social agreement and indeed understanding of these exceedingly complex issues, I believe that it is morally safer to seek gradual improvement in our current methods of trying to reconcile the competing moral concerns—to seek ways of 'muddling through elegantly' as Hunter advocates, rather than to be seduced by systems that seek to convert these essentially moral choices into apparently scientific numerical methods and formulae."

Conclusion

This short discourse on rationing health care has sought to counsel against adopting a system of explicit rationing that is not without its own particular flaws and weaknesses. Rationing is a wicked issue. As Stewart defines them, wicked issues are 'deeply intractable' and "imperfectly understood and to which solutions are not clear" (Stewart, 1998, p. 19). Health economists' techniques may be seductive in their attempt at precision and simplicity but they reduce the complexity and messiness of real-life policy puzzles and decisions in ways that ultimately are self-defeating.

We should resist abandoning an admittedly imperfect though still workable irrationality in favour of a spurious and possibly risky rationality for the reasons set out above. The goal should be to *satisfice* rather than to optimize. As Mechanic (1995, p. 1659) argues, "interest in making rationing explicit arises from the illusion that optimisation is possible". Because there is no realistic alternative to *satisficing*, whether from a practical, political or moral standpoint, a strategy of muddling through elegantly may hold particular appeal grounded as it is in pragmatic sensibility backed by a set of procedural rights governing the way in which individuals are treated and informed about decisions affecting them.

References

Aaron, H.J. and Schwartz, W.B. (1984) *The Painful Prescription: Rationing Hospital Care.* Washington: The Brookings Institution.

British Medical Association (1995) *Rationing Revisited: A Discussion Paper.* Health Policy and Economic Research Unit Discussion Paper No. 4. London: BMA.

Bynoe, I. (1996) *Beyond the Citizen's Charter.* London: Institute for Public Policy Research.

Califano, J.A. (1992) Rationing health care—the unnecessary solution. *University of Pennsylvania Law Review*, 140, 1525–1538.

Carr-Hill, R.A. (1989) Assumptions of the QALY procedure. *Social Science and Medicine*, 28, 469–77.

Cooper, L., Coote, A., Davies, A. and Jackson, C. (1995) *Voices Off: Tackling The Democratic Deficit*. London: Institute for Public Policy Research.

Coote, A. and Hunter, D.J. (1996) *New Agenda for Health*. London: Institute for Public Policy Research.

Coulter, A. and Ham, C. (eds) (2000) *The Global Challenge of Health Care Rationing*. Buckingham: Open University Press.

Doyal, L. and Gough, I. (1991) *A Theory Of Human Need*. London: Macmillan.

Eddy, D. (1994) Health systems reform: will controlling costs require rationing services? *Journal of the American Medical Association*, 272, 324–328.

Gillon, R. (1994) Introduction. In: Gillon, R. (ed.), *Principles of Health Care Ethics*. Chichester: Wiley & Sons

Grimley Evans, J. (1993) Summary. In: Grimley Evans, J., Goldacre, M.J., Hodkinson, H.M., Lamb, S. and Savory, M. *Health and Function in the Third Age*. Papers prepared for the Carnegie Inquiry into the Third Age. London: Nuffield Provincial Hospitals Trust.

Ham, C. and Coulter, A. (2000) Conclusion: where are we now? In: Coulter, A. and Ham, C. (eds), *The Global Challenge of Health Care Rationing*. Buckingham: Open University Press.

Harrison, S. and Hunter, D.J. (1994) *Rationing Health Care*. London: Institute for Public Policy Research.

House of Commons Health Committee (1995). *Priority-setting in the NHS: Purchasing*. First report, session 1994–95, volume II, minutes of evidence and appendices, HC 134-II. London: HMSO.

Hughes, D. and Griffiths, L. (1996) "But if you look at the coronary anatomy . . .": risk and rationing in cardiac surgery. *Sociology of Health and Illness*, 18, 172–197.

Hunter, D.J. (1993) *Rationing Dilemmas in Health Care*. Research paper number 8. Birmingham: National Association of Health Authorities and Trusts.

Hunter, D.J. (1998) *Desperately Seeking Solutions: Rationing Health Care*. Harlow: Longman.

Klein, R. (1992) Dilemmas and decisions. *Health Management Quarterly*, xiv, 2–5.

Klein, R. (1995). *The New Politics of the NHS*, 3rd edn. Harlow: Longman.

Klein, R. (1997) Defining a package of healthcare services the NHS is responsible for: the case against. *British Medical Journal*, 314, 506–509.

Klein, R., Day, P. and Redmayne, S. (1996) *Managing Scarcity: Priority-setting and Rationing in the NHS*. Buckingham: Open University Press.

Lenaghan, J. (1997) Citizens juries: towards best practice. *British Journal of Health Care Management*, 3, 20–22.

Loughlin, M. (1996) Rationing, barbarity and the economist's perspective. *Health Care Analysis*, 4, 146–156.

Mechanic, D. (1995) Dilemmas in rationing health care services: the case for implicit rationing. *British Medical Journal*, 310, 1655–1659.

Ministry of Welfare, Health and Cultural Affairs (1992) *Choices in Health Care*. A report by the Government Committee on Choices in Health Care. Rijswijk: The Netherlands. Ministry of Welfare, Health and Cultural Affairs.

Moore, W. (1996) *Hard Choices: Priority-setting in the NHS*. Birmingham: National Association for Health Authorities and Trusts.

New, B. and Le Grand, J. (1996) *Rationing in the NHS: Principles and Pragmatism*. London: King's Fund.

Richardson, A. (1997) Determining priorities for purchasers: the public response to rationing within the NHS. *Journal of Management in Medicine*, 11, 222–232.

Roberts, C., Crosby, D., Dunn, R., Evans, K., Grundy, P., Hopkins, R., Jones, J.H., Lewis, P., Vetter, N. and Walker, P. (1995) Rationing is a desperate measure. *Health Service Journal*, 105, 15.

Smith, R. (1995) Editorial: rationing: the debate we have to have. *British Medical Journal*, 310, 686.

Stewart, J. (1998) Advance or retreat from the traditions of public administration to the new public management and beyond. *Public Policy and Administration*, 13, 12–27.

Stewart, J., Kendall, E. and Coote, A. (1994) *Citizens' Juries*. London: Institute for Public Policy Research.

Wildavsky, A. (1979) *The Art and Craft of Policy Analysis*. London: Macmillan.

World Health Organisation (1996) *European Health Care Reform: Analysis Of Current Strategies*. Copenhagen: WHO Regional Office for Europe.

Zimmern, R. (1996) Beyond effectiveness: the appropriateness of clinical care—what needs to happen now. Transcript of a speech to the National Medical Directors and Directors of Public Health Meeting, November.

45 | Treatment pressures, coercion and compulsion

G. Szmukler and P. Appelbaum

Introduction

In the last half of the 20th century, psychiatrists and other mental health clinicians became increasingly sensitive to the effects and implications of treatment that was not fully consensual. The number of psychiatric in-patients declined by more than two-thirds during that period, much of this accounted for by a diminution in the use of long-term involuntary hospitalization. Many countries have tightened their procedures and standards for involuntary commitment, making it harder to hospitalize patients against their will (Appelbaum, 1997). Mental health systems have worked harder to protect patients' liberty interests, and to avoid circumstances in which non-consensual treatment occurs.

Nonetheless, the nature of mental illness—with patients frequently manifesting denial of their disorder or of a need for care—and the public's concerns about the propensity of mentally ill persons to injure others or themselves, will probably make it impossible for non-consensual treatment ever to be abandoned completely. Indeed, with the movement to community care, new mechanisms for exerting pressures on patients have developed in such services as assertive community treatment (ACT) (Sledge *et al.*, 1995; Meuser *et al.*, 1998; Stein and Santos, 1998). A major focus of ACT—usually targeted at persons with chronic mental illness who are thought likely to drift away from care—is to prevent defaulting from treatment, since loss of contact is likely to lead to relapse and readmission to hospital. Treatment is brought assertively *to* the patient making disengagement difficult. 'Compliance'

with medication is often a central issue. In the background also remains the possibility of compulsory admission to hospital.

The degree to which services exert treatment pressures on patients in the community is also influenced by community attitudes to community care (Holloway, 1996). If community care is seen as failing, or the mentally ill are seen as posing a risk to the public, the practice of community mental health teams may shift, perhaps with little awareness, to increasing pressure on patients to accept treatment.

This chapter has three aims:

(i) To outline a spectrum of treatment pressures in contemporary practice, drawing ethically relevant distinctions between them.

(ii) To consider when the exercise of such treatment pressures can be justified.

(iii) To suggest approaches aimed at reducing the need for treatment pressures in psychiatric services.

A range of treatment pressures

The term 'coercion' is often used in a way that makes its meaning almost synonymous with pressures exerted by one person (or organization) on another with the intention of making the latter act in accordance with the wishes of the former. We prefer to use the less moralized term 'treatment pressures'; as we shall see, 'coercion' is best applied to specific types of pressure. Within the concept of 'treatment pressures', we cover the whole range of interventions aimed at inducing patients to accept treatment which they initially have declined or seem likely to decline. Since our purpose is a discussion of ethics in treatment, the key question is whether we can identify morally relevant distinctions within the range of treatment pressures.

The actions of non-professionals such as family members are often included in discussions of coercion. Sometimes the patient's mental disorder itself is called 'coercive' in that it may limit autonomous action. We shall restrict our considerations to the actions of mental health professionals. All relationships can manifest power struggles in one form or another but, since we are concerned with mental health services and the examination of justifiable actions by team members, we exclude family and non-professional relationships (apart from actions which might be instigated by professionals).

A recent volume dealing with coercion and 'aggressive community treatment' contains a series of contributions which, while differing in terminology or detail, all point to a range of pressures on patients to accept treatment (Berg and Bonnie, 1996; Diamond, 1996; Hiday, 1996; Solomon, 1996; Susser and Roche, 1996). We attempt to build on these contributions to outline a hierarchy of pressures for which commensurate justifications must be provided. Our spectrum of pressures is as follows:

- persuasion;
- leverage;
- inducements;
- threats; and
- compulsory treatment (in the community or as an in-patient).

In order to help clarify the distinctions we are making, we present a case vignette. The patient's reluctance to take treatment is followed by a number of possible responses by the patient's keyworker or mental health team representing different types of pressure.

Patient A, aged 36 years, has suffered from an illness diagnosed as schizophrenia for 12 years. He was born in Ghana and came to the UK with his parents at the age of 6. His parents separated when he was 10, his father returning to Ghana. After doing well at a public school, A read Law at a college of London University. It was soon after gaining his degree that he became ill. He subsequently never practised. He lives in a small flat on his own, not far from his mother. A has no friends.

During the early phases of his illness, he suffered from florid symptoms, mainly auditory hallucinations and bizarre persecutory delusions. Over time, negative symptoms have become more prominent, although at times of relapse he shows marked formal thought disorder and loud inappropriate laughter. At these times, he also neglects himself severely and has, presumably because of distractibility, left his gas cooker to burn resulting in the fire brigade being called out on a number of occasions. Consequently, the Council has threatened him with eviction in the past. His flat becomes extremely filthy while A spends most of his time reading poetry or law books. However, at these times, he is unable to give a coherent account of their content.

When taking medication (currently an antipsychotic drug, risperidone) positive symptoms are absent and his self-care is reasonable. A's concentration is much improved and he engages in adult education courses and day centre programmes. He is able to cook simple meals but also visits his mother almost daily for supper.

A has had seven admissions to hospital, most of them on a compulsory order. He is always reluctant to take medication. He denies that he currently suffers from a mental disorder, although he says he may have done so in the past. Medication, he maintains, impairs his sleep and concentration, and slows him down. He argues that he is better off without. His treatment team and his mother are in no doubt that his condition invariably deteriorates when he is off medication.

For 4 years, the same community psychiatric nurse (CPN) has seen A at home, weekly. The relationship is clearly valued by the patient. They talk about everyday stresses as well as A's disappointment at not having lived up to his father's expectations or grief about not having a family of his own. Together, they engage in a variety of practical activities including cleaning, shopping, budgeting and paying bills. Furthermore, the CPN acts as an advocate to help A obtain assistance from social and non-statutory agencies, and regularly accompanies him to his GP or the general hospital for treatment of hypertension and psoriasis. While a psychiatric social worker (PSW) is also involved, A prefers help from the CPN who often acts as an intermediary for the PSW in arranging benefits or a bus pass (which, to the chagrin of the local authority, he regularly loses when unwell). When the CPN goes on leave, A says he misses him and on occasions his behaviour has become more disorganized.

After a relatively stable period of 6 months following a compulsory admission to hospital, A tells his consultant psychiatrist and CPN that he wishes to discontinue medication.

Persuasion

The CPN rehearses the reasons for believing that A suffers from a mental illness. He goes through the past history to show that whenever A discontinues medication, relapse commences 1 or 2 months later. The benefits as well as the side effects of medication are discussed. Possible adjustments of dose are considered. The patient's arguments are heeded and attempts are made to answer them.

Least problematic is *persuasion*, an appeal to reason. The discussion with the patient revolves around an arguably realistic appraisal of the benefits and risks of treatment. There is a respect for the patient's arguments and the treatment is discussed in the context of his or her value system. The process does not go beyond a debate.

Leverage

The CPN looks saddened by A's reluctance to take medication. He sighs, and shakes his head while looking distractedly out of the window. A limp handshake accompanies the CPN's departure. Perhaps they can talk about it some more next time.

Since the clinician (keyworker, case manager), especially in ACT programmes, may have established a relationship with the patient broader in scope and more intimate than a traditional patient–clinician relationship, opportunities for other kinds of pressure arise. Keyworkers engage with patients in their ordinary community settings to help with many basic skills. They may spend long periods with the patient assisting with budgeting, shopping or cooking, attending appointments with the patient to see other professionals, advocating for services, and working closely with carers, housing officers and other key social agencies. The patient may develop a significant degree of emotional dependency on the keyworker. *Leverage* (or 'interpersonal pressure') may be exercised through this dependency. The patient may wish to please someone who has proved helpful, or agree to a clinician's proposal in reaction to signs of disappointment in the clinician when a treatment suggestion is rejected. Although threats are not expressed, patients may fear the loss of valued aspects of their care should they fail to comply with a treatment proposal.

Inducement

The CPN points out that A's furniture looks in need of replacement. A agrees. The CPN says that there is a second-hand furniture store where he has recently taken other patients. The owner is sympathetic to people with mental health problems, offering substantial discounts. If A were to remain well, and this would require his taking medication, the CPN will take him. Perhaps a small grant of money towards buying the furniture could be arranged through a voluntary Trust. Again, A would need to be well to take advantage of this. Also, the CPN has on his own initiative arranged with a top football club for a small number of tickets for a number of games this season. A could have one if he took his medication.

Threat

(i) The CPN reminds A that he might be eligible for a higher rate of his disability allowance. To get it, however, would require help with filling in forms and presenting his case. An appeal might be

necessary if he is rejected the first time. The CPN says he would not be prepared to do this if A does not accept treatment (including medication).

(ii) The CPN then goes on to say that if A will not take medication, there is no point in his visiting so frequently. Efforts to help A must come to naught if A refuses medication. He will monitor his condition monthly. There is no point going on as before.

The next level of pressure arises with the introduction of 'if . . . then' propositions. *If* the patient accepts treatment A, *then* the clinician will do X; or *if* the patient does not accept treatment A, the clinician will do Y. At this point, application of the term *coercion* is likely to be considered. A helpful account by Wertheimer (1993) argues that no simple definition of 'coercion' can be offered. He argues that *threats* coerce but *offers* generally do not:

"The crux of the distinction between threats and offers is that A makes a threat when B will be worse off than in some relevant base-line position if B does not accept A's proposal, but that A makes an offer when B will be no worse off than in some relevant base-line position if B does not accept A's proposal."

Therefore, the key to understanding what counts as a coercive proposal is properly to fix the *moral baseline.* Wertheimer gives an example to clarify this concept: A comes upon B who is drowning. A proposes to rescue B on condition that B pays A a large sum of money. There are no other potential rescuers. Has A made a threat or an offer? The answer depends on where we set the baseline. Under a moral test, the key issue is whether A is *morally required* to rescue B (or whether B has a *right* to be rescued by A). If A is morally required to rescue B, then B's baseline includes a right to being saved by A.. A's proposal is therefore a threat. On the other hand, if A is not morally required to rescue B, then A's proposal is an offer.

A threat thus anticipates making the recipient worse off according to the relevant moral base-line, while an offer—even if declined—typically does not. Threatening to remove something to which the subject is *entitled* (e.g. a housing benefit determined by legal decree) makes the subject worse off if he or she does not accede. An offer of something which is not an entitlement but is in the nature of extra assistance (e.g. a mental health worker having a connection with a second-hand furniture dealer who gives special discounts) made on condition that the patient complies with the treatment would, if rejected, not make the patient worse off compared with the relevant moral base-line—what his or her position would have been if the offer had never been made. On the other hand, conditional access to monetary benefits (statutory entitlements), as occurs when some patients in the USA have a 'representative payee' under Supplemental Security Income/Social Security Disability Insurance (SSI/SSDI) who only gives the patients their benefits when they comply with treatment is on this account coercive. The 'offer' to re-instate an entitlement already withdrawn would also be coercive. These circumstances constitute exceptions to the usual rule that offers cannot coerce.

Wertheimer (1993) describes other, subsidiary features often associated with coercion but which do not define it. These may include the subjective experience of being constrained, a restriction on one's autonomy, a reduction of choice and the mitigation of moral or legal responsibility (including freely given consent).

Allied to threats is *deception.* Failing to correct a patient's misconception about the consequences of not accepting treatment could be construed as coercive. It is possible that some out-patient commitment orders depend for their effectiveness on a patient's misapprehension concerning the consequences of failing to comply. The patient may falsely believe that transgression of the order will result in rehospitalization or enforced treatment, but it may in fact only permit the conveying of the patient to a treatment facility or an assessment for compulsory in-patient treatment (Munetz *et al.,* 1997).

In our hierarchy of pressures, we thus place *offers* (or inducements) before *threats.* Only the latter would count as *coercive,* as would presumably the exercise of compulsion in treatment described below.

An important corollary follows in respect of complex mental health services such as those operating in the community today. Defining the moral baseline requires that a mental health service defines a patient's entitlements to various components of health care as well as help to be offered in accessing social and other forms of care. Threats should then be more easily distinguished from offers. Such 'entitlements' could be spelt out in a service's or community mental health team's objectives, operational policies and statements about its relationships with other agencies. Given the large variety of interventions offered by community mental health teams and an ethos which prizes innovation and problem solving, such a task could be a daunting one. However, our analysis would indicate that it is necessary. Another interesting consequence arises. The greater the range of services a community mental health team offers its patients, the greater the scope for coercive threats. It might further be asked whether it is fair, or on what basis, some patients should be offered inducements and not others.

Although the law may give a community mental health team discretion to make entitlements conditional on treatment, there remain other considerations of an ethical kind as to whether it is right to do so.

In many instances, perhaps the majority, where a patient is reluctant to accept treatment, a variety of pressures of the types described above may be exerted in the course of an interview with the patient; combinations of persuasion, leverage, inducements and threats may be employed. In such cases, the level of pressure might be best characterised as residing at the highest level reached within our hierarchy.

Compulsion

New legislation has recently been introduced establishing a form of involuntary out-patient treatment, 'community treatment orders' (CTOs). After discontinuing medication, A soon starts to relapse. Again he is involuntarily admitted to hospital in a severely neglected state. He continues to deny he is ill or that he needs treatment. This time he is discharged on a CTO that requires that he take medication in the community. Failure to do so will lead to his recall to hospital.

Next in our hierarchy of pressures is *compulsion* (backed up by force supported by legal statute). As the locus of treatment has shifted to the community and concerns about non-adherence to treatment have grown, a number of jurisdictions have introduced *out-patient commitment* orders. Three major types can be discerned:

(i)   As a substitute for hospital admission: the out-patient commitment order is considered a less restrictive alternative to compulsory in-patient admission, when alternatives to compulsory treatment have been exhausted.

(ii) To facilitate earlier discharge from hospital (a form of conditional discharge): although the patient may not be well enough for full discharge and requires continued treatment under compulsion, this can be obtained in the community as an alternative to the hospital.

(iii) To prevent relapse: this type of order is applied where there is a proven history of relapse secondary to discontinuation of treatment, usually medication, and relapse is believed to be associated with significant risk to the patient or others.

Out-patient commitment orders carry varying powers. Some allow recall of the patient for compulsory treatment as an in-patient. Others are limited to forced medication 'in the community', usually achieved by conveying the patient to a clinic where an injection is administered. Still others only permit non-compliant patients to be brought involuntarily to a clinic to be subject to persuasion, leverage or inducements; coercive treatment *per se* is not authorized. Out-patient commitment orders also vary in the range of conditions attached to the order (e.g. specification of clinician, clinic, frequency of reviews, treatments, residence) and their duration (Hiday, 1996). Finally, there is the option of compulsory admission to hospital.

Objective and subjective 'coercion'

An important dimension in thinking about treatment pressures, including coercion, involves the distinction between 'objective' and 'subjective' aspects (Hiday, 1992; Rogers, 1993; Lidz *et al.*, 1995; Hoge *et al.*, 1997). The subjective experience of feeling coerced may not follow an 'objective' schema such as the one outlined above (Hiday, 1992). From the patient's perspective, this may be the most important issue in coercion, and services should aim to minimise subjective coercion. Approaches to reducing the need for coercion, to be discussed later, may also be effective in minimising subjective coercion.

However, for the clinician seeking to act ethically in pressing a reluctant patient to accept treatment, there is a need to use morally relevant distinctions of an 'objective' kind to help him or her make justifiable decisions. The hierarchy we have outlined is an attempt to meet this need, but it will require adjustment to take account of a particular patient's preferences and values. For example, a patient may regard a long-term outpatient commitment order, say lasting a year, aimed at preventing relapse and demanding medication associated with troubling side effects as being more 'coercive' than a shorter period, say of 4 weeks, of compulsory treatment as an in-patient. Some of the subsidiary characteristics of coercion as described by Wertheimer (1993) could be of relevance here. Within the domain of *compulsory treatment*, there may be variations in restrictions on autonomy or of choice, as well as the subjective experience of constraint.

Research on 'coercion' and compulsory treatment

Although the main purpose of this chapter is to examine coercion from an ethical point of view, a brief account of research in this area will remind us that there are relevant empirical questions that also need to be addressed. Compulsory treatment might be justified at times in the interests of the patient's health or safety, for which the patient may later be grateful, but there may, on the other hand, also be negative consequences. These include alienation of the patient from the service with less likelihood of his or her agreeing to treatment later and therefore ultimately suffering a poorer outcome; the possibility of treatment being less effective if it is imposed against the patient's wishes; and a threatening treatment environment which, because of fears of coercion, may discourage other patients from seeking help from which they, as well as society as a whole, might benefit. (Winick, 1997).

Most research to date has focused on involuntary hospitalization. There is a substantial literature examining changes in attitude to compulsory in-patient treatment, before and after (see comprehensive review by Hiday, 1992). A general finding is that the majority of patients develop a positive attitude to the treatment, but a sizeable minority do not. However, most studies suffer from significant methodological deficiencies, including non-representative patient groups and retesting while the patient is still an in-patient, thus introducing the possibility that the patient may be responding positively to questions about non-consensual treatment out of a wish to please in the hope that discharge will occur sooner. Positive attitudes at discharge are associated with a greater expectation of improvement at the time of admission and a better response to treatment during admission. Whether patients are less likely to engage in follow-up care or to have poorer outcomes following a compulsory admission is not known. Of course, many if not most patients could never ethically be randomized in a controlled trial to compare the effects of voluntary and involuntary care.

Recent studies, funded by the Research Network on Mental Health and the Law of the John D. and Catherine T. MacArthur Foundation, have clarified the distinction between 'subjective' and 'objective' aspects of 'coercion' (Lidz *et al.*, 1995; Hoge *et al.*, 1997; Hiday *et al.*, 1997; Lidz *et al.*, 1998). Valid research instruments have been developed, and their application has shown that the experience of coercion during the admission process is strongly associated with the degree of 'procedural justice' experienced by the patient (Lidz *et al.*, 1995). Patients are likely to feel less coerced if they believe that others act out of concern for them, treat them fairly and with respect, give them a chance to tell their side of the story, and consider what was said in making the decision. 'Negative' pressures, such as threats or force, engender more perceived coercion than 'positive' pressures, such as persuasion and inducements (Hoge *et al.*, 1997; Lidz *et al.*, 1998). Research increasingly is focusing on whether perceived coercion may be an important predictor of long-term outcome. There is evidence that patients perceiving high coercion in their admission to hospital are more likely at follow-up to have negative attitudes to services, to use them less, to have poor expectations of treatment and to have poorer symptomatic outcomes (Kaltiala-Heino *et al.*, 1997).

Coercion in community treatment has been little studied. Luckstead and Coursey (1995) found that a large proportion of patients, in retrospect, felt that being pressured into treatment was justified. ACT studies generally have found that patient satisfaction is reported as being higher than with in-patient treatment, but measures of satisfaction have tended to be weak (Gerber and Prince, 1999).

A series of out-patient commitment studies, uncontrolled and using before versus after comparisons, have found that following out-patient commitment, patients are admitted less often and experience fewer days as in-patients (reviewed by Swartz *et al.*, 1995; Hiday, 1996). However, the concomitant introduction of out-patient commitment and significant service changes, including a greater emphasis on community treatment and reduction in bed use, may make it difficult to identify the actual cause of the changes observed. Perhaps these service changes on their own were responsible for the positive outcomes attributed to out-patient commitment (Swartz *et al.*, 1995; Swanson *et al.*, 1997). If community services are poor, out-patient commitment is ineffective (Bar El *et al.*, 1998). When attempts have been made to match patients subjected to out-patient commitment with those having similar characteristics but not committed, differences tend to shrink (Geller *et al.*, 1998). Two recent randomized controlled trials comparing out-patient commitment with the same range of services offered without compulsion reached somewhat discrepant findings. A New York study found no differences in outcome

measures (including arrest, rehospitalization and quality of life) between the two groups (Policy Research Associates, 1998). A study in North Carolina also revealed no significant differences between the two groups as a whole, but did find, on secondary analysis, significantly reduced rates of rehospitalization and violence for the group receiving out-patient commitment, as long as commitment was sustained beyond 6 months, and service intensity exceeded three contacts per month (Swanson, *et al.*, 2000; Swartz, *et al.*, 2000). Definitive conclusions will have to await extension and attempted replication of these findings. A majority of patients may report satisfaction with out-patient commitment, but appear to make these ratings in comparison with hospital treatment (Hiday, 1992, 1996; Scheid-Cook, 1993).

Justifications for treatment pressures, coercion or compulsion

Two types of justification are usually offered for applying treatment pressures on a patient who declines:

- treatment is in the patient's 'best interests' (or 'health or safety'); or
- treatment is needed for the protection of others.

If a hierarchy of treatment pressures on reluctant patients is defined as above, then one would ask for a stronger justification the more coercive the pressure to be exerted.

Justification in the best interests of the patient

Before the focus on treatment in the community, the major form of treatment pressure revolved around compulsory treatment in hospital, or its threat. Criteria for involuntary admission embodied in mental health legislation generally rely on evidence of substantial dangers to the patient's health or safety that leave no alternative to inpatient care. In the community, however, a wider spectrum of risks or degrees of danger are identified by professionals in closer proximity to the daily lives of their patients. Patients may be caring for themselves poorly and living in dreadful conditions. They may suffer from physical disorders that require treatment they are incapable of seeking. A hard-won tenancy may be jeopardized by the patient's failure to take care of an apartment. Significant supportive relationships may be on the verge of breaking down. The patient may be vulnerable to exploitation by others or incapable of managing an already meagre budget. Criteria of the type set down in mental health legislation governing involuntary hospitalization are simply not sensitive to the broader range of risk encountered in community settings. Nor are they sensitive to value and cultural differences in the complex multi-cultural societies of today, and their role in determining what is in the 'best interests' of a person.

Linking justifications for treatment pressures in the spectrum outlined above to the spectrum of risks seen in the community thus requires a broader, more flexible ethical framework. It must be able to deal with questions of value that often loom large. For example, one might ask whose values are being served by the emphasis on avoiding hospital admissions—the patient's, or the mental health services'?

We outline two 'best interests' frameworks, one deriving from an analysis of paternalistic actions and the other from an analysis of capacity (or mental competence).

A framework based on 'paternalism'

Culver and Gert (1982) propose that a person is acting paternalistically towards another if his action benefits the other; his action involves violating a moral rule with regard to the other; and his action does not have the other's past, present or immediately forthcoming consent.

Agreement between clinicians on when paternalistic actions are appropriate may be difficult to achieve. Beauchamp and Childress (1994) have characterized the difficulties thus:

"The problem of medical paternalism is the problem of putting just the right specification and balance of physician beneficence and patient autonomy in the patient-physician relationship. It is a messy complicated problem, and coherence is difficult to achieve. Paternalistic intervention requires persons of good judgement as well as persons with well developed principles able to confront contingent conflicts."

The approach to 'paternalistic' actions of Culver and Gert (1982) may be helpful. In justifying a paternalistic act, a series of pertinent questions can be asked:

(i)   What are the moral rules that would be violated if the clinician were to act against the patient's wishes (e.g. limiting freedom of choice, causing psychological pain)? What thus are the evils to be perpetrated on the patient and for how long will they last?

(ii) What is the seriousness of the evils to be avoided through the paternalistic intervention (e.g. death, disability, worsening of the psychiatric disorder), and what is their likelihood?

(iii) How does the clinician rank the two sets of evils compared with the patient?

(iv) Is the patient's preference when comparing the evils to be avoided with the evils to be incurred, irrational, i.e. does the patient have a rational reason to prefer an outcome with apparently greater evils?

(v)   Can the clinician advocate publicly for his or her ranking of the evils to be perpetrated compared with those to be avoided? Would most rational people agree that this kind of moral violation should in such circumstances be universally allowed?

A decision to exercize a specific treatment pressure in a specific circumstance would depend on a balance informed by the answers to these questions, although no algorithm exists to allow these determinations to be made in a rigorous (or possibly even replicable) way.

A framework based on 'capacity' and 'best interests'

'Mental incapacity' is assuming an increasing emphasis in justifying interventions against a patient's will, in psychiatry as well as in general medicine where it has been long established (Law Commission, 1995; Eastman and Peay, 1998; Grisso and Appelbaum, 1998; Szmukler and Holloway, 1998). As for physical disorders, it is difficult in psychiatry to argue for treatment against a person's wishes unless that person lacks the capacity (or 'competence', used by us synonymously) to make treatment decisions for themselves. Definitions of capacity vary, but common elements are the ability to understand and retain information relevant to the decision (including the consequences of deciding one way or the other), and the ability to use that information to make a decision. The latter includes the ability to appreciate that the information applies to the patient's predicament, the ability to reason with that information and the ability to exercise a choice (Law Commission, 1995; Grisso and Appelbaum, 1998).

Only if the patient fails on capacity, would treatment against a patient's wishes be considered (so-called 'soft paternalism'); but a further test must be passed—that treatment is in the patient's 'best interests'. Definitions of 'best interests' are difficult (McCubbin and Weisstub, 1998), but the UK Law Commission (1995) has proposed useful, practical guidance for deciding on the matter. Regard should be given to the following:

- the ascertainable past and present wishes and feelings of the person concerned, and the factors that person would consider if able to do so;
- the need to permit and encourage the person to participate or improve his or her ability to participate as fully as possible in anything done for and any decision affecting him or her;
- the views of other persons whom it is appropriate and practical to consult about the person's wishes and feelings and what would be in his or her best interests; and
- whether the purpose for which any action or decision is required can be achieved as effectively in a manner less restrictive of the person's freedom of action.

The two approaches described above, 'paternalistic' and 'capacity' based, are not as far apart as may appear at first sight. Most of the questions in the Culver and Gert analysis relate to determining what is in the patient's best interests. The fourth question concerns capacity—choosing what appears to presage a poor outcome, but for reasons which may be related to unconventional values. Within this context, the choice may be 'rational' or 'non-rational' (e.g. based on a set of religious beliefs).

We are not necessarily advocating adherence to either of the above frameworks. However, we insist that if community mental health teams are to exercise their powers to intervene in patients' lives in an ethical manner, an appropriate framework is required. Professionals should be as well versed in using such a framework as they are in assessing 'technical' problems, for example the likely benefits of interventions such as medication or psychological treatments.

The application of a framework such as one described above suggests that the degree of pressure to be used should be the minimum necessary, and that the justification should be stronger the more one moves along the spectrum from persuasion to direct force.

These principles should also be considered in relation to involuntary out-patient commitment. As discussed above, blunt criteria similar to those used in mental health legislation are difficult to apply when a wide spectrum of risk is identified by professionals in close and frequent contact with patients in the community. If out-patient commitment is an alternative to admission to hospital or is used to facilitate earlier discharge, *criteria for terminating the order* are essential. There is evidence that community treatment orders under the 'less restrictive alternative' concept continue long after the patient would have been discharged from hospital (McDonnell and Bartholomew, 1997). The criteria for termination of the order could be based on one of the frameworks above. For example, recovery of capacity to make treatment decisions or the compulsory treatment no longer being in the best interests of the patient would be appropriate.

The use of out-patient commitment to prevent relapse in patients with a history of persistent non-compliance and an illness which puts them at risk needs the most careful of justifications. Such orders are likely to be prolonged. Again, a justification in terms of *continuing incapacity* (or capacity which is 'fragile', i.e. only retained for brief periods) would, in our view, be the soundest. Furthermore, by framing justifications in terms of capacity to make treatment decisions, other options for non-consensual treatment also present themselves (e.g. advance directives, appointment of surrogate decision makers, court appointed managers; see Law Commission, 1995).

Justification based on protection of others

'Protection of others' is a common criterion for involuntary hospitalization, and generally also for out-patient commitment. However, in a community setting, the definition of risk to others is in danger of becoming elastic; in the same way as there is a spectrum of degrees of risk to the well-being of the patient, so is there one for risk to others. Expectations of community members may be based on the expected impact of interventions on community life, not necessarily on physical danger. For example, a community mental health team may be asked to intervene by neighbours or shopkeepers when a person's behaviour is disturbing or a nuisance. In a climate of concern that community care is failing and that the safety of the public is threatened, pressures to intervene intensify. Patients may become subject to treatment pressures not primarily in their own best interests, but in the context of a potentially broad interpretation of the 'protection of others'.

The 'protection of others' is often confused with 'best interests.' Unhelpful in this regard is their usual co-habitation in mental health legislation. However, they are logically distinct (Culver and Gert, 1982). When others ask to be allowed to determine what is in a patient's best interests, the legitimacy of their request depends on the patients' capacity to make treatment decisions for

themselves. It is the patient's welfare or health care needs which are at issue. In contrast, the protection of others does not turn on capacity to make treatment decisions, but on factors such as the magnitude of the risk of harm and the potential seriousness of the harm. The justification for coercive actions on the grounds of danger to others must rest on the accuracy with which that danger can be predicted.

Viewed thus, the fact that 'preventive' detention on the grounds of dangerousness to others is generally restricted only to those with a mental disorder is difficult to defend. After all, the mentally disordered are responsible for a very small proportion of serious violence (Taylor and Gunn, 1999). The likelihood of serious violence is higher in many non-mentally disordered persons, for example those who regularly become assaultative when intoxicated with drugs, or who habitually perpetrate domestic violence. Yet we do not force preventive interventions on such persons before they have been convicted of an offence. It has been argued that separate generic 'dangerousness' legislation is the most appropriate measure for preventing violence if that is deemed a significant societal goal. According to this approach, only *after* a court finds an unacceptable risk of dangerous behaviour based on sound evidence pertaining to the risks should questions about mental disorder or treatment arise. Current procedures, by reversing this sequence, discriminate against those suffering from a mental illness (Campbell and Heginbotham, 1991; Rosenman, 1994; Szmukler and Holloway, 1998).

Predicting serious violence also suffers from a major limitation carrying significant ethical implications. Despite the public's fears, incidents of serious violence are rare. The prediction of rare events inherently lacks accuracy. A predictive test even with extremely high 'sensitivity' (the proportion of violent people accurately predicted by the test) and 'specificity' (the proportion of non-violent people accurately predicted to be non-violent) will seriously err in the direction of false-positives (persons predicted by the test to be violent who are not) if the base rate of predicted events is low in the population being considered. This was demonstrated, for example, by a study involving patients of a community mental health team in South London (Shergill and Szmukler, 1997). Seventy three of 320 patients seen in 1 month were assessed by clinicians as posing a 'moderate' or 'severe' risk of violence to others over the next 6 months. Based on an expected rate of 20 violent incidents in 6 months and using the best available predictive statistics, seven of the 73 patients were likely to be violent. So also were 10 of the 245 low-risk patients. For grave offences such as homicide, the positive predictive value of even a hypothetical test with outstanding sensitivity and specificity is likely to be less than 1 in a 1000. If the risk of violence were to lead to coercive interventions, the moral cost of unnecessarily infringing the liberty of a large number of patients in order to prevent harm by a few needs justification.

We are left with some thorny issues. Society demands a degree of social control from mental health services. As services move into the community and see at close quarters the lives of their patients and those around them, dilemmas around risk may become especially problematic. Mental health professionals may accept an obligation to notify appropriate authorities if there is a *serious* risk of harm to others, but what is *serious* and who should instigate or implement coercive responses is a matter for debate. The potential for community mental health teams to expand activities directed at social control must be recognized. A dialogue between those advocating on behalf of patients with mental illness and a community often fearful of such persons in its midst is essential (and urgent) if abuses are to be avoided.

Reducing the need for pressure and coercion in treatment

Services can employ measures to reduce the need for exerting pressures on patients to accept treatment.

Make services as acceptable and attractive to users as possible

Traditionally, mental health service users have had little say in how services ostensibly created to help them are actually implemented. For services to become more responsive to patients' needs requires an active, not token, involvement of service users in their planning (Pilgrim and Waldron, 1998). Judgements of their quality must also give due attention to users' views and satisfaction. Users can make crucial contributions as members of management committees where they ensure that discussion, service developments and evaluations of quality and outcomes are seen from a users' as well as a providers' perspective. Advocacy services may also contribute in this regard, as well as systems for reviewing patient complaints. Some services have employed users and ex-users as workers with patients, claiming that they have more success in engaging reluctant patients than professional keyworkers.

In the 'real world' of mental health services, though, the limits of such an approach must be acknowledged. Improvement of services is often vitally dependent on public resources, and funding for mental health is rarely at the top of the governmental list of priorities. Thus, some amount of coercive care is likely to continue to take place that could be avoided by a more generous allocation of funds.

Enhance patients' involvement in planning their own care

Patients are likely to feel less coerced the more they play an active role in determining their treatment. Some recent initiatives are worth exploring further. In the UK, 'crisis cards' originated as a service user/voluntary sector initiative to facilitate access to an advocate and to state patients' preferences for care during an emergency when they might be too unwell to express their wishes clearly. 'Crisis cards' can be designed to be carried by the patient and can contain useful information about persons to contact, the patient's care plan and statements about the patient's wishes for treatment in a crisis. 'Crisis cards' have often been drawn up by the patient alone, without discussion with the mental health team. There is scope for this idea to be developed into what we have termed 'joint crisis plans' (Sutherby and Szmukler, 1998). Here the content of the card, though ultimately still determined by the patient, is negotiated with the treatment team when the patient is well enough to make competent judgements about what is in his or her best interests. The aim is to reach a joint agreement on the care plan.

Sutherby *et al.* (1999) have reported on the introduction of crisis cards and joint crisis plans in Camberwell, South London. Participation was offered to patients with a psychotic illness who were at high risk of relapse. During the limited study period, a substantial proportion, 40%, wished to develop a card. They chose to include a wide range of information including diagnosis, current treatment, contact information for carers and professionals, first signs of relapse and the preferred treatment for these, treatment preferences and refusals for established relapses, indications for admission and practical requests (e.g. who should ensure that domestic arrangements are not neglected in the case of admission). Independent assessment showed that patients experienced the process as non-coercive and believed that their views were respected. Follow-up, 6–12 months later, showed that the card was consulted in most crises. The information was considered helpful by patients and mental health professionals. A majority of the patients reported feeling empowered in determining details of their care. Thus a joint crisis plan could serve both a manifest, practical function in a crisis—to provide important information when patients are too ill to do so—as well as a latent, psychological one—exerting positive effects on patients' attitudes to their mental health problems and their treatment, and on their relationship with the clinical team.

Informal cards such as these also have the potential for further transformation into legally binding psychiatric 'advance directives' (Appelbaum, 1991; Backlar, 1995; Srebnick and La Fond, 1999). Such directives, anticipating relapse of a psychosis, embody the concept of the 'living will'. They could reconcile two apparently contradictory themes in the current practice of psychiatry—on the one hand, the need to provide non-consensual treatment in the community, and on the other, the promotion of patient autonomy. They could, for some, be an alternative to outpatient commitment orders. Challenges to their implementation are discussed by Backlar (1997) and Halpern and Szmukler (1997) and include the problem of evaluating the patient's competence—when it is adequate to make a directive, sufficiently inadequate to trigger its application and adequate enough to revoke a directive; ensuring the absence of coercion in drawing up the directive; mechanisms for appeal in cases of dispute; resource implications; mechanisms for making the directives available when treatment decisions need to be made; and clarifying relationships between advance directives and existing mental health legislation. Psychiatric advance directives are possible now in some jurisdictions in the USA. All states permit advance directives to be written for health care in general, and four states (Hawaii, Minnesota, Oregon and Wyoming) have statutes creating specific provisions for psychiatric advance directives. Data on utilization are limited, but the difficulties in the application of advance directives appear to have restricted their use (Backlar and McFarland, 1996). Despite this, advance directives might still find a place for some groups of seriously mentally ill patients.

'Crisis cards' and their variants could significantly reduce the number of situations in which clinicians find themselves needing to act against a patient's competent preferences. Many of the ethical dilemmas discussed above occur precisely at such times of crisis.

Advocacy services can help improve the dialogue between patients and clinicians and foster a better working relationship based on better mutual understanding. They can play a significant role in 'crisis card' planning and formulating advance statements.

Use approaches to de-escalate potentially coercive situations

Applying the principles derived from studies such as the MacArthur Foundation *coercion* project (Lidz *et al.*, 1995; Hoge *et al.*, 1997), though so far untested, may reduce the need for actual coercion as well as reduce patients' 'perceived' coercion. Where situations with the potential for coercive interactions arise, principles of 'procedural justice' can be borne in mind—treating the patient with respect and fairness, giving him or her a 'voice' and taking seriously what is said, and avoiding 'negative pressures' such as threats or force. It must be recognized, however, that such practices have the potential for 'sugar-coating' coercive measures, i.e. rendering them less objectionable to patients without reducing the amount of interference with their lives. This may lead to even more widespread use of coercive measures and demonstrates that attempts to reduce subjective coercion may constitute a double-edged sword.

Use pressure or coercion only when it is necessary

Applying pressures or coercive measures on patients only when justified and to a degree commensurate with the risks to the patient's best interests as discussed above should minimize their use. The multi-disciplinary team is an invaluable resource for ethical decision making of this kind since proposed interventions can be tested across a range of team members' perspectives on the values at stake. The views of informal and other formal care-givers should also be considered.

Conclusions

The scope for exerting pressures for treatment on reluctant patients is probably as great in the modern era of community care as it ever was. New forms exist, while ways of thinking about compulsory treatment hallowed by time and convention are not adequate to the task of dealing with the subtle gradations of risk and distinctions between interventions relevant to the practice of community psychiatry. We strongly suggest that being adept at dealing with an ethical framework for deciding when a specific treatment pressure is justified should be a core skill of members of community mental health teams. We have

outlined possible frameworks that can be adopted or form a basis for further thinking. If community mental health services are to flourish within complex, multi-cultural and ever-changing societies, they will need to rest on sound ethical foundations. The history of psychiatry, an enterprise in which questions of value are always to the fore, shows that a swing of the moral pendulum is never far away (Appelbaum, 1994).

References

Appelbaum, P.S. (1991) Advance directives for psychiatric treatment. *Hospital and Community Psychiatry*, 42, 983–984.

Appelbaum, P.S. (1994) *Almost a Revolution: Mental Health Law and the Limits of Change*. New York: Oxford University Press.

Appelbaum, P.S. (1997) Almost a revolution: an international perspective on the law of involuntary commitment. *Journal of the American Academy of Psychiatry and Law*, 25, 135–148.

Backlar, P. (1995) The longing for order: Oregon's medical advance directive for mental health treatment. *Community Mental Health Journal*, 31, 103–108.

Backlar, P. (1997) Anticipatory planning for psychiatric treatment is not quite the same as planning for end-of-life care. *Community Mental Health Journal*, 33, 261–268.

Backlar, P. and McFarland, B.H. (1996) A survey on the use of advance directives for mental health treatment in Oregon. *Psychiatric Services*, 47, 1387–1389.

Bar El, Y.C., Durst, R., Rabinowitz, J., Kalian, M., Teitelbaum, A. and Shlafman, M (1998) Implementation of order of compulsory ambulatory treatment in Jerusalem. *International Journal of Law and Psychiatry*, 21, 65–71.

Campbell, T. and Heginbotham, C. (1991) *Mental Illness: Prejudice, Discrimination and the Law*. Vermont: Dartmouth.

Beauchamp, T.L. and Childress, J.F. (1994) *Principles of Biomedical Ethics*, 4th edn. New York: Oxford University Press.

Berg, J.W. and Bonnie, R.J. (1996) When push comes to shove: aggressive community treatment and the law. In: Dennis, D.L. and Monahan, J. (eds), *Coercive and Aggressive Community Treatment: A New Frontier in Mental Health Law*. New York: Plenum Press, pp. 169–196.

Culver, C.N. and Gert, B. (1982) *Philosophy in Medicine: Conceptual and Ethical Issues in Medicine and Psychiatry*. Oxford: Oxford University Press.

Diamond, R.J. (1996) Coercion and tenacious treatment in the community: applications to the real world. In: Dennis, D.L. and Monahan, J. (eds), *Coercive and Aggressive Community Treatment: A New Frontier in Mental Health Law*. New York: Plenum Press, pp. 51–71.

Eastman, N. and Peay, J. (1998) Bournewood: an indefensible gap in mental health law. *British Medical Journal*, 317, 94–95.

Geller, J., Grudzinskas, A.J., Jr, McDermeit, M., Fisher, W.H. and Lawlor, T. (1998) The efficacy of involuntary outpatient treatment in Massachusetts. *Administration and Policy in Mental Health*, 25, 271–285.

Gerbner, G.J. and Prince, P.N. (1999) Measuring client satisfaction with assertive community treatment. *Psychiatric Services*, 50, 546–550.

Grisso, T. and Appelbaum, P.S. (1998) *Assessing Competence to Consent to Treatment: A Guide for Physicians and Other Health Professionals*. New York: Oxford University Press.

Halpern, A. and Szmukler, G. (1997) Psychiatric advance directives: reconciling autonomy and non-consensual treatment. *Psychiatric Bulletin*, 21, 323–327.

Hiday, A.H. (1996) Outpatient commitment: official coercion in the community. In: Dennis, D.L. and Monahan, J. (eds), *Coercive and Aggressive Community Treatment: A New Frontier in Mental Health Law*. New York: Plenum Press, pp. 29–47.

Hiday, V.A. (1992) Coercion in civil commitment: process, preferences, and outcome. *International Journal of Law and Psychiatry*, 15, 359–377.

Hiday, V.A., Swartz, M.S., Swanson, J. and Ryan Wagner, H. (1997) Patient perceptions of coercion in mental hospital admission. *International Journal of Law and Psychiatry*, 20, 227–241.

Hoge, S.K., Lidz, C.W., Eisenberg, M., Gardner, W., Monahan, J., Mulvey, E., Roth, L. and Bennett, N. (1997) Perceptions of coercion in the admission of voluntary and involuntary psychiatric patients. *International Journal of Law and Psychiatry*, 20, 167–181.

Holloway, F. (1996) Community psychiatric care: from libertarianism to coercion: moral panic and mental health policy in Britain. *Health Care Analysis*, 4, 235–244.

Kaltiala-Heino, R., Laippala, P. and Salokangas, K.R. (1997) Impact of coercion on treatment outcome. *International Journal of Law and Psychiatry*, 20, 311–322.

Law Commission (1995) *Mental Incapacity*. Report No. 231. London: HMSO.

Lidz, C., Hoge, S., Gardner, W., Bennett, N., Monahan, J., Mulvey, E. and Roth, L. (1995) Perceived coercion in mental hospital admission: pressures and process. *Archives of General Psychiatry*, 52, 1034–1039.

Lidz, C.W., Mulvey, E.P., Hoge, S.K., Kirsch, B.L. and Monahan, J. (1998) Factual sources of psychiatric patients' perceptions of coercion in the hospital admission process. *American Journal of Psychiatry*, 155, 1254–1260.

Lucksted, A. and Coursey, R.D. (1995) Consumer perceptions of pressure and force in psychiatric treatments. *Psychiatric Services*, 46, 146–152.

McCubbin, M. and Weisstub, D.N. (1998) Towards a pure best interests model of proxy decision making for incompetent psychiatric patients. *International Journal of Law and Psychiatry*, 21, 1–30.

McDonnell, E. and Bartholomew, T. (1997) Community treatment orders in Victoria: emergent issues and anomalies. *Psychiatry, Psychology and Law*, 4, 25–36.

Meuser, K.T., Bond, G.R., Drake, R.E. and Resnick, S.G. (1998) Models of community care for severe mental illness: a review of research on case management. *Schizophrenia Bulletin*, 24, 37–74.

Munetz, M.R., Grande, T., Kleist, J., Peterson, G.A. and Vuddagiri, S. (1997) What happens when effective outpatient civil commitment is terminated? *New Directions in Mental Health Services*, 75, 49–59.

Pilgrim, D. and Waldron, L. (1998) User involvement in mental health service development: how far can it go? *Journal of Mental Health*, 7, 95–104.

Policy Research Associates.(1998) *Final Report: Research Study Of The New York City Involuntary Outpatient Commitment Pilot Programme (at Bellevue Hospital)*. New York: Policy Research Associates.

Rogers, A. (1993) Coercion and voluntary admission: an examination of psychiatric patient views: voluntary admission under the British medical health law. *Behavioral Sciences and the Law*, 11, 259–267.

Rosenman, S. (1994) Mental health law: an idea whose time has passed. *Australian and New Zealand Journal of Psychiatry*, 28, 560–565.

Scheid-Cook, T.L. (1993) Controllers and controlled: an analysis of participant constructions of outpatient commitment. *Sociology of Health and Illness*, 15, 179–198.

Shergill, S.S. and Szmukler, G. (1998) How predictable is violence and suicide in psychiatric practice? *Journal of Mental Health*, 7, 393–401

Sledge, S.H., Astrachan, B., Thompson, K. *et al.* (1995) Case management in psychiatry: an analysis of tasks. *American Journal of Psychiatry*, 152, 1259–1265.

Solomon, P. (1996) Research on the coercion of persons with severe mental illness. In: Dennis, D.L. and Monahan, J. (eds), *Coercive and Aggressive Community Treatment: A New Frontier in Mental Health Law*. New York: Plenum Press, pp. 129–145.

Srebnik, D.S. and La Fond, J.Q. (1999) Advance directives for mental health treatment. *Psychiatric Services*, 50, 919–925.

Stein, L.I. and Santos, A.B. (1998) *Assertive Community Treatment of Persons with Severe Mental Illness*. New York: Norton.

Susser, E. and Roche, B. (1996) 'Coercion' and leverage in clinical outreach. In: Dennis, D.L. and Monahan, J. (eds), *Coercive and Aggressive Community Treatment: A New Frontier in Mental Health Law*. New York: Plenum Press, pp. 73–84.

Sutherby, K. and Szmukler, G. (1998) Crisis cards and self-help crisis initiatives. *Psychiatric Bulletin*, 22, 4–7.

Sutherby, K., Szmukler, G.I., Halpern, A., Alexander, M., Thornicroft, G., Johnson, C. and Wright, S. (1999) A study of 'crisis cards' in a community psychiatric service. *Acta Psychiatrica Scandinavica*, 100, 56–61.

Swanson, J.W., Swartz, M.S., George, L.K., Burns, B.J., Hiday, V.A., Borum, R. and Wagner, H.R. (1997) Interpreting the effectiveness of involuntary outpatient commitment: a conceptual model. *Journal of the American Academy of Psychiatry and Law*, 25, 5–16.

Swanson, J.W., Swartz, M.D., Borum, R., Hiday, V.A., Wagner, H.R. and Burns, B.J. (2000) Involuntary outpatient commitment and reduction of violent behavior in persons with severe mental illness? *British Journal of Psychiatry*, 176, 324–331.

Swartz, M.S., Burns, B.J., Hiday, V.A., George, L.K. Swanson, J. and Wagner, H.R. (1995) New directions in research on involuntary outpatient commitment. *Psychiatric Services*, 46, 381–385.

Swartz, M.S., Swanson, J.W., Wagner, H.R., Burns, B.J., Hiday, V.A. and Borum, R. (2000) Can involuntary outpatient commitment reduce hospital recidivism?: Findings from a randomised trial with severely mentally ill individuals. *American J Psychiatry*, 156, 1968–1975.

Szmukler, G. and Holloway, F. (1998) Mental health legislation is now a harmful anachronism. *Psychiatric Bulletin*, 22, 662–665.

Taylor, P.J. and Gunn, J. (1999) Homicides by people with mental illness: myth and reality. *British Journal of Psychiatry*, 174, 9–14.

Wertheimer, A. (1993) A philosophical examination of coercion for mental health issues: some basic distinctions: analysis and justification. *Behavioral Sciences and the Law*, 11, 239–258.

Winick, B.J. (1997) Mandatory treatment: an examination of therapeutic jurisprudence. *New Directions in Mental Health Services*, 75, 27–34.

46 | *Privacy and confidentiality*
Patricia Backlar

"The sense of privacy itself, of the area of personal relationships as something sacred in its own right, derives from a conception of freedom which, for all its religious roots, is scarcely older, in its developed state, than the Renaissance or Reformation. Yet its decline would mark the death of a civilisation, of an entire moral outlook."
(Isaiah Berlin, 1998, p. 201)

"The principle of medical confidentiality described in medical codes of ethics and still believed in by patients no longer exists. In this respect it is a decrepit concept."
(Mark Seigler, 1982, p. 1520)

"... in the wake of the rise of radical individualism between 1960 and the 1990s, a new conception of privacy is called for, one that does not privilege privacy over the common good but rather is open to balance with concerns of social responsibilities." (Amitai Etzioni, 1999, p. 188)

Introduction

In recent years, the general public has shown an increased interest and heightened concern about plausible hazards to medical privacy and privacy's ancillary, confidentiality. Apprehension about threats to personal privacy has been intensified by computerized record keeping of medical information, the advent of AIDS and the advancement of genetic research and testing (Seigler, 1982; Appelbaum and Appelbaum, 1990; Gostin, 1995; The Nuffield Council, 1998). In western medicine since the time of the historical Hippocrates, it has been recognized that patients are vulnerable and dependent even in commonplace encounters with physicians. Patients uncover their bodies, disclose personal information and allow the physician—who in many cases may be a virtual stranger—to be privy to their most private selves (Parsons, 1951). Patients trust their physicians and permit them to hold enormous power; in exchange, they expect physicians to be loyal and to act solely in their best interests (Rodwin, 1993). It is presumed that "in the course of treatment, the physician is obligated to the patient and to no one else" (Jonas, 1969, p. 239). By obtaining the doctor's promise to keep medical information private, patients feel less defenceless and more in control. Indeed, in the relationship between physicians and patients, the doctor's obligation to respect confidentiality typically is regarded as second only to the primary goal of providing therapeutic benefits to the patient (Beauchamp and Childress, 1994). In psychiatric practice, which by its nature involves intimate personal revelations from a vulnerable population of patients, providers' ability to keep promises of confidentiality is a significant concern (Stone, 1976; Appelbaum, 1982; Rachlin and Appelbaum, 1983; Backlar, 1996a).

When people with serious mental disorders were cared for in mental hospitals, issues of privacy and confidentiality were little considered (Scull, 1993; Grob, 1994). Today, with the shift in locus of care from long-term custodial institutions to a catch-as-catch-can existence in the community, management of privacy and confidentiality for persons with mental disorders poses moral dilemmas. Problems may occur because of discrete circumstances or a combination of factors involving *where* the care occurs, *who* delivers the services and *what* those services entail. Community living for persons with serious mental disorders can involve supervision by community mental health centre programmes, care by informal care-givers, being alone and homeless or, as is increasingly true in the USA, incarceration in correctional facilities (Isaac and Armat, 1990; Lamb and Shaner, 1993; Carpenter and Buchanan, 1994; Backlar, 1996a). Mental health services are provided in the community in diverse settings: respite facilities, day hospital settings, clinics, jails and prisons, group homes, private offices, private homes, shelters, and on the streets and under bridges (Diamond and Wikler, 1985; Martin, 1994; Backlar, 1996b). Just as the loci of treatment have changed, so has the makeup of the service providers. No longer does the provider cohort consist only of traditionally trained professionals but now includes users of mental health services. The concept of training users to perform work as peer counsellors inside and outside mental health clinic settings and the importance of peer support has become well recognized (Curtis and Hodge, 1994). In addition, the provision of therapy for persons with serious mental disorders living in the community includes not only psychiatric medication, psychotherapy, drug and alcohol abuse treatment, and psychosocial services involving housing and vocational rehabilitation, but also incorporates a mechanism that provides protection for society in general. Mental health providers may be required by law to serve as agents of social control.

Delivering a complex assortment of mental health services to a heterogeneous population, who often have unpredictable needs, in a variety of locations (including public places), is a far cry from conventional medical practice. Mental health providers do not always have the luxury of waiting for patients to come to their door. Also, it is more than likely that they may count among their colleagues-in-care not only their patient's family members and friends—informal care-givers—but their patients who may also serve as peer counsellors. There may be considerable potential for patients' loss of privacy and breaches of confidentiality. Privacy, however, is a contingent concept (Etzioni, 1999, p. 188); it is not an absolute privilege or an absolute good. Determining individual claims to privacy in any particular context is likely to require a "careful evaluation of subjective, variable and competing interests" (Cate, 1997, p. 31).

The different senses of privacy

Privacy has to do with that which we keep to ourselves. We have privacy if others do not have or do not use access to us. What matters or counts as a loss of privacy varies not only from individual to individual but also from culture to culture. The range of things we may wish to keep private may extend from that which is trivial to knowledge which, if obtained by others, may be used to shame us or cause us some real personal harm (Beauchamp and Childress, 1994). As Fried (1968) recognizes, "We may not mind that a person knows a general fact about us, and yet feel that our privacy has been invaded if he knows the details. For instance, a casual acquaintance may comfortably know that I am sick, but it would violate my privacy if he knew the nature of the illness."

In general, we refer to three different senses of 'privacy' (Dworkin, 1993). In one sense, we use the concept of privacy to denote that we are free legitimately to direct our own lives. This liberty to control our personal decisions does not mean that private choices are necessarily hidden. Indeed, often such choices are open to public view—as, for example, where, with whom and how we choose to live (Backlar, 1994). Decisional privacy is recognized as our privilege to control our own acts (Etzioni, 1999). However, the more our choices are dictated by personal needs the less free we become. Conditions of poverty or psychosis may severely limit a person's decisional liberty. People who suffer from mental illness often struggle to maintain the minimum conditions necessary for a worthwhile life.

Raz (1986, p. 156) maintains that "harsh natural conditions can reduce the degree of autonomy to a bare minimum just as effectively as systematic coercive intervention." Perceptions of coercion are subjective and may be less tied to a particular circumstance such as involuntary hospitalization or out-patient commitment, than to whether individuals have been treated with dignity (Szmukler and Holloway, 1998). Not surprisingly, when providers appear to be disinterested in patients' well-being, perceptions of coercion rise. According to Lidz and colleagues

(1995) and Hiday (1997), patients feel excessively coerced when they are excluded from decision making or when threats and physical force are used to hospitalize them. Even for those who live in the community, the freedom to make personal choices may be constrained. Some patients with mental disorders may feel as though their only opportunity to make private choices may be their decisions about how much or how little medication they are willing to take.

In another sense, privacy is understood to be territorial. We speak of a person's condition or state as being protected from unwanted access by others, including access to personal information (Bok, 1984). Etzioni (1999, p. 210) suggests that an effective metaphor here is the image of a 'veil or cloth with which an individual can drape his or her self when there is legitimate reason' to keep something concealed from others. This condition or state is sometimes alluded to as a zone or sphere of personal privacy. Nozick (1974, p. 57) refers to this personal sphere in spatial terms as "an area in moral space around an individual". For persons who are mentally ill and homeless, this moral space may be the only private space available to them. Indeed, it appears that outreach to homeless persons is likely to be successful only when providers are sensitive to and do not brusquely intrude upon this moral space (Martin, 1994).

We use privacy in a third sense to mean that we may keep things to ourselves. We do not have to share with or disclose to others what we are thinking, how we cast our political ballot, what religious beliefs we hold or—other than to the taxman—how much money we have in our bank accounts (Dworkin, 1993). In effect, this sense of privacy is closely related to confidentiality. In human relationships, the difference between what persons reveal to public view and keep secret or divulge "only to intimates is essential to permit creatures as complex as ourselves to interact without constant social breakdown" (Nagel, 1998, p. 15). However, many persons with serious mental disorders who live in the community may not be able to afford the luxury of personal privacy. It is more than likely that many private details of these patients' lives—their financial arrangements, their intimate relationships and, when psychotic, even their innermost private thoughts—may be apparent not only to their formal and informal care-givers, but to their landlords, to their local shopkeepers and to passers-by on the street.

Confidentiality

Privacy and confidentiality, often mentioned in one breath, are discrete concepts even when they overlap. When we speak of confidentiality, we refer to the "boundaries surrounding shared secrets and to the process of guarding these boundaries" (Bok, 1983, p. 119). Usually when confidentiality is invoked it is to keep information from third parties. In the practice of medicine, the patient's claim to privacy and the physician's promise to maintain confidentiality—as described more than 2000 years ago in the Hippocratic Oath—is considered to be the cornerstone to the patient–physician relationship. The goal of medical confidentiality is twofold (Seigler, 1982). First, it acknowledges respect for the patient's dignity and privacy. The patient's personal physical and psychological information are kept confidential in order to minimize a sense of embarrassment and defencelessness. Secondly, the observance of confidentiality allows the goal of medicine to be achieved, which is to better the patient's health. Adequate information is needed for health care providers to be able to make correct diagnoses and prognoses, or suggest suitable treatment (Beauchamp and Childress, 1994).

The promise to maintain confidentiality engenders trust. Trust is essential to and serves to lessen the complexity of all human relationships (Pellegrino, 1991). Without trust, persons who are suffering, ashamed of their disease—and thus particularly vulnerable—might not go to visit doctors. Stigma is a widespread feature of mental disorders. Persons with psychiatric diseases are little understood, often demeaned and unjustifiably feared (Albrecht *et al.*, 1982; The Nuffield Council, 1998). Such persons may be especially reluctant to access health care. The consequence of such reluctance not only can harm the health of individuals, but also has the potential to endanger public health and public safety.

However, questions about confidentiality remain. The moral weight we give to obligations of confidentiality is warranted not merely because of the good inherent in the convention, but because of the good anticipated to ensue. Therefore, as Bok (1984, p. 135) remarks, even though "the premises supporting confidentiality are strong, . . . they cannot support practices . . . that undermine and contradict the very respect for persons and for human bonds that confidentiality was meant to protect."

The limits of confidentiality

The physician's promise to maintain confidentiality, in western societies, is implied and broadly presumed. Patients do not solicit this promise explicitly (McConnell, 1997). Thus, the obligation falls to the provider to inform the patient under what conditions confidentiality will not be maintained.

To invoke a promise of confidentiality, which suggests *prima facie* grounds of obligation, does not put to rest the debate over an oath of secrecy. "Rather, one must go on to ask whether it was right to make the pledge in the first place, and right to accept it; whether the promise is a binding one, and even when it is, what circumstances might nevertheless justify overriding it" (Bok, 1984, p. 121). The obligation to respect confidentiality may be overlooked when patients' interest in safeguarding their confidential information conflicts with their need to secure adequate health care (Backlar, 1996a). Alternatively, in certain circumstances, a physician may be required to breach confidentiality based on societal interests. For example, when a patient: divulges ongoing child abuse, presents with a gunshot wound or is ill with an infectious disease. Additionally, for persons with mental disorders, confidentiality may properly be abrogated relevant to a patient's imminent suicide, civil commitment proceedings or if the patient reveals an intention to murder someone.

Confidentiality and the duty to protect the public interest—the Tarasoff case

"The protective privilege ends where the public peril begins" argued Justice Mathew Tobriner, author of the majority opinion in *Tarasoff v. Regents of the University of California* (1976; Beauchamp and Childress, 1994, p. 511). The *Tarasoff* case has become the classic example of health care professionals' competing obligations to respect patient autonomy and duty to fulfil the requirements of beneficence to the public good or innocent third parties. The case involves the kind of conflicts that mental health providers may face when patients reveal that they wish to harm others.

In, 1969, Prosenjit Poddar, a depressed young man who was a student at the University of California at Berkeley, told his psychotherapist that he planned to kill his former girlfriend, Tatiana Tarasoff. The psychotherapist and his colleagues decided to commit the young man to a mental hospital for observation. A commitment request was sent to the campus police. The police detained the young man briefly, but Poddar promised to stay away from Ms Tarasoff. The police released him because they believed he was 'rational.' When the police reported Poddar's release to the director of psychiatry, he ordered no further action be taken and that the correspondence between the psychotherapists and the police be destroyed. Two months later, Poddar murdered the young woman. Tatiana Tarasoff's parents brought suit against the university, the campus police and the psychotherapists for failing to warn them of Tatiana's peril.

In the majority opinion, Justice Tobriner argued that the obligation to protect public safety overrides the requirement to protect patient confidentiality. The court recognized that confidentiality is an important value, but not an absolute value. The dissenting opinion, written by Justice William Clark, claimed that if psychotherapists breach confidence in like cases, it might deter patients from seeking treatment and the public interest may be open to even greater harm. Indeed, many psychiatrists have argued that the duty to warn potential victims threatens the trust between patient and therapist. Alan Stone (1976) asserts that the duty to warn potential patients about the limits of confidentiality "will deter both patients and therapists from undertaking treatment, thereby further increasing the risk of violence to which society is exposed." Other commentators contend that a mere *threat* of violence does not mean that anything will occur. Furthermore, as some writers note, psychiatrists' abilities reliably to predict an individual's propensity to commit future violence remains an area of controversy (Mulvey, 1994; Swanson *et al.*, 1996). Nevertheless, the question remains: does the psychotherapist's inability to predict accurately mean that the prospect of danger to a potential victim should be ignored?

The *Tarasoff* court decision recognized that therapists are in a confidential relationship with their patients, but that the rule the court adopted might, at times, cause confidentiality to be breached. The court concluded that when "a patient poses a serious threat of violence to others, [the therapist] bears a duty to exercise reasonable care to protect the foreseeable victim of that danger." The *Tarasoff* case is about the duty to protect, not about the duty to warn. The therapists could have protected Ms Tarasoff if they had committed the young man to an in-patient facility. This would have been a more extreme invasion of his freedom and privacy than breaching his confidentiality by warning the young woman of his intentions. Psychiatrists, unlike other physicians, are legally authorized to civilly commit their patients. Indeed, that was the initial purpose of therapists in this case. "The fact that the psychiatrists had the power to control the young man by committing him to a mental hospital puts them in the 'special relationship' that creates a duty to act at all" (Annas *et al.*, 1995, p. 154).

Over the years, since the handing down of the *Tarasoff* decision, there appears to be no evidence that psychiatric treatment has been compromised because patients are warned that in certain situations (threats of violence to others, revelations of child abuse, etc.) the protection of their confidences is not absolute (Beck, 1990, p. 212;

Appelbaum, 1994). Most individuals with mental disorders are far more worried that information in their medical records will in some way become available to others and affect their employment, cause them to lose their insurance, be used to stigmatize them or be scooped up by "privacy merchants, profit-making companies that grow rich by selling information about people's medical condition to all comers" (Etzioni, 1999, p. 182). Indeed, the recent trend in community care to lesser degrees of 'danger to others' being deemed as justifying breaches of confidentiality (Szmukler and Holloway, 2000) appears to support these fears.

In the *Tarasoff* case, it is a mistake to focus the moral concern narrowly on weighing and balancing harms and benefits to breaching confidentiality. The implied promise to keep confidentiality is the *prima facie* obligation. However, there is a competing obligation—the requirement of beneficence—which in this case becomes the actual obligation. Indeed, the facts in this case justify overriding the confidentiality obligation. Tom Beauchamp and Jim Childress (1994, p. 267) correctly observe, "Only a remarkably narrow view of moral obligation would hold that the psychiatrist is under no obligation to protect the woman by contacting her . . . . If morality does not demand this much beneficence, it is hard to see how morality imposes any positive obligations at all." It was wrong not to warn Tatiana Tarasoff.

Confidentiality and the informal care-giver

Patient 'recovery' and the importance of the informal care-giver

The healing function of medicine encompasses both curing and caring, and healing may in a broader sense be possible even in those cases where medicine cannot cure. It can heal by helping a person cope effectively with permanent maladies (Callahan, 1996, p. S12).

Even with improved knowledge about brain chemistry and the expanding availability of novel antipsychotic medications, 'recovery' for mentally ill individuals should not be equated with the realization of cure (Hatfield and Lefley, 1993). Recovery involves a slow rehabilitative process that includes coping and adapting to the disorder. A patient's successful rehabilitation requires daily attention, patience and perseverance. In community psychiatric care, the daily task of helping patients often devolves to families or good friends—if the mentally ill individual is fortunate enough to have a relationship with such persons.

Mental health providers have long recognized the sociological aspects of their patients' needs and the significance of finding and developing patients' natural helping networks (Collins and Pancoast, 1976). Indeed, according to Szmukler and Bloch (1997, p. 401), "the crucial role of [informal] carers in making 'community care' possible is increasingly recognized." Recent legislation in Australia, England and Wales designates a formal status for carers that has implications in terms of a carer's rights to certain types of information about the patient (Szmukler and Holloway, 2000), and practice guidelines in the USA now recommend involving families in all phases of routine care (American Psychiatric Association, 1997).

For more than a decade, there has been substantial research on family care-giving and family burden (Lefley, 1996). Yet, little clinical or research effort has been focused on how to help sustain social networks and support systems for persons with chronic mental illness (Cutler and Tatum, 1983; Twigg and Atkin, 1994). Thus, insufficient policy has been effected to establish a systematic relationship between informal care-givers, the cared for and the formal service practice system. In particular, confusion about the best way to deal with confidentiality relevant to the release of medical information to informal care-givers continues to be a stumbling block to effecting an acceptable relationship between persons with mental disorders, informal care-givers and the formal service system.

Informal care-givers

Who are informal care-givers? They may be kin. They may be significant others, or kind friends.

Szmukler and Holloway (2000) argue that if the connection to the patient is not only familial, but also as a 'carer,' such persons have a special relationship that qualifies them to be classified as informal care-givers. In the best of all possible worlds, informal carers will be characterized by their strong sense of obligation to promote the well-being of the patient. In reality, however, informal care-givers will represent a range of characteristics. Indeed, some carers' own interests may be at cross purposes with the best interests of the patient.

Informal care-givers provide residential services and case management for the majority of persons with mental disorders (Beal, 1994). Yet, the barriers of confidentiality still prevent adequate medical information about the patient from being given to the carers (Krauss, 1992; Petrial and Sadoff, 1992; Backlar, 1994, 1996a). This can be harmful to the health of the patient. When family or kind friends take responsibility for providing patient care, 'common sense and good clinical judgement' require that at a minimum there be an exchange of medical information relevant to treatment (Krauss, 1992, p. 256). Indeed, as noted by Petrial and Sadoff (1992), we would find it odd if patients were discharged from psychiatric hospitals to out-patient clinics or residential care facilities and the discharging psychiatrists did not provide the in-taking agencies with patients' medical information.

A 'recovery' model of care

Rehabilitation is now recognized as an important and growing part of psychiatric patients' treatment in the community. The role of the informal care-giver has come to be viewed as integral to the patient's well-being and recovery process (Pfeiffer and Mostek, 1991; Hatfield and Lefley, 1993; Szmukler, 1999). However, creating a milieu that is beneficial to patients' ongoing 'recovery,' in which clinicians are not only responsible for the care of a heterogeneous group of patients but also for involving informal carers in many phases of the treatment process, is likely to be a demanding charge. Szmukler and Bloch (1997, p. 402) propose a model of care that may be flexible enough both to sustain a therapeutic environment for patients and also be sensitive to the carers' needs. The authors consider this model of care acceptable only when informed consent is obtained from all the stakeholders—patient *and* family.

"While the interests of family members [informal carers] are taken into account, the particular features of the therapeutic situation guide the clinician's responses. Thus, he or she may attend to the patient at one point but switch to other members, for example, the patient's principal carer at another time. The patient is not the chief priority; indeed, satisfactory functioning may sometimes be at the expense of others. Moreover, given that family members' wellbeing may change during treatment, the clinician monitors the welfare of each and adjusts interventions accordingly"

A model of care that balances the interests of the patient with the interests of the informal care-givers gives rise to, at the least, two interrelated concerns. The first concern grows out of our normative notion that physicians, for the most part, are expected to take a special, individual and partisan interest in the patient. The second concern is closely associated with this patient-centred consideration. The establishment of a successful healing environment requires that informal carers receive medical information relevant to the patient's diagnosis, current treatment, expected side effects from medications and effective strategies for coping with the illness. Therefore, this 'recovery' model of care challenges our conventional concept of patient confidentiality (even though it should be noted, there is no need to divulge a patient's private confidences). With few exceptions (as mentioned above, e.g. suspected child abuse, civil commitment proceedings, the obligation to warn potential victims), long-standing custom, professional codes, regulations and laws require patient authorization for the release of medical information.

Patient release of information forms

The tension that exists between psychiatrists' obligations to respect patient confidentiality and informal carers' need to know is not new. A decade ago, Zipple and colleagues (1990)

suggested a strategy to circumvent the confidentiality barrier. They proposed that patient release forms used by clinicians to share information about their patients with other practitioners or agencies should also be used with informal carers. It is common practice for patients to sign a release form giving permission for one provider to impart specified confidential information to another designated provider. Bogart and Solomon (1999) elaborate upon the Zipple recommendation. They suggest that a standardized form, to be used for releasing patient information to informal carers, be designed. The form should: (i) distinguish between the categories of information to be released; (ii) specify whether the information be presented verbally or in writing; and (iii) stipulate the length of time that the form remains valid. The authors propose that standardized release forms be incorporated into routine clinical practice, and routinely presented to the patient upon intake to the mental health centre or to the mental health system. If the patient is too ill to consent, Bogart and Solomon advise that when the patient is stabilized the clinician should reintroduce the form.

Psychiatric anticipatory planning

Anticipatory planning for psychiatric treatment provides another approach that affords a limited waiver of confidentiality between in-patient and out-patient clinicians, and informal carers. Special arrangements, which allow care-givers (who often endure trying burdens of care when the patient is in crisis) to participate with patients in their treatment decisions, are another feature of such advance planning.

Psychiatric advance directives (PADs) are licit documents that allow competent adults to make choices in the present about their future psychiatric treatment should they lose their decision-making capacity (Backlar, 1995, 1997). Twelve states in the USA have laws that specify PADs. 'Crisis cards,' which are used in the UK, are similar documents but with no legal standing (Sutherby and Szmukler, 1998).

PADs are patterned after advance directives (ADs) for end-of-life care. Both types of documents allow autonomous persons to plan ahead for a time when decision-making capacity may be impaired and to put in place protections of their own choosing. However, the two kinds of documents are essentially different. The AD for end-of-life care mainly addresses circumstances preceding a singular event—the principal's death. Such documents were designed to allow autonomous individuals the opportunity to refuse heroic measures at the time of a terminal illness. In contrast, the PAD addresses events that may occur repeatedly—resulting from an ongoing condition and fluctuating capacity to make psychiatric health care decisions. PADs are intended for persons who already have experienced the sort of crisis that they anticipate will recur. Thus, patients may be able to use such previous experience to plan better for similar situations in the future. In short, while ADs prepare for dying, PADs are concerned with restoration and recovery, i.e with living. Indeed, according to opinion studies in the UK (Sutherby *et al.*, 1999; Szmukler, 1999) and the USA (Backlar *et al.*, 1999), the employment of PADs may provide an intangible personal benefit for patients. Patients report that they feel more secure when they are able to plan for their care in advance of a psychiatric crisis.

PADs may be both substantive and procedural. Substantively, patients can use PADs to declare specific preferences for treatment. For example, patients may describe the kinds of medications and treatments that work for them and those that do not, and they may consent in advance to a voluntary admission to a health care facility. PAD instruments also may allow patients to document and describe their past decompensations and prodromal symptoms. Procedurally, these instruments allow individuals to appoint a surrogate decision maker to make mental health decisions for them should they lose their capacity to make decisions for themselves. Surrogates assume such decision-making responsibilities only when patients are incapable, thus allowing for a limited waiver of confidentiality. Optimally, patients will choose someone they know and trust who is familiar with their considered wishes and can be counted upon to protect their welfare. In essence, such legal documents enable patients to

make a projection—a forecast—not only of informed consent and refusal, but also of their values and relationships (National Bioethics Advisory Commission, 1998).

Problems inherent in assessment of patients' decision-making capacity

A release of information form or PAD must be authorized and signed by a patient who is judged to be competent in order for the documents to be considered legal and binding. In general, 'competence' refers to a legal determination, while 'capacity' usually refers to a clinical judgement (Berg and Appelbaum, 1998)—in this chapter, these words are used indiscriminately.

We presume that all persons are capable of making decisions for themselves unless there are specific reasons and conditions to believe otherwise. Our goal is to avoid two kinds of mistakes: we should not prevent competent patients from making their own choices; neither should we fail to protect incompetent patients (patients who are unable to care for their own interests) from making decisions that may be harmful to their health and well-being (Backlar, 1996c). Typically, evaluating a patient's capacity is a matter of subjective judgement. The competency of patients who *disagree* with the clinician making the assessment may be depreciated, while patients who *agree* may have their capacity overestimated (Rhoden, 1992). There are beginning to be some tested approaches for assessing capacity objectively (Grisso and Appelbaum, 1995). Yet, we have no normative agreement on the degree of impairment we are willing to countenance before we deem that an individual lacks adequate decision-making capacity (Appelbaum, 1997).

We use the term 'decision-making capacity' to describe an ability that involves mental and volitional competence. We consider that people have capacity if, for example, they are able: to understand what a particular illness might be; to grasp the consequences of taking a specific medicine; to make a particular choice; and to know when they are engaged in such an action (Appelbaum and Grisso, 1988; Berg *et al.*, 1996). Customarily, decision-making capacity is considered task specific (Culver and Gert, 1982). A person may lack capacity in one area but have the capacity to make decisions in other areas.

Persons with mental disorders whose capacity may fluctuate have intermittent periods when they have decision-making capacity. It is morally correct—and usually possible—to approach persons about signing a release of information form or preparing a PAD when they are competent (e.g. when they are capable of understanding, appreciating, rationally manipulating pertinent information and evincing a choice—the four elements commonly used for competence evaluation—relevant to a particular situation). Conversely, it usually will be quite obvious when patients lack decision-making capacity. Some patients may be flagrantly psychotic. Others may not recognize that they have a serious mental disorder. The illness itself may rob them of the insight necessary to acknowledge their illness (Dickerson *et al.*, 1997). It is unlikely that such persons will have the capacity to give valid consent or refusal.

Typically, the greatest difficulty in making capacity judgements lies with patients who are not easily identified as having or lacking ability to make decisions. Some patients may appear to manage their lives adequately, but suffer from unfounded paranoia. Indeed, such persons may make persuasive arguments—but not rooted in reality—as to why they object to having any information shared with their informal carers. Yet other individuals suffering from a psychiatric crisis may still be capable of knowing who is kind to them and who is not, able to identify persons that they trust and even to name precisely medications or treatments that are appropriate or inappropriate for their care. With patients whose competence is not assessed easily or accurately, it may not be possible to make proper decisions about issues that intimately affect their lives, such as breaching medical confidentiality, if such decisions are to depend *only* on the patient's competent authorization.

Practical guidelines for breaching patient confidentiality

If a 'recovery' model of care involving suitable informal carers is to be effected, sensible guidelines relevant to the sharing of patients' medical information may be necessary. Importantly, new practice standards applicable to breaching patient confidentiality should be acceptable to all the stakeholders and only concern medical information. Private discussions (save for allowed exceptions) between patient and clinician should remain privileged.

We are familiar with changing criteria used for implementing involuntary hospitalization (Appelbaum, 1994) and out-patient commitment (Swanson *et al.*, 1997). In general, such criteria are an assemblage of reasons intended to justify interference with an individual's liberty. In a similar vein, Szmukler and colleagues (Szmukler and Bloch, 1997 p. 403; Szmukler and Holloway, 2000) advance a set of inter-related standards, *predicated on risks to the patient's health*, that would permit medical information to flow to those persons acknowledged to be the patient's authentic informal carers:

(i) *The patient's capacity to make a genuine choice is impaired.* Grounds that warrant breaching confidentiality of medical information may not be invoked when competent patients refuse involvement with informal carers. The proposed guidelines are to be used only when patients are not capable of making autonomous choices.

(ii) *The nature and magnitude of the harms to be avoided must be significant, and there must be a high probability of their occurrence.* Szmukler and Bloch (1997) propose specific grounds that would permit breaching a patient's confidentiality:

"The risk to the patient's health falls short of that warranting compulsory admission. The patient is often in the process of relapse with a likelihood that compulsion will become necessary later. Preventing further deterioration may be an immediate goal. Common risks include severe self-neglect, loss of accommodation, job, money or friends, intense distress, exploitation by others, predictable worsening of symptoms, or deterioration to a point which jeopardises future rehabilitation" (p. 403).

(iii) *No acceptable alternatives are available.* There may be alternatives to the informal carers. Perhaps the patient will not be averse to communicating with other friends or organizations who are willing to provide appropriate help.

(iv) *The ... [informal carers'] values embody mutual concern and assistance.* The normative relationship between patient and informal carers is germane. Szmukler and Bloch (1997) recommend that pertinent questions be asked:

"Following recovery, would the patient be likely to see family involvement as having been desirable? Has previous discussion with patient and family revealed contact would be acceptable, given the current circumstances?" (p. 403).

(v) *The principle of 'the least restrictive' option could apply when ... [informal carers] involvement will reduce the likelihood of a greater restriction on the patient's freedom, especially involuntary hospitalization.*

Conclusion

Any undertaking to engender changes in criteria for breaching a relapsing patient's confidentiality should be approached cautiously. Modifications of long-standing criteria that support confidentiality should not occur in an empirical vacuum. Studies are needed in order to find which paths most satisfactorily serve patients' best interests.

We live in a world in which a plurality of values exist. Reform attempts relevant to breaching patient confidentiality must begin by soliciting input from the various stakeholders—the patients themselves, their families and carers, and their clinicians. There is no single set of interests that should determine new practice and policy with the potential for far-reaching effects on vulnerable

patients. In the words of Isaiah Berlin ([1965], 1999), "Human beings sooner or later realise that they must make do, they must make compromises" (p. 15).

References

Albrecht, G., Walker, V. and Levy, L. (1982) Social distance from the stigmatized: a test of two theories. *Social Science and Medicine*, 16, 1319–1327.
American Psychiatric Association (1997) Practice guidelines for the treatment of patients with schizophrenia. *American Journal of Psychiatry*, 154 (Suppl.), 1–63.
Annas, G.J., Glantz, L.H. and Roche P.A. (1995) Appendix: genetic information and the duty to warn. In *The Genetic Privacy Act and Commentary*,. pp. 142–165. The Final Report of a project entitled 'Guidelines for Protecting Privacy of Information Stored in Genetic Data Banks' which was funded by the Ethical, Legal and Social Implications of the Human Genome Project, Office of Energy Research, US, Department of Energy, No. DE-FG02-93ER61626.
Appelbaum, P.S. (1982) Confidentiality in psychiatric treatment. In: Grinspoon, L. (ed.), *The American Psychiatric Association Annual Review*. American Psychiatric Press, pp. 327–335.
Appelbaum, P.S. (1994) *Almost a Revolution: Mental Health Law and the Limits of Change*. Oxford: Oxford University Press.
Appelbaum, P.S. (1997) Rethinking the conduct of psychiatric research. *Archives of General Psychiatry*, 54, 117–120.
Appelbaum, K. and Appelbaum, P.S. (1990) The HIV antibody-positive patient. In: Beck, J.C. (ed.), *Confidentiality Versus the Duty to Protect: Foreseeable Harm in the Practice of Psychiatry*. Washington, DC: American Psychiatric Press, pp. 121–140.
Appelbaum, P.S. and Grisso, T. (1988) Assessing patients' capacities to consent to treatment. *New England Journal of Medicine*, 319, 1635–1638.
Backlar, P. (1994) *The Family Face of Schizophrenia*. New York: Tarcher/Putnam.
Backlar, P. (1995) The longing for order: Oregon's medical advance directive for mental health treatment. *Community Mental Health Journal*, 31, 103–108.
Backlar, P. (1996a) Confidentiality and common sense. *Community Mental Health Journal*, 32, 513–518.
Backlar, P. (1996b) The three Rs: roles, relationships, and rules. *Community Mental Health Journal*, 32, 505–509.

Backlar, P. (1996c) Assessing decision-making capacity: a slippery business. *Community Mental Health Journal*, 32, 321–325.

Backlar, P. (1997) Anticipatory planning for psychiatric treatment is not quite the same as planning for end-of-life care. *Community Mental Health Journal*, 33, 261–268.

Backlar, P., McFarland, B.H., Swanson, J.W. and Mahler, J. (1999) Patient and provider views on psychiatric advance directives. *XXIV International Congress on Law and Mental Health*, Toronto, Canada, 16 June.

Beal, M.A. (1994) The consequences of invisibility. *NAMI Advocate*, 16, 8.

Beauchamp, T.L. and Childress, J.F. (1994) *Principles of Biomedical Ethics*, 4th edn. Oxford: Oxford University Press.

Beck, J.C. (1990) *Confidentiality Versus the Duty to Protect: Foreseeable Harm in the Practice of Psychiatry*. Washington, DC: American Psychiatric Press.

Berg, J.W. and Appelbaum, P.S. (1998) Subjects' capacity to consent to neurobiological research. In: Pincus, H.A., Lieberman, J.A. and Ferris, S. (eds), *Ethics in Psychiatric Research: A Resource Manual for Human Subjects Protection*. American Psychiatric Association, pp. 81–106.

Berg, J.W., Appelbaum, P.S. and Grisso, T. (1996) Constructing competence: formulating standards of legal competence to make medical decisions. *Rutgers Law Review*, 48, 354–396.

Berlin, I. (1998) Two concepts of liberty. In: Hausheer, H. and Hausheer R. (eds),*The Proper Study of Mankind: An Anthology of Essays*. New York: Farrar, Straus and Giroux, pp. 191–242.

Berlin, I. ([1965] 1999) The Romantics and their roots. *Times Literary Supplement*, February 19, 5003, 13–15.

Bogart, C.H. and Solomon, P. (1999) Procedures to share information among mental health providers, consumers, and families. *Psychiatric Services*, 50 (10), 1321–1325.

Bok, S. (1984). *SECRETS: On the Ethics of Concealment and Revelation*. New York: Vintage Books.

Callahan, D. (1996) The goals of medicine: setting new priorities. *Hastings Center Report*, 26 (Special Supplement), S1–S27.

Carpenter, W.T. and Buchanan, R.W. (1994) Medical progress: schizophrenia. *New England Journal of Medicine*, 330, 681–690.

Cate, F.H. (1997) *Privacy in the Information Age*. Washington, DC: Brookings Institution Press.

Collins, A.H. and Pancoast, D.L. (1976) *Natural Helping Networks: A Strategy For Prevention*. Washington, DC: National Association of Social Workers Publication.

Culver, C.M. and Gert, B. (1982) *Philosophy in Medicine: Conceptual and Ethical Issues in Medicine and Psychiatry*. Oxford: Oxford University Press.

Curtis, L.C. and Hodge, M. (1994) Old standards, new dilemmas: ethics and boundaries in community support services. In: Spaniol, L., Brown, M.A., Blankertz, L. *et al.* (eds), *An Introduction to Psychiatric Rehabilitation*. The International Association of Psychosocial Rehabilitation (IAPSRS), pp. 339–354.

Cutler, D.L. and Tatum, E. (1983) Networks and the chronic patient. In: Cutler, D.L. (ed.), *Effective Aftercare for the 1980s. New Directions for Mental Health Services, No. 19*. San Francisco: Jossey-Bass, pp. 13–22.

Diamond, R.J. and Wikler, D.J., (1985) Ethical problems in community treatment of the chronically mentally ill. In: Stein, L.I. and Test, M.A. (eds), *The Training in Community Living Model: A Decade of Experience. New Directions for Mental Health Services, No. 26*. San Francisco: Jossey-Bass, pp. 85–93.

Dickerson, F.B., Boronow, J.J., Ringel, N. and Parente, F. (1997) Lack of insight among outpatients with schizophrenia. *Psychiatric Services*, 48, 195–199.

Dworkin, R. (1994) *Life's Dominion*. New York: Vintage Books.

Etzioni, A. (1999) *The Limits of Privacy*. New York: Basic Books.

Fried, C. (1968) Privacy a rational context. *The Yale Law Journal*, 77, 475–493.

Gostin, L.O. (1995) Genetic privacy. *Journal of Law, Medicine and Ethics*, 23, 320–330.

Grisso, T. and Appelbaum, P.S. (1995) The MacArthur treatment competence study, III: abilities of patients to consent to psychiatric and medical treatments. *Law and Human Behavior*, 19, 149–174.

Grob, G.N. (1994) *The Mad Among Us: A History of Care of America's Mentally Ill*. New York: The Free Press.

Hatfield, A.B. and Lefley, H.P. (1993) *Surviving Mental Illness: Stress, Coping, and Adaptation*. New York: The Guilford Press.

Hiday, V.A. (1997) Patient perceptions of coercion in mental hospital admission. *International Journal of Law and Psychiatry*, 20, 227–241.

Hollis, M. (1988) A death of one's own. In: Bell, J.M. and Beck, S. (eds), *Philosophy and Medical Welfare*. Cambridge: Cambridge University Press, pp. 1–15.

Isaac, R.J. and Armat, V.C. (1990) *Madness in the Streets: How Psychiatry and the Law Abandoned the Mentally Ill*. New York: The Free Press.

Jonas, H. (1969) Philosophical reflections on experimenting with human subjects. *Daedalus*, 98, 219–247.

Krauss, J.B. (1992) Sorry, that's confidential. *Archives of Psychiatric Nursing*, VI, 255–256.

Lamb, H.R. and Shaner, R. (1993) When there are almost no hospital beds left. *Hospital and Community Psychiatry*, 44, 973–976.

Lefley, H.P., (1996) *Family Caregiving in Mental Illness*. London: Sage Publications.

Lidz, C., Hoge, S., Gardner, W., Bennet, N., Monahan, J., Mulvey, E. and Roth, L. (1995) Perceived coercion in mental hospital admission: pressures and process. *Archives of General Psychiatry*, 52, 1034–1039.

Martin, M. (1994) Slipping through the cracks: failure of the mental health system. In Backlar, P. (ed.), *The Family Face of Schizophrenia*. New York: Tarcher/Putnam, pp. 126–144.

McConnell, T. (1997) *Moral Issues in Health Care*, 2nd edn. Wadsworth Publishing Company.

Mulvey, E.P. (1994) Assessing the evidence of a link between mental illness and violence. *Hospital and Community Psychiatry*, 45, 663–668.

Nagel, T. (1998). The shredding of public privacy: reflections on recent events in Washington. *Times Literary Supplement*, 4975, 17.

National Bioethics Advisory Commission (1998) *Research Involving Persons with Mental Disorders That May Affect Decisionmaking Capacity*. Volume I. Rockville, MD, National Bioethics Advisory Commission

Nozick, R. (1974) *Anarchy, State and Utopia*. New York: Basic Books.

Nuffield Council on Bioethics (1998) *Mental Disorders and Genetics: The Ethical Context*. London: The Nuffield Foundation.

Parsons, T. (1951) The sick role and the role of the physician. *Milbank Quarterly*, 53, 257–278.

Pellegrino, E.D. (1991) Trust and distrust in professional ethics. In: Pellegrino, E.D., Veatch, R.M. and Langan, J.P. (eds), *Ethics, Trust, and the Professions: Philosophical and Cultural Aspects*. Washington, DC: Georgetown University Press, pp. 69–85.

Petrillo, J.P. and Sadoff, R.L. (1992) Confidentiality and the family as caregiver. *Hospital and Community Psychiatry*, 43, 136–139.

Pfeiffer, E.J. and Mostek, M. (1991) Services for families of people with mental illness. *Hospital and Community Psychiatry*, 40, 262–264.

Rachlin, S. and Appelbaum, P.S. (1983) The limits of confidentiality. *Hospital and Community Psychiatry*, 34, 589–590.

Raz, J. (1986) *The Morality of Freedom*. New York: Oxford University Press.

Rhoden, N.K. (1982) Can a subject consent to a 'Ulysses Contract'? *Hastings Center Report*, 12, 26–28.

Rodwin, M.A. (1993). *Medicine, Money, and Morals: Physicians' Conflicts of Interest*. Oxford: Oxford University Press.

Scull, A. (1993) *The Most Solitary of Afflictions: Madness and Society in Britain 1700–1900*. Yale University Press.

Seigler, M. (1982) Confidentiality in medicine: a decrepit concept. *New England Journal of Medicine*, 307, 1581–1521.

Stone, A.A. (1976) The Tarasoff decision: suing psychotherapists to safeguard society. *Harvard Law Review*, 90, 358–378.

Sutherby, K. and Szmukler, G. (1998) Crisis cards and self-help crisis initiatives. *Psychiatric Bulletin*, 22, 4–7.

Sutherby, K., Szmukler, G.I., Halpern, A., Alexander, M., Thornicroft, G., Johnson, C. and Wright, S. (1999) A study of 'crisis cards' in a community psychiatric service. *Acta Psychiatrica Scandinavica*, 100, 56–61.

Szmukler, G. (1999) Ethics in community psychiatry. In: Bloch, S., Chodoff, P. and Green, S.A. (eds), *Psychiatric Ethics*, 3rd. edn. Oxford: Oxford University Press.

Szmukler, G.I. and Bloch, S. (1997) Family involvement in the care of people with psychosis: an ethical argument. *British Journal of Psychiatry*, 171, 401–405.

Szmukler, G. and Holloway, F. (1998) Ethics in community psychiatry. *Current Opinion in Psychiatry*, 11, 549–53.

Szmukler, G., and Holloway, F. (2000) Confidentiality in community psychiatry. In: Cordess, C. (ed.), *Confidentiality*. London: Jessica Kingsley Publisher.

Swanson, J.W., Borum, R., Swartz, M.S. and Monahan, J. (1996) Psychotic symptoms and disorders and the risk of violent behavior in the community. *Criminal Behavior and Mental Health*, 6, 317–338.

Swanson, J.W., Swartz, M.S., George, L.K., Burns, B.J., Hiday, V.A., Borum, R. and Wagner, R.H. (1997) Interpreting the effectiveness of involuntary outpatient commitment. *Journal of the Academy of Psychiatry and Law*, 25, 5–16.

Swartz, M.S., Hiday, V.A., Swanson, J.W., Wagner, H.R., Borum, R. and Burns, B.J. (1999) Measuring coercion under involuntary outpatient commitment: initial results from a randomized controlled trial. In: Morrisey, J. and Monohan, J. (eds), *Research in Community and Mental Health: Coercion in Mental Health Services*, Vol. 10. Stamford, CT: Jai Press, pp. 31–58.

Tarasoff v. Regents of the University of California (decided July 1, 1976). 17 Cal.3d 425. 131 California Reporter. See also in, Beauchamp, T.L. and Childress, J.F. (1994). *Principles of Bioemdical Ethics*. Fourth Edition. Oxford University Press, pp. 509–512.

Twigg, J. and Atkin, K. (1994) *Carers Perceived: Policy and Practice in Informal Care*. Milton Keynes: Open University Press.

Zipple, A.M., Langle, S., LeRoy, S. and Fisher, H. (1990) Client confidentiality and the family's need to know: strategies for resolving the conflict. *Community Mental Health Journal*, 26, 533–545.

Glossary

Accessibility
A service characteristic, experienced by users and their carers, which enables them to receive care where and when it is needed.

Accountability
The complex, dynamic relationships between mental health services and patients, their families and the wider public.

Approved Social Workers (ASWs)
Approved Social Workers are social workers specifically approved and appointed under Section 114 of the Mental Health Act 1983 in England by a local social services authority 'for the purpose of discharging the functions conferred upon them by this Act'. Among these, one of the most important is to carry out assessments under the Act and to function as applicant in cases where compulsory admission is deemed necessary.

Assertive outreach (assertive community treatment, intensive case management)
An active form of treatment delivery: the service can be taken to the service users rather than expecting them to attend for treatment. Care and support may be offered in the service user's home or some other community setting, at times suited to the service user rather than focused on service providers' convenience. Workers would be likely to be involved in direct delivery of practical support, care co-ordination and advocacy as well as more traditional therapeutic input. Closer, more trusting relationships may be developed with the aim of maintaining service users in contact with the service and complying with effective treatments.

Atypical (novel) antipsychotic drugs
Newer and more expensive antipsychotic drugs which have a different range of side effects from the standard antipsychotics, and particularly do not produce the neuromuscular (Parkinsonian) side effects.

Autonomy
A patient characteristic consisting of the ability to make independent decisions and choices, despite the presence of symptoms or disabilities.

Care co-ordinator (or keyworker)
A worker (team member) with responsibility for co-ordinating Care Programme Approach reviews for mental health service users with complex needs and for communicating with others involved in the service user's care. Care co-ordinators usually have the most contact with the service user.

Care management
A system of organizing care to vulnerable adults by local authority social services departments. It involves assessing needs, care planning, the organization of care packages within available resources, monitoring and review, and close involvement with service users and carers. For mental health service users, it should be integrated with the Care Programme Approach.

Care Programme Approach (CPA)
The CPA, introduced in England and Wales in 1991, provides a framework for care co-ordination of service users under specialist mental health services. There are four main elements to the CPA: (i) systematic arrangements for assessing the health and social needs of people accepted by the specialist psychiatric services; (ii) the formulation of a care plan which addresses those needs; (iii) the appointment of a keyworker to keep in close touch with the patient and monitor care; and (iv) regular review, and if need be, agreed changes to

the care plan. Multi-disciplinary and interagency working is stressed. Care plans should be agreed with users and their carers, as far as possible.

Carers

Relatives or friends who voluntarily look after individuals who are sick, disabled, vulnerable or frail.

Clinical governance

A framework through which NHS organizations are accountable for continuously improving the quality of their services and safeguarding high standards of care by creating an environment in which excellence in clinical care will be achieved. This is a recent development in the NHS which places the duty on health care providers to achieve quality on the same level as financial probity. Methods include standard setting through clinical policies, protocols and guidelines, and their monitoring through clinical audit, review of serious untoward incidents and complaints made about care. The National Institute for Clinical Excellence (NICE) and the National Service Framework (NSF) contribute to standard setting at a national level. The Commission for Health Improvement is a national body responsible for overseeing and supporting the implementation of clinical governance and the quality of clinical services.

Commission for Health Improvement (see Clinical governance)

Co-morbidity

The simultaneous presence of two or more disorders, often referring to combinations of severe mental illness, substance misuse, learning difficulties and personality disorder. The term dual diagnosis, co-occurring disorder or complex needs may also be used.

Case registers

Health information systems of a geographically defined area that record contacts between patients and designated services.

Comprehensiveness

A service characteristic, comprising how far a service extends across the range of mental illness severity and patient characteristics (horizontal comprehensiveness), and the availability of the basic components of care and their use by prioritized patient groups (vertical comprehensiveness).

Continuity

The ability of services to offer an uninterrupted series of contacts over time (longitudinal continuity) and between service providers (cross-sectional continuity).

Co-ordination

A service characteristic, manifested by coherent treatment plans for individual patients.

Dual diagnosis

Dual diagnosis or co-occurring disorders are used to describe people with a combination of disorders, usually drug and alcohol misuse and mental illness, but also other combinations such as learning disability and mental illness.

DALY

Disability Adjusted Life Years, the sum of years of life lost because of premature mortality plus the years of life lived with disability, adjusted for the severity of disability.

Effectiveness

The proven, intended benefits of treatments (at the patient level) or services (at the local level) provided in real-life situations.

Efficacy

The outcomes of an intervention under experimental (rather than routine) conditions.

Efficiency

A service characteristic, which minimizes the inputs needed to achieve a given level of outcomes, or which maximizes the outcomes for a given level of inputs.

Equity

The fair distribution of resources.

Health Action Zones (HAZs)

HAZs are designated by the government and help bring together local health services and local authorities, community groups, the voluntary sector and local businesses to establish and foster strategies for improving the health of local people. Twenty six areas with a history of some deprivation and poor health amongst local residents have now been assigned as Health Action Zones.

Health Authorities (HAs)

HAs have the responsibility of commissioning a comprehensive range of services for mentally ill residents of their areas, and for liaising with social services departments over the provision of services to meet these patients' social care needs. HAs also have a statutory responsibility, along with local authorities and in co-operation with relevant voluntary agencies, to secure the provision of aftercare for certain categories of detained patients under Section 117 of the Mental Health Act 1983. Commissioning plans are required to be: (i) *comprehensive*, including in-patient facilities of differing degrees of security, and a range of facilities and services located outside the hospital setting; (ii) *based on agreed assessment of needs* between health, social services and housing agencies; and (iii) *targeted*—those in greatest need should receive the highest priority.

Health and social care community

Local health authority, local authority, NHS Trusts, Primary Care Groups and Trusts, and the independent sector.

Health improvement programmes

Health improvement programmes are the local strategies for improving health and health care. Led by the health authority, a health improvement programme brings together the local NHS with local authorities and others, including the voluntary sector, to set the strategic framework for improving health, tackling inequalities and developing faster, more convenient services of a consistently high standard to meet the needs of local people.

Home Office

British government department dealing with all the internal affairs of state except those specifically assigned to other departments. Responsibilities include the police, the prison service, immigration, race relations and broadcasting. The Home Secretary, the head of the department, holds cabinet rank. In many countries, this part of the government administration is called the Department of Internal Affairs.

Independent sector

Voluntary, charitable and private care providers.

'Internal market' (see National Health Service)

Joint investment plans

Joint investment plans in England are mechanisms for local and health authorities, with key partner agencies, to set out their investment intent together. They aim to promote transparency between statutory services and ensure more coherent investment across sectors.

Local Authorities Social Services Departments

LASSDs have a wide range of duties and responsibilities to provide services for individuals and families, and to facilitate positive mental health. In addition, they have a regulatory function with regard to services provided by the voluntary and private sector, and they may work collaboratively with these bodies. LASSDs have a lead role in purchasing and providing social care services for mentally ill people living in the community. Only a small part of their responsibilities is related directly to the purchasing and provision of mental health services, but many of their activities have implications for mentally ill people. Their main responsibilities in this area are as follows:

- to agree a community care plan for the authority to meet the social care needs of the residents. This must be agreed with the relevant Health Authorities (HAs);
- to assess people in need;
- to design care packages to meet the assessed needs of users and their carers, which are then

monitored in the community (see **Care management**);

- to provide social work support to people with mental health problems, and their carers;
- to provide/purchase a range of personal social services (e.g. residential and day services, domiciliary services, etc);
- to register and inspect residential care homes;
- to liaise with HAs in implementing the Care Programme Approach;
- to provide Section 117 aftercare jointly with HAs, in co-operation with relevant voluntary organizations.

Long-term service agreements
Long-term service agreements are between health authorities and, increasingly, Primary Care Groups and NHS Trusts on the service that should be provided for a local population. All commissioning in the NHS now takes place through long-term service agreements, which replaced annual contracts in April 1999. They run for a minimum of 3 years and are expected to deliver improvements in health and health care. They need to reflect the development of long-term relationships between Primary Care Groups and NHS Trusts, based on a shared view of the outcomes of care that are needed, and covering 'pathways of care' that cross traditional organizational boundaries.

Managed care
Health delivery systems involving a range of financing and payment strategies designed to control the price, volume, delivery site and intensity of provided services. Administrative techniques used include physician gate-keepers to approve access to specialized services, utilization review, case management and standardized criteria. Managed care organizations encompass a variety of types of health plans. These include:

- *Health Maintenance Organization (HMO):* a health care system providing or otherwise ensuring the delivery of defined treatment services to a group of voluntarily enrolled persons. The HMO is reimbursed through a pre-determined, fixed per capita payment without regard to the amount of actual services eventually provided to the enrolled person.

- *Preferred Provider Organization (PPO):* managed care plans that contract with networks of hospitals and physicians to provide health care services at discounted rates in return for expedited claims payment and a relatively predictable market share. Although consumers can use non-PPO providers, financial incentives favour use of PPO providers.

- *Point-of-service plan (POS):* this is a kind of hybrid in which at the time a service is rendered, the insured can elect to receive the service from a provider such as an HMO at a discount or at no out-of-pocket cost, or from a non-network provider subject to higher patient co-payment.

- *Carve-out benefit:* specific benefits which are administered separately from the rest of an organization's basic health insurance package. An intermediary other than the one that administers the firm's basic insurance plan manages carve-out benefits. Mental health and substance abuse are common examples.

Matrix model
A conceptual model (comprising geographical and temporal dimensions) to help formulate service aims and the steps necessary for their implementation (Thornicroft and Tansella, 1999). The temporal dimension of the matrix model comprises input, process and outcome levels:

- *Input phase.* The resources which are put into mental health care, comprising visible (e.g. budget, staff, facilities) and invisible (e.g. skills of staff, organizational arrangements) inputs.
- *Process phase.* Those activities which take place to deliver mental health services, the vehicle for the delivery of health care.
- *Outcome phase.* Changes in the health status of patients (either individually or aggregated), comprising measures before and after a clinical intervention.

The geographical dimension of the matrix model, comprises country/regional, local and patient levels:

- *Country/regional level.* The level with a shared government, which passes mental health laws, sets overall policy and minimum clinical standards, and organizes professional training.
- *Local level.* The catchment area for which an integrated system of care for general adult mental health can be provided.
- *Patient level.* The therapeutic domain, which includes interventions for patients (individually or in groups), families or carers.

Medicaid

A US federally aided, state-operated and administered programme which provides medical benefits for certain indigent or low-income persons in need of health and medical care. It does not cover all of the poor, however, but only persons who meet specified eligibility criteria. Subject to broad Federal guidelines, states determine the benefits covered, programme eligibility, rates of payment for providers and methods of administering the programme.

Medicare

A US health insurance programme for people aged 65 and over, for persons eligible for social security disability payments for 2 years or longer and for certain workers and their dependants who need kidney transplantation or dialysis. Monies from payroll taxes and premiums from beneficiaries are deposited in special trust funds for use in meeting the expenses incurred by the insured.

Mental Health Act (1983)

The Mental Health Act concerns 'the reception, care and treatment of mentally disordered patients, the management of their property and other related matters'. It governs the implementation of involuntary admission and treatment in England.

National Health Service (NHS)

Established in 1948, the NHS is funded predominantly out of central taxation and remains for the most part (with the exception of charges for prescriptions and dental services) free at the point of use. Officially, it continues to have a commitment to its founding principles of universality, comprehensiveness and equity. The NHS has undergone a number of reorganizations, the most radical of which occurred with the NHS and Community Care Act 1990. The NHS changed from an 'administrative' model to a new style 'managerialism', and from a 'control and command' economy to a managed 'internal market'. The former change introduced a system of 'general management'; the latter a splitting of the former District Health Authorities which previously had provided health care services, into purchasers (the new Health Authorities) and providers (NHS Trusts and a wide range of other non-NHS health care providers, including private ones).

National Health Service Executive (NHS Executive)

The executive arm of the Department of Health in England and Wales with offices in each health region. While NHS Trusts and Health Authorities are free-standing bodies, a substantial degree of central control is exercised through policy directives and guidance.

National Institute of Clinical Excellence (NICE)

Established in April 1999, the Institute is responsible for promoting clinical excellence and cost-effectiveness, producing and issuing clinical guidelines (see **Clinical governance**).

National Service Framework for Mental Health

The National Service Framework for Mental Health (NSFMH) is a strategic blueprint for mental health services in England for adults of working age. Its stated aims are to:

- help drive up quality;
- remove the wide and unacceptable variations in provision;
- set national standards and define service models for promoting mental health and treating mental illness;
- put in place underpinning programmes to support local delivery;

- establish milestones and a specific group of high-level performance indicators against which progress within agreed timescales will be measured.

The scope of the framework includes health promotion, primary care services, local mental health and social care services for those with mental health problems and substance misuse, and more specialised mental health services, including all forensic mental health services.

Performance Assessment Frameworks
Performance Assessment Frameworks are designed to give a general picture of NHS or social care performance. Six areas are covered for the NHS: health improvement; fair access to services; effective delivery of health care; efficiency; service users' and carers' experience; and the health outcomes of NHS care. Five areas are covered for social care: national priorities and strategic objectives; cost and efficiency; effectiveness of service delivery and outcomes; quality of services for service users and carers; and fair access.

Primary Care Groups (PCGs)
Groups of family doctors and community nurses with resources for commissioning health care. Their budget is based on their local population's share of available resources for hospital and community health services, the general medical services cash-limited budget, and prescribing. They are subcommittees of health authorities. In time, they will become Primary Care Trusts.

Primary Care Trusts (PCTs)
It is planned that Primary Care Groups will move to become PCTs. This will bring increased autonomy as, unlike Primary Care Groups, Trusts are not subcommittees of health authorities—they are free-standing bodies. The chief executive of a Trust will have the same financial accountability as the chief executives of Health Authorities and NHS Trusts. A Trust will also be directly accountable for clinical governance to the Commission for Health Improvement and have to be clearly responsible for the quality of care delivered by every clinician and every team in the Trust. Trusts

will be able to commission both primary and secondary care, and to buy or build community hospitals and other outreach facilities and own them.

Regional Secure Units (RSUs)
Medium secure units for individuals who are thought to pose special risks, particularly of violence to others (see **Security—medium**).

Royal College of Psychiatrists
The professional and educational body for psychiatrists in the UK and the Republic of Ireland. It conducts the professional examination, visits and approves training positions, and organizes continuing education activities. It also issues statements on policies and issues related to psychiatry.

Royal Commission
A group of people appointed by the British government (nominally by the sovereign) to investigate a matter of public concern and make recommendations on any actions to be taken in connection with it, including changes in the law. In cases where agreement on recommendations cannot be reached, a minority report can be submitted by dissenters.

Security
- Low: some local hospitals have wards with locked doors and above average staff ratios. Also known as intensive care or high dependency units

- Medium: units, including Regional Secure Units, which care for patients whose behaviour is too difficult or dangerous for local hospitals but who do not require the higher levels of security available in special hospitals

- High: provided by the three special hospitals in England—Ashworth, Broadmoor and Rampton. Their patients are often very dangerous and violent and require intensive care, supervision and observation within the most secure surroundings.

Select Committees

Committees set up by British parliament to scrutinize the work of a government department (e.g. health), but have the remit to stray beyond departmental boundaries in pursuit of an issue. Made up by backbench Members of Parliament reflecting the distribution of seats in the House of Commons. It is one of the ways in which the governmental executive branch (ministers and their departmental officials) is checked by parliament.

Service and Financial Frameworks (SaFFs)

Service and Financial Frameworks are annual agreements drawn up by each health authority and partners, such as Primary Care Groups, Primary Care Trusts, NHS Trusts, social service authorities and other local agencies, of the resources and activity needed to deliver the objectives agreed in the local health improvement programme for the year ahead. SaFFs encompass primary care, mental health, community and secondary care. They are examined each year, and refined in consultation with regional offices of the NHS Executive to ensure that they are robust.

Service user(s)

People who need health and social care for their mental health problems. They may be individuals who live in their own homes, are staying in care or are being cared for in hospital. In some countries, service users are referred to as clients, consumers or patients.

Social care

Personal care for vulnerable people, including individuals with special needs which stem from their age or physical or mental disability, and children who need care and protection. Examples of social care services are residential care homes, home helps and home care services. Local authorities have statutory responsibilities for providing social care.

Supervised discharge

Under the 1995 Mental Health (Patients in the Community) Act, consultant psychiatrists may apply for powers of supervision of patients following discharge from hospital. A supervisor, typically a community psychiatric nurse acting as care co-ordinator, has the power to: require the patient to reside in a specified place; require the patient to attend for medical treatment and rehabilitation; and, convey a patient to a place where he or she is to attend for treatment (but cannot force treatment).

Systems approach

An approach to categorising service components, in which each facility or programme is viewed as part of a wider system of care, with inter-relationships explicitly considered, as opposed to the fragmented approach where service components (e.g. community mental health teams) are considered in isolation from each other (see Matrix model).

Trust (NHS Trust)

Following the NHS and Community Care Act 1990, District Health Authorities split into purchasing and provider units. The provider units established themselves as Trusts and became free to operate as independent non-profit organizations responsible to a board comprising both executive and non-executive members. The NHS Executive continues to exercise substantial central influence through policy and other guidance. Trusts own their capital assets but pay capital charges. For a period, general practices could also hold their own budgets and purchase health care services from providers of their choice (known as GP 'fundholding'). Current policy supports the development of Primary Care Groups (PCGs) and eventually primary care trusts (PCTs).

Index